A Comprehensive Guide to Drug Therapy

A Comprehensive Guide to Drug Therapy

Edited by Brendon Krauss

hayle
medical

New York

Hayle Medical,
750 Third Avenue, 9th Floor,
New York, NY 10017, USA

Visit us on the World Wide Web at:
www.haylemedical.com

ISBN: 978-1-63241-524-0

Cataloging-in-Publication Data

A comprehensive guide to drug therapy / edited by Brendon Krauss.
    p. cm.
Includes bibliographical references and index.
ISBN 978-1-63241-524-0
1. Chemotherapy. 2. Drugs. 3. Pharmacology. I. Krauss, Brendon.
RM262 .C66 2018
615.58--dc23

TABLE OF CONTENTS

Preface

Drug therapy or pharmacotherapy is the branch of medicine, which studies the therapeutic use of pharmaceutical drugs. It is unlike any other therapy as it is based on the efficient, safe, economical and optimum use of drugs to treat ailments. This book explores all the important aspects of drug therapy in the present day scenario. It is a compilation of chapters that discuss the most vital concepts and emerging trends in this field. Students, researchers, experts and all associated with drug therapy will benefit alike from this book.

The information shared in this book is based on empirical researches made by veterans in this field of study. The elaborative information provided in this book will help the readers further their scope of knowledge leading to advancements in this field.

Finally, I would like to thank my fellow researchers who gave constructive feedback and my family members who supported me at every step of my research.

Editor

The Impact of Text Message Reminders on Adherence to Antimalarial Treatment in Northern Ghana

Julia R. G. Raifman[1]*, **Heather E. Lanthorn**[2], **Slawa Rokicki**[3], **Günther Fink**[1]

1 Department of Global Health and Population, Harvard School of Public Health, Boston, MA, United States of America, 2 Harvard School of Public Health, Boston, MA, United States of America, 3 Department of Health Policy, Harvard Graduate School of Arts and Sciences, Cambridge, MA, United States of America

Abstract

Background: Low rates of adherence to artemisinin-based combination therapy (ACT) regimens increase the risk of treatment failure and may lead to drug resistance, threatening the sustainability of current anti-malarial efforts. We assessed the impact of text message reminders on adherence to ACT regimens.

Methods: Health workers at hospitals, clinics, pharmacies, and other stationary ACT distributors in Tamale, Ghana provided flyers advertising free mobile health information to individuals receiving malaria treatment. The messaging system automatically randomized self-enrolled individuals to the control group or the treatment group with equal probability; those in the treatment group were further randomly assigned to receive a simple text message reminder or the simple reminder plus an additional statement about adherence in 12-hour intervals. The main outcome was self-reported adherence based on follow-up interviews occurring three days after treatment initiation. We estimated the impact of the messages on treatment completion using logistic regression.

Results: 1140 individuals enrolled in both the study and the text reminder system. Among individuals in the control group, 61.5% took the full course of treatment. The simple text message reminders increased the odds of adherence (adjusted OR 1.45, 95% CI [1.03 to 2.04], p-value 0.028). Receiving an additional message did not result in a significant change in adherence (adjusted OR 0.77, 95% CI [0.50 to 1.20], p-value 0.252).

Conclusion: The results of this study suggest that a simple text message reminder can increase adherence to antimalarial treatment and that additional information included in messages does not have a significant impact on completion of ACT treatment. Further research is needed to develop the most effective text message content and frequency.

Trial Registration: ClinicalTrials.gov NCT01722734

Editor: Laurence Slutsker, Division of Parasitic Diseases and Malaria, Center for Global Health, United States of America

Funding: The Clinton Health Access Initiative funded the study. The funders had no role in study design, data collection and analysis, decision to publish, or preparation of the manuscript.

Competing Interests: The authors have declared that no competing interests exist.

* Email: JuliaRGoldberg@gmail.com

Introduction

Despite massive international efforts over the past decades, malaria continues to be one of the primary causes of mortality worldwide. An estimated 655,000 to 1.24 million people died of malaria in 2010, and more than half of those who died were children younger than five years [1,2]. Of malaria deaths, 92% occurred in sub-Saharan Africa (SSA), where *Plasmodium (P.) falciparum*, the most virulent form of the malaria parasite, is most common. Artemisinin-based combination therapies (ACTs) are recommended by the World Health Organization (WHO) as the first-line treatment for uncomplicated *P. falciparum* malaria in all cases except the first trimester of pregnancy [1]. *P. falciparum* has developed resistance to other treatments, leaving ACTs as the only first-line treatment suitable for use among the general population [3,4]. Aided by a subsidy through the Affordable Medicines

Facility-malaria (AMFm), ACTs became more widely available and affordable in seven pilot SSA countries [5]. Widespread access to ACTs in both the private and the public sectors is crucial for averting death and disability from malaria [6], but also increases the likelihood that *P. falciparum* strains resistant to artemisinin derivatives will emerge in Africa, as has already occurred in Southeast Asia [7,8].

The high frequency of non-adherence to ACTs in SSA is a primary concern for treatment failure and could also lead to drug resistance, particularly in patients with high parasite burdens [4]. In a systematic review of antimalarial adherence studies, Banek et al. found that reported adherence to artemether-lumefantrine (AL) ranged from 38% to 96% and that adherence to artesunate-amodiaquine (AS+AQ) ranged from 48% to 93% [9]. In two studies which included both public and private facilities, Cohen et al. found that 66% of patients adhered to the prescribed dosing of AL in Uganda [10] and Lemma et al. found that 38% of patients adhered to the treatment regimen for AL in Ethiopia [11].

Mobile technologies are increasingly being incorporated into the health sector both in developed and developing countries. Mobile phone ownership in low-income countries increased from 7.9 phones per 100 inhabitants in 2001 to 78.8 phones per 100 inhabitants in 2011, providing a new and relatively inexpensive platform to reach a large proportion of patients in low-income countries [12]. While few studies have examined the effects of text reminders in developing country settings [13,14], two studies indicate that text reminders improved patient adherence to HIV/AIDS treatment in Kenya [15,16] and another study indicates that text reminders improve health worker adherence to treatment guidelines for pediatric malaria [17]. We conducted a randomized trial in northern Ghana to assess the impact of mobile phone-based text message reminders on ACT treatment completion. To our knowledge, this randomized controlled trial is the first attempt to evaluate the impact of text reminders to patients on adherence to malaria treatment [18].

Methods

Design Overview

This randomized trial took place within a one hour driving radius of Tamale, Ghana, the capital of Northern Region, between July and November of 2011. and Checklist S1 contain the trial protocol and CONSORT checklist.

Ethics Statement

The review boards at the Harvard School of Public Health and the Ghana Health Services provided ethics approval. All participants provided written informed consent.

Setting and Participants

The site of the study was the urban area of Tamale, Ghana, and its peri-urban and rural surroundings (see Figure S1 in file S1 for geographic location). Tamale is the capital of Ghana's Northern Region and has a population of 540,000 people [19]. Malaria is endemic in the area, with 48.3% of children in the Northern

Region testing microscopy-positive for malaria in 2011 [20]. While Ghana as a whole is rapidly developing, the Northern region lags behind the rest of the country on literacy and other indicators [19].

The primary ACTs available in Ghana are AL and AS+AQ. AL regimens generally contain six doses, with the number of pills in each dose varying between one and four. AS+AQ regimens contain six tablets taken in three doses. The first dose of both treatments is taken immediately or with the next meal, and subsequent doses are supposed to be taken in 12-hour intervals for AL and in 24-hour intervals for AS+AQ, so that the full treatment course should be completed within 60 hours of treatment initiation, regardless of patient age.

Ghana is also one of seven pilot countries in SSA where ACTs were subsidized through the AMFm, and thus made available at low prices both in the public and private health sectors beginning in August 2010. The average price per adult ACT dose in Ghana fell from $2.74 to $0.94 in public facilities and from $3.42 to $1.13 in private facilities [5]. Ghana's National Health Insurance Scheme also fully covers ACTs for insured patients at registered facilities. The National Health Insurance Authority estimates that 25.5% of individuals in the Northern Region were active members in 2010 [21]. It is likely that individuals living in and around Tamale were more likely to be registered than those in more rural areas.

The target population was defined as all individuals acquiring ACTs. Data enumerators compiled a complete listing of vendors distributing ACTs within a 30-minute drive of Tamale. As shown in Table S1 in file S1, enumerators compiled a list of 217 ACT vendors within 30 minutes driving time from the center of Tamale. The most common vendor types were licensed chemical sellers (177), followed by pharmacies (15), private clinics (7) and public hospitals (6). Daily Patient and ACT volumes were highest at private and public facilities as well as pharmacies – the three categories together accounted for about two thirds of the estimated total daily volume.

We continuously recruited participants from 11 high-volume facilities, which primarily included clinics and hospitals, in order to ensure high enrollment volumes to achieve sufficient power. Data enumerators made additional recruitment efforts – generally

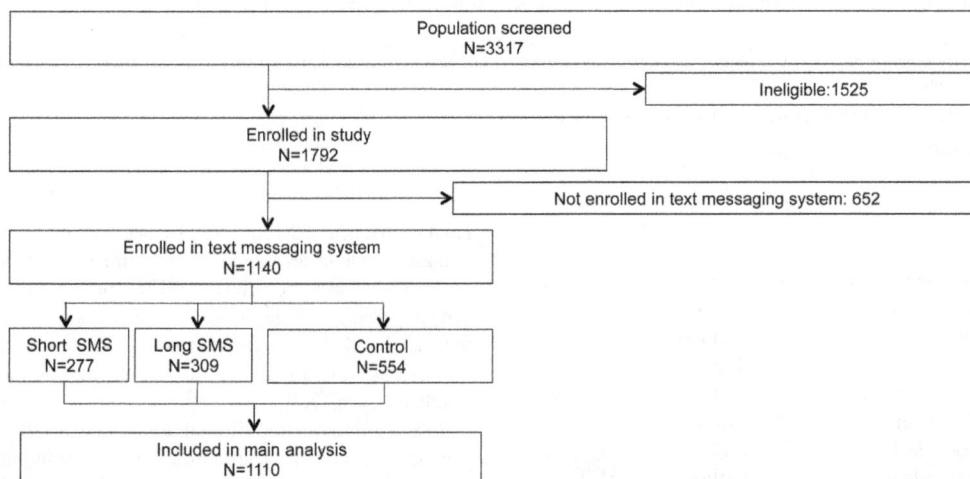

Figure 1. Study Flow. Notes: 1792 of 3317 screened individuals were eligible to participate in the study. The most common reasons for exclusion were living more than a 30-minute drive from the ACT vendor and not having a mobile phone, followed by purchasing drugs for somebody who was not a member of the same household. Of those eligible for study participation, 1140 enrolled with the same mobile phone number that they shared with data enumerators, of whom 554 were randomized to the control group, 277 to the reminder-only message group, and 309 to the reminder and additional information message group. A total of 1110 participants reported on their ACT adherence and were included in the main analysis.

Table 1. Sample Characteristics.

	Control		Treatment		Eligible but without mobile match		Ineligible	
	n	% (SD)	n	% (SD)	n	% (SD)	n	% (SD)
Patient is male	213	46.6 (73.9)	225	44.3 (70.5)	301	40.3 (79.7)		
Patient age <5	76	13.7 (35.2)	97	16.5 (36.6)	94	14.8 (32.3)	239	16.6 (36.4)
Patient age 5–17	90	16.3 (36.6)	124	21.1 (41.0)	110	17.3 (36.6)	304	21.1 (40.0)
Patient age 18–59	350	63.4 (48.3)	329	56.1 (49.6)	390	61.4 (49.9)	800	55.5 (50.0)
Patient age 60+	31	5.6 (23.4)	23	3.9 (20.6)	41	6.5 (23.1)	99	6.9 (24.6)
Male household head	498	89.9 (30.2)	511	87.2 (33.4)	571	87.6 (33.0)	1311	85.9 (34.7)
Head of hh: no education	202	39.8 (48.1)	226	42.1 (48.7)	237	40.5 (48.1)	641	48.8 (49.4)
Head of hh: some education	200	39.4 (48.1)	209	38.9 (47.9)	207	35.4 (46.5)	408	31.1 (44.2)
Head of hh: higher education	106	20.9 (39.4)	102	19.0 (37.9)	141	24.1 (41.2)	264	20.1 (37.8)
Household poorest quintile	107	19.3 (39.5)	102	17.5 (37.9)	99	15.2 (35.9)	352	23.7 (34.7)
Household second quintile	100	18.1 (38.5)	94	16.1 (36.7)	133	20.4 (40.3)	324	21.8 (42.1)
Household third quintile	122	22.1 (41.5)	137	23.5 (42.4)	134	20.6 (40.4)	265	17.8 (40.1)
Household fourth quintile	115	20.8 (40.6)	136	23.3 (42.3)	137	20.1 (40.8)	266	17.9 (37.9)
Household wealthiest quintile	109	19.7 (39.8)	114	19.6 (39.6)	146	21.0 (41.7)	280	18.8 (37.9)
Artemether Lumefantrine	317	51.3 (49.5)	326	55.6 (49.7)	379	58.1 (49.4)	782	51.3 (50.0)
Artesunate Amodiaquine	147	26.5 (44.2)	169	28.8 (45.3)	189	29.0 (45.4)	435	28.5 (45.2)
Private hospital	128	23.4 (42.4)	129	22.3 (41.7)	176	27.8 (44.8)	354	23.9 (42.6)
Private clinic	54	9.9 (29.9)	50	8.7 (28.1)	44	6.9 (25.4)	142	9.6 (29.4)
Public hospital	78	14.3 (35.0)	90	15.6 (36.2)	95	15.0 (35.7)	226	15.2 (40.0)
Public clinic	120	21.9 (41.4)	131	22.7 (41.4)	134	21.1 (40.9)	382	25.8 (43.7)
Pharmacy	13	2.4 (15.2)	11	1.9 (13.7)	12	1.9 (13.6)	23	1.6 (12.4)
Licensed Chemical Seller	139	25.4 (4.4)	152	26.3 (44.1)	168	26.5 (44.2)	311	21.0 (40.7)

Notes: n is the number of participants in each group who have each characteristic, such as age younger than five years. The denominator for each measure differs based on the number of participants for which an answer was recorded. We did not inquire about patient sex in the screening interview and do not have this information for individuals who were not eligible to participate in the study.

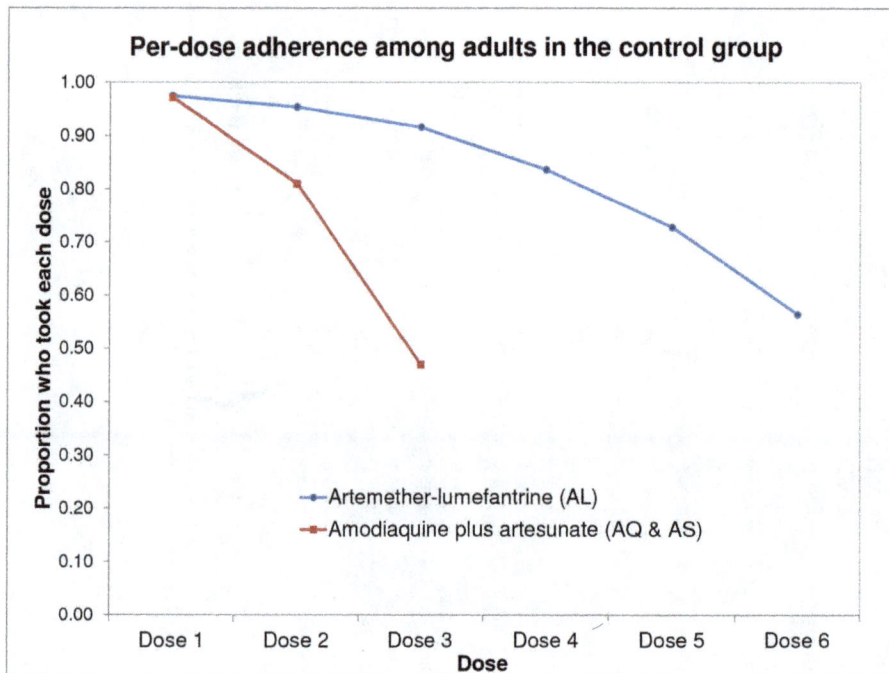

Figure 2. Dose completion among adults in the control group. Notes: Figure 2 indicates the proportion of adults in the control group who reported taking each dose of treatment in the per-dose self-report. Among 239 adults who took AL and reported per-dose adherence, 200 (83.7%) reported taking the fourth dose, 174 (72.8%) reported taking the fifth dose, and 135 (56.5%) reported taking the sixth dose. Among 70 adults in the control group taking AS+AQ, 33 (47.9%) reported completing the full three-dose regimen.

restricted to only a few days – at 73 smaller vendors, which were selected at random from the complete listing of 217 facilities. Figure S2 in file S1 illustrates the spatial distribution of sampled vendors in the larger Tamale region.

Vendor Recruitment

Study staff visited all selected vendors a week prior to participant recruitment to seek vendor consent to participate in the study and to establish a plan for vendor communication with data enumerators. Participant registration in the text messaging system and enrollment in the study then took place in two steps. First, consenting vendors distributed flyers advertising "free text message information about malaria" to all individuals acquiring ACTs. Second, vendors notified data enumerators assigned to each shop of the ACT acquisition, and data enumerators initiated study enrollment.

Participant Recruitment

Participant recruitment for the study took place immediately following acquisition of the malaria treatment and vendor distribution of the flyer. Data enumerators sitting near shop exits approached individuals who acquired anti-malarial treatment when notified of the acquisition by vendors. Data enumerators invited the individuals to participate in a household survey focusing on health and informed them that participating in the household survey would be associated with an interview conducted in their household at a later date; no further information was provided regarding the study's focus on malaria treatment or adherence in order to avoid influencing participants' behavior or reporting.

Study eligibility was restricted to individuals 18 or older, to individuals purchasing malaria medicine for themselves or someone in their household, to individuals living within a

Table 2. Effect of text message treatment on self-reported adherence.

	Percent completed treatment	Adjusted OR (95% CI)
Control Group (n = 538)	61.5	Reference Group
Message A (n = 572)	66.4	1.45**
		(1.03–2.04)
Message B (n = 304)	64.1	0.77
		(0.50–1.20)
Sample size	1110	1110

Notes: Covariates are all those listed in Table 1, including sex and age of the patient, and household characteristics. **p<0.05.

Table 3. Per-protocol Subgroup Analysis.

	Control	Reminder text message		Long message	
	Proportion adhering (%)	Proportion adhering (%)	Adjusted OR (95% CI)	Proportion adhering (%)	Adjusted OR (95% CI)
Age					
Children	71.4	76.9	2.30**	70.5	0.44**
(N)	(164)	(215)	(1.01–5.26)	(112)	(0.20–0.99)
Adults	57.3	60.7	1.26	60.9	0.96
(N)	(373)	(352)	(0.92–1.72)	(189)	(0.64–1.42)
Sex					
Male	63.1	70.5	1.35	70.7	1.05
(N)	(206)	(220)	(0.86–2.13)	(116)	(0.4–1.74)
Female	57,6	66.2	2.11***	60.5	0.58
(N)	(238)	(278)	(1.20–3.75)	(147)	(0.28–1.18)
HH head education					
None	57.9	64.2	2.02**	57.8	0.44**
(N)	(195)	(218)	(1.14–3.56)	(109)	(0.23–0.82)
Some	60.9	66.8	1.23	69.5	1.45
(N)	(197)	(205)	(0.67–2.24)	(105)	(0.63–3.36)
High	71.3	72.0	1.38	66.1	0.46
(N)	(101)	(100)	(0.57–3.37)	(59)	(0.18–1.21)
Wealth Quintile					
Poorest	65.7	69.3	1.02	72.0	1.35
(N)	(105)	(101)	(0.37–2.85)	(50)	(0.43–4.24)
2nd	61.2	69.9	2.55**	66.0	0.47
(N)	(98)	(93)	(1.09–5.96)	(50)	(0.18–1.23)
3rd	58.5	64.1	1.69	65.1	0.91
(N)	(118)	(131)	(0.77–3.69)	(41)	(0.44–1.89)
4th	65.5	64.7	1.77**	57.7	0.40***
(N)	(110)	(133)	(1.05–2.98)	(78)	(0.25–0.66)
Wealthiest	57.6	66.7	1.29	65.8	0.93
(N)	(106)	(111)	(0.63–2.63)	(61)	(0.27–3.16)
Facility					
LCS (N)	58.0	57.1	0.79	62.3	1.51
	(138)	(147)	(0.44–1.40)	(76)	(0.75–3.04)
Private	61.1	75.0	2.07***	70.8	0.73***
Clinic (N)	(54)	(48)	(1.47–2.91)	(24)	(0.60–0.88)
Private	61.5	67.2	2.00***	59.1	0.38***
hospital (N)	(122)	(128)	(1.54–2.60)	(66)	(0.29–0.52)
Public	69.7	77.5	1.69	72.7	0.36***
clinic	(76)	(89)	(0.81–3.53)	(44)	(0.19–0.69)
(N)					
Public	65.3	66.7	1.39	63.8	0.73
hospital	(118)	(126)	(0.91–2.13)	(44)	(0.28–1.85)
(N)					
Treatment					
AL	0.61	0.64	1.51	0.61	0.67
(N)	(305)	(320)	(0.88–2.59)	(174)	(0.34–1.33)
AS+AQ	0.625	0.71	2.25**	0.64	0.41***
(N)	(144)	(163)	(1.17–4.30)	(79)	(0.22–0.78)

Notes: N is the number of people in each subgroup, such as the number of children whose caregivers received the simple reminder message. Covariates are all those listed in Table 1, including sex and age of the patient, and household and facility type. There were fewer than 30 individuals in the main analysis who received ACTs from pharmacies, health posts, CHPs zones, or health professionals' homes. ***p<0.01, **p<0.05.

30-minute drive of the shop, and to individuals able to provide the mobile number for a personal or shared mobile phone. Enumerators informed study participants who met the inclusion criteria about the household interview to take place within the next few months, and, upon consent, enrolled participants in the study. After the initial consent, surveyors conducted a short interview to collect contact information for eligible participants. Both those who were eligible and those who were ineligible completed a short exit interview designed to capture basic demographic information. Individuals who registered in the mobile phone system based on the flyer but who were not eligible for the study received messages but were not enrolled in the study.

Participant registration in the text messaging system

Participants who received flyers from vendors and enrolled in the text-messaging program in response to the flyer used their own phones to enroll and did not receive any assistance from data enumerators. Registration in the text messaging system was possible either by a short ring ("flashing") of the number provided on the flyer or by sending an empty text message to the same number. While flashing is free for the user, phone service providers in Ghana require a non-zero balance to initiate any call, and sending a text message costs between 5 and 10 Ghana pesewas (US\$ 0·03-US\$ 0·06). Registration in the system was confirmed by a text-message stating, "Thanks for registering for Mobile Health Information." Patients who called or sent a text to the system while enrolled received an additional message stating, "You are already registered. To stop receiving messages, text STOP. Thanks." If the system received a "STOP" message, it sent a confirmation ("You will not receive any more messages from Mobile Health") and automatically discontinued sending any further messages.

Message Design

To develop the content of messages, we reviewed the literature on SMS reminders and attention. We shared a variety of possible messages with participants of 8 focus groups and 24 individual interviews with adult male and female participants in rural and peri-urban Tamale in March 2011. Participants provided feedback on clarity, appropriateness, and predicted effectiveness of the various message options. Based on the feedback obtained in interviews and focus groups as well as in a small pilot study conducted in Cape Coast in June 2011, the research team opted for a simple reminder message (message A) and an additional encouragement component (message B), highlighting the importance of finishing the drugs when malaria symptoms become weak or absent – one of the primary obstacles to regimen completion reported in preliminary field work. The final message treatments were as follows:

Message A: "Please take your MALARIA drugs!".

Message A+B: "Please take your MALARIA drugs! Even if you feel better, you must take all the tablets to kill all the malaria."

Randomization of Messages

The text-messaging program was based in the programming language Python version 2.6 and was built on a Django platform (the program is open source and can be found at https://github.com/waveswinger34/pactremind). Participants were sequentially (in order of their enrollment) assigned to treatment and control, with every other enrolled subject assigned to either treatment or control in an alternating manner. The text messaging system then further randomized participants within the treatment condition to receive message A or message A+B with equal probability, based on a pseudo-random number draw.

Message Rollout

All participants in the treatment group received the assigned reminder messages in 12-hour intervals for three days, for a total of 60 hours, overlapping with the typical treatment protocol for ACTs. Participants in the control group received no message during this period. Given that ACT administration is recommended after meals, evening messages were sent at 7pm, while morning messages were sent at 8am. All participants in the control and in the treatment groups received a generic malaria prevention message about bed nets after 120 hours, which ended the text message activities.

Outcomes and Follow-up

Data enumerators conducted follow-up interviews approximately 72 hours after participants enrolled in the study. Individuals who could not be reached for in-person follow-up interviews after three attempts were contacted by phone for short phone interviews. All study materials were printed in English, the standard language used for written communication in Ghana. Enumerators interacting with subjects during the baseline and follow-up interviews were not aware of treatment assignment prior to the interview.

Adherence to antimalarial treatment is generally based on self-report and observation of pill packets [9,14]. The primary outcome variable in this study was self-reported completion of the ACT treatment regimen, with the interviewee reporting whether the patient completed all of their doses. To allow for some delays in treatment initiation, all follow-up interviews were scheduled at least 66 hours after the initial visit; therefore, any unfinished dose found during follow-up visits could be considered as evidence of non-adherence. To address concerns regarding potential recall and social desirability biases associated with self-reports and to validate the robustness of the outcome measure [22,23] study staff collected information on two additional adherence measures.

First, at the beginning of the interview, and before asking patients any questions regarding the preceding illness episode and its treatment, interviewers took a complete inventory of all drugs stored in the households. If participants were willing to show study

Table 4. Self-reported treatment completion and remaining pills or ACT Stock.

	Participant reports treatment completion (N = 711)	Participant reports incomplete treatment (N = 399)
Pills found in blister back (%)	6.4	97.9
ACTs found as part of drug inventory (%)	37.1	72.1

Notes: The proportion of participants who reported adherence and non-adherence and who either had pills remaining in an observed packet or had an ACT stock in the home. Enumerators observed pill packets for 667 (60.1%) participants and drug stocks for 929 (83.7% of) participants.

Table 5. Effect of treatment on still feeling sick.

	Proportion completed treatment %	Adjusted OR (95% CI)
Control Group (n = 538)	29.5	Reference group
Message A (n = 577)	30.9	1.06
		(0.78–1.45)
Message B (n = 303)	30.7	1.02
		(0.79–1.30)
Sample size	1110	1110

Notes: Patients reported still feeling sick at the time of the follow-up interview. Logistic regression includes the full set of covariates listed in Table 1, including sex and age of the patient, household and facility characteristics.

staff their inventories, interviewers noted the total variety of drugs available in the household and documented the presence of ACTs. While this was not a direct measure of adherence, we expected the drug inventory to be correlated with adherence, and for patients who did not finish their pills to be more likely to still have ACTs at their home. After the drug inventory, interviewers asked respondents to report their overall adherence and to complete a detailed self-report module with the exact quantity of each ACT dose.

Second, at the end of the treatment module, surveyors asked patients to see the original blister pack; if participants were willing and able to share the blister pack, data enumerators observed the number of remaining pills. We compared the main self-report outcome to both the household drug inventories and to the observation of the blister packs to assess the strength of the self-report outcome. We did not incorporate pill packet observation into the final outcome measure due to potential bias in which participants shared pill packets.

Statistical Analysis

The study was powered to detect a 10% increase in adherence with power 0.9, assuming an alpha of 0.05 and a control group adherence of 60% based on estimated adherence in a similar study in Uganda [10]. We estimated intent-to-treat (ITT) multiple logistic regression models to estimate the impacts of receiving Message A and Message B relative to the control group, controlling for random patient characteristics that could influence treatment adherence and clustering standard errors by vendor. The covariates included were sex of the patient, patient age, whether the household head was male, educational attainment of the household head, household wealth quintile, and the type of vendor where participants sought treatment. The household wealth index was constructed using principal components analysis based on household cooking arrangements, water source, sanitation, as well as ownership of mobile phones, and air conditioners. Household head educational attainment was classified as no education if the individual had zero years of education, some education if the individual attended primary or secondary school, and higher education if the individual attained undergraduate or other education after secondary school. In addition to the main analysis, we conducted a pre-specified subgroup analysis by age, sex, household head education, wealth, and vendor type using logistic regression. To check the validity of the outcome measure, we tabulated the proportion of patients reporting treatment completion or incompletion against observed pills and observed ACT stock. Finally, we assessed the impact of treatment on still feeling ill during the follow-up interview using logistic regression

with covariates. All analysis was conducted using the Stata 11 statistical software package [24].

Trial Registration

This trial is registered as trial NCT01722734 at clinicaltrials.gov. We regret that we registered the trial late because we were not aware of the requirement to register randomized trials. There are no ongoing trials related to this study, and any future trials related to this study will be registered.

Results

Enrollment

Figure 1 provides an overview of the study. Of 3317 individuals screened for participation, 1525 were ineligible for study participation. The most common reason for exclusion was distance to the facility, with 27% of screened subjects excluded because they lived further than 15 miles from the city of Tamale. Of those who were screened, 11% were excluded because they could not report a mobile phone number at which they could be regularly reached. An additional 18% of those screened were excluded because they bought the drugs for somebody who was not part of their household, because they were under the age of 18, or because they were not willing to participate in the study.

Data enumerators conducted baseline and follow-up interviews with all 1792 eligible participants. Of those eligible, 1140 (63%) enrolled in the SMS system using the same phone number they shared with enumerators. Out of the 652 participants who did not register in the SMS system using the phone number they shared with enumerators, 197 (37%) self-reported successfully enrolling in the system; however, without a matching phone number, we were unable to determine their treatment assignment and did not include them in the analysis. The primary reason subjects reported not being able to register in the mobile system during the follow-up interview was a lack of credit (29%); even though enrollment in the system was designed to be free, "flashing" or texting requires having credit on the phone. The other main reasons for non-enrollment were forgetting the phone at home (23%) and lack of time (14%). Less than ten percent of non-enrollees reported difficulty with the network or phone coverage as the principal reason for not enrolling.

Of the 1140 participants enrolled in the text messaging system using the phone numbers shared with data collectors, 1128 (99.3%) were followed-up in person, 8 (0.7%) were followed up via phone call, and 4 (0.4%) were lost to follow-up. In addition to the 4 lost to follow-up, a further 26 subjects (2.3%) were excluded from the analysis due to missing data on treatment completion, resulting in a total analysis sample of 1110 participants.

Table S1 in file S1 shows enrollment by vendor type. The distribution of the sample population in terms of vendors is fairly similar to the overall patient population of Tamale, with some overrepresentation of patients from public health facilities and underrepresentation of patients from pharmacies.

Descriptive Statistics

Table 1 shows baseline characteristics of the population enrolled in the trial and the populations excluded from the trial. Individuals were excluded from the trial either due to ineligibility or because they did not register for the text messaging system using the phone number that they shared with data enumerators. The characteristics of the control group and the treatment group are similar, though there were minor differences in age structure, with slightly more subjects of age 5–17 years in the treatment group than in the control group and more subjects of age 18–60 in the control group than in the treatment group. The characteristics of individuals who were eligible for the study but did not enroll in the text message system using the phone number shared with providers are similar to those of individuals who were included in the main analysis. Those excluded from the study due to ineligibility were more likely to be in lower wealth quintiles and had household heads with lower educational attainment than those in the main analysis.

While mobile phone ownership was high, with only 11% of individuals screened not able to share a mobile phone number at which they could be reached, text messaging on phones was not widespread. Only 323 (28.3%) of study participants reported sending any text messages within the last week.

Adherence

Figure 2 summarizes basic dose completion patterns for adult participants in the control group. Among 239 adults who took AL and reported per-dose adherence, 92.0% reported completing the first three doses. Adherence to the prescribed treatment rapidly declined starting with the fourth dose. Among adults in the control group, 200 (83.7%) reported taking the fourth dose, 174 (72.8%) reported taking the fifth dose, and 135 (56.5%) reported taking the sixth dose. Among 70 adults in the control group taking AS+AQ, 33 (47.9%) reported completing the full, three-dose regimen.

Message Impact on Adherence

Table 2 shows the main results for the impact of text reminders on self-reported treatment completion. Of 538 participants in the control group, 61.5% report treatment completion. Of 572 participants in the treatment group, 66.4% report treatment completion. According to the ITT analysis, being sent Message A significantly increased the odds of adherence (adjusted OR 1.45, 95% CI [1.03 to 2.04], p-value 0.033). Being in the treatment group to which Message B was also sent did not result in a significant change in the odds of adherence relative to the control group (adjusted OR 0.77, 95% CI [0.50 to 1.20], p-value 0.252).

Pre-specified Subgroup Analysis

Table 3 shows subgroup analysis by age, sex, household head education, household wealth quintile, type of vendor, and type of drug. Baseline levels of adherence differed, particularly by age, household head education, and vendor type. Adherence was greater among children in the control group (71.4%) than adults in the control group (57.6%), as well as among patients whose household heads have higher education (71.3%) than some

education (60.9%) or no education (58.0%). More patients who attended public clinics adhered (69.7%) than those who attended public hospitals (65.3%), private clinics (61.5%), private hospitals (61.1%), or LCSs (58.0%).

Our findings indicate that receiving the simple Message A had a significant impact among children, women, individuals with household heads with no education, individuals living in household in the second lowest wealth quintil, individuals obtaining antimalarial treatment from private hospitals, and individuals taking AS+AQ. Receiving Message B significantly increased adherence among individuals obtaining antimalarial treatment from pharmacies and significantly reduced adherence among children, individuals whose household heads had no education, individuals obtaining antimalarial treatment from private hospitals, and individuals taking AS+AQ.

Reliability of Self-reported Adherence Measures

Study staff collected drug inventories for 929 (83.7%) of 1110 participants included in the analysis. Data enumerators were also able to inspect 667 (60.1%) blister packets. Table 4 shows that data enumerators observed remaining pills for 6.4% of subjects reporting ACT completion and a stock of ACTs for 37.1%, while data enumerators observed remaining pills for 97.9% of participants who did not report completing treatment and a stock of ACTs for 72.1%.

Message impact on patient health

Table 5 shows the associations between treatment and the patient's health status as reported during the follow-up interview. 339 respondents (30.2%) reported that the patient still experienced malaria or fever symptoms when interviewed. Receiving a text reminder did not have a significant impact on the odds of remaining sick during the follow-up interview (adjusted OR 1.06, 95% CI [0.78–1.45], p-value 0.700).

Discussion

The results presented in this paper have two main implications. First, adherence to ACT treatment regimens is low in Ghana, which is consistent with other studies of antimalarial treatment adherence in SSA [9–11]. On average, only 61.0% of patients in the control group reported completing the full regimen of AL, and 62.5% reported completing the full regiment of AS+AQ. The low overall rate of adherence poses a threat to patient health and to the sustainability of current anti-malaria efforts.

Second, the results presented in this paper suggest that receiving a simple reminder stating, "Please take your MALARIA drugs!" significantly increases adherence to antimalarial treatment. The additional message stating, "Even if you feel better, you must take all the tablets to kill all the malaria" did not have a statistically significant impact on adherence. The finding that our message with more content was not more effective than our shorter message is consistent with the results in Pop-Eleches et al. [16]. The power to detect additional message impacts was, however, limited in our setting; further research is necessary to better understand the most effective content of text message reminders for increasing medication adherence.

Third, we find that different message content can play an important role among subgroups. The simple reminder message appeared to be particularly effective in increasing treatment completion among children, women, individuals whose household heads had no education, individuals in the second lowest wealth quintile, individuals acquiring ACTs from private hospitals, and individuals taking AS+AQ. Receiving the additional message about taking all of the tablets significantly reduced treatment completion among children whose parents or caregivers received the message, individuals whose household heads had no education, individuals obtaining antimalarial treatment from private hospitals, and individuals taking AS+AQ. Message A was significantly more effective in increasing treatment completion than Messages A+B for children whose caregivers received the messages, for individuals whose household heads had no education, for individuals acquiring ACTs from private hospitals, and for individuals taking AS+AQ. These results suggest that it is important to understand the mechanisms driving the impact of text message reminders on different subgroups and to carefully design the content of text message reminders based on target populations.

Receiving a text message did not have an impact on the odds of still feeling sick during the follow-up interview. Neither the short message nor the long message impacted still feeling sick during the follow-up interview. This is consistent with the magnitude of the impact of the messages on adherence and the magnitude of the impact of adherence on still feeling sick. The objective of this intervention is not only to improve individual symptoms, but to encourage behaviors beneficial for population health in the long run – in this case, by decreasing the likelihood that artemisinin-resistant parasites may survive and be spread due to patients ending their treatment too early [4].

Strengths and Limitations

One of the main critiques of mobile health programs is that they can be difficult to scale. Our results indicate 63.6% of eligible participants self-enrolled in the mobile health program and that flyers are a feasible method of recruiting participants for a mobile health intervention. Enrolling participants in the text message system through a flyer also implies that individuals not able or unwilling to self-enroll in the mobile information system were excluded from the study and from benefiting from the intervention. In terms of the study population, the self-selected nature of patients in the study means that the results presented do not represent treatment effects for the average (or a representative) population, but rather represent the potential SMS impact on adherence among subjects who would self-enroll in a reminder system.

We also could not match individuals to their treatment unless the phone number they provided matched a phone number in the system. The study would have been strengthened by asking participants if they had multiple phone numbers and through additional methods of tracking randomization assignment.

One of the limitations of this study, and text message programs in similar settings more generally, is the importance of mobile phone literacy. While only 11% of households had to be excluded from the study because of lack of access to phones, only 28.3% of participants had sent a text message within the past week. The effectiveness of the program may have been limited by mobile phone literacy.

The intervention, by nature of its delivery via personal mobile phones, is limited in its ability to reach those of lowest socioeconomic status. Mobile phone ownership among people of low socioeconomic status may increase as mobile service and mobile phones become increasingly ubiquitous. There is promising evidence that the short text message had a greater impact on adherence among patients whose household heads had no education, as well as among females and children. There was, however, no clear trend across wealth quintiles.

It is also worth highlighting that similar interventions may yield different results in other developing country settings. Compared to other developing countries, Ghana has made fast progress both with respect to income and average education levels of its population; nevertheless, education and literacy levels remain low among the adult population, particularly in northern Ghana. Better results seem feasible in settings with higher levels of literacy and more frequent mobile phone use.

Finally, the study is somewhat limited by its use of self-reported adherence as a primary outcome measure. Even though all evidence collected as part of this study suggests that systematic misreporting is likely limited and balanced across treatment groups, self-report does present a risk of inaccuracies due to bias and imperfect memory.

Conclusions

The results of this study suggest that receiving a simple text message reminder can increase adherence to antimalarial treatment. Further research is needed to develop the most effective text message reminder content and frequency.

Supporting Information

File S1 Supporting files. Figure S1, Location of Study Site. **Figure S2,** Each star represents one vendor. Darker stars represent higher patient volumes. **Table S1,** Vendor and Sample Volumes.

Checklist S1 CONSORT checklist.

Protocol S1 Trial protocol.

Acknowledgments

We would like to thank the Clinton Health Access Initiative, Jessica Cohen, Emmanuel Okyere Jr, Jessica Kiessel, Pace Phillips, Suvojit Chattopadhyay, Carolina Corral, Mollie Barnathan, Usamatu Salifu, Becky Antwi, and the entire IPA-Ghana team for their invaluable contributions to the project. We also wish to thank the host vendors and the participants for taking part in the study.

Author Contributions

Conceived and designed the experiments: JR GF HL SR. Performed the experiments: JR GF HL SR. Analyzed the data: JR GF HL. Contributed reagents/materials/analysis tools: JR GF HL SR. Wrote the paper: JR GF SR HL.

References

1. World Health Organization (2011) World Malaria Report. Geneva: World Health Organization.
2. Murray CJ, Rosenfield LC, Lim SS, Andrews KG, Foreman KJ, et al. (2012) Global malaria mortality between 1980 and 2010: A systematic analysis. Lancet 379(9814): 413–31.
3. AMFm Task Force of the Roll Back Malaria Partnership (2007) AMFm Technical Design.
4. White N, Pongtavornpinyo W, Maude R, Saralamba S, Aguas R, et al. (2009). Hyperparasitaemia and low dosing are an important source of anti-malarial drug resistance. Malar J.; 8: 253.
5. Tougher S, Ye Y, Amuasi JH, Kourgueni IA, Thomson R, et al. (2012) Effect of the Affordable Medicines Facility-malaria (AMFm) on the availability, price, and market share of quality-assured artemisinin-based combination therapies in seven countries: a before-and-after analysis of outlet survey data. Lancet 380(9857): 1916–26.

6. Laxminarayan R, Arrow K, Jamison D, Bloom BR (2012) From financing to fevers: lessons of an antimalarial subsidy program. Science 338(6107): 615–6.

7. Pyae Phyo A, Standwell N, Stepniewska K, Ashley EA, Nair S, et al. (2012) Emergence of artemisinin-resistant malaria on the western border of Thailand: a longitudinal study. Lancet 379(9830): 1960–6.

8. Jambou R, Legrand E, Niang M, Khim N, Lim P, et al. (2005) Resistance of Plasmodium falciparum field isolates to in-vitro artemether and point mutations of the SERCA-type PfATPase6. Lancet 366(9501): 1960–3.

9. Banek K, Lalani M, Staedke S, Chandramohan D (2014) Adherence to artemisinin-based combination therapy for the treatment of malaria: a systematic review of the evidence. Malar J 13: 7.

10. Cohen JM, Smith DL, Cotter C, Ward A, Yamey G, et al. (2012) Malaria resurgence: A systematic review and assessment of its causes. Malar J 11: 122.

11. Lemma H, Lofgren C, San Sebastian M (2010) Adherence to a six-dose regimen of artemether lumefantrine among uncomplicated Plasmodium falciparum patients in the Tigray Region, Ethiopia. Malar J.; 10: 349.

12. International Telecommunications Union (2012) Mobile cellular subscriptions per 100 inhabitants, 2001–2011. ICT Data and Statistics.

13. Tomlinson M, Rotheram-Borus MJ, Swartz L, Tsai AC (2013) Scaling Up mHealth: Where Is the Evidence? PLoS Med 10(2): e1001382.

14. Haynes RB, Yao X, Degani A, Kripalani S, Garg A, et al. (2006) Interventions for enhancing medication adherence (Review). Cochrane review: John Wiley & Sons, Ltd.

15. Lester RT, Ritvo P, Mills EJ, Kariri A, Karanja S, et al. (2010) Effects of a mobile phone short message service on antiretroviral treatment adherence in Kenya (WelTel Kenya1): a randomised trial. Lancet 376(9755): 1838–45.

16. Pop-Eleches C, Thirumurthy H, Habyarimana JP, Zivin JG, Goldstein MP, et al. (2011) Mobile phone technologies improve adherence to antiretroviral treatment in a resource-limited setting: a randomized controlled trial of text message reminders. AIDS 25(6): 825–34.

17. Zurovac D, Sudoi RK, Akhwale WS, Ndiritu M, Hamer DH, et al. (2011) The effect of mobile phone text-message reminders on Kenyan health workers' adherence to malaria treatment guidelines: A cluster randomized trial. Lancet 378(9793): 795–803.

18. Zurovac D, Talisuna AO, Snow RW (2012) Mobile phone text messaging: Tool for malaria control in Africa. PLoS Med 9(2).

19. Ghana Statistical Service (2012) 2010 Population and Housing Census. Accra, Ghana.

20. Government of Ghana, Ghana Statistical Service, Ghana Health Service, UNICEF, UNFPA, et al. (2011) Ghana Multiple Indicator Cluster Survey: With An Enhanced Malaria Module and Biomarker.

21. National Health Insurance Authority (2011) Annual Report 2011. Accra, Ghana.

22. Farmer KC (1999) Methods for measuring and monitoring medication regimen adherence in clinical trials and clinical practice. Clin Ther 21(6): 1074–90.

23. Turner BJ, Hecht FM (2001) Improving on a Coin Toss To Predict Patient Adherence to Medications. Ann Intern Med 134(10): 1004–6.

24. StataCorp (2009) Stata Statistical Software: Release 11. College Station, TX: StataCorp LP.

2

Chinese Proprietary Herbal Medicine Listed in 'China National Essential Drug List' for Common Cold

Wei Chen[1], George Lewith[2], Li-qiong Wang[1], Jun Ren[1], Wen-jing Xiong[1], Fang Lu[1], Jian-ping Liu[1]*

1 Centre for Evidence-Based Chinese Medicine, Beijing University of Chinese Medicine, Beijing, China, 2 Primary care and population Sciences, Medical School, University of Southampton, Southampton, United Kingdom

Abstract

Objective: Chinese proprietary herbal medicines (CPHMs) have long history in China for the treatment of common cold, and lots of them have been listed in the 'China national essential drug list' by the Chinese Ministry of Health. The aim of this review is to provide a well-round clinical evidence assessment on the potential benefits and harms of CPHMs for common cold based on a systematic literature search to justify their clinical use and recommendation.

Methods: We searched CENTRAL, MEDLINE, EMBASE, SinoMed, CNKI, VIP, China Important Conference Papers Database, China Dissertation Database, and online clinical trial registry websites from their inception to 31 March 2013 for clinical studies of CPHMs listed in the 'China national essential drug list' for common cold. There was no restriction on study design.

Results: A total of 33 CPHMs were listed in 'China national essential drug list 2012' for the treatment of common cold but only 7 had supportive clinical evidences. A total of 6 randomised controlled trials (RCTs) and 7 case series (CSs) were included; no other study design was identified. All studies were conducted in China and published in Chinese between 1995 and 2012. All included studies had poor study design and methodological quality, and were graded as very low quality.

Conclusions: The use of CPHMs for common cold is not supported by robust evidence. Further rigorous well designed placebo-controlled, randomized trials are needed to substantiate the clinical claims made for CPHMs.

Editor: Chang-Qing Gao, Central South University, China

Funding: This work is supported by a research capacity establishment grant from the State Administration of Chinese Medicine (201207007), the Program for Innovative Research Team of Beijing University of Chinese Medicine (2011-CXTD-09), and research fund for the outstanding young teachers of Beijing University of Chinese Medicine. The funders had no role in study design, data collection and analysis, decision to publish, or preparation of the manuscript.

Competing Interests: The authors have declared that no competing interests exist.

* Email: jianping_l@hotmail.com

Introduction

Common cold is often caused by rhinovirus [1]. Common symptoms include cough, sore throat, runny nose, fever, and etc. It is one of the most widespread illnesses in the world. On average, adults have two to three infections a year [2] and children have six to twelve a year [3]. The common cold is a mild and self-limiting illness that almost always resolves spontaneously. To date there is no effective treatment for common cold and the routine use of antibiotics for the common cold is not recommended [4]. Some alternative treatments are used for common cold; however, there is insufficient scientific evidence to support their use [3]. The recommended first line treatment for common cold is usually medication for symptom control to avoid the unnecessary prescription of antibiotics and the consequent risk of adverse drug reactions and antimicrobial resistance.

Chinese herbal medicines have long history in China for the treatment of common cold. It was recorded more than 2000 years ago in 'Inner Canon of Huangdi', the most acknowledged classics of TCM, that 'pathogenic wind can cause cold' [5]. Traditional Chinese medicine (TCM) practitioners and general public have

deep belief that herbal medicines are effective in alleviating symptoms and shortening the duration of the common cold. Chinese proprietary herbal medicine (CPHMs) is an important component of Chinese herbs. It refers to Chinese herbs that mainly produced by modern manufacturing methods. CPHMs include different formulations such as powder, granule, pastille, tablet, and capsule, and are widely accepted by the Chinese population due to the convenience of application. Until now, More than two hundreds CPHMs have been authorized and listed in the 'China national essential drug list' (EDL), which is approved by the Chinese Ministry of Public Health and is regarded as the accepted reference point for the medicines used in medical institutions in China.

The World Health Organization (WHO) strategy calls for evidence-based TCM. In order to ensure evidence-based practice, we conducted systematic evaluation of all the CPHMs listed in the EDL 2012 for the treatment of common cold. Although RCT was acknowledged as the gold standard for therapeutic evaluation, we didn't want to neglect other designs because they might accounts for a large part of the clinical evidence. Our aim was to provide a well-round clinical evidence assessment of CPHMs for common cold based on a systematic literature search.

Methods

Inclusion criteria

Children and adults with the common cold were included. Typical symptoms include cough, sore throat, runny nose, sneezing, fever, and etc. Colds caused by influenza, acute bronchitis developing from a case of common cold, upper respiratory tract infection caused by bacteria, and patients concurrently suffering from other infectious or febrile diseases were excluded. There was no restriction on age and sex.

The interventions were confined to CPHMs listed in EDL 2012 for common cold. There was no restriction on study design. Systematic reviews (SR), randomized controlled trial (RCT), quasi-randomized controlled trial (Q-RCT), non-randomized controlled trial (NRCT), controlled before-and-after study (CBA), prospective cohort study (PCS), retrospective cohort study (RCS), historically controlled trial (HCT), nested case-control study (NCC), case-control study (CC), cross-sectional study (XS), before-and-after comparison (BA), case reports (CR), and case series (CS) were all identified. In order to reduce misclassification and inconsistencies, we used explicit study design features (as shown in Table S1) to facilitate our judgement on study design. Before assessment, two evaluators (WC, LQW) were trained to apply these standards consistently. Disagreement was resolved by discussion and consensus was reached through a third party (JPL).

For RCT, Q-RCT, NRCT, CBA, PCS, RCS, HCT, NCC, and CC studies, CPHMs compared with no treatment, placebo or conventional medication were included. Studies compared CPHM plus other interventions with other interventions alone were also included. CPHM combined with other TCM therapies (including acupuncture) compared with non-TCM therapies were excluded. Studies that compared different CPHMs were excluded. There was no restriction on language and publication type. Literatures that reported same data were be regarded as multiple publications and excluded.

Search strategy and study selection

The CENTRAL (2012, Issue 12) (http://www.cochrane.org/editorial-and-publishing-policy-resource/cochrane-central-register-controlled-trials-central), MEDLINE (http://www.ncbi.nlm.nih.gov/pubmed/), EMBASE (http://www.elsevier.com/online-tools/embase), SinoMed (Chinese Biomedical Literature Service System) (http://www.sinomed.ac.cn/), Chinese VIP information (VIP) (http://www.cqvip.com/), Chinese National Knowledge Infrastructure (CNKI) (http://www.cnki.net/),, China Important Conference Papers Database (http://www.cnki.net/), and China Dissertation Database (http://www.cnki.net/) were searched from their inception to 31 March 2013. The following search terms were used individually or combined: 'cold', 'nasopharyngitis', 'acute viral rhinopharyngitis', 'acute coryza', 'shang feng (cold in Chinese)', 'wai gan (cold in Chinese)', and 'feng han (cold in Chinese)'.

Website of the clinical trials registry including Chinese clinical trial registry (http://www.chictr.org/) and international clinical trial registry by U.S. national institutes of health (http://clinicaltrials.gov/) were also searched for ongoing registered clinical trials.

Two authors conducted the literature search (LQW, JR), study selection (WJX, FL) and data extraction (WC, LQW) independently. We extracted authors' name and title of study, year of publication, study design (detail of randomization if the study was RCT), sample size, demographic characteristics of the participants, name and component of CPHM, treatment process, detail of the control interventions, outcome and adverse effect for each study. Double check was conducted to reduce inconsistencies. Disagreement was resolved by discussion or through a third party (JPL).

Quality assessment

Two authors (WC, LQW) evaluated the quality of included studies independently. The quality of included RCTs were assessed by using the risk of bias tool according to the 'Cochrane Handbook of Systematic Reviews of Interventions' (Chapter 8) to address the following five criteria: random sequence generation, allocation concealment, blinding of participants and personnel, blinding of outcome assessment, incomplete outcome data, and selective reporting [6]. The quality of all the included trials was categorized to low/unclear/high risk of bias.

For the other study designs, different criteria were used. AMSTAR (A Measurement Tool to Access Reviews) [7] were used to assess the quality of SR, MINORS (Methodological Index for Non-Randomized Studies) [8] was used for NRCT, and NOS (Newcastle-Ottawa Scale) [9] was used for cohort and case-control studies. Due to the lack of acknowledged tool or scale for CR and CS, the quality assessment of these two studies was based on the explicit diagnostic criteria, detailed description of demographic characteristics, intervention, and acknowledged outcome measurements.

Data analysis

SPSS 19.0 statistics software (480c9826941a904069d8) was used for data analyses. Data were summarized using relative risk (RR) with 95% confidence intervals (CI) for binary outcomes or mean difference (MD) with 95% CI for continuous outcomes.

Results

Description of studies

Thirty-three CPHMs were listed in EDL 2012 for the treatment of common cold (the compositions, indications, and dosage of the 33 CPHMs were shown in Table S2). After primary searches, 83 citations were identified. The majority was excluded due to obvious ineligibility (for example, animal experiment, influenza, bacterial infection of the upper respiratory tract, and etc), 46 full text papers were retrieved and 13 studies [10–22] fulfilled the inclusion criteria (Figure 1). The excluded studies and reason for exclusion were listed in Table S3.

Search results showed that only 7 CPHMs had published supporting clinical evidence. These CPHMs were Chaihu injection (5 CSs, 1 RCT), Qingre Jiedu granules (1 CS, 1 RCT), Huoxiang Zhengqi liquid (1 CS), Ganmao Qingre granules (1 RCT), Shuanghuanglian oral liquid (1 RCT), Xiaoer Baotaikang granules 1 RCT), and Xiaoer Resuqing oral liquid (1 RCT). A total of 6 RCTs and 7 CSs were included. No other study design was identified. All the studies were conducted in China, and published in Chinese between 1995 and 2012. The first RCT was published in 1997 [21] and the rest were all published after 2007. No studies report on informed consent or on whether they were properly approved by an IRB. Only one trial [10] revealed funding sources (Taizhou Municipal Science and Technology Project).

The characteristics of included studies were listed in Table S4. A total of 2643 participants with common cold were involved, ranging from 20 to 1560 per study. Eight studies included children [10,11,13,16,19,20,22], 1 study included adults [17], and 4 studies

PRISMA 2009 Flow Diagram

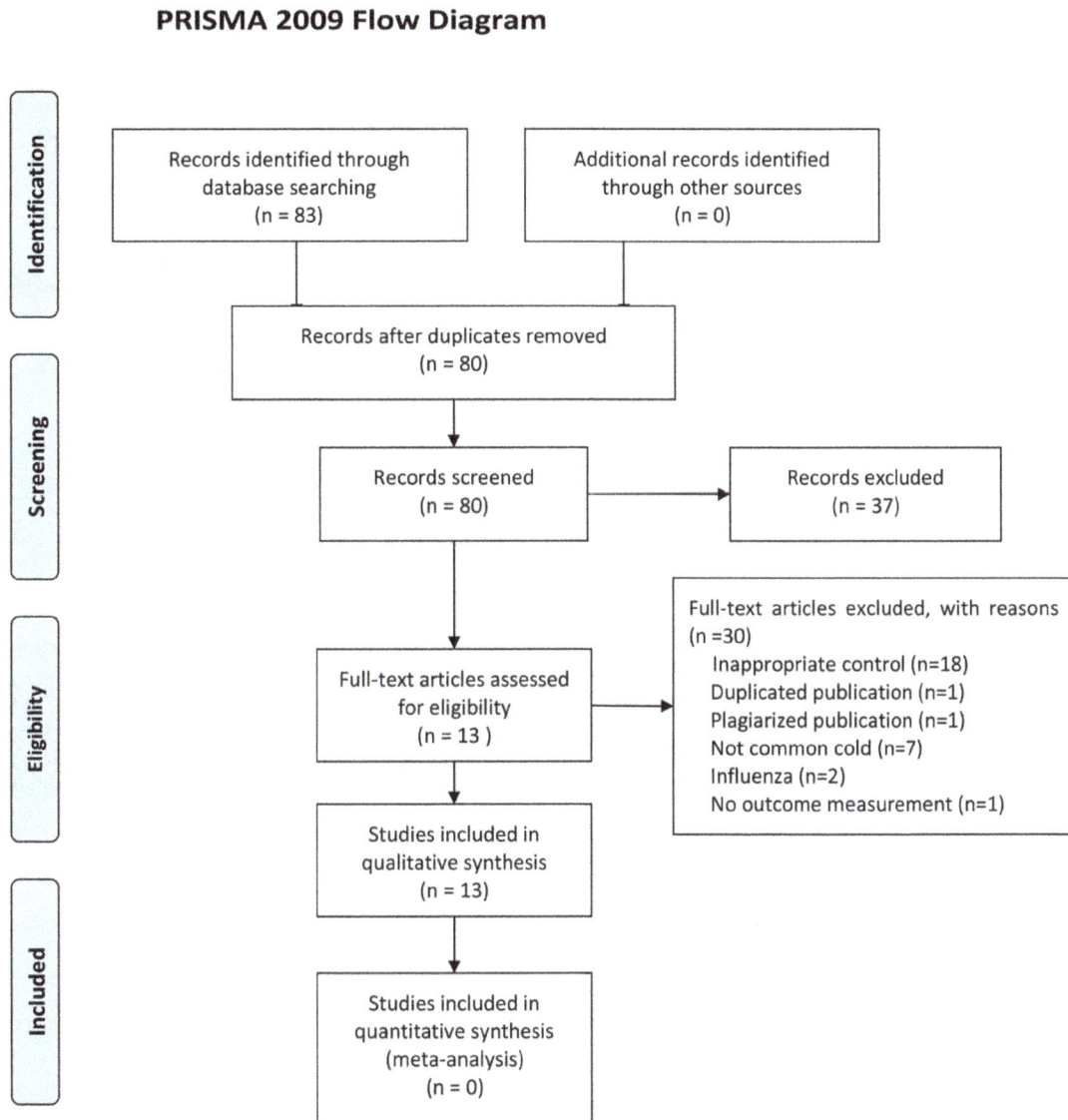

Figure 1. PRISMA 2009 Flow Diagram.

included both children and adults [12,14,15,18]. Five studies provided information on patients' syndrome differentiation (*Bianzheng*, TCM diagnosis) [16–19,21]. One trial used the diagnostic criterion for common cold of textbook 'practical paidonosology' [10], 1 trial used the diagnostic criterion of the China State Administration of Traditional Chinese Medicine, and the other 6 studies did not report their diagnostic criteria [11–15,20].

The routes of administration for CPHMs were quite diverse including oral intake, acupuncture point injection, intramuscular injection, retention enema, and nasal dripping. The treatment period was 3 to 5 days [11,14–17,19,21,22]. Four studies did not provide treatment period [12,13,18,20]. The reported outcomes were duration of fever, body temperature, or clinical symptoms improvement rate within a particular time. Clinical symptoms improvement rate was a composite measurement including a number of symptoms, of which body temperature was the vital one. Adverse events were reported in only 2 studies [12,18]. In Li 1997 [12], no allergic reaction was found. In Jiang 2012 [18], skin flushes, dizziness, and bitter taste in mouth were reported. While in the other 11 studies, the researchers did not reported whether or not they had monitored adverse events.

Therapeutic effects

Because common cold was a mild and self-limiting illness, we could not discriminate its spontaneous recovery with therapeutic effects by using the design of CSs. Therefore, we only calculated the therapeutic effects of CPHMs of RCTs (shown in Table S5). Results showed that Chaihu injection given at acupuncture point (LI 11) could shorten fever duration, Qingre Jiedu granules, Shuanghuanglian oral liquid, and Xiaoer Baotaikang granules had better clinical symptoms improvement rate within 3 days, and that Xiaoer Resuqing oral liquid had better clinical symptoms improvement rate within 5 days.

Methodological quality

Most of the included RCTs were of general poor methodological quality according to the predefined quality assessment criteria. Although 'random allocation' was mentioned in all RCTs, no trial described the methods for random sequence generation. We could not judge whether or not it was conducted properly due to the insufficient information. Allocation concealment and blinding were not reported in any RCT. No trial reported drop-outs or mentioned intention-to-treat analysis. Selective reporting was generally unclear in the RCTs due to the fact that all the RCT did not register before their start and we could not access to their trial protocol.

The included CSs were of very low quality. Most of the CSs did not reported diagnostic criterion, therefore it was possible that patients of influenza or upper respiratory tract infection caused by bacteria were included. Most of CSs did not provide a detailed description of baseline characteristics or treatment strategy. Moreover, most CSs used subjective outcome measurement such as cure rate, which was a self defined criteria and lacked unambiguous definition on outcome. Therefore made it difficult to interpret the effects even if the reported result was positive.

Discussion

In this review, only 7 CPHMs listed in EDL 2012 had clinical evidence to support their use for the common cold, and most of them only had one RCT or CS as supporting evidence. In addition, the evidence quality level of these 7 CPHMs were low due to the limitations in the design and implementation of studies. All studies had a very high likelihood of bias. Therefore the therapeutic effect of CPHM for the common cold should be taken in caution. More importantly, the fact that more than 80% of the CPHMs recommended in the EDL 2012 were not supported by clinical evidence revealed the enormous lack of evidence base that currently underpinned clinical use and policy making in China.

In August 2009, the 'Chinese national essential drug system' was officially launched and implemented. The 'Chinese national essential drug list' (2009 edition) has been issued in the same year [23]. The EDL was adjusted every 3 years and in the year 2012, the newest 2012 edition was published. The EDL 2012 contains 520 medicines, including 317 chemicals and biological products and 203 CPHMs. The CPHMs listed in EDL cover 137 kinds of internal medicine, 11 kinds of surgical medicine, 20 kinds of gynecological medicine, 7 kinds of ophthalmological medicine, 13 kinds of otorhinolaryngological medicine, and 15 kinds of orthopedics and traumatological medicine. The scope and number of CPHMs in the EDL 2012 was listed in Appendix S1. More than 3,100 medical and clinical experts had been assembled to evaluate the safety, effectiveness and economy of CPHMs. The selection process of medicine into EDL was strictly in accordance with the principle that they 'must be preventive and curative, safe and effective, affordable, easy to use, think highly of both Chinese and Western medicine' [24]. The detailed procedure for evaluation was not available because they were confidential files. However, our study demonstrated that they were less likely to be 'evidence-based' and revealed the sharp contrast between the policy and priority given to by the Chinese government to TCM.

In our review, the control interventions included antibiotics, antivirus drugs, and antipyretic and analgesic drugs. It was known that antibiotics had no effect against viral infections. Ribavirin and moroxydine were not recommended treatments for common cold. For mild and self-limiting illness which had no proved effective treatment, like common cold, randomized placebo controlled trial was the best study design to investigate the therapeutic effect.

However, in this review, we did not find placebo controlled RCT. In addition, all the clinical studies were of poor methodology, which frequently happened for Chinese clinical studies. For RCTs, methodology such as randomisation, blinding and placebo controls were not used. No trial reported drop-out or withdrawal, or mentioned intention-to-treat analysis. Poor methodology suggested the positive interpretation of the therapeutic effect of CPHMs could be biased, so claims about their effectiveness should be interpreted with caution. For CSs, we could not discriminate spontaneous recovery with therapeutic effects using the design of CSs due to the lack of comparison. The positive result itself drawn from a CS was not reliable. In addition, all the included CSs had poor methodology quality which was embodied in lack of diagnostic criterion, inadequate description of baseline characteristics or treatment strategy, and inappropriate outcome measurement, and therefore downgraded the reliability of the positive results. We thought part of the reason for the poor quality of TCM studies was that the research training in evidence-based medicine and critical appraisal had only just begun in China. There remains urgent need to train Chinese researchers in conducting unbiased trials in the future. Recently the government had increased the investment in TCM research, and many research activities were on-going in academic institutions and universities. With increasing awareness of the international guidelines for reporting of clinical trials, we hope the picture may change in future.

In the era of EBM, we need better evidence for CPHMs, and to achieve this we need to do thoughtful, placebo-controlled trials with proper randomization and blinding and, above all else, we need to think carefully about inappropriate control and outcome assessment. In the literature searching, a total of 18 trials were excluded due to inappropriate control. As a control, the drug should be definite effective or definite ineffective, or was widely used in clinical practice. During the literature searching, we found lots of trials which compared CPHM with another Chinese herb. We could not prove that the Chinese herb used as control was effective for common cold because we could not find any previous placebo-controlled trials on the treatment of this Chinese herb. Therefore, we have to exclude them. Using two different Chinese herbs as mutual comparison was a common mistake in TCM clinical trials in China and future researchers should be aware of this and make the correction. In our review, all the Chinese studies were so dependent on the presence or absence of fever as opposed to other symptoms, and this was at odds with the way Western medicine tends to design its evaluation of upper and lower respiratory tract infections. Most of the studies used body temperature or duration of fever as the main or exclusive outcome. For the studies that used composite criteria such as 'clinical symptoms improvement rate', body temperature was also a vital component. However, fever is just one of the symptoms and by no means the primary outcome because simple respiratory infections caused a range of symptoms (sore throat, muscle aches, sometimes gastrointestinal upset, runny nose, etc). Our suggestion to the future researchers was to use well validated outcome measurements and to consider all the related symptoms. A patient-reported daily symptom diary including symptom variables giving each symptom a score would be a valuable approach. Patients could also completed Likert scales of how satisfied or concerned they were with different aspects of treatment. These Likert scales have previously been shown to be reliable, have good construct validity, and predict illness duration [25–27].

In our review, we searched all studies assessing the CPHMs for treatment of common cold regardless of study design. However, only CSs and RCTs were identified. The possible reasons might be that in China few TCM practitioners, researchers, and journal editors have received scientific research methodology training [28–30]. Articles based on case series were more acceptable during the l990s and early 2000's as they were closer to clinical practice. Since the year of 2000, with the spread of evidence-based medicine, more and more TCM practitioners began to use RCTs because it was regarded as the gold standard for evaluating therapeutic effects. That was why we did not find other study designs.

In our review, all the included 13 studies were published in 12 different journals. The 12 journals were all legitimate Chinese medical journals. However, only 5 journals were rated as the core journals in China. The grade of journal was thought related to the quality of the trials it published. We suggest the editors of all TCM journals to be trained on clinical research methodology to ensure the scientific scrutiny for published researches.

The report of adverse events of CPHMs was not adequate. One study [12] reported that no allergic reaction was found; one study [18] reported skin flushes, dizzy and bitter taste. However, their reports were too brief to providing useful information. Turner observed that adverse events were often not well-reported in CAM RCTs [31]. In China, it was commonly believed that CPHMs was safer than western medicine. However, the increasing reports of adverse events associated with Chinese herbal medicines have excited attentions [32–34]. More and more TCM researchers began to investigate the specific mechanism of ingredient of Chinese herbs and its safety. TCM investigators for future study should be encouraged to monitor and report adverse events in clinical trials to GCP standards in order to evaluate the potential harms of CPHMs.

We have found that a systematic review titled 'Chinese medicinal herbs for the common cold' has been published in the Cochrane library in 2007 [35]. In this review, the author assessed the effect of Chinese medicinal herbs for the common cold. They only included RCT and included both CPHMs and individually prescribed herbal formulae. Our review is different from Zhang 2007 [35] not only in aim, but also in inclusion criteria, search strategy, analysis, and problem revealed. Our aim was to provide a well-round clinical evidence assessment of state authorized recommended CPHMs for common cold. Therefore we included all study designs and restricted CPHMs as those in the EDL.

The limitation of our review was that there were 6 studies that did not provided their diagnostic criteria, just mentioned that 'common cold patients were included'. We did not exclude them with the intent to providing more information in our review. Thereafter, possibility existed that participants with other acute respiratory infections such as influenza were recruited.

In summary, a confirmative conclusion on the beneficial effect of CPHMs for common cold still cannot be drawn. To ensure evidence-based clinical practice, further rigorous placebo-controlled, randomized trials are warranted. Further TCM researchers should pay more attention to reducing risks of bias and other limitations of trials, and improving the reporting quality by complying with international reporting standards such as the CONSORT [36], in addition, more emphasis should be paid on the selection of control intervention and outcome measurement. Too much dependent on the presence of absence of fever is not recommended.

The rough results of this review have been published in abstract form in the Journal of Alternative and Complementary Medicine as a conference paper for the 2014 International Research Congress on Integrative Medicine and Health [37].

Supporting Information

Table S1   List of study design features.

Table S2   Compositions and indications of 33 CPHMs listed in 'China national essential drug list 2012' for common cold.

Table S3   List of the excluded studies with reasons.

Table S4   The characteristics of included studies.

Table S5   Effect estimations of CPHMs for treatment of common cold in included trials.

Checklist S1   PRISMA 2009 checklist.

Appendix S1   The scope and number of CPHMs in the 'Chinese national essential drug list 2012'.

Author Contributions

Conceived and designed the experiments: WC JPL. Performed the experiments: WC LQW JR WJX FL. Analyzed the data: WC LQW. Wrote the paper: WC. Revised the manuscript: GL.

References

1. Turner RB. (2001) The treatment of rhinovirus infections: progress and potential. Antiviral Research 49: 1–4.
2. Eccles R. (2005) Understanding the symptoms of the common cold and influenza. Lancet Infect Dis 5: 718–725.
3. Simasek M, Blandino DA. (2007) Treatment of the common cold. American Family Physician 75: 515–520.
4. Kenealy T, Arroll B. (2013) Antibiotics for the common cold and acute purulent rhinitis. Cochrane Database Syst Rev 6: CD000247.
5. Yang SS. (1965) Inner Canon of Huangdi·Taisu. Beijing: People's Medical Publishing House.
6. Higgins JPT, Altman DG, Sterne JAC. (editors) (2011) Chapter 8: Assessing risk of bias in included studies. In: Higgins JPT, Green S (editors). Cochrane Handbook for Systematic Reviews of Interventions Version 5.1.0 (updated March 2011). The Cochrane Collaboration, 2011. Available from www.cochrane-handbook.org.
7. Shea BJ, Grimshaw JM, Wells GA, Boers M, Andersson N, et al. (2007) Development of AMSTAR: a measurement tool to assess the methodological quality of systematic reviews. BMC Med Res Methodol 15: 10.
8. Slim K, Nini E, Forestier D, Kwiatkowski F, Panis Y, et al. (2003) Methodological index for non-randomized studies (minors): development and validation of a new instrument. ANZ J Surg 73: 712–716.
9. GA Wells, B Shea, D O'Connell, J Peterson, V Welch, et al. The Newcastle-Ottawa Scale (NOS) for assessing the quality of nonrandomised studies in meta-analyses. Available: http://www.ohri.ca/programs/clinical_epidemiology/oxford.asp. Accessed 24 October 2013.
10. Lv GQ. (2010) Chaihu injection acupoint block in treating pediatric cold and fever. Inner Mongol Journal of Traditional Chinese Medicine 29: 151–152.
11. Dai LH. (1995) Chaihu auricular point injection in treating pediatric cold and fever in 84 cases. Journal of Henan College of Traditional Chinese Medicine 10: 45.
12. Li ZX, Liu XP. (1997) Chaihu injection enema retention in treating cold and fever in 30 cases. Shanxi J of Traditional Chinese Medicine 13: 16.
13. Wang ZY. (2003) Chaihu injection enema retention in treating pediatric cold and fever in 26 cases. Journal of Emergency in Traditional Chinese Medicine 12: 503.
14. Zhang HY, Wang YF. (2009) Chaihu injection nasal dripping in treating cold and fever. Qingdao Medical Journal 36: 431–432.

15. Wang LZ. (1999) Chaihu injection in treating cold and fever. Shandong Journal of Traditional Chinese Medicine 18: 282.

16. Zhao MD. (2012) Clinical research on Qingre Jiedu granules in treating children with viral upper respiratory tract infection in 106 cases. Chinese Community Doctors 14: 223–224.

17. Xu HQ, Zhao JC. (2010) Clinical report of Qingre Jiedu granules in treating wind-heat type of common cold in 90 cases. Medical Journal of Chinese People's Health 22: 132.

18. Jiang XQ, Chen SQ, Yuan JX. (2012) Analysis of 1560 patients taking Huoxiang Zhengqi liquid in our hospital department of traditional Chinese medicine. Guangming Journal of Chinese Medicine 27: 386–387.

19. Di JH. (2012) Clinical observation of Ganmao Qingre granules in treating pediatric wind-cold type of common cold in 30 cases. Chinese Pediatrics of Integrated Traditional and Western Medicine 4: 277–278.

20. Wang HR, Wang YF. (1997) Clinical observation of Shuanghuanglian oral liquid in treating children with upper respiratory tract infection. Qingdao Medical Journal 29: 40.

21. Wu CF, Guan MC, Chi XW. (2012) Clinial observation of Xiaoer Baotaikang granules in treating children with upper respiratory tract infection. Strait Pharmaceutical Journal 24: 239–240.

22. Li QF, Song M. (2007) Clinical observation of Xiaoer Resuqing oral liquid in treating pediatric cold and fever. Shandong Medical Journal 47: 24.

23. The Central People's Government of the People's Republic of China (2009) Healthy ministry: Chinese project of establishing national essential drug system was officially launched. Available: http://www.gov.cn/gzdt/2009-08/18/content_1395565.htm. Accessed 12 May 2014.

24. National Health and Family Planning Commission of the People's Republic of China (2013) The 'Chinese national essential drug list' (2012 edition) has been published. Available: http://www.moh.gov.cn/mohywzc/s3582/201303/b058a4edf14e4dc9a1f6f0f0c71a2cce.shtml. Accessed 12 May 2014.

25. Little P, Rumsby K, Kelly J, Watson L, Moore M, et al. (2005) Information leaflet and antibiotic prescribing strategies for acute lower respiratory tract infection: a randomized controlled trial. JAMA 293: 3029–3035.

26. Little P, Gould C, Williamson I, Moore M, Warner G, et al. (2001) Pragmatic randomised controlled trial of two prescribing strategies for childhood acute otitis media. BMJ 322: 336–342.

27. Williamson IG, Rumsby K, Benge S, Moore M, Smith PW, et al. (2007) Antibiotics and topical nasal steroid for treatment of acute maxillary sinusitis: a randomized controlled trial. JAMA 298: 2487–2496.

28. Zhang Y, An R, He LY, Chen LN, Liu SY, et al. (2010) Investigation and analysis on actuality and demands of scientific researchers in state clinical research facility of TCM. International Journal of Traditional Chinese Medicine 32: 523–524.

29. Han M, Tian N, Yang GY, Liu GH, Chen J, et al. (2013) Survey and Analysis on Basic Status of Clinical Scientific Researchers of the National Chinese Medicine Clinical Research Base. Modernization of Traditional Chinese Medicine-World Science and Technology 15: 1771–1775.

30. An R. (2011) Investigations and analysis of professional work building of the National Chinese Medicine Clinical Research Base. [Dissertation of Master's Degree]: Beijing university of Chinese Medicine.

31. Turner LA, Singh K, Garritty C, Tsertsvadze A, Manheimer E, et al. (2011) An evaluation of the completeness of safety reporting in reports of complementary and alternative medicine trials. BMC Complement Altern Med 11: 67.

32. Gottieb S. (2000) Chinese herb may cause cancer. BMJ 320: 1623.

33. Ishizaki T, Sasaki F, Ameshima S, Shiozaki K, Takahashi H, et al. (1996) Pneumonitis during interferon and/or herbal drug therapy in patients with chronic active hepatitis. European Respiratory Journal 9: 2691–2696.

34. Melchart D, Linde K, Weidenhammer W, Hager S, Shaw D, et al. (1999) Liver enzyme elevations in patients treated with traditional Chinese medicine. JAMA 282: 28–29.

35. Zhang X, Wu T, Zhang J, Yan Q, Xie L, et al. (2007) Chinese medicinal herbs for the common cold. Cochrane Database of Systematic Reviews Issue 1. Art. No.: CD004782. DOI: 10.1002/14651858.CD004782.pub2.

36. Moher D, Hopewell S, Schulz KF, Montori V, Gøtzsche PC, et al, for the CONSORT Group. (2010) CONSORT 2010 Explanation and Elaboration: updated guidelines for reporting parallel group randomised trial. BMJ 340: c869.

37. Chen W, Wang LQ, Liu JP. (2014) Chinese Patent Medicines Listed in China National Essential Drug List for Common Cold: An Evidence Synthesis. The Journal of Alternative and Complementary Medicine. 5: A128–A128.

3

Multi-Targeted Antiangiogenic Tyrosine Kinase Inhibitors in Advanced Non-Small Cell Lung Cancer: Meta-Analyses of 20 Randomized Controlled Trials and Subgroup Analyses

Wenhua Liang[9], Xuan Wu[9], Shaodong Hong[9], Yaxiong Zhang, Shiyang Kang, Wenfeng Fang, Tao Qin, Yan Huang, Hongyun Zhao, Li Zhang*

Sun Yat-sen University Cancer Center, State Key Laboratory of Oncology in South China, Collaborative Innovation Center for Cancer Medicine, Guangzhou, China

Abstract

Background: Multi-targeted antiangiogenic tyrosine kinase inhibitors (MATKIs) have been studied in many randomized controlled trials (RCTs) for treatment of advanced non-small cell lung cancer (NSCLC). We seek to summarize the most up-to-date evidences and perform a timely meta-analysis.

Methods: Electronic databases were searched for eligible studies. We defined the experimental arm as MATKI-containing group and the control arm as MATKI-free group. The extracted data on objective response rates (ORR), disease control rates (DCR), progression-free survival (PFS) and overall survival (OS) were pooled. Subgroup and sensitivity analyses were conducted.

Results: Twenty phase II/III RCTs that involved a total of 10834 participants were included. Overall, MATKI-containing group was associated with significant superior ORR (OR 1.29, 95% CI 1.08 to 1.55, $P = 0.006$) and prolonged PFS (HR 0.83, 0.78 to 0.90, $P = 0.005$) compared to the MATKI-free group. However, no significant improvements in DCR (OR 1.08, 1.00 to 1.17, $P = 0.054$) or OS (HR 0.97, 0.93 to 1.01, P = 0.106) were observed. Subgroup analyses showed that the benefits were predominantly presented in pooled results of studies enrolling previously-treated patients, studies not limiting to enroll non-squamous NSCLC, and studies using MATKIs in combination with the control regimens as experimental therapies.

Conclusions: This up-to-date meta-analysis showed that MATKIs did increase ORR and prolong PFS, with no significant improvement in DCR and OS. The advantages of MATKIs were most prominent in patients who received a MATKI in combination with standard treatments and in patients who had previously experienced chemotherapy. We suggest further discussion as to the inclusion criteria of future studies on MATKIs regarding histology.

Editor: William B. Coleman, University of North Carolina School of Medicine, United States of America

Funding: This study was funded by the National High Technology Research and Development Program of China Molecular classification and individualized diagnosis and treatment of lung cancer (grant numbers: 2012AA02A502) and the role of monitoring circulating tumor cells and drug-resistance-associated molecular in the therapeutic prediction, evaluation and mechanism of drug-resistance in EGFR mutant advanced NSCLC patients receiving EGFR-TKI (grant numbers: Wu Jieping Funds 320.6750.1316). The funders had no role in study design, data collection and analysis, decision to publish, or preparation of the manuscript.

Competing Interests: The authors have declared that no competing interests exist.

* Email: zhangli6@mail.sysu.edu.cn

9 These authors contributed equally to this work.

Introduction

Lung cancer is the leading cause of cancer-related mortality worldwide, with about 85% patients diagnosed with non-small cell lung cancer (NSCLC) [1]. Locally advanced or metastatic NSCLC accounts for 80% patients; for these patients the standard care is systemic chemotherapy [2]. Regardless of the emergence of new agents, however, chemotherapy provides only marginal benefit in overall survival [3].

Another treatment option is to inhibit angiogenesis, a complicated process that is regulated by cellular cues, multiple receptor-mediated signaling networks, and a number of pro- and antiangiogenic factors [4,5]. Antiangiogenic therapy is designed to minimize the acquisition of nutrients and oxygen diffusion to starve tumors. Vascular endothelial growth factor (VEGF) is a key mediator of angiogenesis which has been well studied. Currently, the only antiangiogenic agent approved for patients with NSCLC is bevacizumab, an anti-VEGF monoclonal antibody [6]. However, many other antiangiogenic agents are under clinical development.

VEGF receptor (VEGFR) also plays an important role in the pathways regarding angiogenesis. Multi-targeted antiangiogenic tyrosine kinase inhibitors (MATKIs) are novel agents that target VEGFR-dependent tumor angiogenesis and simultaneously inhibit some other key pathways, such as platelet-derived growth factor (PDGF), fibroblast growth factor (FGF), epidermal growth factor and their associate receptors. Previous studies showed that these small-molecule inhibitors are activitive in a wide variety of cancers [7]. MATKIs could fill in a unique niche for cancer therapeutics, especially in western countries where a relatively small population is suitable for receiving targeted therapies that direct known gene alterations [8]. Recently, these similar MATKIs have showed promising advantages in the treatment of advanced NSCLC [9]. A previous meta-analysis suggested that a regimen of chemotherapy in combination with MATKIs have specific advantages over chemotherapy alone in terms of PFS and ORR, but not in OS [10]. However, it involved only six randomized controlled trials (RCTs) and three agents. Since then, plenty of novel results from phase II/III RCTs have been reported. Thus, we sought to perform a timely meta-analysis to summarize all the evidence including the updated reports. In addition, the abundant data allowed us to carry out some subgroup analyses.

Methods

Search Strategy

PubMed, EMBASE, the Cochrane Library as well as the ASCO and ESMO databases from Jan 2005 to Jan 2014 were searched for eligible trials. Search terms were the combination of "non-small-cell lung cancer" with any of the following: "multitargeted antiangiogenesis tyrosine kinase inhibitors" or "sorafenib", "sunitinib", "cediranib", "vandetanib", "motesanib", "nintedanib", "pazopanib" or "axitinib". The reference lists of the included studies and recent reviews were checked manually as a supplement. No language restriction was applied.

Eligibility Criteria

In order for a study to be included in this analysis, the following criteria should be met: 1) phase II or III RCT; 2) studies that compared at least one MATKI-containing regimen to MATKI-free regimens as any line treatments in patients with advanced NSCLC; 3) studies reporting at least one response or survival endpoints. In cases of overlap reports, we included only the latest results. Trials will be excluded if they were not in accordance with the eligible criteria.

Endpoints

The major endpoints for this meta-analysis were overall survival (OS; defined as the time of randomization to the time of death), progression free survival (PFS; defined as the time of randomization to the time of disease progression or death), objective response rate (ORR, percent of patients whose best response was complete response or partial response according to the Recist 1.1 criteria) and disease control rate (DCR, percentage of patients whose best response was complete response, partial response or stable disease according to Recist 1.1 criteria), as well as adverse events (AEs).

Quality Assessment and Data Extraction

The quality of each eligible study was rated according to the JADAD score [11]. Baseline clinical characteristics, total number of enrolled patients, number of patients who showed complete response, partial response or stable disease, hazard ratio (HR) of median OS and PFS were extracted by two investigators independently. Discrepancies were discussed by the two investigators to reach consensus. In case of missing data, we contacted the primary investigators through emails.

Statistical Analysis

We defined the experimental arm as MATKI-containing group and the control arm as MATKI-free group. Pooled hazard ratios (HRs) for survival outcomes (PFS and OS) and pooled odds ratio (ORs) for dichotomous data (ORR, DCR and toxicities) with 95% confidence intervals (CI) were calculated using the Inverse Variance algorithm and Mantel-Haenszel algorithm. Heterogeneity across studies was assessed with a forest plot and the inconsistency statistic (I^2). An I^2 of 25%, 50% and 75% was considered the cutoff of mild, moderate and severe statistical heterogeneity respectively. A random-effects model was employed in case of the existence of potential heterogeneity; however, both fixed-effect and random effects model were tested. All calculations were performed using STATA 11.0 (StataA Corp, College Station, TX). Subgroup analysis was conducted according to the line of treatment (1st-line vs. 2nd-/3rd-line/maintenance), involved histological type (unselective population vs. selective population for non-squamous carcinoma), the comparison pattern (MATKI + standard treatment/standard treatment vs. MATKI/standard treatment) respectively. Interaction tests were conducted to assess the inter-subgroup differences. Sensitivity analyses were performed. Graphical funnel plots were generated to visually inspect for publication bias. The statistical methods for detecting funnel plot asymmetry were the rank correlation test of Begg and Mazumdar and the regression asymmetry test of Egger [12,13]. For all analyses, P<0.05 was considered statistically significant.

Results

Selection and Features of Included Studies

Six agents (vandetanib, sunitinib, cediranib, sorafenib, motesanib and nintedanib) could be analyzed while trial data for the other agents remain immature. After screening, 20 phase II/III RCTs (7 for vandetanib, 2 for sunitinib, 3 for cediranib, 5 for sorafenib, 2 for motesanib, and 1 for nintedanib) involving a total of 10834 participants [14-33]. Figure 1 showed the flow chart of study selection. The definitions of all studied endpoints were consistent among included studies. Among all studies, 10 trials enrolling patients who previously received chemotherapy while the other 10 included chemo-naïve patients. In addition, five studies limited the eligible histological type to non-squamous carcinoma [18,20,31-33]. The 2007 study by Heymach et al. [24] contained two dose groups (100 mg/d and 300 mg/d) and the 2008 study by Heymach et al. [27] contained two experimental regimens, they were therefore divided into two separate arms for all analyses. Similarly, Blumenschein's study [32] was divided into two arms: motesanib 125 mg arm and motesanib 75 mg arm respectively. Table 1 summarized the characteristics of both the included agents and studies.

Meta-analysis of the MATKI-containing Regimens versus MATKI-free Regimens

When compared to MATKI-free group, MATKI-containing group was associated with significantly superior ORR (OR 1.29, 95% CI 1.08 to 1.55, P = 0.006; Fig. 2A) and longer PFS (HR 0.83, 95% CI 0.78 to 0.90, P = 0.005; Fig. 2C). However, no significant improvement in DCR (OR 1.08, 95% CI 1.00 to 1.17, P = 0.054; Fig. 2B) and OS (HR 0.97, 95% CI 0.93 to 1.01,

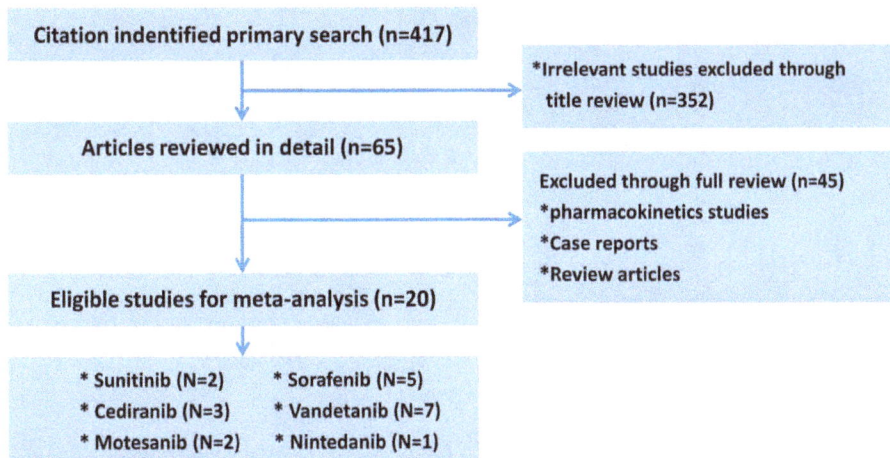

Figure 1. Flow chart of study selection.

P = 0.106; Fig. 2D) was observed. Figure 2 illustrates all results of the overall meta-analyses.

Subgroup Analyses, Sensitivity Analyses and Publication Bias

When stratifying patients according to chemotherapy history, we observed that greater benefits of MATKIs in ORR and DCR were presented in patients who failed the prior chemotherapy than those without any prior chemotherapy regarding all outcomes (2nd-/3rd-line/maintenance vs. 1st-line: ORR, OR 1.547 vs. 1.116, $P_{interaction} = 0.08$; DCR, OR 1.183 vs. 0.956, $P_{interaction} = 0.003$; PFS, HR 0.817 vs. 0.848, $P_{interaction} = 0.60$; OS, HR 0.965 vs. 0.97, $P_{interaction} = 0.92$) (greater OR indicated better ORR or DCR, while smaller HR indicated better PFS or OS). In terms of histology, the pooled results of studies that includes tumors of all histological types (not limited to non-squamous NSCLC) showed a favorable trend in comparison with studies selectively enrolled non-squamous carcinoma especially in ORR and PFS (unselective population vs. selective population: ORR, OR 1.375 vs. 1.140, $P_{interaction} = 0.33$; DCR, OR 1.077 vs. 1.081, $P_{interaction} = 0.97$; PFS, HR 0.811 vs. 0.899, $P_{interaction} = 0.21$; OS, HR 0.965 vs. 0.966, $P_{interaction} = 0.98$). We found that the studies whose experimental arms investigated regimens of adding MATKIs to the regimens in the control arm were associated with greater benefits on PFS (HR 0.798 vs. 0.998, $P_{interaction} = 0.03$). In addition, significance of DCR improvement (OR 1.095, 95% CI 1.016 to 1.180, $P = 0.018$) and OS benefits (HR 0.951, 95% CI 0.907 to 0.998, P = 0.042) were found to be statistically significant, which differed from the overall results and the results of other subgroups. Conversely, we failed to observe any benefit from studies comparing the efficacy of MATKI to the standard regimens in the control arms. All results of the subgroup analyses (including test of interaction) are illustrated in Figure 3 and were summarized in Table S1.

We conducted a sensitivity analysis by using a fixed-effects model (Table S1). We also conducted a sensitivity analysis to examine the pooled results after excluding one study by lee et al. [30] because it compared vindetanib to placebo which differed significantly from all other included trials. The conclusions regarding all outcomes were not altered in sensitivity analyses. In regard to the publication bias, no significant bias was observed in analyses of all endpoints through both Begg's test and Egger's test (P>0.05).

Discussions

The angiogenesis pathways, which play a critical role in the nourishment of both the tumors and metastatic lesions, have been targeted as a therapeutic option. Bevacizumab, a monoclonal antibody that binds to VEGF, is the only antiangiogenic drug approved for the treatment of NSCLC since it showed overall survival improvement when combined with chemotherapy [6]. An alternative approach is to shut down the VEGFR functions. Therefore, several multi-targeted tyrosine kinase inhibitors (MATKIs) that target VEGFR as well as other key pathways concerning angiogenesis and tumor proliferation are being developed. In some solid tumors, such as renal cell carcinoma and hepatocellular carcinoma, MAKTIs did reduce tumor burden and prolong overall survival [7]. Several of these agents have been evaluated in a series of phase II/III clinical trials for NSCLC patients. A previous meta-analysis suggested that regimens of chemotherapy plus MATKIs were superior to chemotherapy alone in terms of PFS and ORR, but not in OS [10]. However, this meta-analysis involved only six RCTs and three agents (sorafenib, sunitinib, and cediranib). There have been more than ten novel studies published afterwards. Thus, we believed it necessary to update the results using the new evidence and explore some novel information.

According to the current results, regimens containing sorafenib, sunitinib, cediranib, vandetanib, motesanib or nintedanib had substantial improvements for ORR and PFS outcomes, when compared with regimens free of these agents. In contrast, benefits in DCR and OS were not statistically significant. Since ORR is a part of DCR, we speculated that the underlying reason for a difference in associated benefits between ORR and DCR was that MATKIs failed to deliver any additional benefit in patients that presented primary resistance to standard treatments (chemotherapies or TKIs). This hypothesis was strengthened by our findings in the subgroup analyses: MATKIs failed to achieve any improvement when using alone. The current results could be explained by a widely accepted hypothesis that anti-angiogenic agents can transiently normalize the abnormal structure and function of tumor vessels to make it more efficient for drug delivery [34]. Therefore, MATKIs could 'rescue' those who actually

Table 1. Features of included agents and studies.

Agents	Targets	Study by Author	Year	Phase	Line	Histology Types	Regimens (Experimental arm)	Regimens (Control arm)
Sunitinib	VEGFR-1, -2, -3; PDGFRβ; c-kit; Flt-3	Socinski[14]	2010	2	1	All	Bevacizumab+TC+Sunitinib	Bevacizumab+TC
		Scagliotti[15]	2012	3	2-3	All	Erlotinib+Sunitinib	Erlotinib
Sorafenib	b-Raf; VEGFR-2, -3; PDGFRβ; Flt-3; c-kit	Spigel[16]	2011	2	2-3	All	Erlotinib+Sorafenib	Erlotinib
		Scagliotti[17]	2010	3	1	All	TC+Sorafenib	TC
		Paz-Ares[18]	2012	3	1	N-S	GP+Sorafenib	GP
		Wang[19]	2011	2	1	All	GP+Sorafenib	GP
		Molina[20]	2011	2	2	N-S	PEM+Sorafenib	PEM
Cediranib	VEGFR-1, -2, -3; PDGFR; FGFR-1; c-kit	Goss[21]	2010	2,3	1	All	TC+Cediranib	TC
		Dy[22]	2013	2	1	All	GC+Cediranib	GC
		Laurie[22]	2012	2,3	1	All	TC+Cediranib	TC
Vandetanib	VEGFR-2, -3; EGFR	Heymach[24]	2007	2	2	All	DOC+Vandetanib 100 mg	DOC
						All	DOC+Vandetanib 300 mg	DOC
		Herbst[25]	2010	3	2	All	DOC+Vandetanib 100 mg	DOC
		deBoer[26]	2011	3	2	All	PEM+Vandetanib 100 mg	PEM
		Heymach[27]	2008	2	1	All	TC+Vandetanib 300 mg	TC
						All	Vandetanib 300 mg	TC
		Natale[28]	2011	3	2	All	Vandetanib 300 mg	Erlotinib
		Natale[29]	2009	2	2	All	Vandetanib 300 mg	Gefitinib
		Lee[30]	2012	3	2	All	Vandetanib 300 mg	Placebo
Motesanib	VEGFR-1, -2, -3; PDFGR; c-kit	Scagliotti[31]	2012	3	1	N-S	TC+Motesanib	TC
		Blumenschein[32]	2011	2	1	N-S	TC+Motesanib 125 mg	TC+Beva
						N-S	TC+Motesanib 75 mg	TC+Beva
Nintedanib	VEGFR 1-3; FGFR 1-3; PDGFR α/β	Martin[33]	2013	3	2	N-S	DOC+Nintedanib	DOC

N-S, non-squamous cell carcinoma; TC, paclitaxel+carboplatin; GP, gemcitabine+cisplatin; DOC, docetaxol; PEM, pemetrxed.

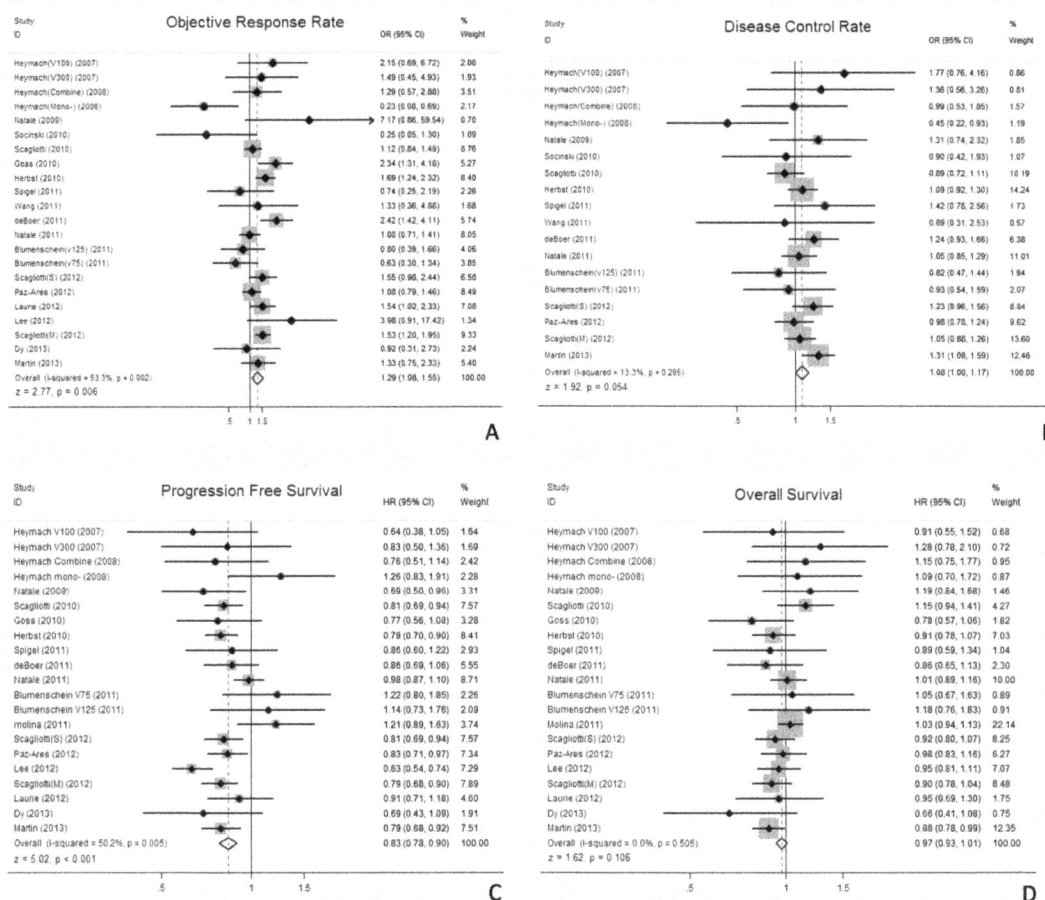

Figure 2. Meta-analyses of MATKIs-containing regimens versus MATKIs-free regimens. A, ORR; B, DCR; C, PFS; D, OS.

respond to chemotherapy but suffered from drug accessibility; this finally translated into significantly improved pooled ORR; however patients who were non-responsive remained the same status, therefore there was no significant increase in DCR. Another hypothesis derived from these results was that regulating the VEGFR pathway might play a more important role than inhibition of other targets (EGFR, PDGFR, etc) in the use of MATKIs when no selection for specific patients was conducted. It implied that MATKIs might have to work in combination with other anti-proliferative agents.

With respect to the survival outcomes, the improvement in PFS of MATKIs failed to translate into overall survival benefits. In the perspective of trial design, this might be attributed to the confounding effects from bias of the subsequent treatments. This speculation was supported by the current subgroup analyses which showed that trials studying the maintenance/2nd-line/3rd-line settings have greater magnitudes of benefits compared with those studying the 1st-line settings. This evidence highlighted the advantages of using MATKIs and highlighted the need for balancing post-trial therapies in the future studies.

Since increased risk of hemoptysis in squamous cell carcinoma was documented during the early trials, bevacizumab is only indicated for non-squamous NSCLC [35]. Similarly, part of trials on MATKIs excluded patients with squamous cell carcinoma. Through subgroup analyses, we observed that these trials did not

reveal any advantages of MATKI-containing regimens over MATKI-free regimens. However, significant differences were presented when pooling the studies that recruited all histological types (including squamous cell carcinoma). It at least suggested that non-squamous NSCLC might not the targeted subpopulation that benefits most from MATKIs. An exploratory analysis revealed an increased pooled incidence of hemorrhage based on two studies including all histological types, while the incidence was similar between the groups based on the other two studies including only non-squamous NSCLC (data not shown). Although our results did not provide direct evidences, they suggested that patients with squamous cell carcinoma might benefit more from MATKI but might be associated with increased risk for hemorrhage compared with non-squamous NSCLC. However, some recent reports argued that the risk of hemorrhage among squamous NSCLC when using anti-angiogenic agents was acceptable [36]. Therefore, the inclusion criteria, in terms of histology, require further discussion for future studies on MATKIs. Of course, direct comparison of histology associated hemorrhage risk should be proposed to clarify this issue.

This is the most up-to-date comprehensive analysis to compare the MATKI-containing to MATKI-free regimens, confirming the true efficacy of MATKIs. Nevertheless, there are several limitations. Firstly, the meta-analysis might suffer from significant clinical heterogeneity. There were various chemotherapeutic

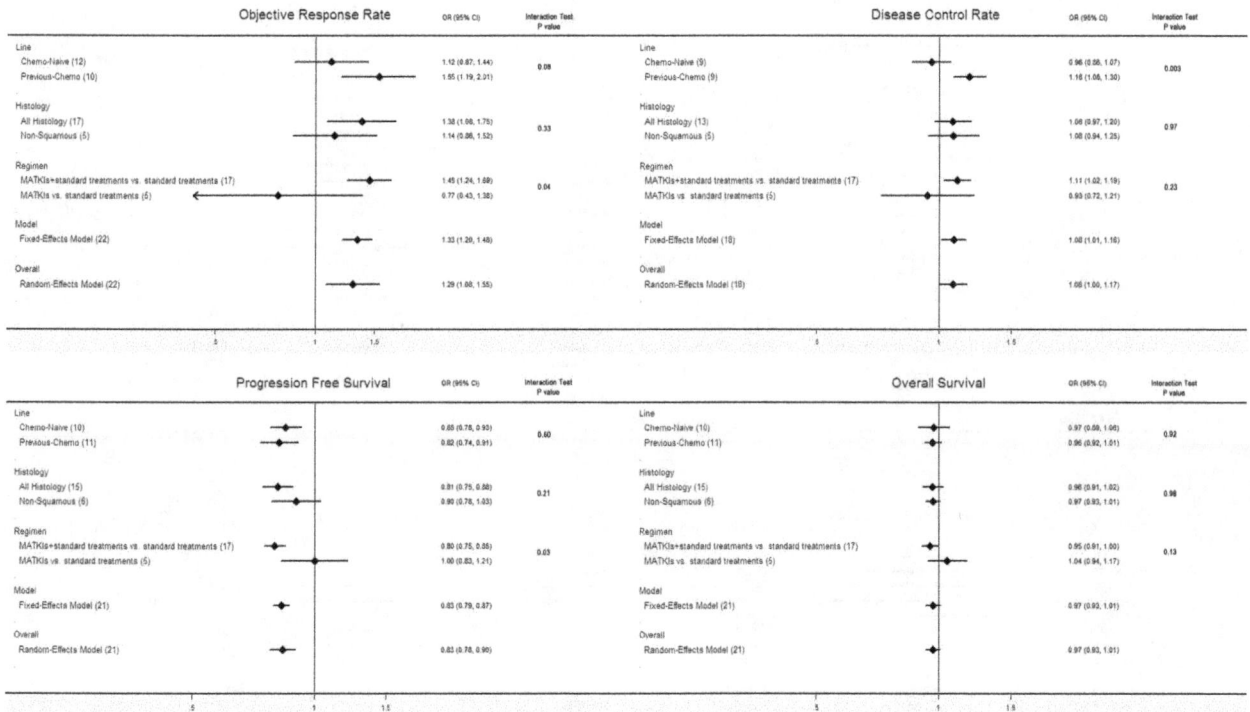

Figure 3. Subgroup analyses of each endpoint (number of studies or arms). A, ORR; B, DCR; C, PFS; D, OS.

regimens and patterns involved but we were unable to evaluate the respective effect of different MATKIs or treatment settings since current data were not sufficient to draw any solid conclusion for each subset. Secondly, only six agents were finally included in the analysis because studies on other agents were still ongoing (http://clinicaltrials.gov). Thirdly, we were unable to conduct this analysis based on individual patient data, which could definitely provide more reliable information especially in subgroup analyses. To be sure, further studies are warranted to complete the information.

In conclusion, regimens consisting of multi-targeted antiangiogenic TKIs were superior to those without these agents in terms of ORR and PFS in patients with advanced NSCLC. However, no significant benefits in DCR or OS were observed. In addition, subgroup analyses provided us some hints to improve future studies and clinical application of MATKIs.

Supporting Information

Table S1   Summary of Subgroup Analyses Results.

Checklist S1   PRISMA checklist.

Flowchart S1   PRISMA flow chart.

Author Contributions

Conceived and designed the experiments: WHL XW SDH LZ. Performed the experiments: WHL XW YXZ SYK. Analyzed the data: WHL SDH WFF TQ. Contributed reagents/materials/analysis tools: WFF YH HYZ. Contributed to the writing of the manuscript: WHL XW YXZ.

References

1. Jemal A, Siegel R, Xu J, Ward E. Cancer statistics, 2010. CA Cancer J Clin 2010; 60: 277–300.
2. National Comprehensive Cancer Network. NCCN Clinical Practice Guidelines in OncologyTM. Non-Small Cell Lung Cancer. V 2.2010. http://www.nccn.org/professionals/physician gls/PDF/nscl.pdf. Accessed April 8; 2010.
3. Ramalingam S, Belani C. Systemic chemotherapy for advanced non-small cell lung cancer: recent advances and future directions. Oncologist 2008; (Suppl. 1): 5–13.
4. Ferrara N, Gerber HP, LeCouter J. The biology of VEGF and its receptors. Nat Med 2003; 9: 669–76.
5. Carmeliet P, Jain RK. Angiogenesis in cancer and other diseases. Nature 2000; 407(6801): 249–57.
6. Sandler A, Gray R, Perry MC, Brahmer J, Schiller JH, et al. Paclitaxel carboplatin alone or with bevacizumab for non-smallcell lung cancer. N Engl J Med 2006; 355: 2542–2550.
7. Ivy SP, Wick JY, Kaufman BM. An overview of small molecule inhibitors of VEGFR signaling. Nat Rev Clin Oncol 2009; 6: 569–579.
8. Dearden S, Stevens J, Wu YL, Blowers D. Mutation incidence and coincidence in non small-cell lung cancer: meta-analyses by ethnicity and histology (mutMap). Ann Oncol 2013; 24(9): 2371–6.
9. Wozniak A. Challenges in the current antiangiogenic treatment paradigm for patients with non-small cell lung cancer. Crit Rev Oncol Hematol. 2012 May; 82(2): 200–12.
10. Xiao YY, Zhan P, Yuan DM, Liu HB, Lv TF, et al. Chemotherapy plus multitargeted antiangiogenic tyrosine kinase inhibitors or chemotherapy alone in advanced NSCLC: a meta-analysis of randomized controlled trials. Eur J Clin Pharmacol 2013; 69(2): 151–9.
11. Jadad AR, Moore RA, Carroll D, Jenkinson C, Reynolds DJ, et al. Assessing the quality of reports of randomized clinical trials: is blinding necessary? Control Clin Trials 1996; 17: 1–12.
12. Egger M, Davey Smith G, Schneider M, Minder C. Bias in meta-analysis detected by a simple, graphical test. BMJ 1997; 315(7109): 629–34.
13. Begg CB, Mazumdar M. Operating characteristics of a rank correlation test for publication bias. Biometrics 1994; 50: 1088–1101.
14. Socinski MA, Scappaticci FA, Samant M, Kolb MM, Kozloff MF. Safety and efficacy of combining sunitinib with bevacizumab + paclitaxel/carboplatin in non-small cell lung cancer. J Thorac Oncol 2010; 5(3): 354–60.
15. Scagliotti GV, Krzakowski M, Szczesna A, Strausz J, Makhson A, et al. Sunitinib plus erlotinib versus placebo plus erlotinib in patients with previously treated advanced non-small-cell lung cancer: a phase III trial. J Clin Oncol 2012; 30(17): 2070–8.

16. Spigel DR, Burris HA 3rd, Greco FA, Shipley DL, Friedman EK, et al. Randomized, double-blind, placebo-controlled, phase II trial of sorafenib and erlotinib or erlotinib alone in previously treated advanced non-small-cell lung cancer. J Clin Oncol 2011; 29(18): 2582–9.
17. Scagliotti G, Novello S, von Pawel J, Reck M, Pereira JR, et al. Phase III study of carboplatin and paclitaxel alone or with sorafenib in advanced non-small-cell lung cancer. J Clin Oncol 2010; 28(11): 1835–42.
18. Paz-Ares LG, Biesma B, Heigener D, von Pawel J, Eisen T, et al. Phase III, randomized, double-blind, placebo-controlled trial of gemcitabine/cisplatin alone or with sorafenib for the first-line treatment of advanced, nonsquamous non-small-cell lung cancer. J Clin Oncol 2012; 30(25): 3084–92.
19. Wang Y, Wang L, Liu Y, Yu S, Zhang X, et al. Randomize trial of cisplatin plus gemcitabine with either sorafenib or placebo as first-line therapy for non-small cell lung cancer. [Article in Chinese] Zhongguo Fei Ai Za Zhi 2011; 14(3): 239–44.
20. Molina JR, Dy GK, Foster NR, Allen Ziegler KL, Adjei A, et al. A randomized phase II study of pemetrexed (PEM) with or without sorafenib (S) as second-line therapy in advanced non-small cell lung cancer (NSCLC) of nonsquamous histology: NCCTG N0626 study. Journal of Clinical Oncology 2011; 29 [Abstract 7513].
21. Goss GD, Arnold A, Shepherd FA, Dediu M, Ciuleanu TE, et al. Randomized, double-blind trial of carboplatin and paclitaxel with either daily oral cediranib or placebo in advanced non-small-cell lung cancer: NCIC clinical trials group BR24 study. J Clin Oncol 2010; 28(1): 49–55.
22. Dy GK, Mandrekar SJ, Nelson GD, Meyers JP, Adjei AA, et al. A randomized phase II study of gemcitabine and carboplatin with or without cediranib as first-line therapy in advanced non-small-cell lung cancer: North Central Cancer Treatment Group Study N0528. J Thorac Oncol 2013; 8(1): 79–88.
23. Laurie SA, Solomon BJ, Seymour L, Ellis PM, Goss GD, et al. A randomized double-blind trial of carboplatin plus paclitaxel (CP) with daily oral cediranib (CED), an inhibitor of vascular endothelial growth factor receptors, or placebo (PLA) in patients (pts) with previously untreated advanced non-small cell lung cancer (NSCLC): NCIC Clinical Trials Group study BR.29. J Clin Oncol 2012; 30 S:abstr 7511.
24. Heymach JV, Johnson BE, Prager D, Csada E, Roubec J, et al. Randomized, placebo-controlled phase II study of vandetanib plus docetaxel in previously treated non small cell lung cancer. J Clin Oncol 2007; 25(27): 4270–7.
25. Herbst RS, Sun Y, Eberhardt WE, Germonpré P, Saijo N, et al. Vandetanib plus docetaxel versus docetaxel as second-line treatment for patients with advanced non-small-cell lung cancer (ZODIAC): a double-blind, randomised, phase 3 trial. Lancet Oncol 2010; 11(7): 619–26.
26. de Boer RH, Arrieta Ó, Yang CH, Gottfried M, Chan V, et al. Vandetanib plus pemetrexed for the second-line treatment of advanced non-small-cell lung cancer: a randomized, double-blind phase III trial. J Clin Oncol 2011; 29(8): 1067–74.
27. Heymach JV, Paz-Ares L, De Braud F, Sebastian M, Stewart DJ, et al. Randomized phase II study of vandetanib alone or with paclitaxel and carboplatin as first-line treatment for advanced non-small-cell lung cancer. J Clin Oncol 2008; 26(33): 5407–15.
28. Natale RB, Thongprasert S, Greco FA, Thomas M, Tsai CM, et al. Phase III trial of vandetanib compared with erlotinib in patients with previously treated advanced non-small-cell lung cancer. J Clin Oncol 2011; 29(8): 1059–66.
29. Natale RB, Bodkin D, Govindan R, Sleckman BG, Rizvi NA, et al. Vandetanib versus gefitinib in patients with advanced non-small-cell lung cancer: results from a two-part, double-blind, randomized phase ii study. J Clin Oncol 2009; 27(15): 2523–9.
30. Lee JS, Hirsh V, Park K, Qin S, Blajman CR, et al. Vandetanib Versus placebo in patients with advanced non-small-cell lung cancer after prior therapy with an epidermal growth factor receptor tyrosine kinase inhibitor: a randomized, double-blind phase III trial (ZEPHYR). J Clin Oncol 2012; 30(10): 1114–21.
31. Scagliotti GV, Vynnychenko I, Park K, Ichinose Y, Kubota K, et al. International, randomized, placebo-controlled, double-blind phase III study of motesanib plus carboplatin/paclitaxel in patients with advanced nonsquamous non-small-cell lung cancer: MONET1. J Clin Oncol 2012; 30(23): 2829–36.
32. Blumenschein GR Jr, Kabbinavar F, Menon H, Mok TS, Stephenson J, et al. A phase II, multicenter, open-label randomized study of motesanib or bevacizumab in combination with paclitaxel and carboplatin for advanced nonsquamous non-small-cell lung cancer. Ann Oncol 2011; 22(9): 2057–67.
33. Reck M, Kaiser R, Mellemgaard A, Douillard JY, Orlov S, et al. Docetaxel plus nintedanib versus docetaxel plus placebo in patients with previously treated non-small-cell lung cancer (LUME-Lung 1): a phase 3, double-blind, randomised controlled trial. Lancet Oncol 2014; 15(2): 143–55.
34. Cesca M, Bizzaro F, Zucchetti M, Giavazzi R. Tumor Delivery of Chemotherapy Combined with Inhibitors of Angiogenesis and Vascular Targeting Agents. Front Oncol 2013; 3: 259.
35. Johnson DH1, Fehrenbacher L, Novotny WF, Herbst RS, Nemunaitis JJ, et al. Randomized phase II trial comparing bevacizumab plus carboplatin and paclitaxel with carboplatin and paclitaxel alone in previously untreated locally advanced or metastatic non-small-cell lung cancer. J Clin Oncol 2004; 22(11): 2184–91.
36. Hellmann MD1, Chaft JE, Rusch V, Ginsberg MS, Finley DJ, et al. Risk of hemoptysis in patients with resected squamous cell and other high-risk lung cancers treated with adjuvant bevacizumab. Cancer Chemother Pharmacol 2013; 72(2): 453–61.

4

Effects of Cytochrome P450 2C19 and Paraoxonase 1 Polymorphisms on Antiplatelet Response to Clopidogrel Therapy in Patients with Coronary Artery Disease

Damrus Tresukosol[1], Bhoom Suktitipat[2,3], Saowalak Hunnangkul[4], Ruttakarn Kamkaew[2], Saiphon Poldee[2], Boonrat Tassaneetrithep[4], Atip Likidlilid[2]*

1 Division of Cardiology, Department of Internal Medicine, Faculty of Medicine, Siriraj Hospital, Mahidol University, Siriraj, Bangkoknoi, Bangkok, Thailand, 2 Department of Biochemistry, Faculty of Medicine, Siriraj Hospital, Mahidol University, Siriraj, Bangkoknoi, Bangkok, Thailand, 3 Integrative Computation BioScience Center (ICBS), Mahidol University, Salaya, Nakhon Prathom, Thailand, 4 Department of Health Research and Development, Faculty of Medicine, Siriraj Hospital, Mahidol University, Siriraj, Bangkoknoi, Bangkok, Thailand

Abstract

Clopidogrel is an antiplatelet prodrug that is recommended to reduce the risk of recurrent thrombosis in coronary artery disease (CAD) patients. Paraoxonase 1 (PON1) is suggested to be a rate-limiting enzyme in the conversion of 2-oxo-clopidogrel to active thiol metabolite with inconsistent results. Here, we sought to determine the associations of CYP2C19 and PON1 gene polymorphisms with clopidogrel response and their role in ADP-induced platelet aggregation. Clopidogrel response and platelet aggregation were determined using Multiplate aggregometer in 211 patients with established CAD who received 75 mg clopidogrel and 75–325 mg aspirin daily for at least 14 days. Polymorphisms in CYP2C19 and PON1 were genotyped and tested for association with clopidogrel resistance. Linkage disequilibrium (LD) and their epistatic interaction effects on ADP-induced platelet aggregation were analysed. The prevalence of clopidogrel resistance in this population was approximately 33.2% (n = 70). The frequencies of CYP2C19*2 and *3 were significantly higher in non-responder than those in responders. After adjusting for established risk factors, CYP2C19*2 and *3 alleles independently increased the risk of clopidogrel resistance with adjusted ORs 2.94 (95%CI, 1.65–5.26; p<0.001) and 11.26 (95%CI, 2.47–51.41; p = 0.002, respectively). Patients with *2 or *3 allele and combined with smoking, diabetes and increased platelet count had markedly increased risk of clopidogrel resistance. No association was observed between PON1 Q192R and clopidogrel resistance (adjusted OR = 1.13, 95%CI, 0.70–1.82; p = 0.622). Significantly higher platelet aggregation values were found in CYP2C19*2 and *3 patients when compared with *1/*1 allele carriers (p = 1.98×10^{-6}). For PON1 Q192R genotypes, aggregation values were similar across all genotype groups (p = 0.359). There was no evidence of gene-gene interaction or LD between CYP2C19 and PON1 polymorphisms on ADP-induced platelet aggregation. Our findings indicated that only CYP2C19*2 and *3 alleles had an influence on clopidogrel resistance. The risk of clopidogrel resistance increased further with smoking, diabetes, and increased platelet count.

Editor: Carmine Pizzi, University of Bologna, Italy

Funding: This study was partly supported by Graduate Thesis Scholarship grant from Faculty of Medicine Siriraj Hospital, Mahidol University to RK. AL and BS were supported by "Chalermphrakiat" grant, Faculty of Medicine Siriraj Hospital, Mahidol University. The funders had no role in study design, data collection and analysis, decision to publish, or preparation of the manuscript.

Competing Interests: The authors have declared that no competing interests exist.

* Email: atip.lik@mahidol.ac.th

Introduction

Acute coronary syndromes (ACS), the leading cause of sudden death worldwide, including Thailand [1], occurs as a result of platelet aggregation (thrombosis) within the human artery. Clopidogrel and aspirin are dual antiplatelet therapy that inhibit platelet function, preventing ischemic events and improving outcomes following ACS and percutaneous coronary intervention (PCI) with stent implantation [2]. Clopidogrel is a thienopyridine prodrug that requires enzymatic biotransformation into the active thiol metabolite to inhibit platelet ADP P2Y12 receptor. Aspirin (acetylsalicylic acid) is a cyclooxygenase-1 (COX-1) inhibitor,

thereby preventing the production of thromboxane A_2, which plays a prominent role in platelet aggregation. Due to the different pathways that clopidogrel and aspirin inhibit platelet aggregation, combined antiplatelet therapy provides additive benefit compared with either agent alone and is considered as a therapy of choice for preventing thrombosis in patients undergoing coronary stenting [3]. However, inter-individual variability in the response to clopidogrel is multifactorial and can be influenced by environmental, clinical, and genetic factors [4–6]. Many investigations have indicated that 4% to 44% of patients fail to attain platelet inhibition after clopidogrel therapy [7–12]. Recent studies have confirmed that *in vivo* bioactivation of clopidogrel is a two-step process which is closely linked to the cytochrome P450 (CYP) 2C19 enzyme [13]. The common genetic variants within the CYP2C19 gene, the loss-of-function hepatic CYP2C19*2 (rs4244285) and *3 (rs4986893) polymorphisms were found to be dominantly associated with a lower clopidogrel responsiveness [14–16] and a higher risk of adverse cardiac events such as the occurrence of stent thrombosis and recurrent myocardial infarction [17–19].

Recently, Bouman et al [20] reported that clopidogrel metabolism involved in two steps of bioactivation. First, clopidogrel undergoes oxidation to 2-oxo-clopidogrel by hepatic CYP450 enzyme. Then, in the second step, PON1 and PON3, the paraoxonases synthesized in the liver associated with HDL, play a crucial role in clopidogrel biotransformation to convert clopidogrel to its thiol active metabolite. Contrary to the prior observations, Bouman identified PON1 Q192R (rs662) as a single key factor for the bioactivation and clinical response of clopidogrel, and found no evidence for CYP2C19 involvement in this step of clopidogrel activation. Specifically, carriers of the QQ genotype were found to have a significantly higher risk of stent thrombosis after PCI as compared with individual with QR or RR genotype with an odds ratio (OR) of 3.3 (95% CI, 1.6–7.9; p = 0.003). However, other investigators had found no association between PON1 Q192R genotype and platelet response to clopidogrel in either Caucasian populations or populations with mixed racial background [21–23]. This may be due to the lower enzymatic activity of Q allele in a dose dependent manner (QQ<QR<RR) [24,25]. Additionally, PON1 also contains the antioxidant property by breaking down biologically active oxidized phospholipids and oxidized cholesteryl esters [26], thereby preventing oxidation of HDL and LDL. Therefore, PON1 has been proposed as an atherosclerotic susceptibility gene. Many studies have reported the association between PON1 Q192R polymorphism and coronary artery disease (CAD) with mixed results. A meta-analysis of 39 studies (10,738 cases and 17,068 controls) reported a pooled OR of 1.10 (95%CI, 1.06–1.13; p<0.001) per R allele for CAD [27]. The prospective REGRESS study in 739 secondary prevention patients reported a hazard ratio (HR) of 1.71 (95%CI, 1.0–2.8; p = 0.03) per Q allele for death due to ischemic disease [28]. The GeneBank study in 1,399 sequential patients undergoing diagnostic coronary angiography reported that the Q allele was associated with an increased risk of major adverse cardiovascular events (HR, 1.48; 95%CI, 1.09–2.03; p = 0.01) [25]. This discrepancy may be due to the PON1 allele frequency which vary greatly across human populations; a relatively high frequency of the PON1 R192 allele is reported in Blacks, Japanese, Chinese and Thai ranging from 58% to 65% [29–31] as compared with Caucasians (25% to 30%) [32]. The frequency of CYP2C19 alleles associated with poor metabolizer phenotype also showed high variability from 2–6% in Caucasians to 13–23% in Asians [33]. Since most studies were in Caucasians, there was a paucity of data in Asian populations who have different genetic background. Therefore, the aim of this study was to investigate the impact and interaction of PON1 Q192R, CYP2C19*2 and CYP2C19*3 genotypes on clopidogrel platelet inhibition using multiple electrode platelet aggregometry (MEA) in Thai population.

Methods

Study population

211 patients who resided in Bangkok with aged-range from 39–94 years were recruited if they had established CAD and were on dual antiplatelet therapy with clopidogrel 75 mg and aspirin 75–325 mg daily at least 14 days prior to enrollment for secondary prevention. Subjects were excluded if they had a history of drug or alcohol abuse, bleeding disorder, current warfarin use, myelodysplastic or myeloproliferative disorders, chronic liver disease or any contraindication against aspirin or clopidogrel. Subjects were also excluded if they were pregnant, if the platelet count was less than 10^5 cell/mm^3 (thrombocytopenia), or if there was prior usage of glycoprotein IIb/IIIa antagonist. Questionnaires and medical records were used to collect family and medical history, smoking habit, platelet count, diabetic status, and physical activities. The study protocols were approved by Siriraj Institutional Review Board, Faculty of Medicine Siriraj Hospital, Mahidol University. Informed consent was signed by all subjects after explanation on aims and benefits of this research project.

Platelet aggregation assays

After 14 days of taking 75 mg clopidogrel combined with 75–325 mg aspirin daily, peripheral venous blood samples were obtained from subjects in a catheterization laboratory prior to the next dose of clopidogrel and aspirin. Platelet aggregation was measured using MEA on the Multiplate analyser (Dynabyte, Munich Germany). Blood was placed in 4.5 ml plastic tubes containing hirudin with a final concentration of 25 μg/ml. The final concentration of ADP (6.5 μM) -induced platelet aggregation was assessed as previously reported [34]. Platelet aggregation measured with MEA was quantified as area under the curve (AUC = AU×min) of aggregation unit (AU). A 10 AU×min corresponds to 1 unit (U). The cut off point for this clopidogrel resistance was 50 U as previously reported [35]. All material used for platelet aggregation study was obtained from the manufacturer.

Genotyping

Genomic DNA was isolated from whole blood by guanidine-HCl methods. Subjects were genotyped for CYP2C19*2 (681 G>A), CYP2C19*3 (636 G>A), and PON1 Q192R (575 A>G) using PCR-RFLP as previously described [36–38]. Sequence specific primers were used to amplify the alleles of interest. Primers 5′ AATTACAACCAGAGCTTGGC 3′ and 5′ TATCACTTTC-CATAAAAGCAAG 3′ were used to amplified the sequence of the CYP2C19*2 in exon 5 of the gene. Primers 5′ AAATTGTTTC-CAATCATTTAGCT 3′ and 5′ ACTTCAGGGCTTGGT-CAATA 3′ were used to amplified the sequence of the CYP2C19*3 in exon 4. Primers 5′ TATTGTTGCTGTGG-GACCTGAG 3′ and 5′ CCTGAGAATCTGAGTAAATC-CACT 3′ were used to amplify the sequence of the PON1 gene containing the Q192R polymorphism in exon 6. PCR cycles for denaturation, annealing and extension were 35 cycles for all polymorphism with initial denaturation at 94°C for 5 min and final extension at 72°C for 5 min. PCR profile of CYP2C19*2 polymorphism was denatured at 94°C for 30 sec, annealing at 60°C for 30 sec and extension at 72°C for 30 sec. PCR profile for CYP2C19*3 polymorphism was denatured at 94°C for 30 sec, annealing at 58°C for 30 sec and extension at 72°C for 30 sec. For PON1 polymorphism, denaturation was at 94°C for 1 min, annealing at 60°C for 1 min, and extension at 72°C for 30 sec. The PCR product for CYP2C19*2, CYP2C19*3 and PON1 were 169, 271 and 238 bp, and were cut by 10 units of SmaI, BamHI, and BspPI restriction enzymes, respectively. Products from SmaI enzyme were 120 and 49 bp for G allele and 169 bp for A allele. For BamHI, the products were 175 and 96 bp for G allele and 271 bp for A allele and the products from BspPI were 175 and 63 bp for R192 allele and 238 bp for Q192 allele. The restriction site cut products were detected by 3.5% agarose gel electrophoresis.

Table 1. Baseline characteristics of study participants.

Parameters	Total (n = 211)	Non-responders (n = 70)	Responders (n = 141)	p-value*
Age	66.25±11.15	64.47±10.51	67.13±11.39	0.102
BMI (kg/m²)	25.54±4.08	25.59±4.13	25.57±4.08	0.970
Female (%)	68 (32.3)	21 (30.0)	47 (33.3)	0.626
Type of CAD				
- Single vessel disease (%)	51 (24.1)	19 (27.1)	32 (22.7)	0.477
- Multi vessel disease (%)	143 (67.8)	46 (65.7)	97 (68.8)	0.757
- Others (%)	17 (8.1)	5 (7.1)	12 (8.5)	0.731
Cardiomyophaty (%)	7 (3.3)	3 (4.3)	4 (2.8)	0.580
Diabetes (%)	97 (46.0)	43 (61.4)	54 (38.3)	0.002*
Hypertension (%)	184 (87.8)	61 (87.1)	123 (87.2)	0.985
Dyslipidemia (%)	149 (70.6)	52 (74.3)	97 (68.8)	0.410
Stroke (%)	14 (6.6)	6 (8.6)	8 (5.7)	0.426
Renal impairment (%)	23 (10.9)	6 (8.6)	17 (12.1)	0.444
Peripheral arterial disorder (%)	13 (6.2)	4 (5.7)	9 (6.4)	0.849
Smoking (%)	85 (40.3)	35 (50.0)	50 (35.5)	0.043*
Medication				
- Proton pump inhibitors (%)	83 (39.3)	30 (42.9)	53 (37.6)	0.461
- Calcium channel blockers (%)	67 (31.8)	22 (31.4)	45 (31.9)	0.943
- Statin (%)	183 (86.7)	65 (92.9)	118 (83.7)	0.065
Platelet count (×10⁵/mm³)	2.55±0.76	2.73±0.84	2.47±0.72	0.033*
ADP platelet aggregation (U)	43.98±26.19	73.33±18.26	28.95±10.42	<0.001

* Variable is significant difference between responders and non-responders at p-value<0.05.

Statistical analyses

Variables were presented as mean ± standard deviation (SD). Chi-square goodness-of-fit test or Fisher's exact test was used to test for a possible deviation of genotype distribution from Hardy-Weinberg equilibrium (HWE) proportions. Normally distributed continuous variables were compared across two groups with the two-sided student's t-test and for genotype group comparisons with the one-way ANOVA test. The differences in allele and genotype frequencies between groups were compared using Chi-square test. A nominal p value <0.05 was considered statistically significant.

Univariable and multivariable logistic regression analyses were applied to examine whether *PON1* Q192R, *CYP2C19**2 and *3 genotypes were associated with clopidogrel resistance after adjusting for age, sex, diabetes, smoking status and platelet count, assuming an additive genetic model coded as the number of mutated allele. Bonferroni's method was used for multiple testing correction considering three genetic loci tests. Statistical significant level was set at p≤0.017.

Interaction between *PON1* variants and *CYP2C19**2 and *3 was performed using Cordell's test for epistatic interactions [39], using models containing two genetic markers with and without interaction term and covariates (age, sex, diabetic status, smoking status, and platelet count). Likelihood ratio test was performed with 10,000 permutations to calculate the empirical significance of the interaction term, and empirical statistically significant level was set to p<0.05. All analyses were performed using SPSS 13 (SPSS Inc. Chicago, IL, USA) and R version 2.14.2. Cordell's test was performed using *scrime* package in R [40,41]. To determine the extent of linkage disequilibrium (LD) in our samples, standardized LD coefficient (D′) and correlation coefficient (r) were calculated for all pairs of polymorphism.

Results

Baseline characteristics of study participants

Based on the result from platelet function test using MEA, the CAD patients were categorized into responders and non-responders to clopidogrel. Among 211 patients included in this study, 70 patients (33.2%) were classified as non-responders and 141 patients (66.8%) as responders. There was no significance between the two groups regarding differences in age, BMI, sex, number of vessel diseases, underlying diseases (cardiomyopathy, hypertension, dyslipidemia, stroke, renal impairment, and peripheral disorder), and concurrent medications (p>0.05). However, clopidogrel non-responders had a significantly higher proportion of diabetes (p = 0.002), smokers (p = 0.043), and higher platelet counts (p = 0.033) as shown in Table 1.

Distribution and allele frequencies of *CYP2C19**2, *3 and *PON1* Q192R genotypes

The distribution of *CYP2C19**2, *3 and *PON1* Q192R genotypes in the clopidogrel responsive and non-responsive groups were summarized in Table 2, which indicates consistency with the Hardy-Weinberg equilibrium (p>0.05). There was no homozygous *CYP2C19**3 genotype detected in the study population, which is consistent with its very rare frequency in Caucasians, Africans, Americans, Japanese and Koreans. Moreover, the high frequency of *PON1* R192 in this study was consistent with the

Table 2. Distribution of CYP2C19*2, *3 and PON1 genotypes in clopidogrel responders and non-responders.

CYP2C19*2 (rs4244285)

Genotype	Non-responders (n = 70)	Responders (n = 141)	Total (n = 211)	p-value*
GG (*1/*1)	27 (38.6%)	85 (60.3%)	112 (53.1%)	$2.9 \times 10^{-3\dagger}$
GA (*1/*2)	31 (44.3%)	53 (37.6%)	84 (35.8%)	0.349
AA (*2/*2)	12 (17.1%)	3 (2.1%)	15 (7.1%)	$1.6 \times 10^{-4\dagger}$
HWE p-value‡	0.549	0.106	0.889	-
Allele frequency				
Allele*2 (95%CI)	0.39 (0.32–0.48)	0.21 (0.16–0.26)	0.27 (0.23–0.31)	$6.3 \times 10^{-5\dagger}$

CYP2C19*3 (rs4986893)

Genotype	Non-responders (n = 70)	Responders (n = 141)	Total (n = 211)	p-value*
GG (*1/*1)	60 (85.7%)	137 (97.2%)	197 (93.4%)	$2.9 \times 10^{-3\dagger}$
GA (*1/*3)	10 (14.3%)	4 (2.8%)	14 (6.6%)	$2.9 \times 10^{-3\dagger}$
AA (*3/*3)	0 (0)	0 (0)	0	-
HWE p-value‡	0.520	0.864	0.618	-
Allele frequency				
Allele*3 (95%CI)	0.07 (0.03–0.11)	0.01 (0.0003–0.03)	0.03 (0.02–0.05)	$3.4 \times 10^{-3\dagger}$

CYP2C19*2 and *3 Combination

Genotype	Non-responders (n = 70)	Responders (n = 141)	Total (n = 211)	p-value*
*1/*1	24 (34.3%)	82 (58.2%)	106 (50.2%)	$1.1 \times 10^{-3\dagger}$
*1/*2	24 (34.3%)	52 (36.9%)	76 (36.0%)	0.712
*1/*3	3 (4.3%)	3 (2.1%)	6 (2.9%)	0.401
*2/*2	12 (17.1%)	3 (2.1%)	15 (7.1%)	$1.6 \times 10^{-4\dagger}$
*2/*3	7 (10.0%)	1 (0.7%)	8 (1.8%)	$2.1 \times 10^{-3\dagger}$
*3/*3	0 (0)	0 (0)	0	-
HWE p-value‡	0.127	0.451	0.083	-
Allele frequency				
Allele*1 (95%CI)	0.54 (0.45–0.62)	0.78 (0.72–0.83)	0.70 (0.65–0.74)	$4.0 \times 10^{-7\dagger}$
Allele*2 (95%CI)	0.39 (0.31–0.47)	0.21 (0.16–0.26)	0.27 (0.23–0.31)	$6.5 \times 10^{-5\dagger}$
Allele*3 (95%CI)	0.07 (0.04–0.10)	0.01 (0.0003–0.02)	0.03 (0.02–0.05)	$3.6 \times 10^{-4\dagger}$

PON1 (Q192R; rs662)

Genotype	Non-responders (n = 70)	Responders (n = 141)	Total (n = 211)	p-value*
GG (RR)	34 (48.6%)	71 (50.4%)	105 (49.8%)	0.807
AG (QR)	29 (41.4%)	55 (39.0%)	84 (39.8%)	0.735
AA (QQ)	7 (10.0%)	15 (10.6%)	22 (10.4%)	0.886
HWE p-value‡	0.824	0.381	0.399	0.886
Allele frequency				
Allele Q (95%CI)	0.31 (0.24–0.38)	0.30 (0.25–0.35)	0.30 (0.26–0.34)	0.904

* Comparison of genotype and allele frequencies between non-responders and responders.
†Statistically significant difference at p<0.05.
‡p-value of Hardy-Weinberg equilibrium.

other reports in Asian populations. The frequencies of both *2/*2 and *2/*3 genotypes (17.10, 10.00 vs 2.10, 0.70%) and *2 and *3 alleles (39.29, 7.14 vs 20.92, 1.42%) were significantly higher in clopidogrel non-responders than those in responders ($p = 1.6 \times 10^{-4}$, $p = 2.1 \times 10^{-3}$ and $p = 6.5 \times 10^{-5}$, $p = 3.6 \times 10^{-4}$, respectively). Similarly, the frequencies of CYP2C19*1 genotype

Table 3. Association between CYP2C19*2, *3, PON1 Q192R and clopidogrel resistance.

CYP2C19*2 (rs4244285)

Genotype	Crude OR (95%CI)	p-value	Adjusted OR (95%CI)[†]	p-value
GG (*1/*1)	1	-	1	-
GA (*1/*2)	1.84 (0.99–3.42)	0.053	2.30 (1.14–4.66)	0.021
AA (*2/*2)	12.59 (3.31–47.96)	<0.001*	13.23 (2.87–60.88)	0.001*
Allele A (*2)	2.57 (1.59–4.14)	<0.001*	2.86 (1.63–5.03)	<0.001*

CYP2C19*3 (rs4986893)

Genotype	Crude OR (95%CI)	p-value	Adjusted OR (95%CI)[†]	p-value
GG (*1/*1)	1	-	1	-
GA (*1/*3)	5.71 (1.72–18.93)	0.004*	10.59 (2.39–46.85)	0.002*
AA (*3/*3)	-	-	-	-
Allele A (*3)	5.71 (1.72–18.93)	0.004*	10.59 (2.39–46.85)	0.002*

CYP2C19*2 and *3 combination

Genotype	Crude OR (95%CI)	p-value	Adjusted OR (95%CI)[†]	p-value
*1/*1	1	-	1	-
*1/*2	1.58 (0.81–3.06)	0.179	2.01 (0.95–4.29)	0.070
*1/*3	3.42 (0.65–18.04)	0.148	3.70 (0.46–30.01)	0.221
*2/*2	13.67 (3.56–52.43)	<0.001*	13.09 (2.83–60.57)	0.001*
*2/*3	23.92 (2.80–204.11)	0.004*	84.06 (6.89–1026.24)	0.001*
Allele *2 [‡]	2.63 (1.62–4.27)	<0.001*	2.94 (1.65–5.26)	<0.001*
Allele *3 [‡]	6.18 (1.80–21.17)	0.004*	11.26 (2.47–51.40)	0.002 *

PON1 (Q192R; rs662)

Genotype	Crude OR (95%CI)	p-value	Adjusted OR (95%CI)[†]	p-value
GG (RR)	1	-	1	-
AG (QR)	1.10 (0.60–2.02)	0.756	1.36 (0.68–2.72)	0.381
AA (QQ)	0.98 (0.36–2.61)	0.959	1.05 (0.35–3.16)	0.925
Allele A (Q)	1.03 (0.67–1.57)	0.907	1.13 (0.70–1.82)	0.622

* Risk is statistical significant when compared to the reference genotype at p-value<0.017.
[†]Adjusted for diabetes, age, sex, history of smoking and platelet count.
[‡]Adjusted for concurrent *2 or *3 allele and covariates (diabetes, age, sex, history of smoking, and platelet count).

and allele (34.30, 53.57 vs 58.20, 77.66%) were significantly lower in non-responders than those in responders (p = 1.1×10^{-3} and 4.0×10^{-7}, respectively). There were no significant differences of PON1 Q192R genotypes and alleles between the two groups (p> 0.05).

Association of CYP2C19 and PON1 Q192R gene polymorphisms and clopidogrel responsiveness

The results of a simple logistic regression model demonstrated that having one copy of CYP2C19*3 was significantly associated with a 5.71 fold higher risk of clopidogrel resistance (95% CI, 1.72–18.93; p = 0.004) as compared with wild type CYP2C19 (*1/*1). Although one copy of CYP2C19*2 was not significantly associated with clopidogrel resistance (p = 0.053), two copy of CYP2C19 (*2/*2) was associated with 12.59 times higher risk of clopidogrel resistance (95%CI, 3.31–47.96; p<0.001). The combined effect of CYP2C19*2 and *3 estimated that both *2/*2 and *2/*3 genotypes significantly increased the risk of clopidogrel resistances with an unadjusted OR of 13.67 (95%CI, 3.56–52.43; p<0.001) and 23.92 (95%CI, 2.80–204.11; p = 0.004), respectively. After adjusting for the co-dominant effects of *2 and *3 alleles,

comparing to *1 allele, *2 was associated with 2.63 times higher risk of clopidogrel resistance (95%CI, 1.62–4.27; p<0.001), and *3 was associated with 6.18 times higher risk of clopidogrel resistance (95%CI, 1.80–21.17; p = 0.004). In contrast, the PON1 Q192R, both genotypes (QQ/QR) and Q allele, did not significantly associate with clopidogrel resistance (p>0.05).

From multivariable logistic regression analysis, assuming a co-dominant allele effect, having one copy of CYP2C19*2 (*1/*2) was associated with 2.30 times higher risk than *1/*1 (95%CI, 1.14–4.66); p<0.021), after adjusted for age, sex, and all variables that differed between responders and non-responders (from Table 1). Similarly, one copy of CYP2C19*3 (*1/*3) was associated with 10.59 times higher risk of clopidogrel resistance compared with *1/*1 (95%CI, 2.39–46.85; p = 0.002). Two copy of CYP2C19*2 (*2/*2) was associated with 13.23 times higher risk of clopidogrel resistance compared with *1/*1 (95%CI, 2.87–60.88; p = 0.001).

The combined effects of CYP2C19*2 and *3, after controlling for additional covariates, compared with *1/*1, CYP2C19*2/*3 was associated with 84.06 times higher risk of clopidogrel resistance (95%CI, 6.89–1026.24; p = 0.001); homozygous

Table 4. Estimated risk of clopidogrel resistance in patients with at least one of the following risk factors: CYP2C19*2, CYP2C19*3, smoking, diabetes mellitus, increase in platelet count adjusted for age and sex.

Risk Factors	Adjusted OR*	95% CI	p-value[†]
*1/*1	1	-	-
*1/*1+Smoking	3.52	1.53–8.09	0.003
*1/*1+DM	3.33	1.62–6.85	0.001
*1/*1+Platelet	1.05	1.00–1.10	0.034
*1/*1+DM+Smoking	7.78	2.68–22.53	<0.001
*1/*1+DM+Platelet	3.26	1.65–6.45	0.001
*1/*1+DM+Smoking+Platelet	8.12	2.82–23.73	<0.001
*1/*2	2.94	1.65–5.26	<0.001
*2/*2	8.78	3.00–25.71	<0.001
*1/*3	11.26	2.47–51.41	0.002
*2/*3	33.15	7.01–156.72	<0.001
*1/*2+Smoking	7.43	2.76–20.05	<0.001
*2/*2+Smoking	22.03	5.44–89.17	<0.001
*1/*3+Smoking	28.06	4.84–162.83	<0.001
*2/*3+Smoking	83.16	12.51–552.97	<0.001
*1/*2+DM	9.19	3.59–23.52	<0.001
*2/*2+DM	27.23	6.90–107.37	<0.001
*1/*3+DM	34.68	6.75–178.06	<0.001
*2/*3+DM	102.77	17.16–615.29	<0.001
*1/*2+Platelet count	3.12	1.82–5.34	<0.001
*2/*2+Platelet count	9.23	3.15–27.03	<0.001
*1/*3+Platelet count	11.76	2.81–49.29	<0.001
*2/*3+Platelet count	34.86	7.30–166.45	<0.001
*1/*2+Smoking+DM	23.05	6.36–83.56	<0.001
*2/*2+Smoking+DM	68.3	12.96–360.05	<0.001
*1/*3+Smoking+DM	86.99	12.30–615.28	<0.001
*2/*3+Smoking+DM	257.79	31.21–2129.62	<0.001
*1/*2+Smoking+DM+Platelet	24.23	6.67–87.95	<0.001
*2/*2+Smoking+DM+Platelet	71.82	13.62–378.77	<0.001
*1/*3+Smoking+DM+Platelet	91.47	12.82–652.52	<0.001
*2/*3+Smoking+DM+Platelet	271.07	32.56–2256.56	<0.001

*Estimated OR for each risk factor category compared to men with no CYP2C19 mutation (wild type), with average age (66.25 year-old), average platelet count (255,900 platelets/mm³), who do not smoke and do not have diabetes. Platelet variable is calculated per ×1,000 platelet increased. Log odds for clopidogrel resistance were calculated using multivariate logistic regression as a function of CYP2C19*2+CYP2C19*3+Smoking+Diabetic Status+increased Platelet Count.
[†]Risk is statistically significant when compared to the reference genotype at p-value<0.05.

CYP2C19*2 (*2/*2) was associated with 13.09 times higher risk of clopidogrel resistance (95%CI, 2.83–60.57; p = 0.001).

For allelic association, after adjusting for the co-dominant effect of *3 allele, *2 allele carrier was associated with 2.94 times higher risk of clopidogrel resistance compared with *1 allele (95%CI, 1.65–5.26; p<0.001). After adjusting for the effects of *2 allele, *3 allele was associated with 11.26 times higher risk of clopidogrel resistance compared with *1 (95%CI, 2.47–51.40; p = 0.002). In contrast, PON1 QR and QQ genotypes and Q allele showed no association with clopidogrel resistance compared with either RR genotype or R allele as references (Table 3).

The estimated effects of *1, *2, and *3 genotypes, combined with smoking, diabetes status, and increase in platelet count using *1/*1 as a reference genotype, markedly increase the risk of clopidogrel resistance in linear trend as summarized in Table 4.

CYP2C19*2, *3 and PON1 Q192R genotypes and platelet aggregation

The ADP-induced platelet aggregation values across CYP2C19*2 and *3 genotypes were shown in Table 5. For CYP2C19*2 genotypes, ADP-induced platelet aggregation significantly differed across genotype groups (p = 2.98×10^{-5}). In the patients who were carriers of at least one *2 allele (*1/*2 or *2/*2), ADP induced-platelet aggregation was also significantly different when compared with *1/*1 genotype (p = 0.004). For CYP2C19*3 genotypes, the ADP-induced platelet aggregation did not differ across genotype groups (p = 0.069). However, when combining CYP2C19*2 and *3, the ADP-induced platelet aggregations across genotypes were significantly different (p = 1.98×10^{-6}). For PON1 Q192R genotypes, the ADP-induced platelet aggregation did not differ across genotype groups (p = 0.359).

Table 5. ADP induced platelet aggregation level by CYP2C19*2, *3 and PON1 Q192R polymorphisms in clopidogrel treated patients with coronary artery disease.

	Genotypes	n	Platelet Aggregation Level
*CYP2C19*2*	GG (*1/*1)	112	39.16±23.28
(rs4244285; 681G>A)	GA (*1/*2)	84	45.20±23.62
	AA (*2/*2)	15	73.07±39.77
	p-value		2.98×10^{-5}
*CYP2C19*3*	GG (*1/*1)	197	43.10±26.36
(rs4986893; 636G>A)	GA (*1/*3)	14	56.29±20.69
	AA (*3/*3)	0	-
	p-value		0.069
*CYP2C19*2*	*1/*1	106	38.90±23.49
*& CYP2C19*3*	*1/*2	76	43.36±23.28
	*1/*3	6	47.67±19.14
	*2/*3	8	62.75±20.54
	*2/*2	15	73.07±39.77
	p-value		1.98×10^{-6}
PON1	GG (RR)	105	42.14±25.43
(rs662; 575A>G)	AG (QR)	84	45.77±27.30
	AA (QQ)	22	45.86±26.08
	p-value		0.359

p-values assuming additive genetic model represent the association between genotype and ADP-induced platelet aggregation (U) at p-value<0.05.

Interaction between *PON1* Q192R polymorphisms and ADP-induced platelet aggregation level after stratification by *CYP2C19*2 and *CYP2C19*3

Since both CYP2C19 and PON1 involve in activation of clopidogrel prodrug as suggested by Bouman et al. [20], the interaction effects between CYP2C19 (*2, *3) and PON1 (Q192R) on ADP-induced platelet aggregation were investigated. After stratification by CYP2C19*2 (Figure 1A) and *3 genotypes (Figure 1B), the effects of PON1 (Q192R) polymorphism on ADP-induced platelet aggregation were not modified by neither *CYP2C19*2* nor *CYP2C19*3* allele. Cordell's test for epistatic interaction showed no statistically significant interaction between *CYP2C19*2* or *3 with PON1 Q192R polymorphisms ($p_{int} = 0.21$ and 0.91, respectively). Similarly, *CYP2C19*3* did not modify the effects of *CYP2C19*2* on ADP-induced platelet aggregation ($p_{int} = 0.65$, Figure 1C). To examine the extent of linkage disequilibrium (LD) in these study samples, standardized LD coefficient (D′) and correlation coefficient (r) were calculated for all pairs of polymorphisms. Table 6 shows the LD matrix generated using D′ and r. No evidence of LD was observed among these three polymorphisms (D′ and r<0.5).

Discussion

Bouman et al's study [20] is the first report to identify that *PON1* Q192R is a major determinant of clopidogrel efficacy using in vitro metabolomic profiling techniques. The PON1 activity was significantly reduced in subjects with homozygous wild type allele (*PON1* QQ192) compared with carriers of the mutant allele. In addition, in a group of patients with stent thrombosis and matched controls without stent thrombosis, *PON1* QQ192 was associated with decreased platelet inhibition by clopidogrel and decreased plasma active thiol metabolite after given a 600 mg clopidogrel loading dose. In addition, *PON1* QQ192 was also associated with an OR of 3.3 for the occurrence of stent thrombosis as compared with QR192 or RR192 genotypes. Later, however, other studies could not document the influence of *PON1* Q192R genotype on clopidogrel antiplatelet aggregation since the publication of the study by Bouman et al [21–23]. In this study, we evaluated the effects of *CYP2C19* and *PON1* genetic polymorphisms on clopidogrel antiplatelet function in Thai population. Similar to the findings from other investigators in African-American and Caucasian populations [21,22], our results have shown that only *CYP2C19*2* and *3 genotypes, but not the *PON1* Q192R genotypes, modified the effect of clopidogrel. The mean aggregation values increased by a strong genetic effect across *CYP2C19* genotype groups in individuals treated with clopidogrel. Also, only *CYP2C19*2* and *3 genotypes but not the *PON1* Q192R genotypes were found to be associated with a higher risk of clopidogrel resistance in CAD patients during treatment with clopidogrel.

The present study was strengthened by testing the influence of these SNPs on platelet aggregation in parallel as measured by MEA assay. Only *CYP2C19*2* and *3 polymorphisms have been demonstrated to be a strong determinant of reduced active clopidogrel metabolite formation corresponding to the studies in Caucasians [14,17,42–52]. Nevertheless, the influence of PON1 on the level of platelet aggregation had a trend towards higher values in QR192 and QQ192 patients (Table 5). This suggested that *PON1* polymorphism may be associated with small differences in platelet inhibition as suggested by the finding of Bouman et al [20]. The small effects of *PON1* Q192R could explain why several reports were unable to confirm this association between *PON1* polymorphism and platelet aggregation in patients who were treated with clopidogrel [21–23,53–57]. Concerning the clinical outcome of patients treated with clopidogrel, our results

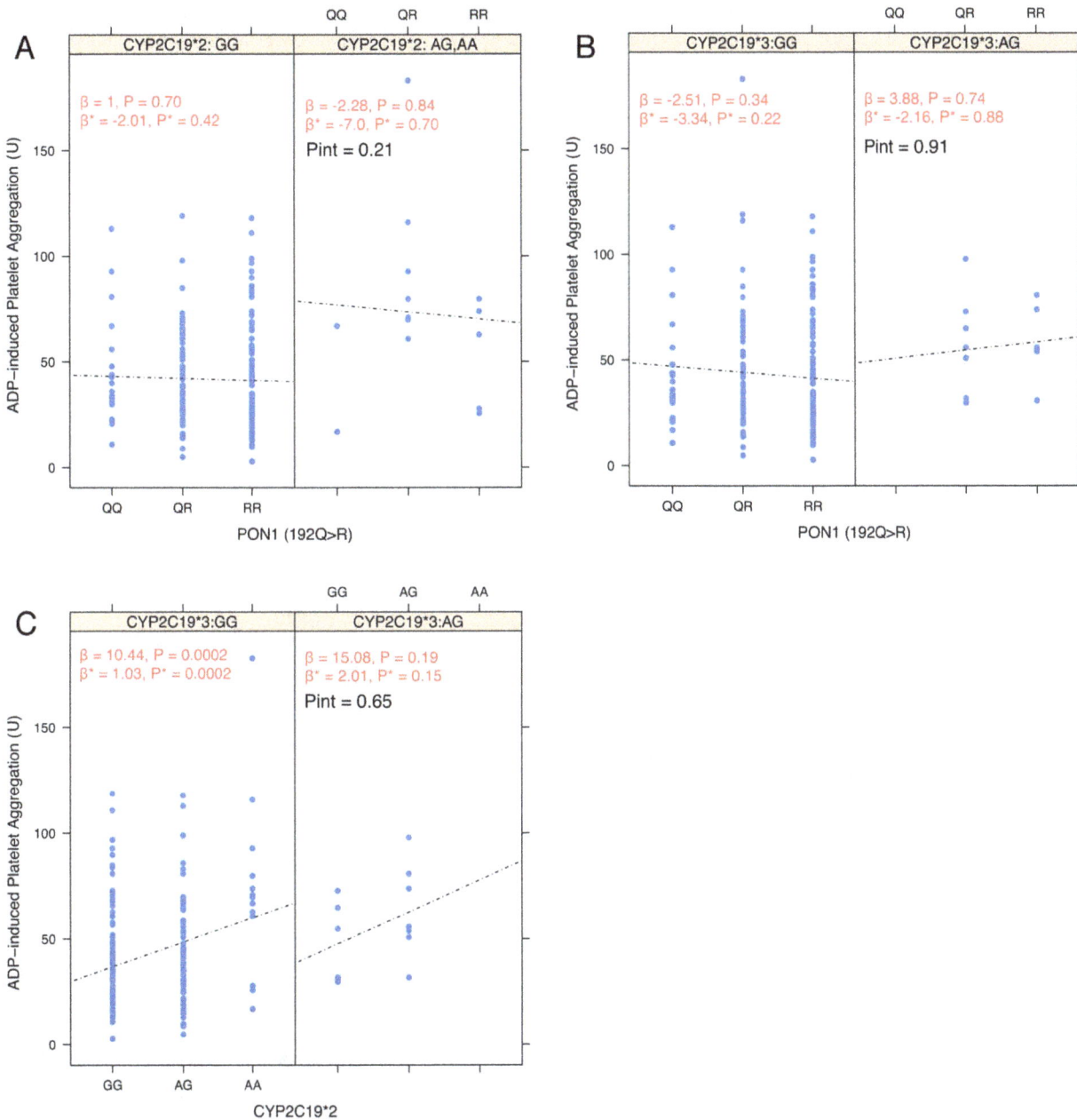

Figure 1. Interaction among polymorphisms in CYP2C19*2, *3 and PON1 Q192R and the effects on ADP-induced platelet aggregation. A) Effects of PON1 Q192R polymorphism on platelet aggregation stratified by *CYP2C19*2* genotype; B) Effects of *PON1* Q192R polymorphism on platelet aggregation stratified by *CYP2C19*3* genotype; C) Effects of *CYP2C19*2* on platelet aggregation stratified by *CYP2C19*3* genotype

Table 6. Standardized linkage disequilibrium coefficient (D′) and correlation coefficient (r) among three polymorphisms in CYP2C19 and PON1.

D′ r	PON1 Q192R	CYP2C19*3	CYP2C19*2
PON1 Q192R	-	−0.0276	0.0089
*CYP2C19*3	0.2258	-	0.0223
*CYP2C19*2	0.0097	0.0731	-

D′ values are shown in the lower triangle, and r values are shown in the upper triangle.

reported here are in agreement with a number of prior studies and confirm the pivotal role of *CYP2C19*2* and *3 as genetic markers for platelet aggregation and clopidogrel response. This present study also demonstrated no association and linkage disequilibrium between *CYP2C19* and *PON1* polymorphisms, which supports the evidence that *CYP2C19* locus, located on chromosome 10, was the only locus which was significantly associated with clopidogrel treatment efficacy in a genome-wide association study (GWAS) [42]. The GWAS did not find evidence for association between SNPs located on or near the *PON1* gene on chromosome 7 and variation in platelet inhibition by clopidogrel [42]. In addition, in a meta-analysis investigating the effect of *CYP2C19* alleles on recurrent stenosis in patients receiving clopidogrel after coronary stenting, the presence of one reduced-function allele was associated with a HR of 2.67, and the presence of two reduced-function alleles was associated with a HR of 3.97 for the recurrence of thrombosis [46]. This study also confirms that the presence of one reduced-function allele of *CYP2C19* was associated with adjusted ORs of 2.94 and 11.26 for *2 and *3, respectively. The presence of two reduced-function alleles was associated with adjusted ORs of 13.09 and 84.06 for *2/*2 and *2/*3, respectively. These findings support the clinical importance of the reduced-function *CYP2C19* polymorphism and clopidogrel resistance on recurrent ischemic events and restenosis after coronary stenting.

In this study, smoking status, diabetes mellitus, and increase in platelet count were shown to be the three major contributing factors that could promote the development of platelet aggregation in CAD patients (Table 4). These conditions have been known to be associated with high oxidative stress, suggesting a possible link between high oxidative stress and response to clopidogrel treatment. This study suggested that not only genetic polymorphisms but also oxidative stress can enhance platelet aggregation to clopidogrel responsiveness in CAD patients.

Limitations of the study include a relatively small sample size, which might contribute to the inability to detect weaker effects of PON1 on clopidogrel response, as compared with the stronger effects of CYP2C19. Although plasma levels of the active metabolite of clopidogrel and PON1 enzyme activity were not measured to confirm the lower level of enzyme activity associated with Q allele, these parameters could be used to indirectly assess the platelet function test as measured by ADP-induced platelet aggregation. Finally, platelet function testing was done with only one single device (Multiplate anslyser), using ADP-induced platelet aggregation, therefore, we could not exclude the possibility that other mechanisms might also explain the clopidogrel resistance as measured by the Multiplate analyser.

Conclusions

This study confirms the impact of *CYP2C19*2* and *3 polymorphisms on antiplatelet effects of clopidogrel in Thai population similar to the results found in Caucasian populations with different genetic background. *PON1* Q192R appeared to have a little modification of efficacy and safety of clopidogrel in CAD patients. A larger study may be needed to confirm the association of the *PON1* Q192 allele with adverse ischemic events in patients receiving clopidogrel treatment. Our results are only relevant to clopidogrel-treated patients; however, knowing the genotypes of *CYP2C19* should aid in selection of antiplatelet therapy. In the future, pharmacogenetic studies may be needed to introduce newer antiplatelet drugs that do not require *CYP2C19* activation and may reduce the overall impact of clopidogrel resistance in patients with CAD.

Acknowledgments

The authors would like to thank Dr. William M. Honsa for English language editorial support. Some parts of this work have been presented in a local meeting at the 39th Congress on Science and Technology of Thailand.

Author Contributions

Conceived and designed the experiments: DT AL BS. Performed the experiments: RK SP AL DT. Analyzed the data: BS SH RK AL. Contributed reagents/materials/analysis tools: DT AL BS. Wrote the paper: AL DT BS SH RK SP BT.

References

1. Moleerergpoom W, Kanjanavanit R, Jintapakorn W, Sritara P (2007) Costs of payment in Thai acute coronary syndrome patients. J Med Assoc Thai 90 Suppl 1: 21–31.

2. Syed FA, Bett J, Walters DL (2011) Anti-platelet therapy for Acute Coronary Syndrome: A review of currently available agents and what the future holds. Cardiovasc Hematol Disord Drug Targets.

3. Smith SC, Jr., Feldman TE, Hirshfeld JW Jr, Jacobs AK, Kern MJ, et al. (2006) ACC/AHA/SCAI 2005 Guideline Update for Percutaneous Coronary Intervention-Summary Article: A Report of the American College of Cardiology/American Heart Association Task Force on Practice Guidelines (ACC/AHA/SCAI Writing Committee to Update the 2001 Guidelines for Percutaneous Coronary Intervention). J Am Coll Cardiol 47: 216–235.

4. Gurbel PA, Tantry US (2006) Drug insight: Clopidogrel nonresponsiveness. Nat Clin Pract Cardiovasc Med 3: 387–395.

5. Gurbel PA, Bliden KP, Hiatt BL, O'Connor CM (2003) Clopidogrel for coronary stenting: response variability, drug resistance, and the effect of pretreatment platelet reactivity. Circulation 107: 2908–2913.

6. Angiolillo DJ, Fernandez-Ortiz A, Bernardo E, Alfonso F, Macaya C, et al. (2007) Variability in individual responsiveness to clopidogrel: clinical implications, management, and future perspectives. J Am Coll Cardiol 49: 1505–1516.

7. Jaremo P, Lindahl TL, Fransson SG, Richter A (2002) Individual variations of platelet inhibition after loading doses of clopidogrel. J Intern Med 252: 233–238.

8. Angiolillo DJ, Fernandez-Ortiz A, Bernardo E, Ramirez C, Sabate M, et al. (2005) Platelet function profiles in patients with type 2 diabetes and coronary artery disease on combined aspirin and clopidogrel treatment. Diabetes 54: 2430–2435.

9. Muller I, Besta F, Schulz C, Massberg S, Schonig A, et al. (2003) Prevalence of clopidogrel non-responders among patients with stable angina pectoris scheduled for elective coronary stent placement. Thromb Haemost 89: 783–787.

10. Mobley JE, Bresee SJ, Wortham DC, Craft RM, Snider CC, et al. (2004) Frequency of nonresponse antiplatelet activity of clopidogrel during pretreatment for cardiac catheterization. Am J Cardiol 93: 456–458.

11. Matetzky S, Shenkman B, Guetta V, Shechter M, Beinart R, et al. (2004) Clopidogrel resistance is associated with increased risk of recurrent atherothrombotic events in patients with acute myocardial infarction. Circulation 109: 3171–3175.

12. Angiolillo DJ, Fernandez-Ortiz A, Bernardo E, Ramirez C, Barrera-Ramirez C, et al. (2005) Identification of low responders to a 300-mg clopidogrel loading dose in patients undergoing coronary stenting. Thromb Res 115: 101–108.

13. Kazui M, Nishiya Y, Ishizuka T, Hagihara K, Farid NA, et al. (2010) Identification of the human cytochrome P450 enzymes involved in the two oxidative steps in the bioactivation of clopidogrel to its pharmacologically active metabolite. Drug Metab Dispos 38: 92–99.

14. Hulot JS, Bura A, Villard E, Azizi M, Remones V, et al. (2006) Cytochrome P450 2C19 loss-of-function polymorphism is a major determinant of clopidogrel responsiveness in healthy subjects. Blood 108: 2244–2247.

15. Brandt JT, Close SL, Iturria SJ, Payne CD, Farid NA, et al. (2007) Common polymorphisms of CYP2C19 and CYP2C9 affect the pharmacokinetic and pharmacodynamic response to clopidogrel but not prasugrel. J Thromb Haemost 5: 2429–2436.

16. Umemura K, Furuta T, Kondo K (2008) The common gene variants of CYP2C19 affect pharmacokinetics and pharmacodynamics in an active metabolite of clopidogrel in healthy subjects. J Thromb Haemost 6: 1439–1441.

17. Simon T, Verstuyft C, Mary-Krause M, Quteineh L, Drouet E, et al. (2009) Genetic determinants of response to clopidogrel and cardiovascular events. N Engl J Med 360: 363–375.

18. Sibbing D, Braun S, Morath T, Mehilli J, Vogt W, et al. (2009) Platelet reactivity after clopidogrel treatment assessed with point-of-care analysis and early drug-eluting stent thrombosis. J Am Coll Cardiol 53: 849–856.

19. Bonello L, Tantry US, Marcucci R, Blindt R, Angiolillo DJ, et al. (2010) Consensus and future directions on the definition of high on-treatment platelet reactivity to adenosine diphosphate. J Am Coll Cardiol 56: 919–933.

20. Bouman HJ, Schomig E, van Werkum JW, Velder J, Hackeng CM, et al. (2011) Paraoxonase-1 is a major determinant of clopidogrel efficacy. Nat Med 17: 110–116.

21. Kreutz RP, Nystrom P, Kreutz Y, Miao J, Desta Z, et al. (2012) Influence of paraoxonase-1 Q192R and cytochrome P450 2C19 polymorphisms on clopidogrel response. Clin Pharmacol 4: 13–20.

22. Sibbing D, Koch W, Massberg S, Byrne RA, Mehilli J, et al. (2011) No association of paraoxonase-1 Q192R genotypes with platelet response to clopidogrel and risk of stent thrombosis after coronary stenting. Eur Heart J 32: 1605–1613.

23. Pare G, Ross S, Mehta SR, Yusuf S, Anand SS, et al. (2012) Effect of PON1 Q192R genetic polymorphism on clopidogrel efficacy and cardiovascular events in the Clopidogrel in the Unstable Angina to Prevent Recurrent Events trial and the Atrial Fibrillation Clopidogrel Trial with Irbesartan for Prevention of Vascular Events. Circ Cardiovasc Genet 5: 250–256.

24. Marsillach J, Aragones G, Beltran R, Caballeria J, Pedro-Botet J, et al. (2009) The measurement of the lactonase activity of paraoxonase-1 in the clinical evaluation of patients with chronic liver impairment. Clin Biochem 42: 91–98.

25. Bhattacharyya T, Nicholls SJ, Topol EJ, Zhang R, Yang X, et al. (2008) Relationship of paraoxonase 1 (PON1) gene polymorphisms and functional activity with systemic oxidative stress and cardiovascular risk. JAMA 299: 1265–1276.

26. Mackness MI, Arrol S, Mackness B, Durrington PN (1997) Alloenzymes of paraoxonase and effectiveness of high-density lipoproteins in protecting low-density lipoprotein against lipid peroxidation. Lancet 349: 851–852.

27. Lawlor DA, Day IN, Gaunt TR, Hinks LJ, Briggs PJ, et al. (2004) The association of the PON1 Q192R polymorphism with coronary heart disease: findings from the British Women's Heart and Health cohort study and a meta-analysis. BMC Genet 5: 17.

28. Regieli JJ, Jukema JW, Doevendans PA, Zwinderman AH, Kastelein JJ, et al. (2009) Paraoxonase variants relate to 10-year risk in coronary artery disease: impact of a high-density lipoprotein-bound antioxidant in secondary prevention. J Am Coll Cardiol 54: 1238–1245.

29. Likidlilid A, Akrawinthawong K, Poldee S, Sriratanasathavorn C (2010) Paraoxonase 1 polymorphisms as the risk factor of coronary heart disease in a Thai population. Acta Cardiol 65: 681–691.

30. Ko YL, Ko YS, Wang SM, Hsu LA, Chang CJ, et al. (1998) The Gln-Arg 191 polymorphism of the human paraoxonase gene is not associated with the risk of coronary artery disease among Chinese in Taiwan. Atherosclerosis 141: 259–264.

31. Imai Y, Morita H, Kurihara H, Sugiyama T, Kato N, et al. (2000) Evidence for association between paraoxonase gene polymorphisms and atherosclerotic diseases. Atherosclerosis 149: 435–442.

32. Ferre N, Tous M, Paul A, Zamora A, Vendrell JJ, et al. (2002) Paraoxonase Gln-Arg(192) and Leu-Met(55) gene polymorphisms and enzyme activity in a population with a low rate of coronary heart disease. Clin Biochem 35: 197–203.

33. Goldstein JA (2001) Clinical relevance of genetic polymorphisms in the human CYP2C subfamily. Br J Clin Pharmacol 52: 349–355.

34. Sibbing D, Braun S, Jawansky S, Vogt W, Mehilli J, et al. (2008) Assessment of ADP-induced platelet aggregation with light transmission aggregometry and multiple electrode platelet aggregometry before and after clopidogrel treatment. Thromb Haemost 99: 121–126.

35. Gerotziafas GT, Zarifis J, Bandi A, Mossialos L, Galea V, et al. (2012) Description of response to aspirin and clopidogrel in outpatients with coronary artery disease using multiple electrode impedance aggregometry. Clin Appl Thromb Hemost 18: 356–363.

36. de Morais SM, Wilkinson GR, Blaisdell J, Nakamura K, Meyer UA, et al. (1994) The major genetic defect responsible for the polymorphism of S-mephenytoin metabolism in humans. J Biol Chem 269: 15419–15422.

37. De Morais SM, Wilkinson GR, Blaisdell J, Meyer UA, Nakamura K, et al. (1994) Identification of a new genetic defect responsible for the polymorphism of (S)-mephenytoin metabolism in Japanese. Mol Pharmacol 46: 594–598.

38. Campo S, Sardo MA, Trimarchi G, Bonaiuto M, Fontana L, et al. (2004) Association between serum paraoxonase (PON1) gene promoter T(-107)C polymorphism, PON1 activity and HDL levels in healthy Sicilian octogenarians. Exp Gerontol 39: 1089–1094.

39. Cordell HJ (2002) Epistasis: what it means, what it doesn't mean, and statistical methods to detect it in humans. Hum Mol Genet 11: 2463–2468.

40. Schwender H, Fritsch A (2013) scrime: Analysis of High-Dimensional Categorical Data such as SNP Data. Available: http://CRAN.R-project.org/package=scrime.

41. R Core Team (2013) R: A language and environment for statistical computing. Vienna, Austria: R Foundation for Statistical Computing. Available: http://www.R-project.org.

42. Shuldiner AR, O'Connell JR, Bliden KP, Gandhi A, Ryan K, et al. (2009) Association of cytochrome P450 2C19 genotype with the antiplatelet effect and clinical efficacy of clopidogrel therapy. JAMA 302: 849–857.

43. Sibbing D, Gebhard D, Koch W, Braun S, Stegherr J, et al. (2010) Isolated and interactive impact of common CYP2C19 genetic variants on the antiplatelet effect of chronic clopidogrel therapy. J Thromb Haemost 8: 1685–1693.

44. Mega JL, Close SL, Wiviott SD, Shen L, Hockett RD, et al. (2009) Cytochrome P450 genetic polymorphisms and the response to prasugrel: relationship to pharmacokinetic, pharmacodynamic, and clinical outcomes. Circulation 119: 2553–2560.

45. Mega JL, Close SL, Wiviott SD, Shen L, Walker JR, et al. (2010) Genetic variants in ABCB1 and CYP2C19 and cardiovascular outcomes after treatment with clopidogrel and prasugrel in the TRITON-TIMI 38 trial: a pharmacogenetic analysis. Lancet 376: 1312–1319.

46. Mega JL, Simon T, Collet JP, Anderson JL, Antman EM, et al. (2010) Reduced-function CYP2C19 genotype and risk of adverse clinical outcomes among patients treated with clopidogrel predominantly for PCI: a meta-analysis. JAMA 304: 1821–1830.

47. Hochholzer W, Trenk D, Fromm MF, Valina CM, Stratz C, et al. (2010) Impact of cytochrome P450 2C19 loss-of-function polymorphism and of major demographic characteristics on residual platelet function after loading and maintenance treatment with clopidogrel in patients undergoing elective coronary stent placement. J Am Coll Cardiol 55: 2427–2434.

48. Trenk D, Hochholzer W, Fromm MF, Chialda LE, Pahl A, et al. (2008) Cytochrome P450 2C19 681G>A polymorphism and high on-clopidogrel platelet reactivity associated with adverse 1-year clinical outcome of elective percutaneous coronary intervention with drug-eluting or bare-metal stents. J Am Coll Cardiol 51: 1925–1934.

49. Sibbing D, Stegherr J, Latz W, Koch W, Mehilli J, et al. (2009) Cytochrome P450 2C19 loss-of-function polymorphism and stent thrombosis following percutaneous coronary intervention. Eur Heart J 30: 916–922.

50. Collet JP, Hulot JS, Pena A, Villard E, Esteve JB, et al. (2009) Cytochrome P450 2C19 polymorphism in young patients treated with clopidogrel after myocardial infarction: a cohort study. Lancet 373: 309–317.

51. Mega JL, Close SL, Wiviott SD, Shen L, Hockett RD, et al. (2009) Cytochrome p-450 polymorphisms and response to clopidogrel. N Engl J Med 360: 354–362.

52. Harmsze AM, van Werkum JW, Ten Berg JM, Zwart B, Bouman HJ, et al. (2010) CYP2C19*2 and CYP2C9*3 alleles are associated with stent thrombosis: a case-control study. Eur Heart J 31: 3046–3053.

53. Simon T, Steg PG, Becquemont L, Verstuyft C, Kotti S, et al. (2011) Effect of paraoxonase-1 polymorphism on clinical outcomes in patients treated with clopidogrel after an acute myocardial infarction. Clin Pharmacol Ther 90: 561–567.

54. Trenk D, Hochholzer W, Fromm MF, Zolk O, Valina CM, et al. (2011) Paraoxonase-1 Q192R polymorphism and antiplatelet effects of clopidogrel in patients undergoing elective coronary stent placement. Circ Cardiovasc Genet 4: 429–436.

55. Fontana P, James R, Barazer I, Berdague P, Schved JF, et al. (2011) Relationship between paraoxonase-1 activity, its Q192R genetic variant and clopidogrel responsiveness in the ADRIE study. J Thromb Haemost 9: 1664–1666.

56. Rideg O, Komocsi A, Magyarlaki T, Tokes-Fuzesi M, Miseta A, et al. (2011) Impact of genetic variants on post-clopidogrel platelet reactivity in patients after elective percutaneous coronary intervention. Pharmacogenomics 12: 1269–1280.

57. Lewis JP, Fisch AS, Ryan K, O'Connell JR, Gibson Q, et al. (2011) Paraoxonase 1 (PON1) gene variants are not associated with clopidogrel response. Clin Pharmacol Ther 90: 568–574.

5

Patient Age and the Prognosis of Idiopathic Membranous Nephropathy

Makoto Yamaguchi[1], Masahiko Ando[2], Ryohei Yamamoto[3], Shinichi Akiyama[1], Sawako Kato[1], Takayuki Katsuno[1], Tomoki Kosugi[1], Waichi Sato[1], Naotake Tsuboi[1], Yoshinari Yasuda[1], Masashi Mizuno[1], Yasuhiko Ito[1], Seiichi Matsuo[1], Shoichi Maruyama[1]*

1 Department of Nephrology, Nagoya University Graduate School of Medicine, Nagoya, Japan, 2 Center for Advanced Medicine and Clinical Research, Nagoya University Hospital, Nagoya, Japan, 3 Department of Geriatric Medicine and Nephrology, Osaka University Graduate School of Medicine, Suita, Japan

Abstract

Background: Idiopathic membranous nephropathy (IMN) is increasingly seen in older patients. However, differences in disease presentation and outcomes between older and younger IMN patients remain controversial. We compared patient characteristics between younger and older IMN patients.

Methods: We recruited 171 Japanese patients with IMN, including 90 (52.6%) patients <65 years old, 40 (23.4%) patients 65–70 years, and 41 (24.0%) patients ≥71 years. Clinical characteristics and outcomes were compared between younger and older IMN patients.

Results: During a median observation period of 37 months, 103 (60.2%) patients achieved complete proteinuria remission, which was not significantly associated with patient age ($P = 0.831$). However, 13 (7.6%) patients were hospitalized because of infection. Multivariate Cox proportional hazards models identified older age [adjusted hazard ratio (HR) = 3.11, 95% confidence interval (CI): 1.45–7.49, per 10 years; $P = 0.003$], prednisolone use (adjusted HR = 11.8, 95% CI: 1.59–242.5; $P = 0.014$), and cyclosporine used in combination with prednisolone (adjusted HR = 10.3, 95% CI: 1.59–204.4; $P = 0.012$) as significant predictors of infection. A <25% decrease in proteinuria at 1 month after immunosuppressive therapy initiation also predicted infection (adjusted HR = 6.72, 95% CI: 1.51–37.8; $P = 0.012$).

Conclusions: Younger and older IMN patients had similar renal outcomes. However, older patients were more likely to develop infection when using immunosuppressants. Patients with a poor response in the first month following the initiation of immunosuppressive therapy should be carefully monitored for infection and may require a faster prednisolone taper.

Editor: Giuseppe Remuzzi, Mario Negri Institute for Pharmacological Research and Azienda Ospedaliera Ospedali Riuniti di Bergamo, Italy

Funding: This study was supported by a Grant-in-Aid for Progressive Renal Diseases Research, Research on Rare and Intractable Disease, from the Ministry of Health, Labor, and Welfare of Japan. The funders had no role in study design, data collection and analysis, decision to publish, or preparation of the manuscript.

Competing Interests: The authors have declared that no competing interests exist.

* Email: marus@med.nagoya-u.ac.jp

Introduction

In Japan, the elderly population (i.e., those aged 65 and over) comprised 24.1% of the total population as of October 2012, a figure that is expected to increase to 39.9% by 2060 [1]. With increases in life expectancy, greater numbers of elderly patients with chronic kidney diseases are surviving longer. Membranous nephropathy (MN) is the most important cause of nephrotic syndrome in elderly patients [2,3]. The incidence of MN is higher in the elderly than in younger adults. Although little information is available regarding the natural course of MN in elderly patients, Zent et al. [4] reported similar clinical presentations between older and younger patients. However, clinical information such as the prevalence of leg edema or pleural effusion was not included. Thus, the clinical severity associated with nephrotic syndrome could not be adequately evaluated.

Most randomized trials of immunosuppressive therapy for MN included few, if any, patients older than 65 [5–9], and only a few retrospective studies and case series specifically reported immunosuppressive therapy outcomes [4,10,11]. Consequently, the optimal immunosuppressive regimen for elderly idiopathic membranous nephropathy (IMN) patients remains controversial.

Based on our clinical experience, our impression is that compared to younger IMN patients, older patients have more severe symptoms associated with nephrotic syndrome and are more susceptible to infection. It can therefore be difficult to weigh the risks and benefits of initiating immunosuppressive therapy, especially among elderly patients.

To understand the clinical characteristics of elderly IMN patients and identify patients at high risk for infection, we conducted a retrospective multicenter observational cohort study that was organized as part of the Nagoya Nephrotic Syndrome

Cohort Study (N-NSCS), a study based in 10 major nephrology centers in Nagoya, Japan.

Subjects and Methods

Study Population and Data Sources

Participants in the present study were included in our previous multicenter retrospective cohort study, N-NSCS, which identified cigarette smoking as a risk factor for kidney dysfunction for IMN [12]. The study design of N-NSCS was described in detail elsewhere [12]. Briefly, this study included patients older than 18 years who were diagnosed with MN based on kidney biopsy results at Nagoya University, Chubu Rosai Hospital, Japanese Red Cross Nagoya Daiichi Hospital, Tsushima City Hospital, Kasugai Municipal Hospital, Nagoya Kyoritsu Hospital, Anjo Kosei Hospital, Ichinomiya Municipal Hospital, Handa City Hospital, or Tosei General Hospital between January 2003 and December 2012. Out of 272 identified MN patients, we excluded those with conditions generally considered to cause secondary MN [10]. Furthermore, we excluded seven patients (3.9%) because of loss to follow-up (n = 6) and missing data (n = 1). Ultimately, 171 (62.9%) IMN patients were enrolled and followed up until September 2013.

Our study was conducted by using linkable anonymous data set. No informed consent was obtained. The study protocol and consent procedure were approved by the ethics committees of Nagoya University, Chubu Rosai Hospital, Japanese Red Cross Nagoya Daiichi Hospital, Tsushima City Hospital, Kasugai Municipal Hospital, Nagoya Kyoritsu Hospital, Anjo Kosei Hospital, Ichinomiya Municipal Hospital, Handa City Hospital, and Tosei General Hospital.

Data Collection

Baseline characteristics were collected retrospectively from patients' medical records. Clinical characteristics at the time of kidney biopsy were considered to represent baseline if the patient had not received immunosuppressive therapy or received immunosuppressive therapy only after a kidney biopsy. For patients who received immunosuppressive therapy before biopsy, the clinical characteristics at the time of initiating immunosuppressive therapy were used as baseline. Baseline characteristics included age, gender, body mass index, systolic and diastolic blood pressure, serum total cholesterol, serum creatinine, glomerular filtration rate [GFR; estimated using the equation recently developed by the Japanese Society of Nephrology: eGFR (mL/min/1.73 m^2) $= 194 \times Scr^{-1.094} \times Age^{-0.287} \times 0.739$ (if female) (13)], serum albumin, 24-hour urinary protein excretion or urinary protein/creatinine ratio, smoking status, antihypertensive drug use, and initial use of corticosteroids and/or other immunosuppressive agents.

Antihypertensive drugs used in this cohort included angiotensin-converting enzyme (ACE) inhibitors or angiotensin II receptor blockers (ARB), calcium channel blockers, β-blockers, and thiazides. Information regarding therapeutic interventions was also collected, including the use of ACE inhibitors/ARBs and corticosteroids or other immunosuppressive agents that were prescribed during the observation period.

Nephrotic syndrome was defined as a urinary protein excretion ≥3.5 g/day (or a urinary protein/creatinine ratio ≥3.5) and a serum albumin level <3.0 mg/dL.

Complete remission (CR) from proteinuria was defined as a urinary protein excretion <0.3 g/day, a urinary protein/creatinine ratio <0.3, and/or a negative/trace result for urinary protein on a dipstick test. Partial remission (PR) from proteinuria was

defined as a urinary protein excretion <3.5 g/day and a urinary protein/creatinine ratio <3.5. Relapse was defined as a urinary protein excretion ≥1.0 g/day, a urinary protein/creatinine ratio ≥1.0, or a urinary protein dipstick result ≥2+ on at least two occasions after CR had been achieved.

The rate of eGFR decline per year (mL/min per 1.73 m^2/year) was determined by plotting eGFR against the observation time.

The anonymous data set is available in the **Table S7 in File S2**.

Outcomes

Our primary outcome was the first CR. Secondary outcomes were hospitalization due to infection and a 30% decline in the eGFR before end-stage renal disease (ESRD). Patients who died before achieving either outcome were censored at the time of death. The eGFR was measured as required for each patient at 1–3 month intervals. Patients were followed up until September 2013 and censored at the time of their death before ESRD or as of their last serum creatinine measurement before September 2013.

Statistical Analyses

We stratified patients into three age categories: <65, 65–70, and ≥71 years old. Clinical characteristics were compared between these three groups using a Wilcoxon rank-sum test or Fisher's exact test. To determine predictors independently associated with each outcome, potential covariates were assessed using a log-rank test and/or univariate and multivariate Cox proportional hazards (CPH) models. For continuous variables, a Wilcoxon rank-sum test was used to assess the significance of intergroup differences. Results for categorical variables were expressed as percentages and compared by using Fisher's exact test. The cumulative probabilities of achieving a first CR and hospitalization due to infection were determined using the Kaplan-Meier method and log-rank tests. Predictors of these outcomes were identified using univariate and multivariate CPH models. The proportional hazards assumption for covariates was tested using scaled Schoenfeld residuals. A −2 log likelihood value for fitting a model with all explanatory variables was determined for individual CPH models that included 25%, 50%, or 75% decreases in proteinuria in the first month after initial immunosuppressive therapy, and was used to compare the performance of these three models. A likelihood ratio test was used to determine whether the fit of a model that included a 25% decrease rate was the best model for the present study. The trend in the outcome with respect to the decreases in proteinuria in the first month after initial immunosuppressive therapy was examined statistically by scoring ≥50% decrease as 0 and 25–50% decrease, 0–25% decrease, and exacerbation as 1, 2, and 3, respectively; the resulting scores were then included in the regression model. Least squares mean±95% confidence intervals for urinary protein and eGFR during follow-up period were compared between three age categories using linear mixed-effect models.

The level of statistical significance was set at $P<0.05$. All statistical analyses were performed using JMP version 10.0.0 (SAS Institute, Cary, NC, USA; www.jmp.com), SAS version 9.4 (SAS Institute, Cary, NC; www.sas.com), and STATA version 13.0 (STATA Corp, www.stata.com).

Results

Clinical Characteristics

A total of 171 patients were diagnosed with IMN after appropriate clinical and laboratory screening for secondary causes.

Table 1. Baseline characteristics of 171 IMN patients.

	<65 years	65–70 years	≥71 years	P-value
Number	90	40	41	
Baseline characteristics				
Age (years)	57 (50–62)	68 (66–69)	75 (74–78)	
Male [n (%)]	63 (70.0)	28 (70.0)	27 (65.9)	0.882
Body mass index (kg/m²)	23.2 (21.2–25.8)	23.2 (22.0–25.7)	22.6 (21.1–24.6)	0.440
Systolic blood pressure (mmHg)	129 (120–140)	135 (125–158)	138 (122–147)	0.028
Diastolic blood pressure (mmHg)	77 (70–86)	80 (70–86)	76 (70–84)	0.502
Serum creatinine (mg/dL)	0.77 (0.68–0.90)	0.80 (0.68–0.99)	0.95 (0.7–1.2)	0.011
eGFR (mL/min/1.73 m²)	81 (70–97)	73 (58–86)	59 (46–81)	<0.001
Serum albumin (g/dL)	2.8 (2.1–3.5)	2.5 (2.0–3.1)	2.3 (1.9–2.8)	0.014
Urinary protein (g/day)	4.2 (2.6–7.0)	3.6 (2.6–7.6)	5.1 (3.3–7.7)	0.275
Urinary protein >3.5 (g/day) [n (%)]	29 (32.2)	17 (42.5)	11 (26.8)	0.310
Total cholesterol (mg/dL)	279 (229–382)	284 (239–400)	297 (249–367)	0.859
Leg edema [n (%)]	64 (71.1)	29 (72.5)	38 (92.7)	0.020
Pleural effusion [n (%)]	12 (13.3)	8 (20.0)	13 (31.7)	0.048
Treatment				
ACE inhibitor or ARB therapy [n (%)]	80 (88.9)	39 (97.5)	47 (90.2)	0.268
Immunosuppressive therapy				0.893
No immunosuppressants	36 (40.0)	17 (42.5)	17 (41.5)	
Prednisolone [n (%)]	17 (18.9)	10 (25.0)	8 (19.5)	
Prednisolone+Cyclosporine [n (%)]	37 (41.1)	13 (32.5)	16 (39.0)	
Observational period (months)	44 (20–86)	31 (15–63)	25 (11–54)	0.021

NOTE: Median (interquartile range), Conversion factors for units: SCr in mg/dL to μmol/L, ×88.4; eGFR (mL/min/1.73 m2) = 194×Scr$^{-1.094}$×Age$^{-0.287}$×0.739 (if female), total cholesterol in mg/dL to mmol/L, ×0.02586.
Abbreviations: IMN, idiopathic membranous nephropathy; eGFR, estimated glomerular filtration rate; ACE inhibitor/ARB, angiotensin-converting enzyme inhibitor/angiotensin receptor blocker.

Baseline characteristics stratified by the three age categories are shown in Table 1.

The cohort included 90 (52.6%) patients <65 years old, 40 (23.4%) aged 65–70 years, and 41 (24.0%) ≥71 years old. Compared with younger patients, older patients had lower serum albumin levels (P = 0.014), lower eGFRs (P<0.001), higher serum creatinine levels (P = 0.011), higher systolic blood pressure (P = 0.028), and a higher prevalence of leg edema and pleural effusion (P = 0.020 and P = 0.048, respectively). This suggested a greater severity of symptoms associated with nephrotic syndrome in older patients than in younger patients. The prevalence of pleural effusion was determined by chest radiography results at the time of kidney biopsy. No trends were found for initial immunosuppressive therapy among the different age categories. The observation periods were shorter in the elderly group (P = 0.021).

Treatment During the Observation Period

During follow-up, 156 (91.2%) patients used ACE inhibitors or ARBs. Patients were divided into three groups according to the type of treatment they received during the observation period: (1) a prednisolone group comprising 35 patients (20.5%) who received prednisolone alone; (2) a cyclosporine group comprising 66 patients (38.6%) who received prednisolone and cyclosporine; and (3) a supportive therapy group comprising 70 patients (40.9%) who did not receive prednisolone or other immunosuppressive drugs. One patient in the cyclosporine group (0.6%) developed a

50% serum creatinine increase over baseline and was prescribed mizoribine.

The median initial prednisolone dose was 30 mg (interquartile range: 20–40 mg/day) and was tapered according to treatment response. Most patients in the cyclosporine group were started on cyclosporine at 1–2 mg/kg and prednisolone at 0.4–0.6 mg/kg. Cyclosporine dosing was modified by monitoring whole-blood trough levels, while prednisolone was tapered according to treatment response. The time from kidney biopsy to immunosuppressive therapy initiation was 0.7 months (interquartile range: 0.3–3.3 months).

Outcomes

Primary outcome: first complete remission. Outcome data are shown in Table 2. The median observation period for the entire cohort was 37 months (interquartile range: 15–72 months). CR from proteinuria was achieved by 103 (60.2%) patients. The mean time to CR was 14 months (interquartile range: 6–25 months).

The cumulative probabilities of achieving a CR within 1, 5, and 10 years were, respectively, 0.37, 0.74, and 0.81 for patients <65 years old; 0.45, 0.79, and 0.79 for those 65–70 years old; and 0.32, 0.86, and 0.86 for those ≥71 years old. There were no significant differences in CR from proteinuria according to patient age (P = 0.831; **Figure 1**).

Furthermore, the changes in average proteinuria over time did not differ among the various age groups (P = 0.458; **Figure S1**).

Table 2. Outcomes of 171 IMN patients.

	<65 years	65–70 years	≥71 years	P-value
Number	90	40	41	
30% reduction in eGFR [n (%)]	17 (18.9)	9 (22.5)	11 (26.8)	0.591
Decline in eGFR (mL/min per 1.73 m² per year)	2.37 (0.25–7.43)	3.06 (−2.17–8.33)	4.10 (−0.58–8.31)	0.956
ESRD [n (%)]	1 (1.1)	0 (0.0)	1 (2.4)	1.000
Death [n (%)]	1 (1.1)	3 (7.5)	7 (17.1)	0.003
Death due to infection [n (%)]	0 (0.0)	1 (2.5)	6 (14.6)	<0.001
Hospitalization due to infection [n (%)]	2 (2.2)	3 (7.5)	8 (19.5)	0.003
Hospitalization due to cardiovascular disease [n (%)]	1 (1.1)	0 (0.0)	2 (4.9)	0.197
Venous thrombotic events [n (%)]	0 (0.0)	0 (0.0)	0 (0.0)	1.000
Malignancy [n (%)]	2 (2.2)	2 (5.0)	1 (2.4)	0.671
Steroid psychosis [n (%)]	1 (1.1)	1 (2.5)	1 (2.4)	0.756
Use of antidiabetic agents [n (%)]	8 (8.9)	3 (7.5)	2 (4.9)	0.724
Aseptic osteonecrosis with surgical treatment [n (%)]	0 (0.0)	0 (0.0)	0 (0.0)	1.000
Remission				
Complete remission [n (%)]	56 (62.2)	26 (65.0)	21 (51.2)	0.383
Partial remission [n (%)]	81 (90.0)	36 (90.0)	33 (80.5)	0.270
Relapse [n (%)]	17 (24.3)	2 (6.7)	7 (21.9)	0.120

NOTE: Median (interquartile range), Conversion factors for units: SCr in mg/dL to μmol/L, ×88.4; eGFR (mL/min/1.73 m2) = 194×Scr$^{-1.094}$×Age$^{-0.287}$×0.739 (if female), total cholesterol in mg/dL to mmol/L, ×0.02586.
Abbreviations: IMN, idiopathic membranous nephropathy; eGFR, estimated glomerular filtration rate; ESRD, end-stage renal disease.

Among patients who achieved a first remission, 26 (25.2%) relapsed at least once.

Secondary outcomes: hospitalization due to infection and a 30% decline in eGFR level. During follow-up, 37 (21.6%) patients developed a 30% decline in eGFR before ESRD. In all 37 patients, eGFR levels did not improve by the last follow-up visit.

Although there were no significant differences according to patient age in 30% eGFR declines and eGFR decline rates, the average eGFR over time in patients <65 years old was

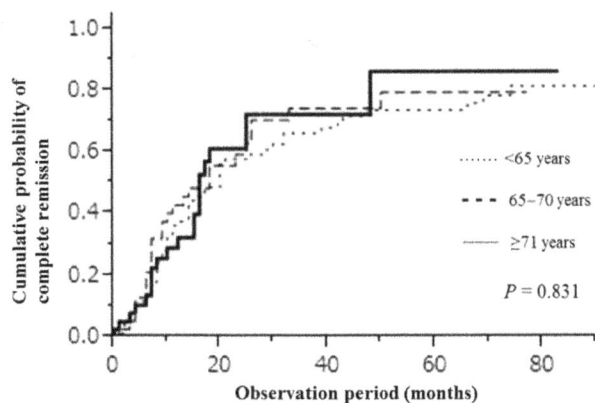

Number at risk

<65 years	90	34	17	13	6
65–70 years	40	12	5	2	0
≥71 years	41	8	3	2	1

Figure 1. Cumulative probability of complete remission in 171 IMN patients stratified by age.

significantly higher than that in ≥71 years old (P = 0.046; **Figure S2**).

Infection caused 13 (7.6%) individual patient hospitalizations and 7 (4.1%) deaths. The older age categories were significantly associated with hospitalization and death due to infection (P = 0.003). The cumulative probabilities of hospitalization due to infection within 1, 5, and 10 years were, respectively, 0.02, 0.02, and 0.02 for those <65 years old; 0.05, 0.08, and 0.08 for those 65–70 years old; and 0.16, 0.28, and 0.28 for those ≥71 years old. There were significant differences in hospitalization due to infection according to patient age (P = 0.002; **Figure 2**).

Causes of infection were tuberculosis pleuritis (n = 1), bacterial pneumonia (n = 7), *Pneumocystis jiroveci* pneumonia (n = 1), vertebral osteomyelitis (n = 1), methicillin-resistant *Staphylococcus aureus* bacteremia (n = 1), fungemia (n = 1), and pyelonephritis (n = 1).

After excluding seven patients who died because of infection, the remaining causes of death were acute subdural hematoma (n = 1), traffic accident (n = 1), sudden death (n = 1), and intestinal bleeding (n = 1). Malignancy occurred in five (2.9%) patients, whose diagnoses included esophageal cancer (n = 1), stomach cancer (n = 1), colon cancer (n = 1), prostate cancer (n = 1), and malignant lymphoma (n = 1). Only three (1.8%) patients were hospitalized for cardiovascular disease, and no patient had a venous thromboembolic event.

Treatment and clinical characteristics: comparison of patients in different treatment groups

Clinical characteristics of the three groups including (1) the prednisolone monotherapy group, (2) the combined cyclosporine group, and (3) the supportive therapy group are shown in **Tables S1 and S2 in File S1**. The serum albumin level in the supportive therapy group was significantly higher than that in the immuno-

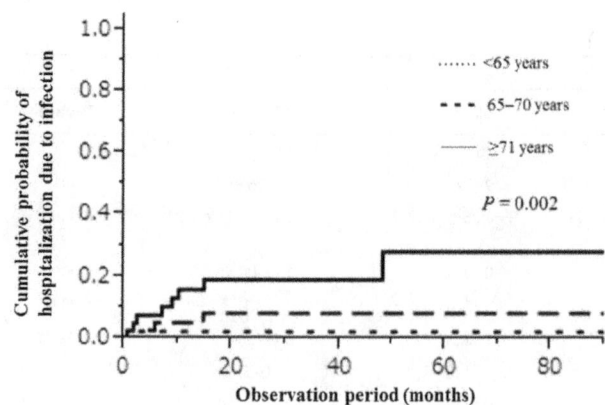

Figure 2. Cumulative probability of hospitalization due to infection in 171 IMN patients stratified by age.

suppressive therapy groups (prednisolone monotherapy and combined cyclosporine groups) ($P<0.001$), and the urinary protein level in the supportive therapy group was significantly lower than that in the immunosuppressive therapy group ($P<0.001$). With respect to outcomes, the proportion of patients achieving a 30% eGFR decrease was not significantly different among the three groups ($P = 0.591$), whereas the proportion of patients achieving CR and the rate of hospitalization due to infection were significantly higher in the immunosuppressive therapy groups than the supportive group ($P = 0.031$ and $P = 0.032$, respectively).

Predictors of First Complete Remission

Univariate CPH models showed that a lower serum creatinine level, initial use of prednisolone monotherapy, and initial use of cyclosporine in combination with prednisolone were significantly associated with a first CR from proteinuria (**Table 3**). After adjusting for clinically relevant factors, the initial use of prednisolone monotherapy [adjusted hazard ratio (HR) = 1.78, 95% confidence interval (CI): 1.01–3.10; $P = 0.045$) and cyclosporine in combination with prednisolone (adjusted HR = 1.95. 95% CI: 1.16–3.26; $P = 0.011$) remained as significant predictors of a first CR from proteinuria.

Predictors of Infection

A total of 13 (7.6%) patients had at least one infection that required hospitalization. Of these, 12 (92.3%) received immunosuppressive therapy before developing an infection. The median time from immunosuppressive therapy initiation to first hospitalization due to infection was 3 months (interquartile range: 1–5 months). When examining all hospitalizations due to infections, univariate analyses identified several statistically significant predictors of increased infection risk: older age, higher serum creatinine levels, and immunosuppressive therapy use, namely prednisolone monotherapy and cyclosporine combination therapy (**Table 4**).

After adjusting for clinically relevant factors, older age (adjusted HR = 3.11, 95% CI: 1.45–7.49; $P = 0.003$), prednisolone use (adjusted HR = 11.8, 95% CI: 1.59–242.5; $P = 0.014$), and cyclosporine used in combination with prednisolone (adjusted

HR = 10.3, 95% CI: 1.59–204.4; $P = 0.012$) were identified as significant predictors for the development of infection. This suggests that among older IMN patients, immunosuppressive therapy was a more important predictor of infection risk.

Because immunosuppressive therapy use may have been affected by patient age, biasing our estimate of the predictive power of age, we assessed potential associations between patient age and immunosuppressive therapy during the observation period, i.e., the cumulative dose of prednisolone and cyclosporine used during the observation period.

Compared with younger patients, the cumulative dose of prednisolone was lower in elderly patients at 3, 6, and 12 months ($P<0.001$, $P<0.001$, and $P = 0.002$, respectively; **Table S3 in File S1**). No significant trend between patient age and cyclosporine use emerged at 1, 3, 6, and 12 months ($P = 0.163$, $P = 0.740$, $P = 0.447$, and $P = 0.387$, respectively).

The median times to reach doses of 20, 15, 10, and 7.5 mg/day were shorter in elderly patients than in younger patients ($P = 0.015$, $P = 0.006$, $P<0.001$, and $P<0.001$, respectively; **Table S4 in File S1**). The cumulative doses of prednisolone to reach 20, 15, 10, and 7.5 mg/day were also lower in elderly patients than in younger patients ($P = 0.006$, $P = 0.005$, $P<0.001$, and $P<0.001$, respectively).

These results strongly suggest that the higher incidence of infections in elderly patients was not attributable to the prednisolone dose or to the type of immunosuppressive therapy.

Predictors of Infections in Patients who Received Immunosuppressive Therapy

In patients who received immunosuppressive therapy (n = 101), we evaluated predictors of infection using clinical data obtained within 1 month from initial immunosuppressive therapy including age, sex, serum creatinine, serum albumin, urinary protein at the time of initiating immunosuppressive therapy, use of immunosuppressive therapy within 1 month after treatment, initial daily dose of prednisolone, and a <25% decrease in proteinuria in the first month after immunosuppressive therapy initiation (**Table 5**).

Univariate CPH models showed that age, serum creatinine, and a <25% decrease in proteinuria in the first month after immunosuppressive therapy initiation were significant risk factors for developing infection. A multivariate CPH model adjusted for age, sex, creatinine, proteinuria at the time of initiating immunosuppressive therapy, use of immunosuppressive therapy within 1 month after starting therapy, and initial daily dose of prednisolone, was then applied. In the multivariate analysis, older age (adjusted HR = 2.80, 95% CI: 1.20–7.83; $P = 0.016$) and a < 25% decrease in proteinuria in the first month after immunosuppressive therapy initiation (adjusted HR = 7.27, 95% CI: 1.74–37.7; $P = 0.007$) were identified as significant risk factors. The −2 log likelihood values with all explanatory variables were 39.32, 39.93, and 39.96, respectively, for Cox models that included a 25% decrease, 50% decrease, and 75% decrease in proteinuria in the first month after immunosuppressive therapy initiation. Because the degrees of freedom were the same for these three models, these results indicate that the Cox model that included a 25% decrease in proteinuria was the best fit to the observed infection events.

We further stratified the decreasing rate of proteinuria in the first month after the initial multivariate analysis, and found that patients with a poor response to initial therapy had a nearly linear high risk for infection ($P = 0.006$, **Table 6**).

Because the decrease in proteinuria in the first month after initial immunosuppressive therapy may have affected subsequent treatment, resulting in bias, we evaluated the associations between

Table 3. Predictors of first CR.

	Univariate model		Multivariate model	
	HR (95% CI)	P-value	HR (95% CI)	P-value
Age (per 10 years)	0.99 (0.83–1.19)	0.886	0.98 (0.79–1.23)	0.759
Male (versus female)	0.69 (0.46–1.04)	0.075	0.77 (0.47–1.27)	0.302
Systolic blood pressure (per 10 mmHg)	1.00 (0.91–1.09)	0.959	1.06 (0.96–1.17)	0.276
Serum albumin (per 1.0 g/dL)	0.86 (0.67–1.11)	0.249	1.04 (0.74–1.45)	0.818
Serum creatinine (per 1.0 mg/dL)	0.47 (0.21–0.96)	0.037	0.25 (0.03–1.68)	0.163
Urinary protein excretion (per 1.0 g/day)	1.01 (0.95–1.06)	0.730	1.16 (0.29–4.18)	0.823
ACE inhibitor or ARB therapy	0.66 (0.44–1.02)	0.061	0.56 (0.26–1.31)	0.170
Immunosuppressive treatment during follow-up period				
No immunosuppressive agents	Reference		Reference	
Prednisolone	1.76 (1.00–2.96)	0.048	1.78 (1.01–3.10)	0.045
Prednisolone+cyclosporine	2.18 (1.41–3.36)	<0.001	1.95 (1.16–3.26)	0.011

NOTE: HR, hazard ratio; CI, confidence interval.
Data are the HR, 95% CI, and P-value from Cox proportional hazard regression analyses.
Adjusted for baseline characteristics (age, sex, systolic pressure, serum albumin level, serum creatinine level, urinary protein, use of immunosuppressive therapy).
Abbreviations: CR, complete remission; IMN, idiopathic membranous nephropathy.

proteinuria decreases (<25% vs. ≥25%) and immunosuppressive therapy during the observation period, namely, the cumulative dose of prednisolone and immunosuppressive agent use during the observation period (**Table S5 in File S1**). There were no significant differences between patients achieving <25% and ≥ 25% decreases in proteinuria with respect to the initial prednisolone dose, cyclosporine use in the first month, and the cumulative dose of prednisolone at 3, 6, and 12 months (P = 0.164, P = 0.553, and P = 0.678, respectively). No significant trend was between age and cyclosporine use was observed at 3, 6, and 12 months (P = 0.526, P = 0.139, and P = 0.675, respectively).

The median times to reach 20, 15, 10, and 7.5 mg/day doses did not between the two groups (P = 0.143, P = 0.349, P = 0.431, and P = 0.650, respectively; **Table S6 in File S1**). The cumulative doses of prednisolone to reach 20, 15, 10, and

7.5 mg/day were not different between these two groups (P = 0.138, P = 0.277, P = 0.958, and P = 0.871, respectively).

These results suggest that patients with a <25% decrease in proteinuria at 1 month did not subsequently receive a higher dose of prednisolone.

Discussion

In the current study, we investigated the clinical characteristics and outcomes of older IMN patients as compared with younger IMN patients. Furthermore, this is the first study to have examined predictors of infection in a large cohort of IMN patients.

Consistent with a previous study [2], we found that the remission rate, a 30% decline in eGFR, and the rate of decline in renal function after the onset of MN were similar in older and

Table 4. Predictors of hospitalization due to infection (n = 171).

	Univariate model		Multivariate model	
	HR (95% CI)	P-value	HR (95% CI)	P-value
Age (per 10 years)	3.07 (1.56–6.58)	<0.001	3.11 (1.45–7.49)	0.003
Male (versus female)	1.49 (0.45–6.63)	0.533	1.34 (0.37–6.29)	0.666
Serum albumin (per 1.0 g/dL)	0.73 (0.33–1.50)	0.394	1.24 (0.47–3.21)	0.662
Serum creatinine (per 1.0 mg/dL)	5.27 (1.81–12.5)	0.004	2.62 (0.83–7.70)	0.098
Urinary protein excretion (per 1.0 g/day)	0.96 (0.79–1.12)	0.613	0.92 (0.71–1.13)	0.468
Immunosuppressive treatment during follow-up period				
No immunosuppressive agents	Reference		Reference	
Prednisolone	9.54 (1.54–182.6)	0.014	11.8 (1.59–242.5)	0.014
Prednisolone+cyclosporine	7.26 (1.29–135.8)	0.022	10.3 (1.59–204.4)	0.012

NOTE: HR, hazard ratio; CI, confidence interval.
Data are the HR, 95% CI, and P-value from Cox proportional hazard regression analyses.
Adjusted for baseline characteristics (age, sex, systolic pressure, serum albumin level, serum creatinine level, urinary protein, use of immunosuppressive therapy).
Abbreviations: IMN, idiopathic membranous nephropathy.

Table 5. Predictors of hospitalization due to infection in patients treated with immunosuppressive therapy.

	Univariate model		Multivariate model	
	HR (95% CI)	P-value	HR (95% CI)	P-value
Age (per 10 years)	2.71 (1.42–5.55)	0.002	2.80 (1.20–7.83)	0.016
Male (versus female)	1.16 (0.34–5.21)	0.827	1.65 (0.39–8.46)	0.500
Serum albumin (per 1.0 g/dL)	1.12 (0.46–2.55)	0.792	2.15 (0.64–7.99)	0.217
Serum creatinine (per 1.0 mg/dL)	4.15 (1.42–9.53)	0.013	1.15 (0.31–3.88)	0.830
Urinary protein excretion (per 1.0 g/day)	0.92 (0.73–1.09)	0.374	0.94 (0.70–1.19)	0.633
Immunosuppressive treatment within 1 month after kidney biopsy				
Prednisolone	Reference		Reference	
Prednisolone+cyclosporine	1.45 (0.46–4.89)	0.524	3.22 (0.74–16.9)	0.119
Initial dose of PSL/mg/day	0.97 (0.92–1.01)	0.162	1.00 (0.94–1.07)	0.943
25% decrease of proteinuria within 1 month after initial immunosuppressive therapy	5.78 (1.67–26.4)	0.005	7.27 (1.74–37.7)	0.007

NOTE: HR, hazard ratio; CI, confidence interval.
Data are the HR, 95% CI, and P-value from Cox proportional hazard regression analyses.
This analysis is based on data from 100 patients because the decrease rate of proteinuria was missing for one patient.
Adjusted for baseline characteristics (age, sex, systolic/diastolic pressure, serum albumin level, serum creatinine level, urinary protein, use of immunosuppressive therapy, initial dose of PSL (mg)/day, 25% decrease of proteinuria within 1 month after initial immunosuppressive therapy).
Abbreviations: IMN, idiopathic membranous nephropathy.

younger IMN patients. However, our elderly patients may have died before developing a 30% decline in eGFR because the relationship between age and renal dysfunction may have been underestimated.

Our study included older patients than previously published cohort studies. Nevertheless, both remission and renal survival rates in the present study were higher than those reported by Ponticelli et al. and Jha et al. [5,6]. This indicates that Japanese patients achieve a benign course compared to patients in other countries.

Unlike previous studies [4,10], we observed that compared to younger patients, older patients presented with more severe clinical findings such as lower serum albumin levels, leg edema, and pleural effusion. In elderly patients, edema is often attributed to heart failure or venous insufficiency of the lower limbs. Edema occurs more readily in elderly patients because of reduced

elasticity of the skin and interstitial tissues. Thus, edema may coincide with higher serum albumin levels in the elderly [14].

With regard to immunosuppressive therapy, the recently published Kidney Disease Improving Global Outcomes (KDIGO) guidelines for IMN recommended a restrictive treatment strategy for IMN patients [15]. According to these guidelines, initial therapy should be started only if proteinuria is persistently >4 g/day after 6 months of conservative therapy and does not show a tendency to decline, if the serum creatinine concentration increases by >30%, or if severe, disabling, or life-threatening symptoms related to nephrotic syndrome are present. However, the KDIGO recommendations were based on studies that included only a small number of elderly patients. Therefore, the optimal immunosuppressive regimen for elderly IMN patients remains unclear.

Two retrospective studies involving 115 patients older than 60–65 years found little evidence for the benefits of glucocorticoid

Table 6. Predictors of hospitalization due to infection.

	Univariate model		Multivariate model	
	HR (95% CI)	P-value	HR (95% CI)	P-value
Decrease of proteinuria within 1 month (%)				
≥50% decrease	Reference		Reference	
25–50% decrease	0.60 (0.03–3.17)	0.609	2.27 (0.10–25.3)	0.535
0–25% decrease	7.98 (1.56–57.6)	0.014	6.52 (0.99–54.3)	0.051
Exacerbation	6.05 (1.18–43.6)	0.031	14.4 (1.87–145.6)	0.011
Test for trend		0.011		0.006

NOTE: HR, hazard ratio; CI, confidence interval.
Data are the HR, 95% CI, and P-value from Cox proportional hazard regression analyses. This analysis is based on data from 100 patients because the decrease rate of proteinuria was missing for one patient. Adjusted for baseline characteristics (age, sex, systolic/diastolic pressure, serum albumin level, serum creatinine level, urinary protein, use of immunosuppressive therapy, initial dose of PSL (mg)/day, 25% decrease of proteinuria within 1 month after initial immunosuppressive therapy).

monotherapy along with a higher incidence of adverse effects such as infection, peptic ulcer, and gastrointestinal disturbances [4,16]. Furthermore, many patients with mild-to-moderate disease achieve a spontaneous remission [17]. These studies therefore suggest that in older patients, immunosuppressive therapy should be considered only for those who are at high risk for progression and only after maximum conservative therapy has failed [11,18,19]. However, these studies provide no information regarding clinical presentation, including the prevalence of pleural effusion or the corticosteroid dose used during the follow-up period, which are important points for consideration in the elderly.

In the present study, the time from kidney biopsy to immunosuppressive therapy initiation was shorter than that recommended in the KDIGO guidelines [15]. However, our results show that elderly patients had more clinically severe symptoms than younger patients. Thus, Japanese doctors may consider that in patients with clinically severe symptoms, immunosuppressive therapy should be started as soon as possible, exhibiting different practice patterns than those observed in other countries.

As in previous studies, our elderly patients were significantly predisposed to infection. The infection incidence in our cohort did not greatly differ from those observed previously [20,21]. We found that the higher incidence of infection among elderly patients was unlikely to be due to more intensive immunosuppressive therapy because the cumulative corticosteroid dose in this age group was lower than that in younger patients. Elderly IMN patients were found to be at a higher risk for infection than younger patients.

Interestingly, we found that a <25% decrease in proteinuria at 1 month after starting immunosuppressive therapy was a significant predictor of infection. Furthermore, the higher incidence of infection associated with a <25% decrease in proteinuria in the first month after initial immunosuppressive therapy was not attributable to the prednisolone dose or the type of immunosuppressive therapy. These results suggest that poor responders after the first month of immunosuppressive therapy are vulnerable to the development of infection.

Therefore, it might be well advised to taper prednisolone more quickly among patients with a poor response to 1 month of initial immunosuppressive therapy.

However, it has also been postulated that severe nephrotic syndrome is associated with an immunologic deficit that predisposes to the development of infection. Susceptibility to bacterial infections in patients with a nephrotic syndrome has been attributed to decreased levels of IgG and the alternative complement factor B [11]. Compared with younger patients, older IMN patients had more severe symptoms of nephrotic syndrome, which may contribute to subsequent infections after the initiation of immunosuppressive therapy. Admittedly, this is a complicated subject, and it is unlikely that this retrospective analysis can address all the issues necessary to reach a conclusion whether the treatment should be intensified or not.

Our study had several limitations. First, our patients may not be representative of IMN patients in other countries. Therefore, we advise caution when interpreting and generalizing our results. Second, due to the retrospective nature of this study, the criteria used to select patients' therapeutic regimens are unknown. Selected regimens may vary across different centers, eras, or physicians. These potential biases should be included in the analyses. In actuality, we could carry out only patient-level analysis adjusted for clinically relevant factors but could not carry out a facility-level analysis to reduce confounding by indication concerning therapy selection. This is because the present study included as many as 10 nephrology centers, some of which treated a patient number too small to evaluate using Cox proportional hazard models. Furthermore, it was difficult to add era as a covariate in our models. Third, our practice patterns are different from those recommended by the KDIGO guidelines. Namely, we often use cyclosporine in combination with corticosteroids for the first-line treatment of IMN patients. The 2012 KDIGO clinical practice guidelines for IMN recommend a cytotoxic agent (cyclophosphamide) for patients at high risk of progression [15]. However, no patients in our study were treated with cyclophosphamide. Therefore, our results should be interpreted carefully. Fourth, because the time from IMN diagnosis to immunosuppressive therapy initiation was relatively short, we did not evaluate whether nephrotic syndrome itself would predispose to infection by observing patients without immunosuppressive therapy.

Allowing for these methodological issues, our study has several advantages. It is one of the largest multicenter adult Japanese MN cohorts ever reported. Additionally, to the best of our knowledge, this is the first study to evaluate predictors of infection in IMN patients.

In conclusion, our retrospective cohort study of IMN patients showed that elderly patients were similar to younger patients in terms of renal outcomes. However, the use of immunosuppressive therapy and poor response to initial immunosuppressive therapy were significant predictors of infection among elderly IMN patients. Therefore, care should be taken when selecting a treatment strategy for these patients.

Supporting Information

Figure S1 The course of proteinuria during the follow-up period (comparison of the three age categories).

Figure S2 The course of eGFR during the follow-up period (comparison of the three age categories).

File S1 Table S1 in File S1, Baseline characteristics of 171 IMN patients: comparison of patients in different treatment groups. **Table S2,** Outcomes of 171 IMN patients: comparison of patients in different treatment groups. **Table S3,** Immunosuppressive treatment during the observation period (comparison of the three age categories). **Table S4,** Duration and cumulative dose of prednisolone (comparison of the three age categories). **Table S5,** Immunosuppressive treatment during the observation period (comparison of the decrease in proteinuria (<25% vs. ≥ 25%) in the first month after starting immunosuppressive therapy). **Table S6,** Duration and cumulative dose of prednisolone (comparison of the decrease in proteinuria (<25% vs. ≥25%) in the first month after starting immunosuppressive therapy).

File S2 Table S7, The anonymous data set of 171 patients with IMN.

Acknowledgments

We are grateful for the time and efforts of the nephrologists who supported the present study: Dr. Shizunori Ichida, Dr. Hideaki Shimizu, Dr. Junichiro Yamamoto, Dr. Tomohiko Naruse, Dr. Hirofumi Tamai, Dr. Kei Kurata, Dr. Hirotake Kasuga, Dr. Arimasa Shirasaki, and Dr. Makoto Mizutani.

Author Contributions

Conceived and designed the experiments: MY MA SK S. Maruyama. Performed the experiments: MY MA RY SA SK T. Katsuno T. Kosugi WS NT YY MM YI S. Matsuo S. Maruyama. Analyzed the data: MY MA RY. Contributed reagents/materials/analysis tools: MY MA RY SK S. Maruyama. Contributed to the writing of the manuscript: MY MA S. Maruyama.

References

1. White Book of Aging from the Government of Japan. Available: http://www8.cao.go.jp/kourei/whitepaper/w-2013/gaiyou/pdf/1s1s.pdf.
2. Cameron JS (1996) Nephrotic syndrome in the elderly. Semin Nephrol 16: 319–329.
3. Yokoyama H, Sugiyama H, Sato H, Taguchi T, Nagata M, et al. (2012) Renal disease in the elderly and the very elderly Japanese: analysis of the Japan Renal Biopsy Registry (J-RBR). Clin Exp Nephrol 16: 903–920.
4. Zent R, Nagai R, Cattran DC (1997) Idiopathic membranous nephropathy in the elderly: a comparative study. Am J Kidney Dis 29: 200–206.
5. Ponticelli C, Zucchelli P, Passerini P, Cesana B, Locatelli F, et al. (1995) A 10-year follow-up of a randomized study with methylprednisolone and chlorambucil in membranous nephropathy. Kidney Int 48: 1600.
6. Jha V, Ganguli A, Saha TK, Kohli HS, Sud K, et al. (2007) A randomized, controlled trial of steroids and cyclophosphamide in adults with nephrotic syndrome caused by idiopathic membranous nephropathy. J Am Soc Nephrol 18: 1899.
7. Ponticelli C, Altieri P, Scolari F, Passerini P, Roccatello D, et al. (1998) A randomized study comparing methylprednisolone plus chlorambucil versus methylprednisolone plus cyclophosphamide in idiopathic membranous nephropathy. J Am Soc Nephrol 9: 444.
8. Cattran DC, Appel GB, Hebert LA, Hunsicker LG, Pohl MA, et al. (2001) North America Nephrotic Syndrome Study Group Cyclosporine in patients with steroid-resistant membranous nephropathy: a randomized trial. Kidney Int 59: 1484.
9. Cattran DC, Greenwood C, Ritchie S, Bernstein K, Churchill DN, et al. (1995) A controlled trial of cyclosporine in patients with progressive membranous nephropathy. Canadian Glomerulonephritis Study Group. Kidney Int 47: 1130.
10. Hofstra JM, Wetzels JF (2012) Management of patients with membranous nephropathy. Nephrol Dial Transplant 27: 6–9.
11. Rollino C, Roccatello D, Vallero A, Basolo B, Piccoli G (1995) Membranous glomerulonephritis in the elderly. Is therapy still worthwhile? Geriatr Nephrol Urol 5: 97–104.
12. Makoto Y, Masahiko A, Ryohei Y, et al. (2014) Smoking is a risk factor for the progression of idiopathic membranous nephropathy. PLoS One, in press.
13. Matsuo S, Imai E, Horio M, Yasuda Y, Tomita K, et al. (2009) Collaborators developing the Japanese equation for estimated GFR. Revised equations for estimated GFR from serum creatinine in Japan. Am J Kidney Dis 53: 982–992.
14. Deegens JK, Wetzels JF (2007) Membranous nephropathy in the older adult: epidemiology, diagnosis and management. Drugs Aging 24: 717–732.
15. KDIGO Working Group: (2012) KDIGO clinical practice guideline for glomerulonephritis. Kidney Int Suppl 2 186–197.
16. Passerini P, Como G, Viganò E, Melis P, Pozzi C, et al. (1993) Idiopathic membranous nephropathy in the elderly. Nephrol Dial Transplant 8: 1321.
17. Philibert D, Cattran D (2008) Remission of proteinuria in primary glomerulonephritis: we know the goal but do we know the price? Nat Clin Pract Nephrol 4: 550.
18. Glassock RJ (1998) Glomerular disease in the elderly population. Geriatr Nephrol Urol 8: 149–154.
19. Bernard DB (1988) Extrarenal complications of the nephrotic syndrome. Kidney Int 33: 1184–1202.
20. Eriguchi M, Oka H, Mizobuchi T, Kamimura T, Sugawara K, et al. (2009) Long-term outcomes of idiopathic membranous nephropathy in Japanese patients treated with low-dose cyclophosphamide and prednisolone. Nephrol Dial Transplant 24: 3082–3088. doi: 10.1093/ndt/gfp251. Epub 2009 May 22.
21. Yoshimoto K, Yokoyama H, Wada T, Furuichi K, Sakai N, et al. (2004) Pathologic findings of initial biopsies reflect the outcomes of membranous nephropathy. Kidney Int 65: 148–153.

6

The Impact of Prophylactic Dexamethasone on Nausea and Vomiting after Thyroidectomy: A Systematic Review and Meta-Analysis

Zhenhong Zou[1¶], Yuming Jiang[1¶], Mingjia Xiao[2], Ruiyao Zhou[3]*

1 Department of General Surgery, Nanfang Hospital, Southern Medical University, Guangzhou City, Guangdong Province, China, 2 Department of Hepatobiliary Surgery, Wuxi People's Hospital of Nanjing Medical University, Wuxi, Jiangsu Province, China, 3 Department of General Surgery, The Third Affiliated Hospital of Wenzhou Medical University, Ruian City, Zhejiang Province, China

Abstract

Background: We carried out a systematic review and meta-analysis to evaluate the impact of prophylactic dexamethasone on post-operative nausea and vomiting (PONV), post-operative pain, and complications in patients undergoing thyroidectomy.

Methods: We searched Pubmed, Embase, and Cochrane Library databases for randomized controlled trials (RCTs) that evaluated the prophylactic effect of dexamethasone versus placebo with or without other antiemetics for PONV in patients undergoing thyroidectomy. Meta-analyses were performed using RevMan 5.0 software.

Results: Thirteen RCTs that considered high quality evidence including 2,180 patients were analyzed. The meta-analysis demonstrated a significant decrease in the incidence of PONV (RR 0.52, 95% CI 0.43 to 0.63, $P<0.00001$), the need for rescue anti-emetics (RR 0.42, 95% CI 0.30 to 0.57, $P<0.00001$), post-operative pain scores (WMD −1.17, 95% CI −1.91 to −0.44, $P=0.002$), and the need for rescue analgesics (RR 0.65, 95% CI 0.50–0.83, $P=0.0008$) in patients receiving dexamethasone compared to placebo, with or without concomitant antiemetics. Dexamethasone 8–10 mg had a significantly greater effect for reducing the incidence of PONV than dexamethasone 1.25–5 mg. Dexamethasone was as effective as other anti-emetics for reducing PONV (RR 1.25, 95% CI 0.86–1.81, $P=0.24$). A significantly higher level of blood glucose during the immediate post-operative period in patients receiving dexamethasone compared to controls was the only adverse event.

Conclusions: Prophylactic dexamethasone 8–10 mg administered intravenously before induction of anesthesia should be recommended as a safe and effective strategy for reducing the incidence of PONV, the need for rescue anti-emetics, post-operative pain, and the need for rescue analgesia in thyroidectomy patients, except those that are pregnant, have diabetes mellitus, hyperglycemia, or contraindications for dexamethasone. More high quality trials are warranted to define the benefits and risks of prophylactic dexamethasone in potential patients with a high risk for PONV.

Editor: Richard E. Burney, University of Michigan, United States of America

Funding: The authors have no support or funding to report.

Competing Interests: The authors have declared that no competing interests exist.

* Email: doctor_zry@126.com

¶ These authors are co-first authors on this work.

Introduction

Post-operative nausea and vomiting (PONV) is a common and distressing complication associated with surgery. The overall incidence of PONV ranges from 20 to 30% in general surgery and up to 80% in high-risk surgical patients when no prophylactic anti-emetic is given [1,2]. For patients undergoing thyroidectomy, PONV is a risk factor for post-operative bleeding [3,4], and prophylactic anti-emetics may be beneficial.

Previous studies have shown that prophylactic dexamethasone has anti-emetic and analgesic effects. Glucocorticoids are anti-inflammatory and immunosuppressive agents, and dexamethasone may exert its therapeutic actions through central inhibition of prostaglandin synthesis, by decreasing serotonin turnover in the central nervous system, and by influencing the systemic inflammatory response in favor of anti-inflammatory mediators [5–9].

A systematic review demonstrated that prophylactic dexamethasone was safe and effective for reducing the incidence of PONV and post-operative pain in patients undergoing laparoscopic cholecystectomy compared to placebo [10]. In patients undergoing thyroidectomy, a previous meta-analysis demonstrated a significant reduction of PONV in patients treated with a single dose of dexamethasone versus placebo [11]. However, the relatively small sample size included in this review precluded the authors from drawing definitive conclusions, and the optimal dose and timing of dexamethasone administration, and efficacy of combining dexamethasone with other anti-emetics, remains unclear.

The objective of the current study was to confirm, and continue to investigate the impact of prophylactic corticosteroid administration on PONV, post-operative pain, and complications following thyroidectomy.

Methods

This systematic review and meta-analysis is reported in accordance with the recommendations of the PRISMA statement [12].

2.1 Outcome measures

2.1.1 Primary outcome measure

1. Incidence of PONV during the immediate 24 h post-operative period, dichotomized as no nausea versus others; this was evaluated according to a 3-point ordinal scale: no nausea; nausea; retching and/or vomiting

2.1.2 Secondary outcome measures

1. Post-operative pain scores
2. Need for rescue anti-emetic or analgesic agent(s)

3. Incidence of steroid-related complications, including hyperglycemia, wound infection, delayed wound healing, headaches, dizziness, facial flushing, constipation, and abdominal pain

2.2 Data collection and analysis

2.2.1 Searches. We searched PubMed, Embase, and Cochrane Library databases from their inception to October 1, 2013 using Cochrane Highly Sensitive Search Strategies to identify randomized controlled trials (RCTs) for potential inclusion in our review [13]. We used the following MeSH terms and keywords: thyroid surgery OR thyroidectomy AND corticosteroid, glucocorticoid, steroid, OR dexamethasone. The search strategy is summarized in Table S1. Authors' names were entered as search terms in the PubMed database to check for additional studies. Trials were also identified using the "related articles" function in PubMed. We hand-searched reference lists from articles identified by the electronic search and from previous meta-analyses. This process was performed iteratively until no additional articles could be identified.

2.2.2 Inclusion and Exclusion Criteria. We included RCTs that: evaluated the prophylactic effect of dexamethasone versus placebo without other anti-emetics, dexamethasone versus placebo plus concomitant administration of a different anti-emetic, dexamethasone versus a different anti-emetic, and comparisons using different doses of dexamethasone for PONV in patients

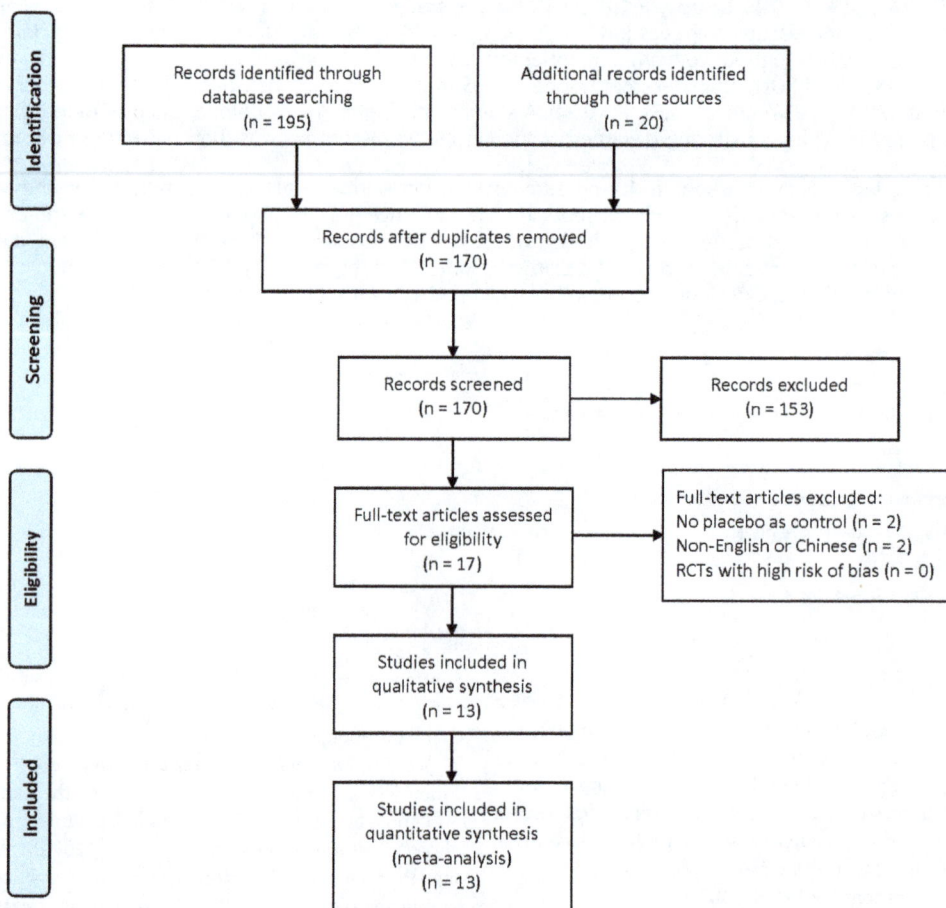

Figure 1. Flow chart for selecting the trials. On the basis of the search strategy, 195 articles were identified by the initial search, and 17 required further assessment. Finally, 13 articles were included in this review.

Table 1. Characteristics of trials included in the meta-analysis.

Study	Sample size	Interventions	Studies divided
Wang 1999 [18]	120	D 10 mg vs. Droperidol 1.25 mg vs. Placebo, all IV at 1 minute before induction	Wang 1999 D 10: D 10 mg vs. Placebo; Wang 1999: D 10 mg vs. Droperidol 1.25 mg
Wang 2000 [19]	225	D 10 mg vs. D 5 mg vs. D 2.5 mg vs. D 1.25 mg vs. Placebo, all IV immediately after induction	Wang 2000 D 10: D 10 mg vs. Placebo; Wang 2000 D 5: D 5 mg vs. Placebo; Wang 2000 D 2.5: D 2.5 mg vs. Placebo; Wang 2000 D 1.25: D 1.25 mg vs. Placebo
Lee 2001 [20]	135	D 8 mg vs. D 5 mg vs. Placebo, all IV before anesthesia	Lee 2001 D 8: D 10 mg vs. Placebo; Lee 2001 D 5: D 5 mg vs. Placebo
Fujji 2007 [21]	75	D 8 mg vs. D 4 mg vs. Placebo, all IV at the end of surgery	Fujji 2007 D8: D 8 mg vs. Placebo; Fujji 2007 D4: D 4 mg vs. Placebo
Worni 2008 [22]	70	D 8 mg vs. Placebo, both IV at 45 minutes before anesthesia	Worni 2008 D8: D 8 mg vs. Placebo
Feroci 2010 [23]	102	D 8 mg vs. Placebo, both IV at 20 minutes before induction	Feroci 2010 D8: D 8 mg vs. Placebo
Doksrod 2012 [24]	120	D 0.3 mg/kg vs. D 0.15 mg/kg vs. Placebo, all IV within 10 min after induction	Doksrod 2012 D18: D 0.3 mg/kg vs. Placebo; Doksrod 2012 D9: D 0.15 mg/kg vs. Placebo
Song 2013 [25]	123	D 10 mg vs. Ramosetron 0.3 mg vs. Placebo, both IV immediately after anesthesia	Song 2013 D 10: D10: D 10 mg vs. Placebo; Song 2013: D 10 mg vs. Ramosetron 0.3 mg
Barros 2013 [26]	40	D 4 mg vs. Placebo, both IV immediately after induction	Barros 2013 D4: D 4 mg vs. Placebo
Schietroma 2013 [27]	328	D 8 mg vs. Placebo, both IV at 90 minutes before skin incision	Schietroma 2013 D8: D 8 mg vs. Placebo
Zhou 2012 [28]	150	D 8 mg + T 5 mg vs. D 8 mg vs. T 5 mg, all IV immediately before induction	Zhou 2012 Tropisetron: D 8 mg + T 5 mg vs.T 5 mg; Zhou 2012: D 8 mg vs. T 5 mg
Bononi 2010 [29]	562	D 4 mg +O 4 mg vs. O 4 mg, D IV at induction and ondansetron IV at 15 minutes before tracheal extubation	Bononi 2010 Ondansetron: D 4 mg +O 4 mg vs. O 4 mg
Fujji 2000 [30]	130	D 8 mg + G 40 ug/kg vs. G 40 ug/kg, both IV immediately before induction	Fujji 2000 Granisetron: D 8 mg + G 40 ug/kg vs. G 40 ug/kg

IV: intravenous; ASA, American Society of Anesthesiologists; D: dexamethasone; T: tropisetron; O: ondansetron; G: Granisetron.

undergoing thyroidectomy. The included trials reported at least one of our outcome measures, and clearly reported patient inclusion and exclusion criteria, anesthetic technique, protocols for administration of the experimental drugs, and a definition and evaluation of nausea and vomiting. Studies were excluded if they were not RCTs, included patients who were undergoing other surgical procedures concomitantly, reported insufficient data, or were duplicate studies.

2.2.3 Selection of studies. Two reviewers (ZH Zou and YM Jiang) independently examined titles and abstracts to select eligible RCTs. We removed records that were ongoing or unpublished studies, or were published as abstracts or conference proceedings. Where datasets were overlapping or duplicated, only the most recent information was included. We retrieved the full text of potentially relevant studies. Two reviewers (ZH Zou and YM Jiang) independently examined the full text records to determine which studies met the inclusion criteria. We resolved disagreements about selection of studies by discussion and consensus.

2.2.4 Data extraction and management. Two reviewers (ZH Zou and YM Jiang) independently extracted data from eligible RCTs including details describing study population,

interventions, and outcomes. We resolved disagreements about data extraction by discussion and consensus.

2.2.5 Assessment of quality of evidence in included studies. Two reviewers (ZH Zou and YM Jiang) independently assessed RCT quality and risk of bias using tools provided by the Cochrane Collaboration [14]. The reviewers examined six domains including sequence generation, allocation concealment, double-blind evaluation (blinding), complete outcome data, selective outcome reporting, and baseline comparability of groups. The risk of bias was categorized as low, high, or unclear. RCTs with high risk of bias in at least three of six domains were not included in the meta-analysis. Baseline comparability of groups was assessed using seven matching criteria: age, sex, history of motion sickness, previous post-operative emesis, anesthetic technique, operation type (partial or total thyroidectomy), and duration of surgery. Baseline incomparability was defined as non-matching in at least three of the seven criteria. We resolved disagreements about quality of evidence by discussion and consensus.

2.2.6 Statistical analysis. Statistical analyses were performed using RevMan (ver. 5.0; The Cochrane Collaboration, Oxford, UK) software and STATA (ver. 11.2; STATA Corpora-

Table 2. Details of anesthetic technique, and rescue analgesics and anti-emetics in the included trials.

Study	Anesthetic technique	Rescue analgesics	Rescue antiemetics
Wang 1999 [18]	Propofol 2.0–2.5 mg/kg, glycopyrrolate 0.2 mg, fentanyl 2.0 ug/kg IV maintained with 1.0%–2.5% isoflurane in oxygen	Diclofenac 75 mg IM q12h	Ondansetron 4 mg IV
Wang 2000 [19]	Propofol 2.0–2.5 mg/kg, glycopyrrolate 0.2 mg, fentanyl 2.0 ug/kg IV maintained with 1.0%–2.5% isoflurane in oxygen	Diclofenac 75 mg IM q12h	Ondansetron 4 mg IV
Lee 2001 [20]	Glycopyrrolate 0.2 mg, fentanyl 2 ug/kg, thiopental 5 mg/kg IV maintained with desflurane in oxygen	Ketorolac 15 mg IV q6h	Droperidol 1.25 mg IV
Fujji 2007 [21]	Propofol 2 mg/kg, fentanyl 2 ug/kg, vecuronium 0.1 mg/kg IV maintained with 1–3% sevoflurane in oxygen	Indomethacin 50 mg rectally	Ranitidine 150 mg orally
Worni 2008 [22]	Propofol/thiopental, atracurium, isoflurane, or sevoflurane and fentanyl 5–10 ug/kg	Acetaminophen 4 g/day; second-line metamizole 1g or morphine	Ondansetron 4 mg IV; second-line droperidol 0.625 mg IV
Feroci 2010 [23]	Propofol 2 mg/kg, fentanyl 2 ug/kg, vecuronium 0.1 mg/kg IV maintained with sevoflurane in oxygen	Paracetamol 1000 mg IV q8 h; second-line ketorolac 30 mg IV q12h	Metoclopramide 10 mg IV; second-line ondansetron 4 mg IV
Doksrod 2012 [24]	Propofol, fentanyl, vecuronium IV maintained with desflurane (4–8%) and itrous oxide (60%) in oxygen	Oxycodone 5 mg orally; second-line metamizole or morphine 2.5 mg IV	Metoclopramide 20 mg IV; second-line ondansetron 4 mg IV
Song 2013 [25]	Remifentanil 1 ug/kg, propofol 1–2 mg/kg, rocuroniumin 0.9 mg/kg IV, maintained with desflurane in oxygen–air mixture	Ketorolac 30 mg IV	Metoclopramide 10 mg IV
Barros 2013 [26]	Propofol, fentanyl 2.0 ug/kg, cisatracurium 0.15 mg/kg, maintained with sevoflurane in oxygen	Ketorolac 30 mg or parecoxib 40 mg IV	Ondansetron 4 mg IV
Schietroma 2013 [27]	Sodium thiopental 5 mg/kg, atracurium besylate 0.5 mg/kg, maintained with oxygen in air, sevoflurane, and remifentanil hydrochloride	Ketorolac tromethamine 30 mg IV q6h	Ondansetron hydrochloride 4 mg IV
Zhou 2012 [28]	Propofol 1.5–2.5 mg/kg, midazolam 0.1–0.2 mg/kg, fentanyl 1.0–2.0 ug/kg, maintained with 1.0–3.0% sevoflurane in oxygen	Pethidine 25 mg IV	Metoclopramide 10 mg IV; second-line tropisetron 5 mg IV
Bononi 2010 [29]	Not stated[a]	Not stated	Not stated
Fujji 2000 [30]	Thiopentone 5 mg/kg, fentanyl 2 ug/kg, vecuronium 0.2 mg/kg maintained with isoflurane (1.0%–3.0%) and nitrous oxide (66%) in oxygen	Indomethacin 50mg rectally for moderae pain and buprenorphiine 0.2 mg IM for severe pain	Domperidone retally

IV, intravenous; IM, intramuscular; [a]no difference.

Table 3. Quality of evidence in included studies.

Included studies	Country	Sequence generation	Allocation concealment	Double blinding	Complete outcome data	No selective reporting	Baseline comparability	Risk of bias
Wang 1999 [18]	China	Adequate	Unclear	Yes	Yes	Yes	Yes	Low
Wang 2000 [19]	China	Adequate	Unclear	Yes	Yes	Yes	Yes	Low
Lee 2001 [20]	China	Adequate	Adequate	Yes	Yes	Yes	Yes	Low
Fujii 2007 [21]	Japan	Adequate	Adequate	Yes	Yes	Yes	Yes	Low
Worni 2008 [22]	Switzerland	Adequate	Adequate	Yes	Yes	Yes	Yes	Low
Feroci 2011 [23]	Italy	Adequate	Adequate	Yes	Yes	Yes	Yes	Low
Doksrod 2012 [24]	Norway	Adequate	Adequate	Yes	Yes	Yes	Yes	Low
Song 2013 [25]	Korea	Adequate	Adequate	Unclear	Yes	Yes	Yes	Low
Barros 2013 [26]	Portugal	Adequate	Adequate	Yes	Yes	Yes	Yes	Low
Schietroma 2013 [27]	Italy	Adequate	Adequate	Yes	Yes	Yes	Yes	Low
Zhou 2012 [28]	China	Adequate	Adequate	Unclear	Yes	Yes	Yes	Low
Bononi 2010 [29]	Italy	Adequate	Adequate	Unclear	Yes	Yes	Yes	Low
Fujii 2000 [30]	Japan	Adequate	Adequate	Yes	Yes	Yes	Yes	Low

tion, College Station, TX, USA) software. Weighted mean differences (WMDs) with 95% confidence intervals (CIs) were calculated for continuous variables, and risk ratios (RRs) with 95% CIs were calculated for dichotomous variables. A random-effects model was used to pool studies with significant heterogeneity, as determined by the chi-squared test ($P \leq 0.10$) and the inconsistency index ($I^2 \geq 50\%$). Potential sources of statistical heterogeneity were explored by carrying out subgroup and sensitivity analyses. Subgroup analyses were performed by stratifying patients according to dose of corticosteroid and timing of dexamethasone administration; sensitivity analyses explored the impact of excluding outlying results. The presence of publication bias was comprehensively assessed using Begg's funnel plot and Begg's rank correlation test of asymmetry. Publication bias was thought to be present when the continuity-corrected $Pr > |z|$ value was ≤ 0.1 [15]. The GRADE system was used to summarize the overall quality of evidence [16,17].

Results

3.1 Trial identification

The searches identified 195 articles. We screened titles and abstracts, and 17 were identified as potentially eligible for inclusion. We retrieved the full text articles. After analyzing the full text articles, 4 studies were excluded and 13 RCTs [18–30] were found eligible for inclusion according to our criteria for considering studies in this review (Fig. 1).

3.2 Characteristics of included studies

The characteristics of the included studies are shown in Table 1. The 13 eligible RCTs included 2,180 patients who underwent general anesthesia for thyroidectomy. The majority of RCTs included patients classified as American Society of Anesthesiologists (ASA) class I or II. Exclusion criteria were: pregnant women, patients with insulin-dependent diabetes mellitus, obesity, and patients with a high risk for PONV. Dexamethasone was administered intravenously in a single or combination dose ranging from 1.25–18 mg. Timing of administration varied from 90 minutes before skin incision to the end of surgery. Controls included placebo, droperidol, granisetron, ondansetron, tropisetron or a combination of these medications. Confounders such as anesthetic technique and rescue analgesics and anti-emetics were standardized within studies (Table 2). Risk of bias was low across all RCTs (Table 3).

3.3 Treatment effects

3.3.1 Primary outcome. *Incidence of PONV: Dexamethasone versus placebo, with or without concomitant anti-emetics* - Data reporting on the incidence of PONV in thyroidectomy patients treated with dexamethasone versus placebo with or without concomitant anti-emetics are described in 11 RCTs [18–25,28–30]. The meta-analysis demonstrated a significant decrease in the incidence of PONV in patients receiving dexamethasone compared to placebo, with or without concomitant anti-emetics (RR 0.52, 95% CI 0.43 to 0.63, $P < 0.00001$; Fig. 2). There was evidence of significant heterogeneity between studies ($P = 0.003$, $I^2 = 56\%$). The dose-response gradient may have caused most of the variation between RCTs (Fig. 3; Fig.S1).

Incidence of PONV: Dexamethasone versus a different anti-emetic - Data reporting on the incidence of PONV in thyroidectomy patients treated with dexamethasone versus a different anti-emetic, including droperidol, granisetron, or tropisetron, are described in three RCTs [18,25,28]. The meta-analysis demonstrated no significant difference in the incidence of PONV in

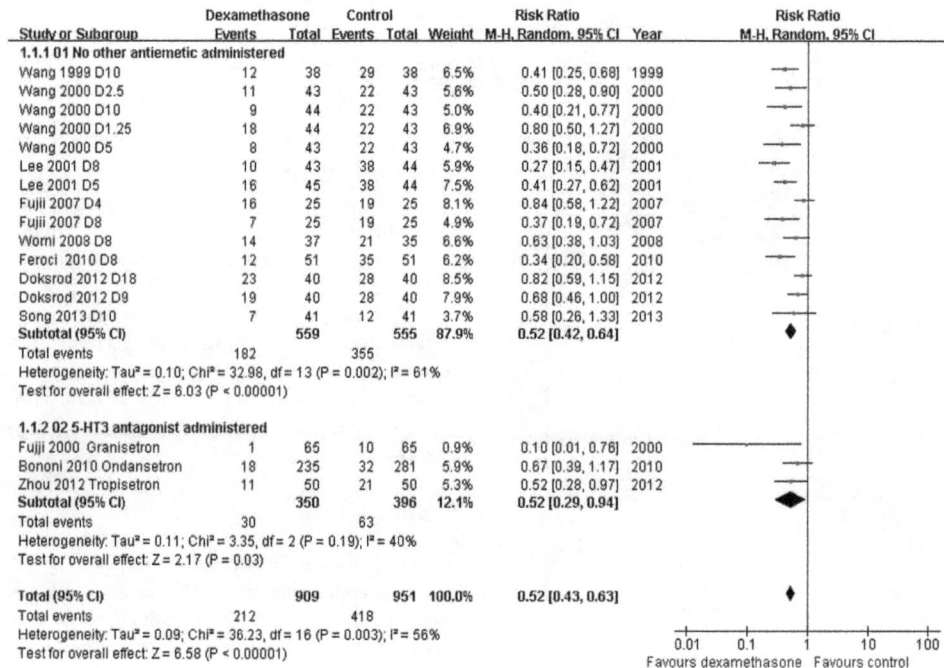

Figure 2. Incidence of PONV grouped by concomitant anti-emetics. Eleven studies described the incidence of PONV in thyroidectomy patients treated with dexamethasone versus placebo with or without concomitant anti-emetics (RR 0.52, 95% CI 0.43 to 0.63, $P<0.00001$). There was evidence of significant heterogeneity between studies ($P=0.003$, $I^2=56\%$).

patients receiving dexamethasone compared to these different anti-emetics (RR 1.25, 95% CI 0.86–1.81, $P=0.24$; Fig. 4). There was no evidence of significant heterogeneity between RCTs ($P=0.27$, $I^2=23\%$).

3.3.2 Secondary outcomes. *Postoperative pain scores and need for rescue analgesia: Dexamethasone versus placebo with or without concomitant anti-emetics* - Data reporting on postoperative pain scores in thyroidectomy patients treated with dexamethasone versus placebo with or without concomitant anti-emetics are described in six RCTs [18,20,22,23,25,26]. Pain scores were evaluated based on visual analogue scales (VAS) completed by patients 24 h post-operatively. Four RCTs [22,23,25,26] reported data as means ± standard deviations (SDs); two RCTs [18,20] reported data as medians (range) converted to estimated means and SDs [31]. The meta-analysis demonstrated a significantly lower post-operative VAS score in patients receiving dexamethasone compared to placebo, with or without concomitant anti-emetics (WMD –1.17, 95% CI –1.91 to –0.44, $P=0.002$; Fig. 5). There was evidence of significant heterogeneity between RCTs ($P<0.00001$, $I^2=94\%$). The doses of dexamethasone may have caused most of the variation between RCTs. The need for rescue analgesia was significantly less frequent in the patients that received dexamethasone (RR 0.65, 95% CI 0.50–0.83, $P=0.0008$; Fig. 6); there was no evidence of significant heterogeneity between RCTs ($P=0.25$, $I^2=25\%$).

Need for rescue anti-emetic: Dexamethasone versus placebo with or without concomitant antiemetics - Data reporting on the need for rescue anti-emetics in thyroidectomy patients treated with dexamethasone versus placebo with or without concomitant anti-emetics are described in six studies [19,25–28,30]. The meta-analysis demonstrated a significant decrease in the need for rescue anti-emetics in patients receiving dexamethasone compared to placebo, with or without concomitant anti-emetics (RR 0.42,

95% CI 0.30 to 0.57, $P<0.00001$; Fig. 7). There was no evidence of significant heterogeneity between RCTs ($P=0.43$, $I^2=0\%$).

Incidence of adverse events: Dexamethasone versus placebo with or without concomitant anti-emetics - Data reporting on blood glucose levels in thyroidectomy patients treated with dexamethasone are described in two RCTs. A significantly higher level of blood glucose was observed in patients receiving dexamethasone compared to controls during the first 8 hours post-operatively [23,24]. No statistical differences in symptomatic transient hypocalcemia and asymptomatic transient hypocalcemia were present [23]. One RCT [27] reported that dexamethasone administration prevented recurrent laryngeal nerve palsy; however, this effect was not described elsewhere [23]. There were no significant differences in the incidences of extrapyramidal signs including headache, dizziness, constipation, and muscle pain, and other adverse events such as wound infection and delayed wound healing, in patients receiving dexamethasone compared to controls.

3.4 Subgroup analyses

Incidence of PONV: Dose of dexamethasone. Subgroup analyses stratified by dose of dexamethasone (range, 1.25 mg to 18 mg) demonstrated that dexamethasone 4–5 mg and 8–10 mg significantly reduced the incidence of PONV compared to controls (1.25–5 mg: RR 0.59, 95% CI 0.44 to 0.79; 8–10 mg: RR 0.45, 95% CI 0.35–0.57), while dexamethasone 18 mg did not (RR 0.82, 95% CI 0.59–1.15) (Fig. 3). Dexamethasone 8–10 mg had a significantly greater effect for reducing the incidence of PONV than dexamethasone 1.25–5 mg (1.25–5 mg RR 0.40, 95% CI 0.28 to 0.55; 8–10 mg: RR 0.23, 95% CI 0.18–0.31; P=0.02; Fig. S1).

Incidence of PONV: Timing of dexamethasone administration. The RCTs included in this review varied with regard to timing of dexamethasone administration. Some patients

Study or Subgroup	Dexamethasone Events	Total	Control Events	Total	Weight	Risk Ratio M-H, Random, 95% CI	Year
1.2.1 Dexamethasone 18mg							
Doksrod 2012 D18	23	40	28	40	8.5%	0.82 [0.59, 1.15]	2012
Subtotal (95% CI)		40		40	8.5%	0.82 [0.59, 1.15]	
Total events	23		28				
Heterogeneity: Not applicable							
Test for overall effect: Z = 1.15 (P = 0.25)							
1.2.2 Dexamethasone 8-10mg							
Wang 1999 D10	12	38	29	38	6.5%	0.41 [0.25, 0.68]	1999
Fujii 2000 Granisetron	1	65	10	65	0.9%	0.10 [0.01, 0.76]	2000
Wang 2000 D10	9	44	22	43	5.0%	0.40 [0.21, 0.77]	2000
Lee 2001 D8	10	43	38	44	5.9%	0.27 [0.15, 0.47]	2001
Fujii 2007 D8	7	25	19	25	4.9%	0.37 [0.19, 0.72]	2007
Worni 2008 D8	14	37	21	35	6.6%	0.63 [0.38, 1.03]	2008
Feroci 2010 D8	12	51	35	51	6.2%	0.34 [0.20, 0.58]	2010
Doksrod 2012 D9	19	40	28	40	7.9%	0.68 [0.46, 1.00]	2012
Zhou 2012 Tropisetron	11	50	21	50	5.3%	0.52 [0.28, 0.97]	2012
Song 2013 D10	7	41	12	41	3.7%	0.58 [0.26, 1.33]	2013
Subtotal (95% CI)		434		432	52.7%	0.45 [0.35, 0.57]	
Total events	102		235				
Heterogeneity: Tau² = 0.05; Chi² = 14.29, df = 9 (P = 0.11); I² = 37%							
Test for overall effect: Z = 6.64 (P < 0.00001)							
1.2.3 Dexamethasone 4-5mg							
Wang 2000 D5	8	43	22	43	4.7%	0.36 [0.18, 0.72]	2000
Lee 2001 D5	16	45	38	44	7.5%	0.41 [0.27, 0.62]	2001
Fujii 2007 D4	16	25	19	25	8.1%	0.84 [0.58, 1.22]	2007
Bononi 2010 Ondansetron	18	235	32	281	5.9%	0.67 [0.39, 1.17]	2010
Subtotal (95% CI)		348		393	26.2%	0.56 [0.37, 0.85]	
Total events	58		111				
Heterogeneity: Tau² = 0.12; Chi² = 9.02, df = 3 (P = 0.03); I² = 67%							
Test for overall effect: Z = 2.72 (P = 0.006)							
1.2.5 Dexamethasone 1.5-2.5mg							
Wang 2000 D1.25	18	44	22	43	6.9%	0.80 [0.50, 1.27]	2000
Wang 2000 D2.5	11	43	22	43	5.6%	0.50 [0.28, 0.90]	2000
Subtotal (95% CI)		87		86	12.5%	0.66 [0.41, 1.04]	
Total events	29		44				
Heterogeneity: Tau² = 0.04; Chi² = 1.54, df = 1 (P = 0.21); I² = 35%							
Test for overall effect: Z = 1.81 (P = 0.07)							
Total (95% CI)		909		951	100.0%	0.52 [0.43, 0.63]	
Total events	212		418				
Heterogeneity: Tau² = 0.09; Chi² = 36.23, df = 16 (P = 0.003); I² = 56%							
Test for overall effect: Z = 6.58 (P < 0.00001)							

Favours dexamethasone   Favours control

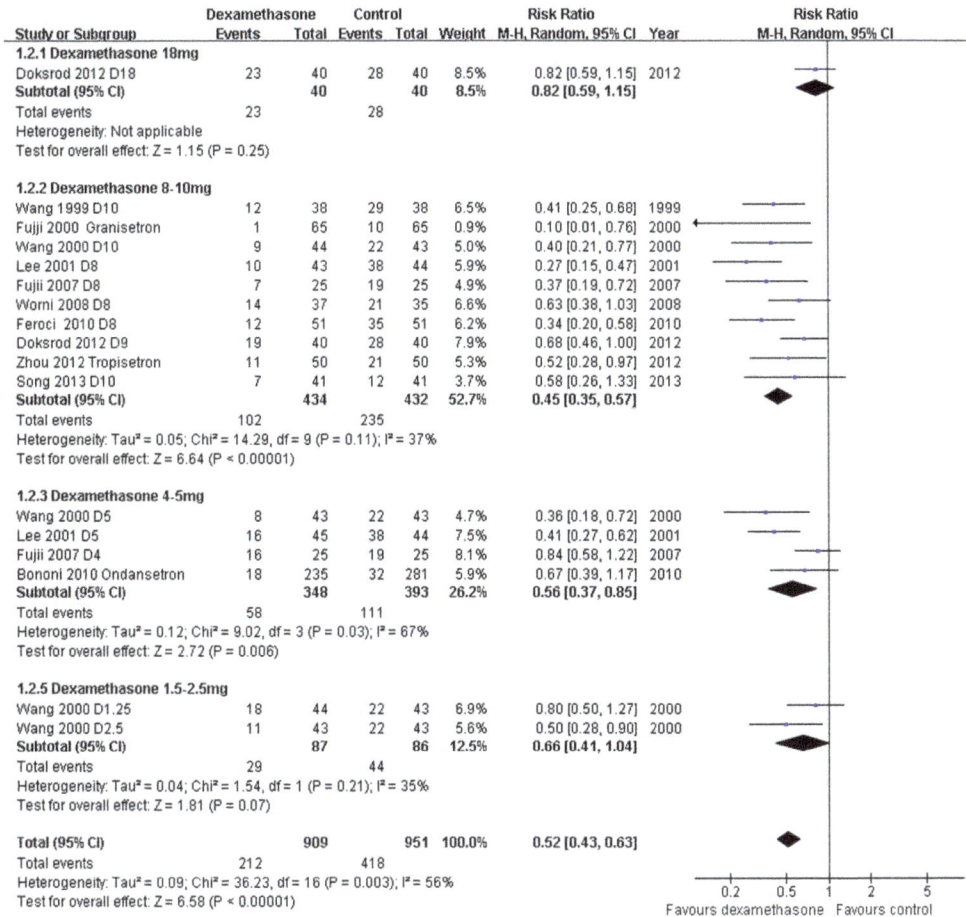

Figure 3. PONV according to dexamethasone dose. Higher dexamethasone doses (8–10 mg) were significantly more effective than lower dexamethasone doses (1.25–5 mg) (P = 0.02).

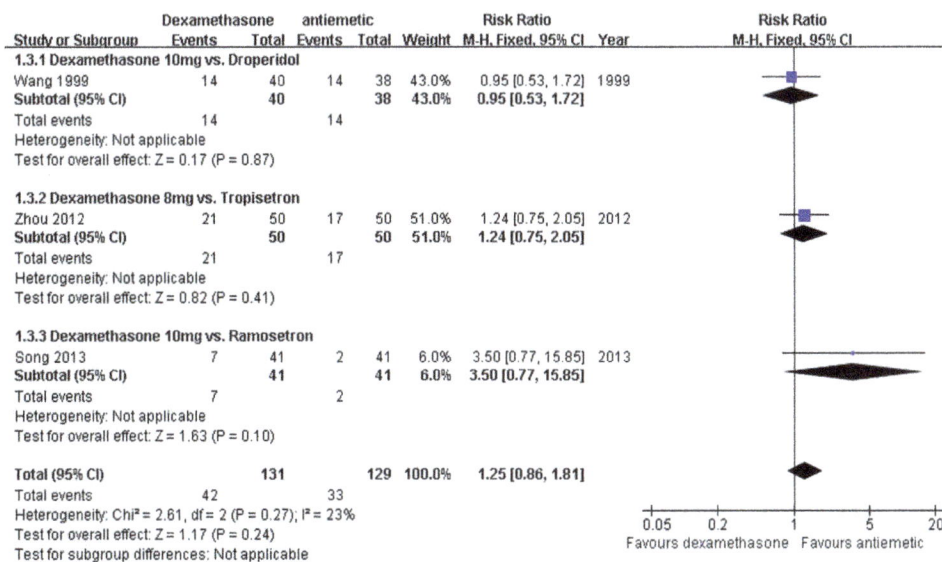

Study or Subgroup	Dexamethasone Events	Total	antiemetic Events	Total	Weight	Risk Ratio M-H, Fixed, 95% CI	Year
1.3.1 Dexamethasone 10mg vs. Droperidol							
Wang 1999	14	40	14	38	43.0%	0.95 [0.53, 1.72]	1999
Subtotal (95% CI)		40		38	43.0%	0.95 [0.53, 1.72]	
Total events	14		14				
Heterogeneity: Not applicable							
Test for overall effect: Z = 0.17 (P = 0.87)							
1.3.2 Dexamethasone 8mg vs. Tropisetron							
Zhou 2012	21	50	17	50	51.0%	1.24 [0.75, 2.05]	2012
Subtotal (95% CI)		50		50	51.0%	1.24 [0.75, 2.05]	
Total events	21		17				
Heterogeneity: Not applicable							
Test for overall effect: Z = 0.82 (P = 0.41)							
1.3.3 Dexamethasone 10mg vs. Ramosetron							
Song 2013	7	41	2	41	6.0%	3.50 [0.77, 15.85]	2013
Subtotal (95% CI)		41		41	6.0%	3.50 [0.77, 15.85]	
Total events	7		2				
Heterogeneity: Not applicable							
Test for overall effect: Z = 1.63 (P = 0.10)							
Total (95% CI)		131		129	100.0%	1.25 [0.86, 1.81]	
Total events	42		33				
Heterogeneity: Chi² = 2.61, df = 2 (P = 0.27); I² = 23%							
Test for overall effect: Z = 1.17 (P = 0.24)							
Test for subgroup differences: Not applicable							

Favours dexamethasone   Favours antiemetic

Figure 4. Comparison of dexamethasone with other anti-emetics. Three studies described the incidence of PONV in thyroidectomy patients treated with dexamethasone versus other anti-emetics (RR 1.25, 95% CI 0.86–1.81, P = 0.24). There was no evidence of significant heterogeneity between RCTs (P = 0.27, I² = 23%).

Study or Subgroup	Dexamethasone Mean	SD	Total	Placebo Mean	SD	Total	Weight	Mean Difference IV, Random, 95% CI	Year	Mean Difference IV, Random, 95% CI
3.3.3 Dexamethasone 8-10mg										
Wang 1999 D10	3.1	0.525	38	5.7	0.95	38	18.0%	-2.60 [-2.95, -2.25]	1999	
Lee 2001 D8	1.9	0.45	43	2.8	0.5	44	18.5%	-0.90 [-1.10, -0.70]	2001	
Worni 2008 D8	1.544	1.587	37	2.424	2.058	35	15.0%	-0.88 [-1.73, -0.03]	2008	
Feroci 2010 D8	1.71	1.976	51	3.27	2.016	51	15.5%	-1.56 [-2.33, -0.79]	2010	
Song 2013 D10	3.2	0.87	41	3.95	0.95	41	17.8%	-0.75 [-1.14, -0.36]	2013	
Subtotal (95% CI)			210			209	84.9%	-1.35 [-2.15, -0.55]		

Heterogeneity: Tau² = 0.75; Chi² = 78.05, df = 4 (P < 0.00001); I² = 95%
Test for overall effect: Z = 3.30 (P = 0.0010)

3.3.4 Dexamethasone 4-5mg										
Barros 2013 D4	2.2	1.5	17	2.4	0.9	17	15.1%	-0.20 [-1.03, 0.63]	2013	
Subtotal (95% CI)			17			17	15.1%	-0.20 [-1.03, 0.63]		

Heterogeneity: Not applicable
Test for overall effect: Z = 0.47 (P = 0.64)

| Total (95% CI) | | | 227 | | | 226 | 100.0% | -1.17 [-1.91, -0.44] | | |

Heterogeneity: Tau² = 0.74; Chi² = 83.81, df = 5 (P < 0.00001); I² = 94%
Test for overall effect: Z = 3.14 (P = 0.002)

(scale: -2, -1, 0, 1, 2; Favours dexamethasone — Favours placebo)

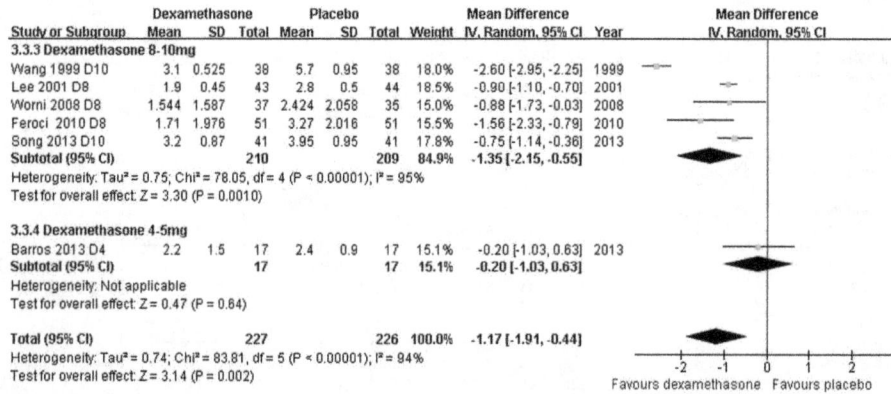

Figure 5. VAS post-operative pain score grouped by dexamethasone dose. Six studies described post-operative pain scores in thyroidectomy patients treated with dexamethasone versus placebo with or without concomitant anti-emetics (WMD -1.17, 95% CI -1.91 to -0.44, $P = 0.002$). There was evidence of significant heterogeneity between RCTs ($P<0.00001$, $I^2 = 94\%$).

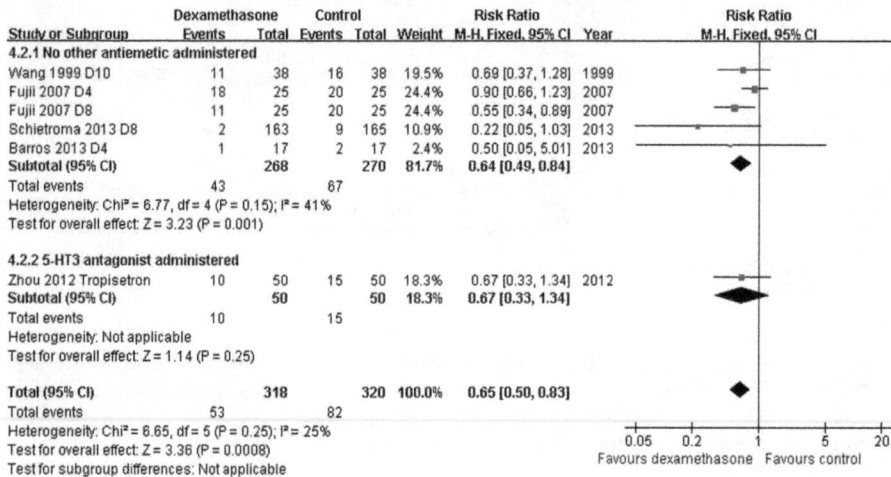

Study or Subgroup	Dexamethasone Events	Total	Control Events	Total	Weight	Risk Ratio M-H, Fixed, 95% CI	Year	Risk Ratio M-H, Fixed, 95% CI
4.2.1 No other antiemetic administered								
Wang 1999 D10	11	38	16	38	19.5%	0.69 [0.37, 1.28]	1999	
Fujii 2007 D4	18	25	20	25	24.4%	0.90 [0.66, 1.23]	2007	
Fujii 2007 D8	11	25	20	25	24.4%	0.55 [0.34, 0.89]	2007	
Schietroma 2013 D8	2	163	9	165	10.9%	0.22 [0.05, 1.03]	2013	
Barros 2013 D4	1	17	2	17	2.4%	0.50 [0.05, 5.01]	2013	
Subtotal (95% CI)		268		270	81.7%	0.64 [0.49, 0.84]		
Total events	43		67					

Heterogeneity: Chi² = 6.77, df = 4 (P = 0.15); I² = 41%
Test for overall effect: Z = 3.23 (P = 0.001)

4.2.2 5-HT3 antagonist administered								
Zhou 2012 Tropisetron	10	50	15	50	18.3%	0.67 [0.33, 1.34]	2012	
Subtotal (95% CI)		50		50	18.3%	0.67 [0.33, 1.34]		
Total events	10		15					

Heterogeneity: Not applicable
Test for overall effect: Z = 1.14 (P = 0.25)

| Total (95% CI) | | 318 | | 320 | 100.0% | 0.65 [0.50, 0.83] | | |
| Total events | 53 | | 82 | | | | | |

Heterogeneity: Chi² = 6.65, df = 5 (P = 0.25); I² = 25%
Test for overall effect: Z = 3.36 (P = 0.0008)
Test for subgroup differences: Not applicable

(scale: 0.05, 0.2, 1, 5, 20; Favours dexamethasone — Favours control)

Figure 6. Need for rescue analgesics grouped by concomitant anti-emetics. Six studies described the need for rescue analgesics in thyroidectomy patients treated with dexamethasone versus placebo with or without concomitant anti-emetics (RR 0.65, 95% CI 0.50–0.83, $P = 0.0008$). There was no evidence of significant heterogeneity between RCTs ($P = 0.25$, $I^2 = 25\%$).

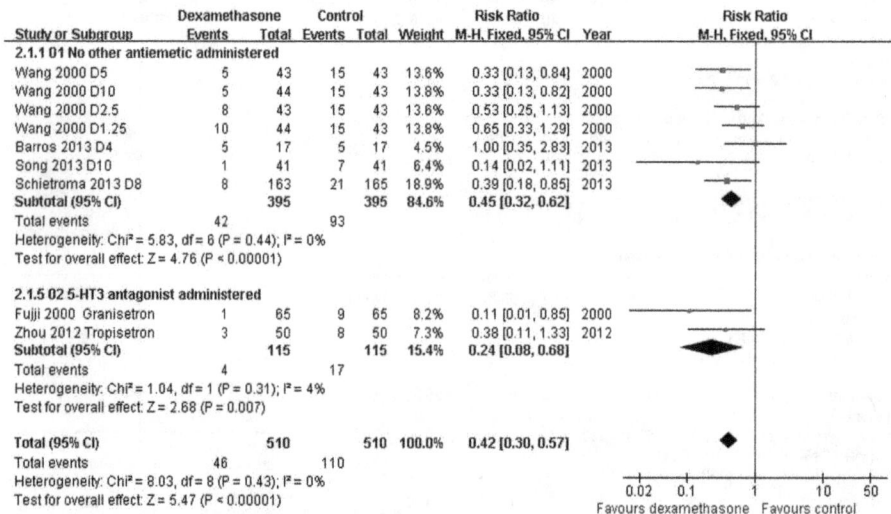

Study or Subgroup	Dexamethasone Events	Total	Control Events	Total	Weight	Risk Ratio M-H, Fixed, 95% CI	Year	Risk Ratio M-H, Fixed, 95% CI
2.1.1 01 No other antiemetic administered								
Wang 2000 D5	5	43	15	43	13.6%	0.33 [0.13, 0.84]	2000	
Wang 2000 D10	5	44	15	43	13.8%	0.33 [0.13, 0.82]	2000	
Wang 2000 D2.5	8	43	15	43	13.6%	0.53 [0.25, 1.13]	2000	
Wang 2000 D1.25	10	44	15	43	13.8%	0.65 [0.33, 1.29]	2000	
Barros 2013 D4	5	17	5	17	4.5%	1.00 [0.35, 2.83]	2013	
Song 2013 D10	1	41	7	41	6.4%	0.14 [0.02, 1.11]	2013	
Schietroma 2013 D8	8	163	21	165	18.9%	0.39 [0.18, 0.85]	2013	
Subtotal (95% CI)		395		395	84.6%	0.45 [0.32, 0.62]		
Total events	42		93					

Heterogeneity: Chi² = 5.83, df = 6 (P = 0.44); I² = 0%
Test for overall effect: Z = 4.76 (P < 0.00001)

2.1.5 02 5-HT3 antagonist administered								
Fujii 2000 Granisetron	1	65	9	65	8.2%	0.11 [0.01, 0.85]	2000	
Zhou 2012 Tropisetron	3	50	8	50	7.3%	0.38 [0.11, 1.33]	2012	
Subtotal (95% CI)		115		115	15.4%	0.24 [0.08, 0.68]		
Total events	4		17					

Heterogeneity: Chi² = 1.04, df = 1 (P = 0.31); I² = 4%
Test for overall effect: Z = 2.68 (P = 0.007)

| Total (95% CI) | | 510 | | 510 | 100.0% | 0.42 [0.30, 0.57] | | |
| Total events | 46 | | 110 | | | | | |

Heterogeneity: Chi² = 8.03, df = 8 (P = 0.43); I² = 0%
Test for overall effect: Z = 5.47 (P < 0.00001)

(scale: 0.02, 0.1, 1, 10, 50; Favours dexamethasone — Favours control)

Figure 7. Need for rescue antiemetics grouped by concomitant antiemetics. Six studies described the need for rescue antiemetics in thyroidectomy patients treated with dexamethasone versus placebo with or without concomitant antiemetics (RR 0.42, 95% CI 0.30 to 0.57, $P<0.00001$). There was no evidence of significant heterogeneity between RCTs ($P = 0.43$, $I^2 = 0\%$).

Table 4. GRADE evidence.

Outcomes	Illustrative comparative risks* (95% CI)		Relative effect (95% CI)	No of Participants (studies)	Quality of the evidence (GRADE)
	Assumed risk	**Corresponding risk**			
	Placebo	**Dexamethasone**			
Dexamethasone versus placebo (in addition to other antiemetics): PONV	**440 per 1000**	**229 per 1000** (189 to 277)	**RR 0.52** (0.43 to 0.63)	1860 (17 studies)	⊕⊕⊕⊕ **high**[1]
Dexamethasone versus placebo (in addition to other antiemetics): rescue antiemetics	**216 per 1000**	**91 per 1000** (65 to 123)	**RR 0.42** (0.3 to 0.57)	1020 (9 studies)	⊕⊕⊕ **high**
Dexamethasone comparison of doses: PONV	**440 per 1000**	**229 per 1000** (189 to 277)	**RR 0.52** (0.43 to 0.63)	1860 (17 studies)	⊕⊕⊕⊕ **high**[2]
Dexamethasone versus placebo: VAS pain score		The mean dexamethasone versus placebo: vas pain score in the intervention groups was **1.17 lower** (1.91 to 0.44 lower)		453 (6 studies)	⊕⊕⊕⊖ **moderate**[3]
Dexamethasone versus placebo (in addtion to other antiemetics): resuce analgesic	**256 per 1000**	**167 per 1000** (128 to 213)	**RR 0.65** (0.5 to 0.83)	638 (6 studies)	⊕⊕⊕⊖ **moderate**[4]
Dexamethasone versus a different antiemetic: PONV	**256 per 1000**	**320 per 1000** (220 to 463)	**RR 1.25** (0.86 to 1.81)	260 (3 studies)	⊕⊕⊕⊕ **high**

*The basis for the **assumed risk** (e.g. the median control group risk across studies) is provided in footnotes. The **corresponding risk** (and its 95% confidence interval) is based on the assumed risk in the comparison group and the **relative effect** of the intervention (and its 95% CI). **CI**: Confidence interval; **RR**: Risk ratio.
GRADE Working Group grades of evidence. **High quality:** Further research is very unlikely to change our confidence in the estimate of effect. **Moderate quality:** Further research is likely to have an important impact on our confidence in the estimate of effect and may change the estimate. **Low quality:** Further research is very likely to have an important impact on our confidence in the estimate of effect and is likely to change the estimate. **Very low quality:** We are very uncertain about the estimate.
[1]Although the PONV results demonstrated significant heterogeneity ($P = 0.003$, $I^2 = 56\%$), it was partly explained by the dose of dexamethasone. [2]Downgraded by not comparing higher dose with lower dose directly, but upgraded by the dose-response gradient. [3]Although there was significant heterogeneity ($P<0.00001$, $I^2 = 94\%$), it was partly explained by the dose of dexamethasone. [4]Publication bias as $Pr>|z| = 0.06$.
PONV: post-operative nausea and vomiting; VAS: visual analogue scales.
Patient or population: patients undergoing thyroidectomy. **Settings:** evidence from China, Japan, Korea, Italy, Switzerland, Norway, Portugal. **Intervention:** dexamethasone. **Comparison:** placebo.

received dexamethasone 90 minutes before skin incision, while others received dexamethasone postoperatively. Wang et al [32] demonstrated that dexamethasone administered before anesthesia was more effective in decreasing early PONV compared to dexamethasone administered after anesthesia. These observations are in accordance with data showing that the onset time of dexamethasone on anti-emesis is approximately 2 hours. In the current study, subgroup analysis stratified by the timing of dexamethasone administration showed that dexamethasone was most effective in preventing PONV when administered before rather than after induction of anesthesia ($P = 0.0002$; Fig. S2).

3.5 Sensitivity analysis

To explore the effects of individual RCTs on the pooled OR estimates, we performed a sensitivity analysis omitting one study at a time. No single RCT significantly affected the overall results of the meta-analysis.

3.6 Publication bias

Visual inspection of a Funnel plot, Egger's test, and Begg's rank correlation test revealed no significant publication bias (Begg's rank correlation test, continuity-corrected $Pr>|z| >0.1$), except for RCTs reporting on the need for rescue anti-emetic in patients receiving dexamethasone versus placebo, with or without concomitant antiemetics ($Pr>|z| = 0.06$), (Table S2).

3.7 Quality of evidence

Quality of available evidence from RCTs, which was downgraded by inconsistency (heterogeneity between studies), indirectness (variations in study setting), or publication bias, and upgraded by dose-response gradient, varied from moderate to high (Table 4).

Discussion

PONV is a common and distressing complication for patients undergoing thyroidectomy; therefore, prophylactic anti-emetics may be beneficial. An optimal anti-emetic regimen should be capable of decreasing the incidence of PONV without increasing the risk for adverse events. However, most of the currently used anti-emetics, including anti-histamines, butyrophenones, and dopamine receptor antagonists cause occasional undesirable adverse events, such as excessive sedation, hypotension, dry mouth, dysphoria, hallucinations, and extrapyramidal signs [33]. 5-HT3 antagonists are effective for preventing and treating PONV in patients undergoing various types of surgery [34]. However, the use of prophylactic anti-emetic therapy with 5-HT3 antagonists has been criticized for being too expensive [35].

Our meta-analysis of 13 RCTs demonstrated that prophylactic dexamethasone is effective in reducing the incidence of PONV, post-operative pain scores, and the need for rescue analgesia and anti-emetics compared to placebo administered with or without contaminant anti-emetics in patients undergoing thyroidectomy. In addition, our findings showed that dexamethasone is as effective as other anti-emetics for reducing PONV in this patient population. However, the benefits of administering dexamethasone as a more cost-effective anti-emetic and efficacious analgesic drug[35] should be weighed against the potential side effects. Our study indicated that dexamethasone administration is associated with an increase in blood glucose during the immediate post-operative period, but with no other serious adverse events.

For optimal dose and timing of dexamethasone administration, subgroup analyses showed that higher doses of dexamethasone (8–10 mg) are more effective than lower doses (1.5–5 mg), and dexamethasone is most effective in preventing PONV when administered before rather than after induction of anesthesia.

In terms of populations eligible for treatment, the RCTs in the current study mostly included healthy patients, and excluded pregnant women, patients with insulin-dependent diabetes mellitus, those who were obese, and patients with a high risk for PONV. As such, the impact of prophylactic dexamethasone on outcomes in high-risk patients is not known. A larger sample size and well-performed RCTs including high risk patients are required for further investigations.

This review has several limitations. First, data reporting on the effects of prophylactic dexamethasone on post-operative pain scores and need for rescue analgesics in thyroidectomy patients were limited by substantial heterogeneity and publication bias,

respectively. Second, the studies in this systematic review included patients across various age groups receiving dexamethasone according to very different protocols.

Conclusion

The present meta-analysis shows that prophylactic dexamethasone is safe and effective for reducing the incidence of PONV, post-operative pain, and the need for rescue analgesia and anti-emetics in thyroidectomy patients. Prophylactic dexamethasone 8–10 mg administered before induction of anesthesia should be recommended for patients undergoing thyroidectomy except for those that are pregnant, have diabetes mellitus, hyperglycaemia or contraindications for corticosteroids. More high quality trials are warranted to define the benefits and risks of prophylactic dexamethasone in potential patients with high risk for PONV.

Supporting Information

Figure S1 Incidence of PONV stratified according to dexamethasone dose: 8–10 mg and 1.25–5 mg.

Figure S2 Incidence of PONV stratified by timing of dexamethasone administration.

Table S1 Search strategy from its inception to October 1, 2013.

Table S2 Begg's rank correlation test for publication bias.

Checklist S1 PRISMA 2009 Checklist.

Author Contributions

Conceived and designed the experiments: RZ ZZ MX. Performed the experiments: ZZ YJ. Analyzed the data: ZZ YJ. Contributed reagents/materials/analysis tools: ZZ YJ. Contributed to the writing of the manuscript: RZ MX.

References

1. Sonner JM, Hynson JM, Clark O, Katz JA (1997) Nausea and vomiting following thyroid and parathyroid surgery. J Clin Anesth 9(5): 398–402.
2. Kranke P, Eberhart LH (2011) Possibilities and limitations in the pharmacological management of postoperative nausea and vomiting. Eur J Anaesthesiol 28: 758–765.
3. Matory YL, Spiro RH (1993) Wound bleeding after head and neck surgery. J Surg Oncol 53(1): 17–19.
4. Schwartz AE, Clark OH, Ituarte P, Lo Gerfo P (1998) Therapeutic controversy: thyroid surgery–the choice. J Clin Endocrinol Metab 83(4): 1097–1105.
5. Fredrikson M, Hursti T, Fürst CJ, Steineck G, Börjeson S, et al. (1992) Nausea in cancer chemotherapy is inversely related to urinary cortisol excretion. Br J Cancer 65: 779–780.
6. Aapro MS, Plezia PM, Alberts DS, Graham V, Jones SE, et al. (1984) Double-blind crossover study of the antiemetic efficacy of high-dose dexamethasone versus high-dose metoclopramide. J Clin Oncol 2: 466–471.
7. Sapolsky RM, Romero LM, Munck AU (2000) How do glucocorticoids influence stress responses? Integrating permissive, suppressive, stimulatory, and preparative actions. Endocr Rev 21: 55–89.
8. Hargreaves KM, Costello A (1990) Glucocorticoids suppress levels of immunoreactive bradykinin in inflamed tissue as evaluated by microdialysis probes. Clin Pharmacol Ther 48: 168–178.
9. Hong D, Byers MR, Oswald RJ (1993) Dexamethasone treatment reduces sensory neuropeptides and nerve sprouting reactions in injured teeth. Pain 55: 171–181.
10. Karanicolas PJ1, Smith SE, Kanbur B, Davies E, Guyatt GH (2008) The Impact of Prophylactic Dexamethasone on Nausea and Vomiting After Laparoscopic

Cholecystectomy A Systematic Review and Meta-Analysis. Ann Surg 248(5): 751–762.
11. Chen CC, Siddiqui FJ, Chen TL, Chan ES, Tam KW (2012) Dexamethasone for prevention of postoperative nausea and vomiting in patients undergoing thyroidectomy: meta-analysis of randomized controlled trials. World J Surg 36: 61–68.
12. Moher D, Liberati A, Tetzlaff J, Altman DG, PRISMA Group (2010) Preferred reporting items for systematic reviews and meta-analyses: the PRISMA statement. Int J Surg 8: 336–341.
13. Lefebvre C, Manheimer E, Glanville J (2011) Chapter 6: searching for studies. In: Higgins JPT, Green S (editors). Cochrane Handbook for Systematic Reviews of Interventions Version 5.1.0 [updated March 2011]. The Cochrane Collaboration, 2011. Available: www.cochrane-handbook.org.
14. Higgins JPT, Altman DG, Sterne JAC (2011) Chapter 8: assessing risk of bias in included studies. In: Higgins JPT, Green S (editors). Cochrane Handbook for Systematic Reviews of Interventions Version 5.1.0 [updated March 2011]. The Cochrane Collaboration, 2011. Available: www.cochrane-handbook.org.
15. Begg CB, Mazumdar M (1994) Operating characteristics of a rank correlation test for publication bias. Biometrics 50(4): 1088–1101.
16. Atkins D, Best D, Briss PA, Eccles M, Falck-Ytter Y, et al GRADE Working Group (2004) Grading quality of evidence and strength of recommendations. BMJ 328: 1490–1494.
17. Guyatt G, Gutterman D, Baumann MH, Addrizzo-Harris D, Hylek EM, et al. (2006) Grading strength of recommendations and quality of evidence in clinical guidelines. Chest 129: 174–181.
18. Wang JJ, Ho ST, Lee SC, Liu YC, Liu YH, et al. (1999) The prophylactic effect of dexamethasone on postoperative nausea and vomiting in women undergoing

thyroidectomy: a comparison of droperidol with saline. Anesth Analg 89: 200–203.

19. Wang JJ, Ho ST, Lee SC, Liu YC, Ho CM (2000) The use of dexamethasone for preventing postoperative nausea and vomiting in females undergoing thyroidectomy: a dose-ranging study. Anesth Analg 91: 1404–1407.

20. Lee Y, Lin PC, Lai HY, Huang SJ, Lin YS, et al. (2001) Prevention of PONV with dexamethasone in female patients undergoing desflurane anesthesia for thyroidectomy. Acta Anaesthesiol Sin 39: 151–156.

21. Fujii Y, Nakayama M (2007) Efficacy of dexamethasone for reducing postoperative nausea and vomiting and analgesic requirements after thyroidectomy. Otolaryngol Head Neck Surg 136: 274–277.

22. Worni M, Schudel HH, Seifert E, Inglin R, Hagemann M, et al. (2008) Randomized controlled trial on single dose steroid before thyroidectomy for benign disease to improve postoperative nausea, pain, and vocal function. Ann Surg 248: 1060–1066.

23. Feroci F, Rettori M, Borrelli A, Lenzi E, Ottaviano A, et al. (2011) Dexamethasone prophylaxis before thyroidectomy to reduce postoperative nausea, pain, and vocal dysfunction: a randomized clinical controlled trial. Head Neck 2011; 33: 840–846.

24. Doksrød S, Sagen Ø, Nøstdahl T, Ræder J (2012) Dexamethasone does not reduce pain or analgesic consumption after thyroid surgery; a prospective, randomized trial. Acta Anaesthesiol Scand 56: 513–519.

25. Song YK, Lee C (2013) Effects of ramosetron and dexamethasone on postoperative nausea, vomiting, pain, and shivering in female patients undergoing thyroid surgery. J Anesth 27: 29–34.

26. Barros A, Vale CP, Oliveira FC, Ventura C, Assunção J, et al. (2013) Dexamethasone effect on postoperative pain and tramadol requirement after thyroidectomy. Pharmacology 91: 153–157.

27. Schietroma M, Cecilia EM, Carlei F, Sista F, De Santis G, et al. (2013) Dexamethasone for the prevention of recurrent laryngeal nerve palsy and other complications after thyroid surgery: a randomized double-blind placebo-controlled trial. JAMA Otolaryngol Head Neck Surg 139: 471–478.

28. Zhou H, Xu H, Zhang J, Wang W, Wang Y, et al. (2012) Combination of dexamethasone and tropisetron before thyroidectomy to alleviate postoperative nausea, vomiting, and pain: randomized controlled trial. World J Surg 36: 1217–1224.

29. Bononi M, Amore Bonapasta S, Vari A, Scarpini M, De Cesare A, et al. (2010) Incidence and circumstances of cervical hematoma complicating thyroidectomy and its relationship to postoperative vomiting. Head Neck 32: 1173–1177.

30. Fujii Y, Tanaka H, Kobayashi N (2000) Granisetron/dexamethasone combination for the prevention of postoperative nausea and vomiting after thyroidectomy. Anaesth Intensive Care 28: 266–269.

31. Hozo SP, Djulbegovic B, Hozo I (2005) Estimating the mean and variance from the median, range, and the size of a sample. BMC Med Res Methodol 5: 13.

32. Wang JJ, Ho ST, Tzeng JI, Tang CS (2000) The effect of timing of dexamethasone administration on its efficacy as a prophylactic antiemetic for postoperative nausea and vomiting. Anesth Analg 91(1): 136–9.

33. Watcha MF, White PF (1992) Postoperative nausea and vomiting: its etiology, treatment, and prevention. Anesthesiology 77: 162–84.

34. Kovac AL (2000) Prevention and treatment of postoperative nausea and vomiting. Drugs 59: 213–43.

35. White PF, Watcha MF (1993) Are new drugs cost-effective for patients undergoing ambulatory surgery? Anesthesiology 78(1): 2–5.

7

Codelivery of Chemotherapeutics via Crosslinked Multilamellar Liposomal Vesicles to Overcome Multidrug Resistance in Tumor

Yarong Liu[1]❾, Jinxu Fang[1]❾, Kye-Il Joo[1], Michael K. Wong[2], Pin Wang[1,3,4]∗

1 Mork Family Department of Chemical Engineering and Materials Science, University of Southern California, Los Angeles, California, United States of America, 2 Division of Medical Oncology, Norris Comprehensive Cancer Center, Keck School of Medicine, University of Southern California, Los Angeles, California, United States of America, 3 Department of Biomedical Engineering, University of Southern California, Los Angeles, California, United States of America, 4 Department of Pharmacology and Pharmaceutical Sciences, University of Southern California, Los Angeles, California, United States of America

Abstract

Multidrug resistance (MDR) is a significant challenge to effective cancer chemotherapy treatment. However, the development of a drug delivery system that allows for the sustained release of combined drugs with improved vesicle stability could overcome MDR in cancer cells. To achieve this, we have demonstrated codelivery of doxorubicin (Dox) and paclitaxel (PTX) *via* a crosslinked multilamellar vesicle (cMLV). This combinatorial delivery system achieves enhanced drug accumulation and retention, in turn resulting in improved cytotoxicity against tumor cells, including drug-resistant cells. Moreover, this delivery approach significantly overcomes MDR by reducing the expression of P-glycoprotein (P-gp) in cancer cells, thus improving antitumor activity *in vivo*. Thus, by enhancing drug delivery to tumors and lowering the apoptotic threshold of individual drugs, this combinatorial delivery system represents a potentially promising multimodal therapeutic strategy to overcome MDR in cancer therapy.

Editor: Bing Xu, Brandeis University, United States of America

Funding: This work was supported by National Institutes of Health grants (R01AI068978, R01CA170820 and P01CA132681), a translational acceleration grant from the Joint Center for Translational Medicine, the National Cancer Institute (P30CA014089), and a grant from the Ming Hsieh Institute for Research on Engineering Medicine for Cancer. The funders had no role in study design, data collection and analysis, decision to publish, or preparation of the manuscript.

Competing Interests: The authors have declared that no competing interests exist.

∗ Email: pinwang@usc.edu

❾ These authors contributed equally to this work.

Introduction

The development of multidrug resistance (MDR) against a variety of conventional and novel chemotherapeutic agents has been a major impediment to the success of cancer therapy [1,2]. One of the most important mechanisms involved in MDR is the overexpression of P-glycoprotein (P-gp) in the plasma membrane of various cancer cells. P-gp, an active drug efflux transporter, is capable of effluxing a broad range of anticancer agents, such as taxanes and anthracyclines [3]. For example, the efficacy of doxorubicin (Dox) and paclitaxel (PTX), two of the most widely used agents for the treatment of various cancers, is often compromised by P-gp-mediated MDR [4,5]. Therefore, a strategy to inhibit P-gp expression has been developed to overcome MDR. For instance, a large number of P-gp inhibitors and siRNAs targeting the gene encoding P-gp have been delivered in combination with anticancer agents to downregulate P-gp expression, thereby enabling drugs to reach sufficient concentrations to induce cytotoxicity [6,7]. However, P-gp inhibitors, either functional inhibitors or siRNA, have yielded disappointing clinical trials resulting from their high systemic toxicities and enhanced side effects of chemotherapy in normal cells [8,9].

Combination therapy with multiple chemotherapeutics provides an alternative strategy to suppress MDR. Different drugs may attack cancer cells at varying stages of their growth cycles, thus decreasing the concentration threshold for individual drugs that is otherwise required for cytotoxicity [10]. It has been reported that various drug combinations have successfully induced synergistic antitumor activities and prevented disease recurrence [11,12]. For example, a Dox and PTX cocktail is now considered a standard anthracycline-taxane combination treatment for various tumors by their ability to overcome drug resistance [13,14,15]. However, a major challenge of combination therapy is coordinating the pharmacokinetics and cellular uptake of combined therapeutics. This obstacle has limited the clinical success of combination therapy [16,17].

To overcome this challenge, novel strategies that allow loading of multiple therapeutics into a single drug-delivery vehicle for concurrent delivery at the site of action have been extensively explored [18,19]. Several drug delivery systems have been able to intercalate multiple drugs for site-specific delivery to tumors and, hence, improve antitumor activities, potentially overcoming drug resistance, while, at the same time, reducing the dosage of individual drugs [20,21,22]. Indeed, nanoparticle delivery systems are known to deliver therapeutics efficiently to the tumor sites through the enhanced permeability and retention (EPR) effect, thereby enhancing the concentration of therapeutics in tumors [23,24]. Moreover, these nanoparticles can enter cancer cells through endocytosis in a manner independent of the P-gp pathway, thereby enhancing cellular accumulation of therapeutics [25,26,27]. Thus, a nanoparticle delivery system capable of mediating high efficiency of cellular entry and subsequent triggering of intracellular release of multiple anticancer drugs to overcome MDR is highly desirable.

Liposomes are one of the most popular nanoparticle delivery systems for combinatorial delivery of multiple drugs based on their ability to efficiently load both hydrophilic and hydrophobic drugs [24,28]. We previously developed a robust crosslinked multi-lamellar liposomal vesicle (cMLV), with enhanced vesicle stability, to efficiently codeliver hydrophilic (Dox) and hydrophobic (PTX) drugs and induce ratio-dependent synergistic antitumor activity, both *in vitro* and *in vivo* [29,30,31]. Moreover, it was shown that cMLV particles are mainly internalized by cells through caveolin-dependent endocytosis and are then trafficked through the endosome-lysosome network for release of drugs [30]. In this study, we have examined the potential of cMLV as a combinatorial delivery system aimed at overcoming P-gp-mediated drug resistance, both *in vitro* and *in vivo*. Indeed, we have demonstrated that the combination of Dox and PTX, when administered at 1:1 weight ratio in cMLV formulations, shows significant enhancement of cytotoxicity and antitumor activities. Combining these drugs through the use of cMLV formulations contributes to these antitumor activities by enhancing systemic delivery efficiency and lowering tumor apoptotic threshold.

Materials and Methods

Mice

Female BALB/c mice (6–10 weeks old) were purchased from Charles River Breeding Laboratories (Wilmington, MA). All mice were held under specific pathogen-reduced conditions in the Animal Facility of the University of Southern California (USA). All experiments were performed in accordance with the guidelines set by the National Institutes of Health and the University of Southern California on the Care and Use of Animals. This study was approved by the Committee on the Ethics of Animal Experiments of the University of Southern California.

Cell culture

B16 tumor cells (B16–F10, ATCC number: CRL-6475) and 4T1 tumor cells (ATCC number: CRL-2539) were maintained in a 5% CO_2 environment with Dulbecco's modified Eagle's medium (Mediatech, Inc., Manassas, VA) supplemented with 10% FBS (Sigma-Aldrich, St. Louis, MO) and 2 mM of L-glutamine (Hyclone Laboratories, Inc., Omaha, NE). B16-R and 4T1-R cells were produced by continuously treating B16 and 4T1 cells with 5 μg/ml PTX for 4 days. The cells were then recovered by replacing medium with fresh medium without drugs for 7 days. The remaining cells formed drug resistance for PTX. JC cells (ATCC number: CRL-2116) were used as a model drug-resistant tumor cell line because it has been shown that JC cells overexpress P-gp and exhibit a drug-resistant phenotype, both *in vitro* and *in vivo* [32].

Synthesis of cMLVs

Liposomes were prepared based on the conventional dehydra-tion-rehydration method. All lipids were obtained from the NOF Corporation (Japan). 1.5 μmol of lipids 1,2-dioleoyl-sn-glycero-3-

phosphocholine (DOPC), 1,2-dioleoyl-sn-glycero-3-phospho-(1'-rac-glycerol) (DOPG), and maleimide-headgrouplipid1,2-dio-leoyl-sn-glycero-3-phosphoeth-anolamine-N-[4-(p-maleimidophe-nyl) butyramide (MPB-PE) were combined in chloroform at a molar lipid ratio of DOPC:DOPG:MPB = 4:1:5, and the organic solvent in the lipid mixture was evaporated under argon gas. The lipid mixture was further dried under vacuum overnight to form dried thin lipid films. To prepare cMLV(PTX) and cMLV(Dox+ PTX) at a molar ratio of 0.2:1 (drugs:lipids), paclitaxel in organic solvent was mixed with the lipid mixture to form dried thin lipid films. The resultant dried film was hydrated in 10 mM Bis-Tris propane at pH 7.0 with (cMLV(Dox) or cMLV(Dox+PTX)) or without doxorubicin (cMLV(PTX)) at a molar ratio of 0.2:1 (drugs:lipids) with vigorous vortexing every 10 min for 1 h, followed by applying 4 cycles of 15-s sonication (Misonix Microson XL2000, Farmingdale, NY) on ice in 1-min intervals of each cycle. To induce divalent-triggered vesicle fusion, $MgCl_2$ was added at a final concentration of 10 mM. The resulting multilamellar vesicles were further crosslinked by addition of Dithiothreitol (DTT, Sigma-Aldrich) at a final concentration of 1.5 mM for 1 h at 37°C. The resulting vesicles were collected by centrifugation at 14,000 g for 4 min and then washed twice with PBS. For pegylation of cMLVs, the particles were incubated with 1 μmol of 2 kDa PEG-SH (Laysan Bio Inc., Arab, AL) for 1 h at 37°C. The particles were then centrifuged and washed twice with PBS. The final products were stored in PBS at 4°C. The mean diameter of all cMLVs is around 220 nm determined by dynamic light scattering (DLS), and around 160 nm estimated by cryo-electron microsco-py. The loading efficiency, and stability of cMLVs were similar to that demonstrated previously [30,31].

In vitro cytotoxicity and data analysis

B16-F10, 4T1, B16–R, 4T1-R, and JC cells were plated at a density of 5×10^3 cells per well in D10 media in 96-well plates and grown for 6 h. The cells were then exposed to a series of concentrations of cMLV (single drug) or cMLV (drug combina-tions) for 48 h. The cell viability was assessed using the Cell Proliferation Kit II (XTT assay) from Roche Applied Science according to the manufacturer's instructions. Slope m and IC_{50} were obtained from median effect model, and IIP_{Cmax} was calculated via the following equation: $IIP_{Cmax} = \log (1+(Cmax/IC_{50})^m)$. Cmax is the maximum plasma drug concentrations for the commonly recommended dose for each drug.

Cellular uptake of doxorubicin and paclitaxel in cells

4T1 cells were seeded in 24-well plates at a density of 2×10^5 cells per well and grown overnight. The cells were then exposed to empty cMLVs (control), cMLV(Dox), cMLV(PTX), cMLV(Dox+ PTX), and Dox+PTX. The final concentrations of Dox and PTX were 1 μg/ml for each group. JC cells were seeded at a density of 10^5 cells per well in D10 media in 96-well plates. The cells were exposed to empty cMLVs, cMLV(Dox), cMLV(PTX), cMLV(Dox+PTX), and Dox+PTX. The final concentrations of Dox and PTX were 5 μg/ml for each group. At 48 h after treatment, the cells were washed twice with PBS and lysed with PBS containing 1% Triton X-100. Doxorubicin and paclitaxel in cell lysates were extracted by 1:1 (v/v) Chloroform/isopropyl alcohol or ethyl acetate, respectively. Paclitaxel concentrations in cell lysates were measured by HPLC C18 column and detected at 227 nm (flow rate 1 ml/min), and doxorubicin was detected by fluorescence with 480/550 nm excitation/emission. The concen-trations of Dox and PTX were normalized for protein content as measured with BCA assay (Pierce).

In vivo antitumor activity study

BALB/c female mice (6–10 weeks old) were inoculated subcutaneously with 0.2×10^6 4T1 breast tumor cells. The tumors were allowed to grow for 8 days to a volume of ~50 mm³ before treatment. After 8 days, the mice were injected intravenously through the tail vein with cMLV(2 mg/kg Dox), cMLV(2 mg/kg PTX), cMLV(2 mg/kg Dox)+cMLV(2 mg/kg PTX), or cMLV(2 mg/kg Dox + 2 mg/kg PTX) every three days (six mice per group). Tumor growth and body weight were monitored for 40 days or to the end of the experiment. The length and width of the tumor masses were measured with a fine caliper every three days after injection. Tumor volume was expressed as $1/2 \times$ (length $\times$ width²). Survival end point was set when the tumor volume reached 1000 mm³. The survival rates are presented as Kaplan-Meier curves. The survival curves of individual groups were compared by a log-rank test.

Immunohistochemistry of tumors and confocal imaging

BALB/c female mice (6–10 weeks old) were inoculated subcutaneously with 0.2×10^6 4T1 or JC tumor cells. The tumors were allowed to grow for 20 days to a volume of ~500 mm³ before treatment. On day 20, the mice were injected intravenously through the tail vein with cMLV (5 mg/kg Dox), cMLV(5 mg/kg PTX), 5 mg/kg Dox + 5 mg/kg PTX, or cMLV(5 mg/kg Dox + 5 mg/kg PTX). Three days after injection, tumors were excised, fixed, frozen, cryo-sectioned, and mounted onto glass slides. Frozen sections were fixed and rinsed with cold PBS. After blocking and permeabilization, the slides were washed by PBS and then incubated with TUNEL reaction mixture (Roche, Indianapolis, Indiana) for 1 h. For P-gp expression, the slides were stained after permeabilization with mouse monoclonal anti-P-gp antibody (Abcam, Cambridge, MA) for 1 h, followed by staining with Alexa488-conjugated goat anti-mouse immunoglobulin G (IgG) antibody (Invitrogen, Carlsbad, CA) and counterstaining with DAPI (Invitrogen, Carlsbad, CA). Fluorescence images were acquired by a Yokogawa spinning-disk confocal scanner system (Solamere Technology Group, Salt Lake City, UT), using a Nikon Eclipse Ti-E microscope. Illumination powers at 405, 491, 561, and 640 nm solid-state laser lines were provided by an AOTF (acousto-optical tunable filter)-controlled laser-merge system with 50 mW for each laser. All images were analyzed using Nikon NIS-Elements software. To quantify TUNEL and P-gp-positive cells, 4 regions of interest (ROI) were randomly chosen per image at ×2 magnification. Within one region, area of TUNEL or P-gp-positive nuclei, and area of nuclear staining were counted by Nikon NIS-Element software. The data are expressed as % total nuclear area stained by TUNEL or P-gp in the region.

Hematoxylin and Eosin staining of heart sections

Mice bearing 4T1 tumors were i.v. injected with 5 mg/kg Dox + 5 mg/kg PTX or cMLV(5 mg/kg Dox+5 mg/kg PTX). Three days after injection, heart tissues were harvested and fixed in 4% formaldehyde. The tissues were frozen, cut into sections, and mounted onto glass slides. The frozen sections were stained with hematoxylin and eosin. Histopathologic specimens were examined by light microscopy.

Statistics

Differences between two groups were determined with Student's t test. The differences among three or more groups were determined with a one-way ANOVA.

Results

In vitro efficacy study by XTT assay

To achieve combination delivery of doxorubicin (Dox) and paclitaxel (PTX), a previously developed crosslinked multilamellar liposomal vesicle (cMLV) was used to incorporate PTX in the lipid membrane and encapsulate Dox in the aqueous core at a 1:1 ratio to form cMLV(Dox+PTX) [30]. We chose this combination ratio because our previous study showed that it could induce synergy combination effect both *in vitro* and *in vivo* [31]. It has been reported that drug combinations can overcome drug resistance that would otherwise limit the potential application of various monotherapeutics [10]. To determine whether codelivery of Dox and PTX could overcome drug resistance, an *in vitro* cytotoxicity assay was performed at a wide range of concentrations of single drug-loaded or dual drug-loaded cMLVs. As shown in Figure 1A and 1B (left panel), both B16 cells and 4T1 cells developed drug resistance to single drug-loaded cMLVs, but this resistance was inhibited by applying the combined formulation, cMLV(Dox+ PTX). The maximal cytotoxicity of single drug-loaded cMLV observed in these two tumor cells was between 60%–80%, while cells treated with dual drug-loaded cMLV(Dox+PTX) showed significantly more growth inhibition (~95%).

To further confirm the efficiency of dual drug-loaded cMLVs in overcoming drug resistance, drug-resistant cell lines B16-R and 4T1-R were generated by continuously treating parental B16 or 4T1 with a high concentration of paclitaxel (5 µg/ml). Various concentrations of single drug-loaded cMLV and dual drug-loaded cMLV(Dox+PTX) were incubated with these two drug-resistant cell lines for 48 h, and the cytotoxicity was measured by a standard XTT assay. As shown in Figure 1D and 1E, both B16-R and 4T1-R cells showed a high tolerance when treated with cMLV(PTX) or cMLV(Dox), indicating that multidrug resistance had been developed in these cells. In contrast, cMLV(Dox+PTX) triggered significantly more cell death (90–100%) compared to that of single drug-loaded cMLVs, confirming that a codelivery system could overcome drug resistance induced by a high concentration of single drug. Furthermore, *in vitro* cytotoxicity studies demonstrated therapeutic efficacy of cMLV(Dox+PTX) in JC cells, a model drug-resistant tumor cell line, corroborating the weaker potency of single drug-loaded cMLVs compared to the dual drug-loaded cMLVs. As shown in Figure 1C (left panel), the maximal cytotoxicity of cMLV(Dox) and cMLV(PTX) was in the range of 60–70%, while peak cMLV(Dox+PTX) cytotoxicity was about 90% in JC cells.

IC_{50}, which indicates drug concentration that causes 50% inhibitory effect on cell proliferation, can provide information on the efficacy of drugs. The IC_{50} values of the individual drugs and combined drugs through cMLVs in B16, 4T1 and JC cells are provided in Figure S1. However, it has also been reported that slope m, a parameter mathematically analogous to the Hill coefficient, may also have a significant effect on cytotoxicity [33,34]. Therefore, a new model has been developed to evaluate drug activity by incorporating three parameters (IC_{50}, drug concentration, and m) from the median effect model into a single-value IIP (potential inhibition) with an intuitive meaning, i.e., the log reduction in inhibitory effect [34]. Accordingly, to increase the trustworthiness of our experiment, IIP was used to evaluate the efficiency of dual drug-loaded cMLVs on cell viability. As shown in Figure 1A to 1C (middle and right panels), Dox and PTX in the dual drug-loaded cMLVs displayed a significantly larger IIP_{Cmax} value in the cell lines studied compared to that of the single drug-loaded cMLVs, indicating that

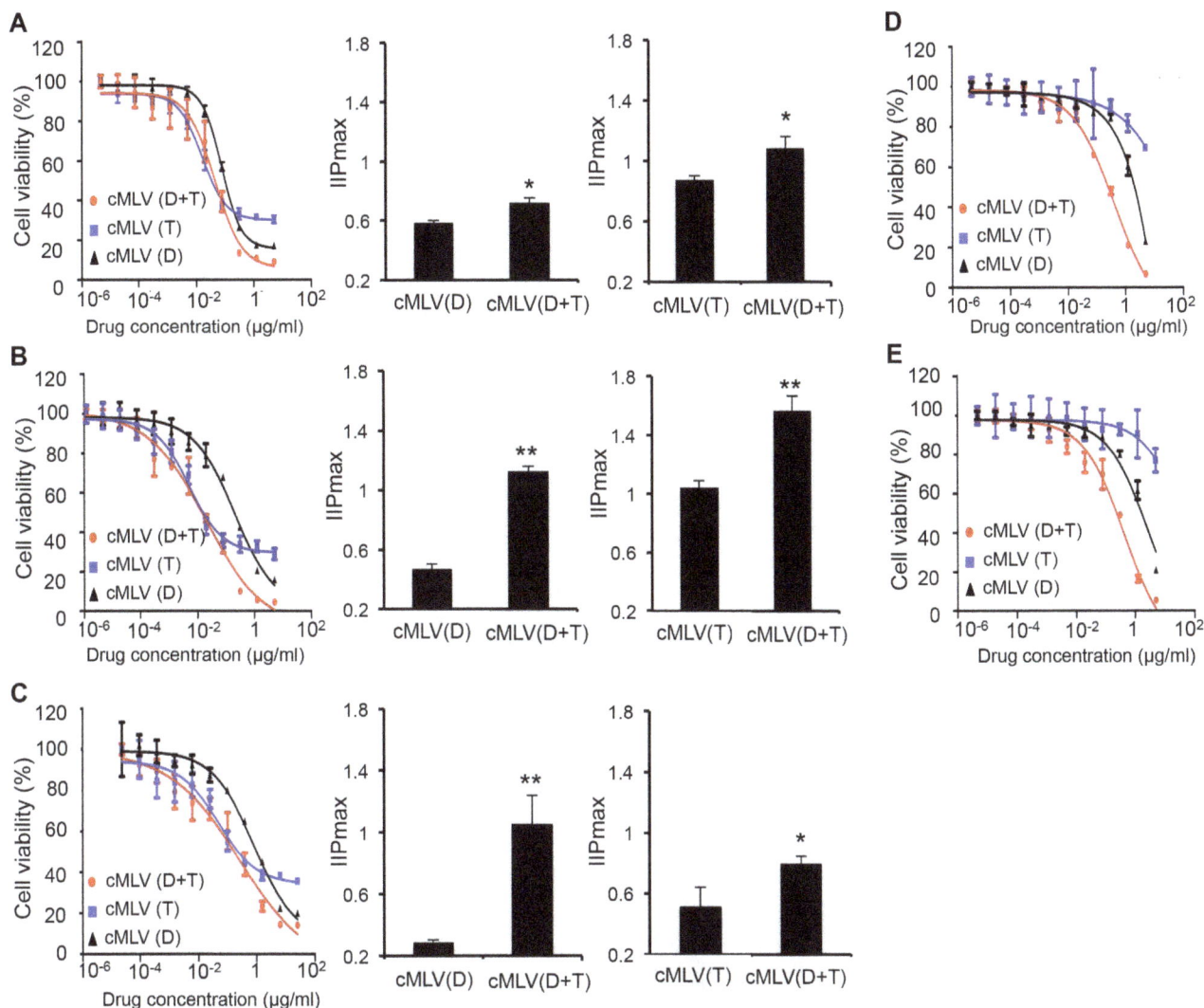

Figure 1. Overcoming drug resistance by codelivery of Dox and PTX via cMLVs (D: Dox; T: PTX). (A, B) *In vitro* cytotoxicity of cMLV(single drug) and cMLV(drug combinations) in B16 melanoma tumor cells (A) and 4T1 breast tumor cells (B). (C, D, E) *In vitro* cytotoxicity of cMLV(single drug) and cMLV(drug combinations) in drug-resistant JC cells (C), B16-R cells (D) and 4T1-R cells (E). IIP_{Cmax} was determined by incorporating three parameters (IC_{50}, D and m) in the median effect model into the following equation: $IIP_{Cmax} = log (1+(Cmax/IC_{50})^{m})$. Data are represented as mean $\pm$ SD (n = 3). Asterisks indicate statistical significance between two groups (*$P < 0.05$, **$P < 0.01$).

combinatorial cMLVs were more potent in cancer treatment than single drug-loaded cMLVs.

Cellular uptake study of doxorubicin and paclitaxel

To investigate the mechanism of enhanced cytotoxicity observed with cMLV combination therapy, we evaluated the effect of dual drug-loaded cMLVs on rates of drug influx/efflux in cells. The intracellular accumulation of Dox and PTX was examined by HPLC in 4T1 cells following exposure to Dox (1 µg/ml) and PTX (1 µg/ml) in cMLVs, both individually and in combination, and in JC cells with higher dose of Dox and PTX (5 µg/ml). After 3 h incubation, the extracellular medium was discarded, and intracellular drug (Dox or PTX) accumulation was quantitatively determined by drug concentration in the cell lysates, normalized by total cellular protein content of the cells. As seen in Figure 2A and 2B, cMLV(Dox+PTX) significantly increased both Dox and PTX accumulation in 4T1 cells compared to that of single drug-loaded cMLVs ($p < 0.05$), suggesting that combination

treatments may overcome drug resistance. In addition, compared to the administration of drug in solution, cMLV combination treatment resulted in higher cellular accumulation of Dox and PTX, an outcome most likely resulting from the internalization of cMLVs by cells through endocytosis [30] and, consequently, effectively bypassing the P-gp efflux pumps. The enhanced cellular accumulation of drugs in dual drug-loaded cMLVs was also observed in drug-resistant JC cells (Figure 2C and 2D) compared to single drug-loaded cMLVs and drug combination in solution. These data suggest that cMLV(Dox+PTX) significantly enhanced the intracellular accumulation of anticancer drugs through mechanisms involving both combination treatment and nanoparticle delivery.

Effect of codelivered nanoparticles on P-gp expression

Having shown that dual drug-loaded cMLVs enhance cellular accumulation of drugs, we next sought to verify that this did, indeed, result from the modulation of membrane pumps, which

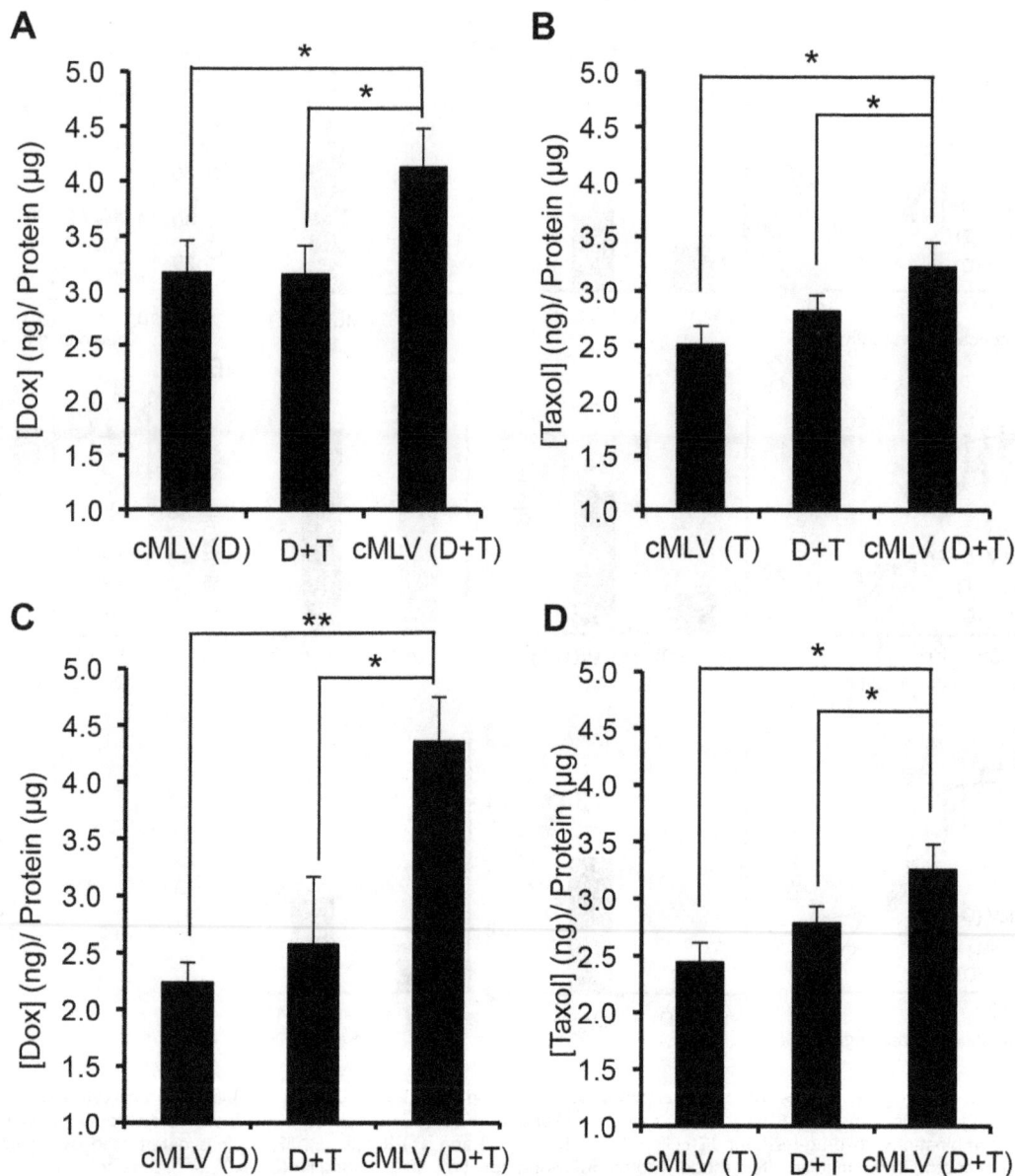

Figure 2. Cellular uptake of Dox and PTX (D: Dox; T: PTX). (A, B) Total cellular uptake of Dox (A) and PTX (B) into 4T1 cells. 4T1 cells were exposed to cMLV(D), cMLV(T), cMLV(D+T), and D+P in solution. The final concentrations of Dox and PTX were 1 µg/ml for each group. (C, D) Total cellular uptake of Dox (C) and PTX (D) in JC cells. JC cells were exposed to cMLV(D), cMLV(T), cMLV(D+T), and D+T. The final concentrations of Dox and PTX were 5 µg/ml for each group. The uptake of Dox and PTX was normalized to protein content measured with the BCA assay. All data are shown as the means of triplicate experiments from three different nanoparticle preparations. Asterisks indicate statistical significance between two groups (*$P < 0.05$, **$P < 0.01$).

are responsible for multidrug resistance. We first measured the expression of P-gp by flow cytometry in 4T1 cells treated with various nanoparticle formulations for 48 h to test if these cMLV formulations were responsible for altering P-gp involvement in multidrug resistance, along with decreased drug accumulation, in cells [3,35]. As shown in Figure 3A, with the single drug-loaded cMLV treatment, the expression of P-gp (in terms of integrated mean fluorescence intensity) increased significantly in 4T1 cells ($p < 0.01$), possibly leading, in turn, to the development of drug resistance in 4T1 cells. However, dual drug-loaded cMLVs significantly inhibited expression of P-gp when compared to that of the single drug-loaded cMLVs and drug combination in

solution ($p < 0.01$), suggesting that the combinatorial delivery of Dox and PTX *via* cMLVs could efficiently suppress P-gp expression, thereby overcoming MDR. We next investigated whether cMLV(Dox+PTX) could inhibit multidrug resistance in JC cells, which exhibit drug-resistant phenotype by overexpression of P-gp [32]. As shown in Figure 3B, the expression of P-gp decreased after 48 h of incubation with JC cells ($p < 0.05$) when treated with single drug-loaded cMLV, indicating that the nanoparticle drug delivery system could, at least partially, suppress MDR. However, the codelivery formulation of cMLV(Dox+PTX) significantly inhibited P-gp expression compared to that of single drug-loaded cMLVs and drug combination in solution ($p < 0.01$).

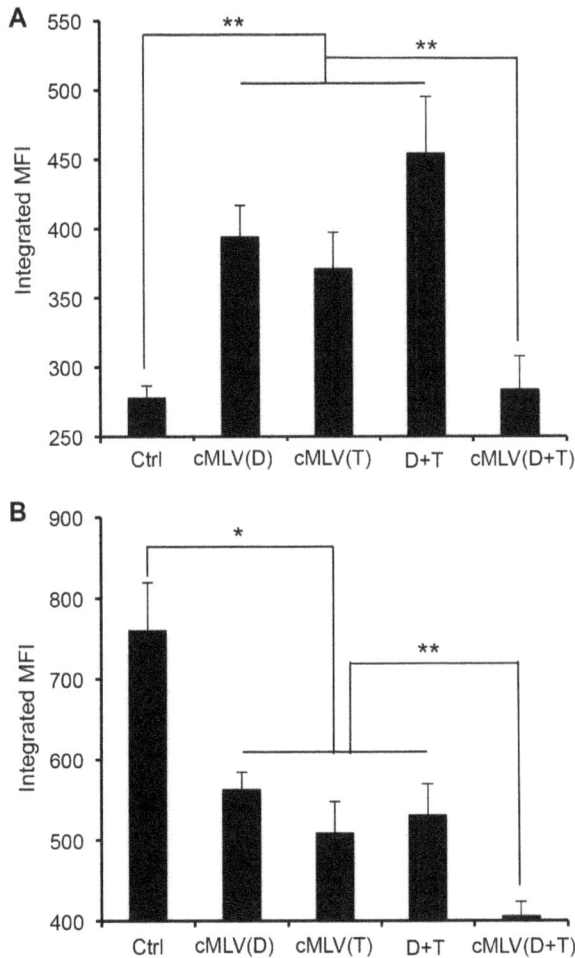

Figure 3. Effect of codelivered nanoparticles on P-gp expression (D: Dox; T: PTX). (A) 4T1 cells were exposed to empty cMLVs (Ctrl), cMLV(D), cMLV(T), cMLV(D+T), and D+T with the same concentration of Dox and PTX (1 µg/ml). (B) JC cells were exposed to empty cMLVs (Ctrl), cMLV(D), cMLV(T), cMLV(D+T), and D+T with the same concentration of Dox and PTX (5 µg/ml). P-gp expression was detected by P-gp-specific antibody *via* flow cytometry. Data are represented as mean ± SD (n = 3). Asterisks indicate statistical significance between two groups (*P < 0.05, **P < 0.01).

Taken together, these results indicated that the codelivery of Dox and PTX via cMLVs could inhibit the expression of P-gp and increase cellular accumulation of drugs, leading to enhanced drug action in cells, including drug-resistant cells.

Efficacy of dual drug-loaded cMLVs against a murine breast cancer model

It has been demonstrated that codelivery of Dox and PTX via cMLVs is able to overcome drug resistance *in vitro*. However, since the *in vivo* environment is considerably more complicated, it remains unknown if this effect could be translated to an animal cancer model. Therefore, in this experiment, a mouse breast tumor model was used to evaluate the therapeutic efficacy of dual drug-loaded cMLVs compared with that of single-drug liposomal formulations. At day 0, BALB/c mice were inoculated subcutaneously with 4T1 breast tumor cells. On day 8, mice bearing tumors were randomly sorted into six groups, and each group was treated with one of the following: PBS (control), cMLV(2 mg/kg

Dox), cMLV(2 mg/kg PTX), cMLV(2 mg/kg Dox)+ cMLV(2 mg/kg PTX), or cMLV(2 mg/kg Dox + 2 mg/kg PTX) every three days. Tumor growth and body weights were monitored until the end of the experiment (Figure 4A).

As shown in Figure 4B, mice in groups receiving cMLV(Dox), cMLV (PTX) or cMLV(Dox)+cMLV(PTX) exhibited tumor inhibition compared to those in the control group ($p < 0.01$). Even more significantly, cMLV(Dox+PTX) treatment induced a greater inhibition than that of cMLV encapsulating a single drug and that of cMLV(Dox)+cMLV(PTX), indicating that codelivery of Dox and PTX through single nanoparticle is essential for overcoming drug resistance ($p < 0.01$). As one indication of systemic toxicity, no weight loss was seen for the cMLV formulation over the duration of the experiment (Figure 4C). The *in vivo* efficacy of dual drug-loaded cMLVs against the 4T1 tumor model was further confirmed by a survival test. As shown in Figure 4D, the groups treated with cMLV(Dox), cMLV(PTX), or cMLV(Dox)+cMLV(PTX) had a prolonged lifespan compared to the control group, while the mice in the group treated with cMLV(Dox+PTX) had a significantly increased lifespan compared to the groups treated with single drug-loaded cMLVs and the group treated with cMLV(Dox) + cMLV(PTX) ($p < 0.01$).

Histology study

To study the antitumor mechanism *in vivo*, a TUNEL assay was carried out to detect tumor cell apoptosis in tumors treated with Dox (5 mg/kg) and/or PTX (5 mg/kg) in various formulations for 3 days. As shown in Figure 5A and Figure 5C, 4T1 tumors treated with cMLV(Dox), cMLV(PTX), and Dox+PTX in solution showed significantly more apoptotic cells compared with controls ($p < 0.01$). The apoptosis index was also significantly higher in the cMLV(Dox+PTX)-treated group as compared with other groups ($p < 0.05$). Thus, the efficacy of cMLV(Dox+PTX) as an antitumor treatment could be explained by data suggesting increased tumor cell apoptosis. To further confirm the induction of cell apoptosis in treated groups, the TUNEL assay was performed in drug-resistant JC tumors treated with various formulations for 3 days. As shown in Figure 5B and 5D, cMLV(Dox), cMLV(PTX), and Dox+PTX induced more apoptotic cells compared to control JC tumors ($p < 0.01$). Dual drug-loaded cMLV-treated JC tumors showed a remarkably higher apoptosis index compared with other groups ($p < 0.01$), again confirming the enhanced antitumor activity of cMLV(Dox+PTX).

To further investigate the innate characteristics of treated tumors, both 4T1 and JC tumor sections from each treatment group were analyzed for the expression of P-gp protein. As shown in Figure 6A, P-gp expression level was moderate in the control group. There appeared to be a significant enhancement of P-gp expression in the cMLV(Dox) and cMLV(PTX) groups, with an even more significant enhancement in Dox+PTX group compared to controls. However, a marked decrease was observed in the cMLV(Dox+PTX)-treated group when compared to the cMLV(Dox), cMLV(PTX), and Dox+PTX groups, as further confirmed by the quantification data in Figure 6C ($p < 0.01$). Interestingly, P-gp was very high in the JC tumor control group, as shown in Figure 6B. However, a significant decrease appeared in the cMLV(Dox), cMLV(PTX), and Dox+PTX groups, as further confirmed by the quantification data in Figure 6D ($p < 0.05$). An even more significant decrease of P-gp expression was seen in the cMLV(Dox+PTX) group ($p < 0.01$), indicating that dual drug-loaded cMLVs might be able to alter the innate characteristics of the multidrug-resistant tumor cells such as JC cells. Taken together, these data show that drug-loaded nanoparticles can partially bypass the P-gp efflux

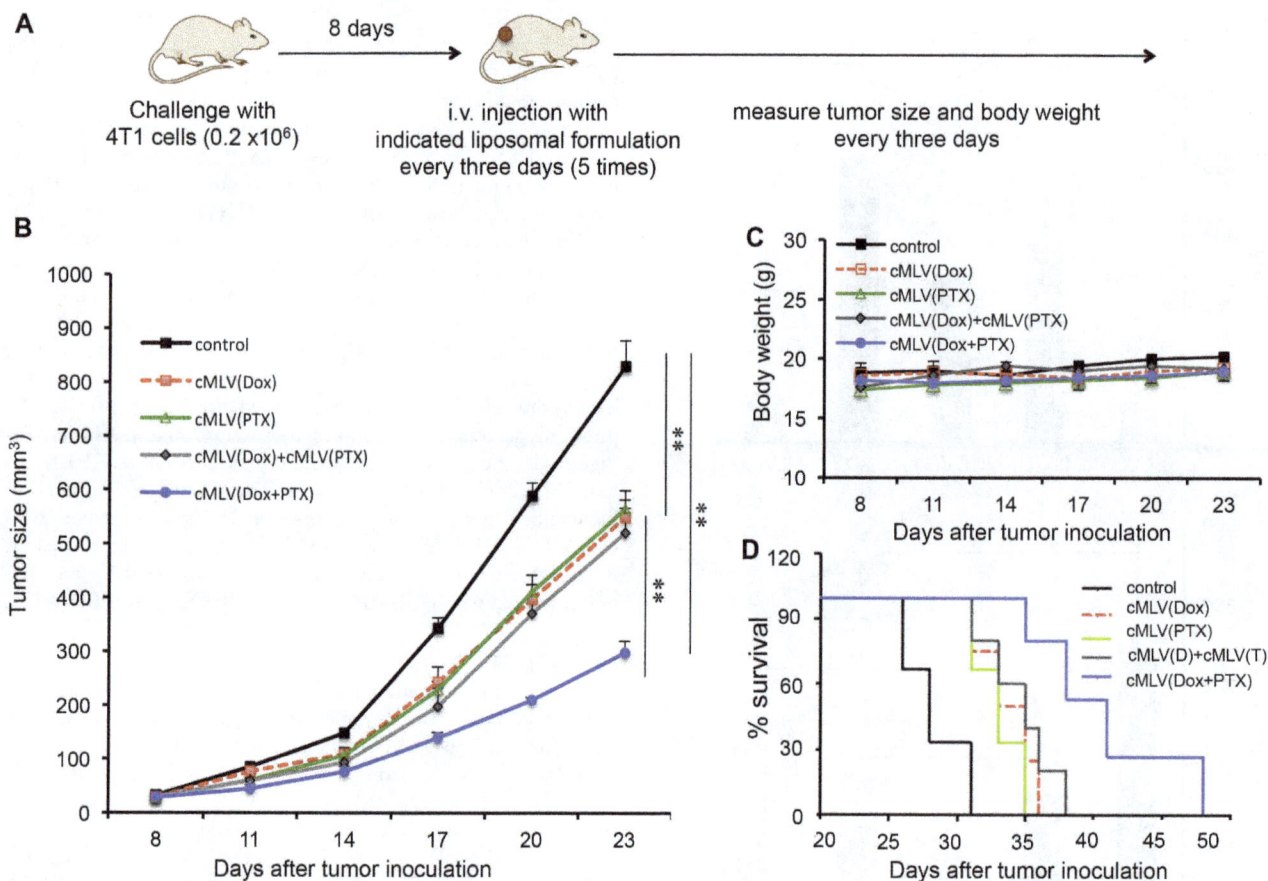

Figure 4. *In vivo* **efficacy of drug combinations** *via* **cMLVs in a 4T1 tumor model.** (A) Schematic diagram of the experimental protocol for *in vivo* 4T1 tumor study in BALB/c mice. (B) Tumor growth was measured after treatment with PBS (control, black solid line), cMLV (2 mg/kg Dox) (red dashed line), cMLV (2 mg/kg PTX) (green solid line), cMLV(2 mg/kg Dox)+cMLV(2 mg/kg PTX) (grey solid line), or cMLV (2 mg/kg Dox+2 mg/kg PTX) (blue solid line). Error bars represent standard error of the mean, n = 6 for each treatment group (**$p < 0.01$). (C) Average mouse weight loss over the duration of the experiment. (D) Survival curves for 4T1-bearing mice treated with PBS (black solid line), cMLV 2 mg/kg Dox) (red dashed line), cMLV (2 mg/kg PTX) (green solid line), cMLV(2 mg/kg Dox)+cMLV(2 mg/kg PTX) (grey solid line), or cMLV (2 mg/kg Dox+2 mg/kg PTX) (blue solid line). Survival end point was set when the tumor volume reached 1000 mm³. The survival rates were presented as Kaplan-Meier curves. The survival curves of individual groups were compared by a log-rank test.

pumps to increase cellular uptake of Dox and PTX, sufficiently inducing cytotoxicity in cancer cells.

It has been reported that Dox treatment results in severe irreversible cardiotoxicity, leading to myocyte apoptosis [36]. In addition, cardiac toxicity, an unexpected clinical outcome of combinatorial Dox and PTX treatment, has been reported [37]. Therefore, systemic toxicity of free Dox+PTX and cMLV(Dox+PTX) was evaluated to determine whether codelived cMLVs could decrease this side effect of combination drug treatment. To accomplish this, a single intravenous dose of either Dox+PTX in solution or cMLV(Dox+PTX) was administered to mice bearing 4T1 tumors. Next, hematoxylin and eosin-stained cardiac tissue sections from each treatment group were examined (Figure S2). Treatment with free Dox (5 mg/kg) and PTX (5 mg/kg) in solution did cause cardiac toxicity, as indicated by myofibril loss, disarray, and cytoplasmic vacuolization. However, when cMLV(5 mg/kg Dox+5 mg/kg PTX) was administered under the same experimental conditions *via* cMLVs, no visible loss of myocardial tissue was observed.

Discussion

Chemotherapeutics are crucial to combating a variety of cancers; however, clinical outcomes are always poor, as cancer cells develop a multidrug resistance (MDR) phenotype after several rounds of exposure to the chemotherapeutics. Many efforts have been made to develop a therapeutic strategy to overcome tumor MDR through the use of combined therapeutics to enhance the efficiency of systemic drug delivered to the tumor site and lower the apoptotic threshold. In this study, we have examined augmentation of therapeutic efficacy upon co-administration of Dox and PTX using a crosslinked multilamellar liposomal vesicle (cMLV) in breast cancer cells and drug-resistant JC cells. We demonstrated that combination therapy of Dox and PTX, especially when codelivered in cMLV formulations, was effective in enhancing the cytotoxicity in both wild-type and drug-resistant cells by elevating the cellular accumulation and retention of the drugs. We also showed that the dual therapeutic strategy efficiently suppressed tumor growth by enhancing apoptotic response.

P-glycoprotein (P-gp), a membrane-bound active drug efflux pump, is considered one of the most important mechanisms involved in MDR [3,35]. As a result, growing interest has been

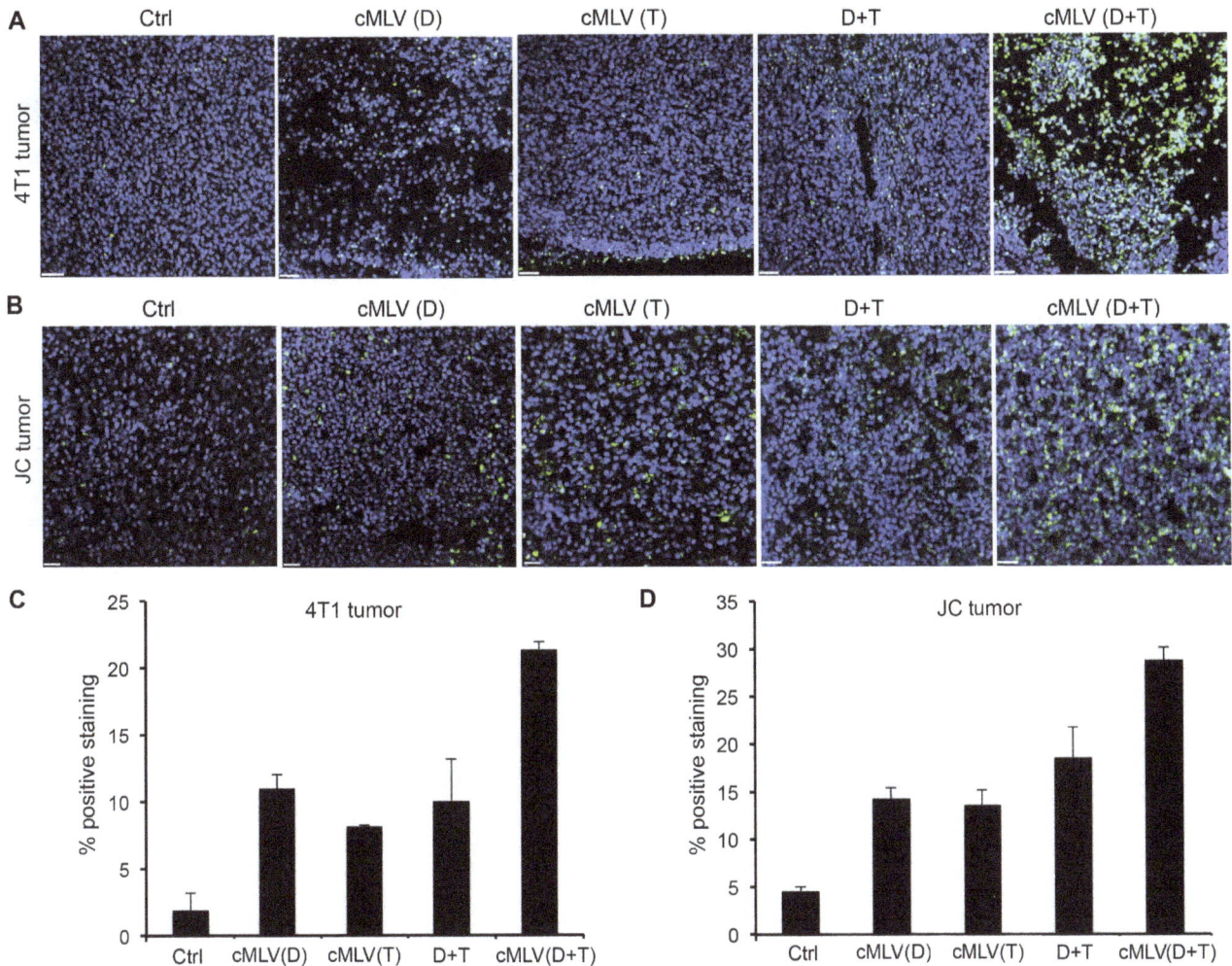

Figure 5. Effect of codelivered cMLVs on tumor apoptosis (D: Dox; T: PTX). (A, B) Mice bearing either 4T1 tumor (A) or multidrug-resistant JC tumor (B) were injected intravenously through the tail vein with cMLV (5 mg/kg Dox), cMLV (5 mg/kg PTX), 5 mg/kg Dox + 5 mg/kg PTX, or cMLV (5 mg/kg Dox+5 mg/kg PTX). Three days after injection, tumors were excised. Apoptotic cells were detected by a TUNEL assay (green), followed by nuclear costaining with DAPI (blue). Scale bar represents 50 μm. (C, D) Quantification of apoptotic cells in 4T1 (C) and JC (D) tumors. To quantify TUNEL-positive cells, 4 regions of interest (ROI) were randomly chosen per image at ×2 magnification. Within one region, area of TUNEL-positive nuclei and area of nuclear staining were counted. The data are expressed as % total nuclear area stained by TUNEL in the region. Data are represented as mean ± SD (n = 3).

shown in the development of nanoparticle drug delivery systems to overcome MDR. With their unique properties, nanoparticles are able to passively target the tumor mass through the enhanced permeability and retention (EPR) effect, enhancing the accumulation of chemotherapeutics at target sites [23,24]. In addition, nanoparticles can enter cells through the endocytosis pathway, which is thought to be independent of the P-gp pathway, thus increasing the cellular uptake and retention of therapeutics in resistant cancer cells [26,27]. Previously, we demonstrated the advantage of cMLVs in cancer therapy over conventional liposomal formulations based on their sustained drug release, enhanced vesicle stability and improved drug release, resulting in improved therapeutic activity with reduced systemic toxicity [30]. Further investigation of this novel liposomal formulation showed that it enable to translate the synergistic combination effect from in vitro to in vivo antitumor efficiency [31]. Moreover, cMLVs are internalized by tumor cells through caveolin-mediated endocytosis [30], suggesting that cMLVs could be an efficient drug carrier to overcome MDR. In this study, our *in vitro* and *in vivo* results

demonstrated that the co-administration of Dox and PTX at the synergistic ratio (1:1) *via* cMLVs efficiently suppressed P-gp expression in both wild-type and drug-resistant cancer cells.

In addition to nanodelivery, another potential strategy to overcome MDR has resulted from combining multiple drugs. For example, the combination of Dox and PTX in a cocktail is a standard anthracycline-taxane treatment regimen and was found to be efficacious in treating a variety of tumors by reducing the individual drug concentration that would otherwise be required to achieve cytotoxicity, thus overcoming drug resistance [13,14,15]. However, its clinical outcome was limited by the un-coordinated biodistribution of combined drugs [16,17] and increase in cardiac cytotoxicity [37]. In this study, the pharmacokinetics of Dox and PTX was unified through the encapsulation of both drugs into a single cMLV particle, resulting in dual drug-loaded cMLVs which successfully reduced P-gp expression, increased the cellular accumulation of drugs, and enhanced cytotoxicity in cancer cells, including drug-resistant cells, as compared to single drug-loaded cMLVs. Moreover, combination therapy of Dox and PTX

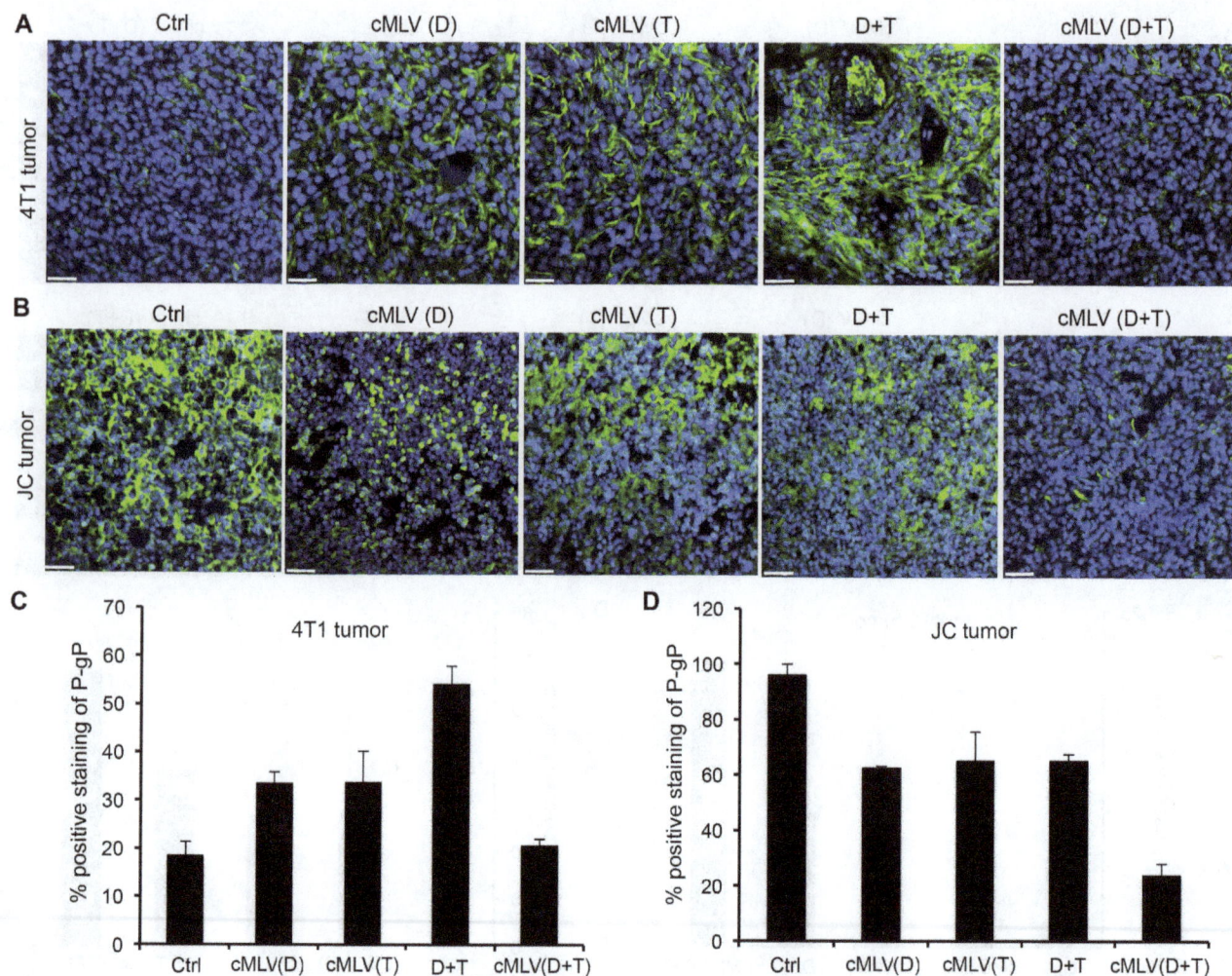

Figure 6. Effect of codelivered cMLVs on P-gp expression in tumors. (A, B) Mice bearing 4T1 tumor (A) and multidrug-resistant tumor JC (B) were injected intravenously through the tail vein with cMLV (5 mg/kg Dox), cMLV (5 mg/kg PTX), 5 mg/kg Dox + 5 mg/kg PTX, or cMLV (5 mg/kg Dox+5 mg/kg PTX). Three days after injection, tumors were excised, and stained by P-gp-specific antibody (green), followed by nuclear costaining with DAPI (blue). Scale bar represents 50 μm. (C, D) Quantification of P-gp-positive cells in 4T1 (C) and JC (D) tumors. To quantify P-gp-positive cells, 4 regions of interest (ROI) were randomly chosen per image at ×2 magnification. Within one region, area of P-gp-positive nuclei and area of nuclear staining were counted. The data are expressed as % total nuclear area that is P-gp-positive in the region. Data are represented as mean ± SD (n = 3).

administered in cMLV formulations showed increased efficacy over cMLV monotherapy in the suppression of tumor growth by promoting apoptotic response *in vivo*.

Conclusion

In summary, we have developed a multimodal therapeutic strategy to overcome tumor MDR by codelivery of Dox and PTX *via* a crosslinked multilamellar liposomal vesicle. We demonstrated that such combinatorial delivery system increased therapeutic efficacy by enhancing delivery efficiency to tumors and lowering the apoptotic threshold of individual drugs, thus overcoming drug resistance. The properties of cMLVs, such as improved stability and sustained release of drugs, enable the nanoparticles to sufficiently accumulate at tumor sites, subsequently entering tumor cells *via* endocytosis to release therapeutics, thus potentially bypassing the P-gp pathway to enhance cellular retention of therapeutics. Moreover, cMLVs enable multidrug delivery to the same action site, thereby lowering the tumor apoptotic threshold of individual therapeutics and potentially inhibiting the MDR.

Taken together, this dual drug-loaded cMLV approach shows promise for reducing MDR in cancer therapeutics.

Supporting Information

Figure S1 IC50 values of cMLV(Dox), cMLV(PTX) and cMLV(Dox+PTX) in B16 melanoma, 4T1 breast tumor cells, or drug-resistant JC cancer cells.

Figure S2 Histologic appearance (hematoxylin and eosin staining) of heart tissues by light microscopy isolated on day 3 after a single intravenous injection of PBS (left), 5 mg/kg Dox+5 mg/kg PTX in solution (middle) and cMLV(5 mg/kg Dox+5 mg/kg PTX) (right).

Acknowledgments

We thank the USC NanoBiophysics Core Facility. We also thank Jennifer Rohrs for critical reading of the manuscript.

Author Contributions

Conceived and designed the experiments: YL PW. Performed the experiments: YL JF KJ. Analyzed the data: YL JF KJ. Contributed reagents/materials/analysis tools: MW PW. Contributed to the writing of the manuscript: YL PW.

References

1. Szakács G, Paterson JK, Ludwig JA, Booth-Genthe C, Gottesman MM (2006) Targeting multidrug resistance in cancer. Nat Rev Drug Discov 5: 219–234.
2. Teicher BA (2009) Acute and chronic in vivo therapeutic resistance. Biochem Pharmacol: 1665–1673.
3. Fletcher JI, Haber M, Henderson MJ, Norris MD (2010) ABC transporters in cancer: more than just drug efflux pumps. Nat Rev Cancer 10: 147–156.
4. Schöndorf T, Kurbacher C, Göhring U, Benz C, Becker M, et al. (2002) Induction of MDR1-gene expression by antineoplastic agents in ovarian cancer cell lines. Anticancer Res 22: 2199–2203.
5. Lespine A, Ménez C, Bourguinat C, Prichard RK (2012) P-glycoproteins and other multidrug resistance transporters in the pharmacology of anthelmintics: Prospects for reversing transport-dependent anthelmintic resistance. Int J Parasitol Drugs Drug Resist 2: 230–270.
6. Chen Y, Bathula SR, Li J, Huang L (2010) Multifunctional nanoparticles delivering small interfering RNA and doxorubicin overcome drug resistance in cancer. J Biol Chem 285: 22639–22650.
7. Xu D, McCarty D, Fernandes A, Fisher M, Samulski RJ, et al. (2005) Delivery of MDR1 small interfering RNA by self-complementary recombinant adeno-associated virus vector. Mol Ther 11: 523–530.
8. Hubensack M, Müller C, Höcherl P, Fellner S, Spruss T, et al. (2008) Effect of the ABCB1 modulators elacridar and tariquidar on the distribution of paclitaxel in nude mice. J Cancer Res Clin Oncol 134: 597–607.
9. Liu Y, Rohrs J, Wang P (2014) Development and challenges of nanovectors in gene therapy. Nano LIFE 4: 1441007.
10. Lehar J, Krueger AS, Avery W, Heilbut AM, Johansen LM, et al. (2009) Synergistic drug combinations tend to improve therapeutically relevant selectivity. Nat biotechnol 27: 659–666.
11. Calabrò F, Lorusso V, Rosati G, Manzione L, Frassinet iL, et al. (2009) Gemcitabine and paclitaxel every 2 weeks in patients with previously untreated urothelial carcinoma. Cancer 115: 2652–2659.
12. Mamounas EP, Sledge GW Jr (2001) Combined anthracycline-taxane regimens in the adjuvant setting. Semin Oncol 28: 24–31.
13. Dean-Colomb W, Esteva F (2008) Emerging agents in the treatment of anthracycline- and taxane-refractory metastatic breast cancer. Semin Oncol 35(2 Suppl 2): S31–38.
14. De Laurentiis M, Cancello G, D'Agostino D, Giuliano M, Giordano A, et al. (2008) Taxane-based combinations as adjuvant chemotherapy of early breast cancer: a meta-analysis of randomized trials. J Clin Oncol 26: 44–53.
15. Kataja V, Castiglione M (2008) ESMO Guidelines Working Group Locally recurrent or metastatic breast cancer: ESMO clinical recommendations for diagnosis, treatment and follow-up. Ann Oncol 19(2 suppl): ii11–ii13.
16. Grasselli G, Viganò L, Capri G, Locatelli A, Tarenzi E, et al. (2001) Clinical and pharmacologic study of the epirubicin and paclitaxel combination in women with meta-static breast cancer. J Clin Oncol 19: 2222–2231.
17. Gustafson DL, Andrea L Merz, Long ME (2005) Pharmacokinetics of combined doxorubicin and paclitaxel in mice. Cancer Letters 220: 161–169.
18. Ahmed F, Pakunlu RI, Brannan A, Bates F, Minko T, et al. (2006) Biodegradable polymersomes loaded with both paclitaxel and doxorubicin permeate and shrink tumors, inducing apoptosis in proportion to accumulated drug. J Control Release 116: 150–158.
19. Sengupta S, Eavarone D, Capila I, Zhao G, Watson N, et al. (2005) Temporal targeting of tumour cells and neovasculature with a nanoscale delivery system. Nature 436: 568–572.
20. Wang H, Zhao Y, Wu Y, Hu Y-l, Nan K, et al. (2011) Enhanced anti-tumor efficacy by co-delivery of doxorubicin and paclitaxel with amphiphilic methoxy PEG-PLGA copolymer nanoparticles. Biomaterials 32: 8281–8290.
21. Gao H, Zhang Z, Yu Z, He Q (2014) Cell-penetrating peptide based intelligent liposomal systems for enhanced drug delivery. Curr Pharm Biotechnol 15: 210–219.
22. Yu Z, Schmaltz RM, Bozeman TC, Paul R, Rishel MJ, et al. (2013) Selective tumor cell targeting by the disaccharide moiety of bleomycin. J Am Chem Soc 135: 2883–2886.
23. Cho K, Wang X, Nie S, Chen ZG, Shin DM (2008) Therapeutic nanoparticles for drug delivery in cancer. Clin Cancer Res 14: 1310–1316.
24. Ferrari M (2005) Cancer nanotechnology: opportunities and challenges. Nat Rev Cancer 5: 161–171.
25. Dobson PD, Kell DB (2008) Carrier-mediated cellular uptake of pharmaceutical drugs: an exception or the rule? Nat Rev Drug Discov 7: 205–210.
26. Hillaireau H, Couvreur P (2009) Nanocarriers' entry into the cell: relevance to drug delivery. Cell Mo Life Sci 66: 2873–2896.
27. Sahay G, Alakhova DY, Kabanov AV (2010) Endocytosis of nanomedicines. J Control Release 145: 182–195.
28. Torchilin VP (2005) Recent Advances with Liposomes as Pharmaceutical Carriers. Nat Rev Drug Discov 4: 145–160.
29. Liu Y, Ji M, Wong MK, Joo K-I, Wang P (2013) Enhanced therapeutic efficacy of iRGD-conjugated crosslinked multilamellar liposomes for drug delivery. BioMed Research International 2013: 378380.
30. Joo K, Xiao L, Liu S, Liu Y, Lee C, et al. (2013) Crosslinked multilamellar liposomes for controlled delivery of anticancer drugs. Biomaterials 34: 3098–3109.
31. Liu Y, Fang J, Kim Y-J, Wong MK, Wang P (2014) Codelivery of doxorubicin and paclitaxel by cross-linked multilamellar liposome enables synergistic antitumor activity. Mol Pharmaceutics 11: 1651–1661.
32. Lee B, French K, Zhuang Y, Smith C (2003) Development of a syngeneic in vivo tumor model and its use in evaluating a novel P-glycoprotein modulator, PGP-4008. Oncol Res 14: 49–60.
33. Goutelle S, Maurin M, Rougier l, Barbaut X, Bourguignon L, et al. (2008) The Hill equation: a review of its capabilities in pharmacological modelling. Fundam Clin Pharmacol 22: 633–648.
34. Shen L, Peterson S, Sedaghat AR, McMahon MA, Callender M, et al. (2008) Dose-response curve slope sets class-specific limits on inhibitory potential of anti-HIV drugs. Nat Med 14: 762–766.
35. Robey RW, To KK, Polgar O, Dohse M, Fetsch P, et al. (2009) ABCG2: a perspective. Adv Drug Deliv Rev 61: 3–13.
36. Rahman AM, Yusuf SW, Ewer MS (2007) Anthracycline-induced cardiotoxicity and the cardiac-sparing effect of liposomal formulation. Int J Nanomedicine 2: 567–583.
37. Bird B, Swain S (2008) Cardiac toxicity in breast cancer survivors: review of potential cardiac problems. Clin Cancer Res 14: 14–24.

8

Presumptive Treatment of Malaria from Formal and Informal Drug Vendors in Nigeria

Chinwoke Isiguzo[1]*, Jennifer Anyanti[2], Chinazo Ujuju[1], Ernest Nwokolo[3], Anna De La Cruz[4], Eric Schatzkin[4], Sepideh Modrek[5], Dominic Montagu[6], Jenny Liu[4]

1 Research and Evaluation Division, Society for Family Health, Abuja, Nigeria, 2 Technical Services Division, Society for Family Health, Abuja, Nigeria, 3 Global Fund Malaria Division, Society for Family Health, Abuja, Nigeria, 4 The Global Health Group, University of California San Francisco, San Francisco, California, United States of America, 5 General Medical Disciplines, Stanford University School of Medicine, Palo Alto, California, United States of America, 6 Epidemiology and Biostatistics, University of California San Francisco, San Francisco, California, United States of America

Abstract

Background: Despite policies that recommend parasitological testing before treatment for malaria, presumptive treatment remains widespread in Nigeria. The majority of Nigerians obtain antimalarial drugs from two types of for-profit drug vendors—formal and informal medicine shops—but little is known about the quality of malaria care services provided at these shops.

Aims: This study seeks to (1) describe the profile of patients who seek treatment at different types of drug outlets, (2) document the types of drugs purchased for treating malaria, (3) assess which patients are purchasing recommended drugs, and (4) estimate the extent of malaria over-treatment.

Methods: In urban, peri-urban, and rural areas in Oyo State, customers exiting proprietary and patent medicine vendor (PPMV) shops or pharmacies having purchased anti-malarial drugs were surveyed and tested with malaria rapid diagnostic test. A follow-up phone survey was conducted four days after to assess self-reported drug administration. Bivariate and multivariate regression analysis was conducted to determine the correlates of patronizing a PPMV versus pharmacy, and the likelihood of purchasing an artemisinin-combination therapy (ACT) drug.

Results: Of the 457participants who sought malaria treatment in 49 enrolled outlets, nearly 92% had diagnosed their condition by themselves, a family member, or a friend. Nearly 60% pharmacy customers purchased an ACT compared to only 29% of PPMV customers, and pharmacy customers paid significantly more on average. Multivariate regression results show that patrons of PPMVs were younger, less wealthy, waited fewer days before seeking care, and were less likely to be diagnosed at a hospital, clinic, or laboratory. Only 3.9% of participants tested positive with a malaria rapid diagnostic test.

Conclusions: Poorer individuals seeking care at PPMVs are more likely to receive inappropriate malaria treatment when compared to those who go to pharmacies. Increasing accessibility to reliable diagnosis should be explored to reduce malaria over-treatment.

Editor: Henk D. F. H. Schallig, Royal Tropical Institute, Netherlands

Funding: The authors wish to acknowledge ExxonMobil for financial support of this study as well as the Global Fund to Fight AIDS, Tuberculosis and Malaria for provision of RDTs and ACTs for the study. The funders had no role in study design, data collection and analysis, decision to publish, or preparation of the manuscript.

Competing Interests: This study was funded in part by ExxonMobil. There are no patents, products in development or marketed products to declare.

* Email: cisiguzo@sfhnigeria.org

Introduction

Nigeria bears one of the world's highest burdens of malaria, accounting for a quarter of all cases in Africa [1]. It is estimated that over half of Nigeria's population experiences at least one episode of malaria each year, accounting for approximately 20% of all hospital admission, 30% of outpatient visits, and 10% of hospital deaths [2]. This burden of disease strains the resources of the health system as spending on malaria treatment and prevention accounts for nearly 50% of all health expenditures in Nigeria [3].

To effectively diagnose and treat malaria, the World Health Organization (WHO) currently recommends a confirmatory blood test for all suspected cases of malaria and prescription of artemisinin-based combination therapy (ACT) upon confirmation of malaria positivity [4]. ACTs are currently the most effective antimalarial treatment and are becoming more widely available in Nigeria [5]. However, many health care providers in Nigeria continue to prescribe less-effective drugs, such as chloroquine (CQ) and sulfadoxine-pyrimethamine (SP), for uncomplicated cases of malaria [6]. Despite the increased availability of malaria rapid diagnostic tests (RDTs) to facilitate point-of-care diagnosis elsewhere in sub-Saharan Africa [7–11], RDTs are not yet widely available in Nigeria [12] and presumptive diagnosis continues to be the most common method for determining a patient's malaria status [13].

This study aims to better characterize the practice of presumptive treatment of malaria in Nigeria and determine where interventions for malaria treatment delivery should be targeted. Nearly 60% of Nigerians seek treatment for malaria at drug shop outlets in the private healthcare sector [14]. Of these vendors, the minority is composed of licensed pharmacies, which are either owned or staffed by formally trained pharmacists, and which are mainly found in urban centers. The majority of vendors are informally trained, loosely regulated proprietary and patent medicine vendors (PPMVs), which are frequently the only source of drugs in rural areas [14–16]. While both types of vendors mainly operate as drug retailers, the quality of health services offered can vastly differ. PPMVs are legally permitted to only sell a number of medications over-the-counter, including antimalarial medications, but recent assessments show that they often do not stock ACTs, and have limited knowledge of malaria symptoms and recommended treatment guidelines [17]. In contrast, pharmacists are perceived to offer higher-quality malaria care services than PPMVs [18], although little empirical evidence exists to corroborate these views.

When choosing the type of facility at which to seek care, patients may prioritize convenience, availability of familiar drugs, and affordability [18]. While hospitals and clinics may provide higher quality care and testing, long wait and travel times often drive patients to accessible, nearby drug vendors. Similarly, there is little demand for confirmatory malaria microscopy testing, leading many people to bypass hospital/clinics or costly independent diagnostic laboratories [19].

Because private sector drug vendors are the source for such a large proportion of Nigeria's population seeking malaria care, it is important to understand the extent to which individuals seeking treatment for malaria are able to receive accurate diagnosis and treatment at pharmacies and PPMVs [20]. It is also important to understand what types of consumers may be at most risk for receiving poor quality services. Consequently, this study seeks to (1) describe and compare the profile of patients who seek treatment at PPMVs versus pharmacies, (2) document the types of drugs purchased for treating malaria, (3) assess which patients are purchasing recommended ACTs, and (4) estimate the extent of malaria over-treatment [21]. Implications of findings for targeting appropriate diagnostic and treatment interventions are discussed.

Materials and Methods

Ethical considerations

The Nigerian Health Research Ethical Review Committee (NHREC Approval Number NHREC/01/01/2007-30/08/2012) and the University of California, San Francisco's Committee for Human Research approved all study protocols. Data collectors obtained written informed consent from study participants and shop proprietors where the customers were recruited. Written consent was obtained from shop proprietors via signature and customers via signature or fingerprint for non-literate customers. The consent procedure was approved by the Nigerian Health Research Ethical Review Committee and the University of California, San Francisco's Committee for Human Research. Funding sponsors for the study did have any role in the study design, execution, or publication.

Study area and sample selection

The study was conducted in Oyo State, located in the Southwest geopolitical zone of Nigeria, comprised of about 4.5million people (predominantly of Yoruba descent) [13]. Four local government areas (LGAs) were purposefully selected for the study to include urban, semi-urban, and rural areas: Ibadan South East (urban) andEgbeda (semi-urban) in and around the Ibadancity area, whileOgbomosho South and OgoOluwa were selected in and around the Ogbomosho town area (rural). All PPMV and pharmaceutical shops were first enumerated within the four selected LGAs and a total number of 236 PPMVs and 24 pharmaceutical shops were identified during the enumeration exercise. Interviewers used a questionnaire that captured the names, addresses, location (urban, seri-urban, rural), LGA, GPS coordinates, notable landmarks, and size of outlets ('small' for outlets with two shelves of medicines; 'medium' for outlets with three to four shelves of medicine; 'large' for outlets with more than five shelves).

From the complete list of shops, a total of fifty pharmacies and PPMVs were randomly selected, stratified by the size of medicinal stock (i.e. small, medium, and large). Selected shops were visited to inform shop owners of the study aims and obtain permission to recruit exiting customers into the study. Enrolled study sites were later modified to exclude 24 small PPMV drug retailers in Ibadan whose main business was not medicinal sales (thus participants were not able to be recruited) and replaced with randomly selected PPMV shops in Ibadan North East LGA. Using a standard script, 49 out of 50 selected private sector retailers (42shop in/around Ibadan, 7shops in/around Ogbomosho) agreedto havetheir shop used for participant recruitment and were enrolled into the study; only one pharmacy declined to participatefor reasons not stated. The final roster of recruitment sites consisted of 21 pharmacies and 23 PPMVs. All seven shops enrolled in Ogbomosho were PPMVs as the city did not have any pharmacies during site enumeration.

Two members of the survey team, one trained nurse and one researcher, were stationed at enrolled PPMVs and pharmacies on randomly selected days of the week (excluding Sunday) and approached customers as they exited the drug store to assess eligibility. The inclusion criteria were as follows: the participant must be a non-pregnant adult having purchased treatment for malaria for him-or herself and be willing to complete a 15-minute survey. Malaria "treatment" was defined to mean any drug purchased by the customer that s/he intended to take for their current episode of suspected malaria, which may include inappropriate drugs for malaria and not necessarily an antimalarial drug. While seeking consent, the participant was informed that if they qualified, they would be offered a RDT and would be compensated for their time with a small mobile phone credit of 200 Naira (~US$1.20) for participating in the interview.

Data collection

Two surveys were conducted, one at the time of enrollment and testing (i.e. baseline) and one after four days of the initial encounter via telephone call(i.e. follow-up). All data were collected concurrently. At baseline, the eligible participant was offered a RDT performed by a trained nurse at the beginning of the survey. While the RDT result was pending (about 15 minutes), a detailed survey was conducted designed to capture information on the background demographics and socioeconomic stats, symptoms experienced, and care-seeking actions taken for the current and past episodes of suspected malaria. Contact information was also collected during enrollment to facilitate later follow-up. At the end of the survey, the participant was provided with the result of his or her test.

Nurses were instructed to provide participants with standard advice according to their RDT results. If the participant tested positive for malaria, he/she was told that the positive result suggests the presence of malaria. Per ethical considerations to ensure that the participants testing positive had a quality-assured anti-malaria drug, a free course of ACTs was provided and participants were instructed to take it according to the recommended dosage protocol. If the test was negative, the participant was told that the negative result indicates the absence of malaria and that anti-malarial drugs they purchased were not needed. Regardless of the test result, all participants were referred to local clinics and hospitals where they could seek care if their condition was not malaria, or if their illness became worse. All participants were told to expect a short 5–10 minute follow up phone call in four days to check on the status of their illness and that they would be compensated with a small phone credit of 100 Naira (~US$0.60)for taking the call.

Four days after the baseline survey, a nurse called the participants and conducted a phone survey to obtain information on the state of their health and the drugs they had used. A total of 465 adults were enrolled in the baseline survey, but eight were excluded due to survey numbering errors, and 424 participated in the follow-up phone survey—a follow-up retention rate of 92.8%. No differences in individual characteristics between attritted and retained participants were detected; detailed sample attrition are described elsewhere [22].

Data Analysis

Descriptive data analysis. Descriptive analysis was used for the study to review the sample for basic socio demographic characteristics, reasons for choosing the drug shop, and drugs purchased and taken. Wealth distribution was assessed using standard principal components analysis (PCA) [23] in two ways. First, to compare the representativeness of the study sample to the overall state and national sample, weights associated with PCA component items generated from the 2010 Nigeria Malaria Indicator Survey (MIS) were applied to comparable asset indicators collected in the study sample to compute a wealth index that reflected the national wealth distribution. This index was then converted to quintile categorical indicators for comparing external sample representativeness. A second wealth index was created using only the study sample via the same PCA technique and converted to quintile indicators to obtain an even, within-sample distribution of wealth.

Regression Analysis. Two types of regression analyses were conducted. First, we estimated bivariate and multivariate logistic regressions to assess differences in the types of individuals that patron different types of drug shops—PPMVs versus pharmacies. The likelihood that a PPMV was chosen was predicted by the individual's age, sex, educational attainment, marital status, and wealth. In addition to basic socio demographics, employment status (i.e. full-time wage worker, part-time wage worker, self-employed, and unemployed) was included as shop owners indicated that customers tend to stop at drug shops on their way to and from work. Self-reported symptoms felt for the current illness episode, the number of days waited before seeking care, and where the recognition of the illness as malaria came from (i.e. myself/relative/friend, a hospital/clinic/diagnostic laboratory, or at a drug retailer) were also included because these factors may influence the choice of drug shop type based on perceived severity, need for drug administration, or recommendations by diagnosticians. Second, the likelihood of buying an ACT was predicted

using logistic regression analysis. In addition to individual characteristics described above, the type of shop (i.e. PPMV vs. pharmacy) was included as a risk factor for receiving the recommended first-line malaria drug. In both analyses, only statistically significant explanatory variables at the 5% level in bivariate analysis were included in the multivariate model. To account for autocorrelation between individuals recruited at the same shop, standard errors were clustered at the shop level. Odds ratios are reported.

Findings

Sample characteristics

Of the 457participants who sought malaria treatment from the 49enrolled shops, 71.1% (n = 325) were recruited in Ibadan, 55.6% (n = 254) were under the age of 40 (median = 37; range: 18–82), 50.8% were male (n = 232), and 68.1% (n = 311) were married. Only 22.5% (n = 103) had primary education or less; 39.8% (n = 182) completed secondary education and 37.6% (n = 172) had some tertiary level education. Among those interviewed, 31.3% (n = 143) were employed either on a full-time or part-time basis; 53.6% were self-employed (n = 245) and 15.1% were unemployed (n = 69). Participants reported feeling a variety of symptoms during their current episode of illness. Fever was most commonly reported (74.6%, n = 341), followed by body aches, chills, or convulsions (57.5%, n = 263), feeling weak, fatigued, or having little appetite (55.8%, n = 255). Nearly half of participants waited one day (18.7%, n = 79) or less (28.7%; n = 122) before seeking care; 34.3% (n = 146) waited three days or more. Nearly 92% (n = 423) of the participants reported that they had diagnosed the episode of malaria by themselves, a family member, or a friend. See Table 1 for a summary of the sample characteristics.

When comparing the wealth distribution between sampled individuals to that of the state and national populations captured by the 2010 MIS, those in the wealthiest quintile are disproportionately represented in the study sample. Based on the composite asset ownership measure, no individuals in the study sample were from the lowest two wealth quintiles of nation as seen in Figure 1. Although the population of Oyo State, and particularly in urban areas, is also comprised of households that are much wealthier than the nation as a whole, the study sample's wealth composition is even more concentrated among the wealthiest.

Types of medicines purchased for malaria treatment

Table 2 summarizes the types of drugs purchased at PPMVs and pharmacies for the current episode of suspected malaria among participants who agreed to have their drugs examined by the study nurse (n = 423). A significantly higher percentage of the patrons of pharmacies (57.4%, n = 132/230) purchased an ACT compared to only 28.5% (n = 55/193) of PPMV patrons (p<0.01). Of non-ACT antimalarials purchased, significantly more customers at PPMVs (47.7%; n = 92/230) purchased SP than customers of pharmacies (28.7%, n = 66/193; p<0.05). A higher percentage of PPMV customers also bought a non-malaria drug (70.1%, n = 136/194) compared to pharmacy customers (54.7%, n = 129/236). Significantly fewer analgesics (76.0%, n = 98/230), but more vitamins/supplements (85.3%, n = 110/230) and antibiotics (20.9%, n = 27/230) were purchased at pharmacies than at PPMVs (respectively: 92.6%, n = 126/193; 60.3%, n = 82/193; 5.9%, n = 8/193). More patrons of pharmacies bought only an antimalarial (45.3%, n = 107/230) compared to those at PPMVs (29.9%, n = 58/193). However, pharmacy customers paid significantly more for all of their drugs than those purchasing at PPMVs on average.

Table 1. Customer demographic and socioeconomic variables (N = 457).

Variable		N	%
Site	Ogbomosho	132	28.9
	Ibadan	325	71.1
Age of respondents	18–29	127	27.8
	30–39	127	27.8
	40–49	100	21.9
	50+	103	22.5
Sex	Male	232	50.8
	Female	227	49.2
Education	No education	130	28.4
	Primary education	13	2.8
	Secondary education	245	53.6
	Higher education	69	15.1
Marital status	Not married	146	31.9
	Married	311	68.1
Employment status	Employed full time	130	28.4
	Employed part time	13	2.8
	Self-employed	245	53.6
	Unemployed	69	15.1
Wealth quintile[1]	Poorest	90	19.7
	Second	92	20.1
	Third	93	20.4
	Fourth	90	19.7
	Richest	92	20.1
Symptoms reported			
Fever, headache, dizziness	Yes	341	74.6
	No	116	25.4
Body aches, chills, convulsions	Yes	263	57.5
	No	194	42.5
Weak, fatigue, no appetite	Yes	255	55.8
	No	202	44.2
Bitter taste in the mouth	Yes	62	13.6
	No	395	86.4
Congestion, shallow breathing	Yes	58	12.7
	No	399	87.3
Vomiting, diarrhea	Yes	54	11.8
	No	403	88.2
Other: blisters, dark urine, yellow eyes	Yes	63	13.8
	No	394	86.2
Number of days waited before seeking care[2]	<1 day	122	28.7
	1 day	79	18.7
	2 days	77	18.2
	3–5 days	104	24.5
	6 days or more	42	9.8
Source of diagnosis	Self-diagnosis	418	91.5
	Hospital/clinic/lab	20	4.4
	Pharmacy/PPMV	19	4.2

[1]Result of within-sample principle components analysis.
[2]N = 424.

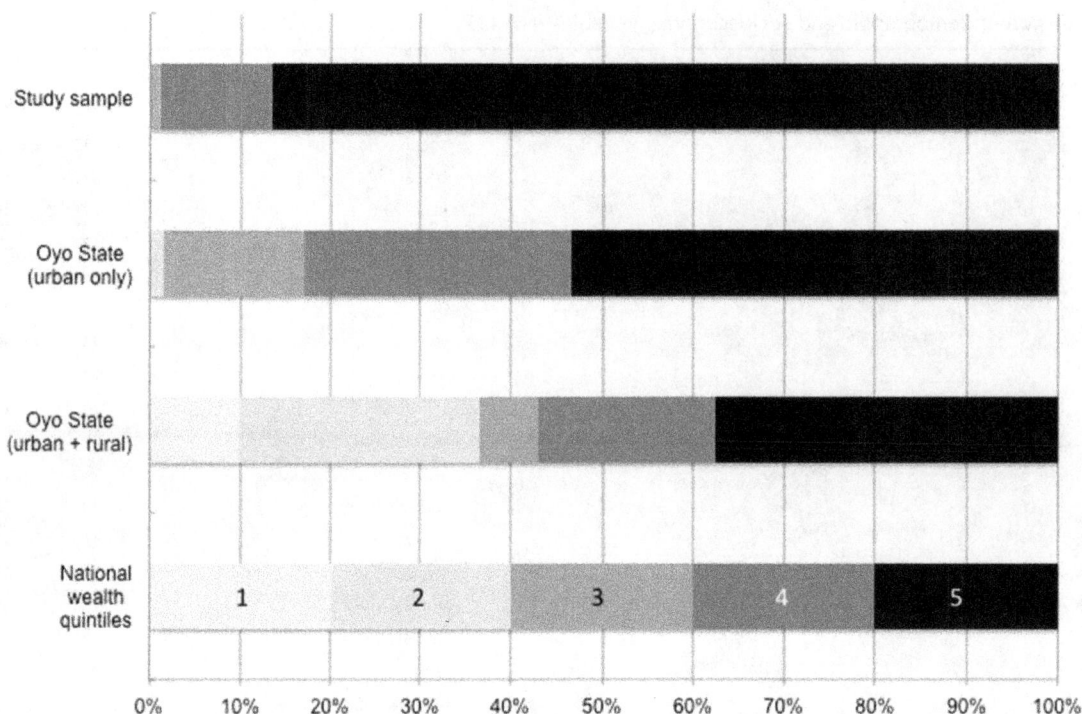

Figure 1. Wealth distribution of enrolled participants versus state and national populations. When comparing the wealth distribution between sampled individuals to that of the state and national populations captured by the 2010 MIS, those in the wealthiest quintile are disproportionately represented in the study sample. Based on the composite asset ownership measure, no individuals in the study sample were from the lowest two wealth quintiles of nation. Although the population of Oyo State, and particularly in urban areas, is also comprised of households that are much wealthier than the nation as a whole, the study sample's wealth composition is even more concentrated among the wealthiest. Source: 2010 Nigeria Malaria Indicators Survey.

Correlates of seeking care at a PPMV versus a pharmacy

Results of logistics regressions predicting the likelihood of going to a PPMV versus a pharmacy for malaria treatment are summarized in Table 3. In bivariate analyses, customers going to different shop types were significantly different in terms of their age, educational attainment, employment status, and wealth. Significant differences were also registered for a number of symptoms (i.e. fever, headache, or dizziness; feeling weak, fatigues, or no appetite; having congestion or shallow breathing; and other symptoms including blusters, dark urine, and yellow eyes), days waited before seeking care, and the source of diagnosis. In multivariate analyses, older individuals are about half as likely to patron a PPMV (age 30–39: OR = 0.416, 95% CI: 0.230–0.752; age 50+: OR = 0.461, 95% CI: 0.229–0.929) than those under age 30. A strong wealth gradient emerges with the individuals in progressively richer wealth quintiles increasingly less likely to go to a PPMV compared to those in the poorest quintile. Those reporting other types of symptoms (i.e. blisters, dark urine, yellow eyes) were more than three times as likely to go to a PPMV (OR = 3.138, 95% CI: 1.381–7.128) while those reporting fever, headache, or dizziness (OR = 2.589, 95% CI: 1.501–4.465) and weakness, fatigue, and lack of appetite (OR = 1.951, 95% CI: 1.043–3.649) were about twice as likely to go to a PPMV. When individuals waited one day before seeking care, they were twice as likely to go to a PPMV (OR = 2.070, 95% CI: 1.256–3.411) compared to those who sought treatment the same day; the likelihood of PPMV patronage progressively declined as the number of days waited increased, but these were not statistically significant. Diagnosis coming from a hospital, clinic, or laboratory was associated with a large and significantly lower likelihood of

going to a PPMV (OR = 0.022, 95% CI: 0.137–1.311). Education and employment status were no longer statistically significant after adjusting for all confounders.

When asked for reasons why they chose the particular drug shop, most respondents stated reasons of habit and convenience (see Figure 2). A significantly higher percentage of participants at PPMVs said that the shop was convenient and had the drugs that s/he needed. In similar percentages, both types of outlets were cited for their prices.

Predictors of purchasing an ACT

The logistic regression results predicting the likelihood of purchasing an ACT over other types of antimalarial drugs are listed in Table 4. In bivariate analyses, shop type, wealth, and the source of diagnoses were the only factors that were significantly associated with the likelihood of buying an ACT. In adjusted regressions, customers who went to PPMVs were significantly less likely to buy an ACT (OR = 0.371, 95% CI: 0.168-0.821). While having a diagnosis from a hospital, clinic, or laboratory was associated with increased likelihood of ACT purchase, this was only marginally significant at the 10% level. Differences in wealth were no longer significant in the multivariate specification, although a gradient was still observed.

RDT results and self-reported drug administration

Of the 457 enrolled participants, 3.9% (n = 18) were RDT-positive as seen in Table 5. During the phone follow-up survey, 97.9% (n = 415/424) of those reached reported that they felt better than the day they were enrolled into the study and 5.9% (n = 25/

Table 2. Drugs purchased to treat malaria.

	Pharmacies		PPMVs		Total		
	n	%	n	%	n	%	P-value
Type of anti-malarial drug[1]							
ACT	132	57.4	55	28.5	187	44.2	0.003
SP	66	28.7	92	47.7	158	37.4	0.022
CQ	46	20.0	33	17.1	79	18.7	0.545
Other	21	9.1	16	8.3	37	8.7	0.830
Purchased non-malaria drug							
Yes	129	54.7	136	70.1	265	61.6	0.068
No	107	45.3	58	29.9	165	38.4	
Type of non-malaria drugs							
Analgesic	98	76.0	126	92.6	224	84.5	0.003
Vitamin/supplement	110	85.3	82	60.3	192	72.5	0.007
Antibiotic	27	20.9	8	5.9	35	13.2	0.019
Other	16	12.4	11	8.1	27	10.2	0.251
Purchase combinations							
Anti-malarial only	107	45.3	58	29.9	167	38.6	0.056
Non-malaria drug only	6	1.3	1	0.3	7	0.8	
Both anti-malarial and non-malaria drug	123	26.2	135	34.9	259	30.1	
	n	median	n	median	n	median	P-value
Total amount paid (median)	234	445	193	140	427	240	0.000

[1] Pharmacies N = 230; PPMVs N = 193; Total N = 423. Not all participants purchased an anti-malarial drug.

Table 3. Logistic regression of the likelihood of buying drugs from a PPMV (versus a pharmacy).

		Pharmacy		PPMV			Bivariate			Multivariate		
		n=245	%	n=212	%	P-value	OR¹	95% CI	P-val	OR¹	95% CI	P-val
Age of respondents	18–29 (reference)	52	21.2	74	34.9	0.005	1.000			1.000		
	30–39	78	31.8	49	23.1		0.441***	0.275–0.709	0.001	0.416***	0.230–0.752	0.004
	40–49	56	22.9	44	20.8		0.552	0.268–1.139	0.108	0.564	0.255–1.249	0.158
	50+	59	24.1	45	21.2		0.524**	0.292–0.939	0.030	0.461**	0.229–0.929	0.030
Sex	Male	125	51.0	106	50.0	0.893	0.969	0.615–1.528	0.893			
	Female (reference)	120	49.0	106	50.0		1.000					
Education	No education (reference)	10	4.1	28	13.2	0.012	1.000			1.000		
	Primary education	24	9.8	42	19.8		0.610	0.247–1.504	0.283	0.984	0.319–3.033	0.977
	Secondary education	102	41.6	79	37.3		0.277**	0.102–0.749	0.012	0.470	0.157–1.407	0.177
	Higher education	109	44.5	63	29.7		0.206***	0.064–0.667	0.008	0.607	0.136–2.712	0.514
Marital status	Not married (reference)	66	26.9	80	37.7	0.089	1.000					
	Married	179	73.1	132	62.3		0.616*	0.352–1.077	0.089			
Employment status	Employed full time (reference)	83	33.9	47	22.3	0.012	1.000			1.000		
	Employed part time	8	3.3	5	2.4		1.104	0.240–5.078	0.899	0.463	0.085–2.520	0.373
	Self-employed	111	45.3	134	63.0		2.116***	1.205–3.717	0.009	1.337	0.627–2.849	0.452
	Unemployed	43	17.6	26	12.3		1.068	0.581–1.962	0.833	0.761	0.299–1.940	0.567
Wealth quintile	Poorest (reference)	21	8.6	68	32.1	0.000	1.000			1.000		
	Second	38	15.5	54	25.5		0.439***	0.235–0.819	0.010	0.430**	0.205–0.900	0.025
	Third	53	21.6	40	18.9		0.233***	0.126–0.431	0.000	0.205***	0.087–0.487	0.000
	Fourth	59	24.1	32	15.1		0.162***	0.072–0.368	0.000	0.152***	0.056–0.413	0.000
	Richest	74	30.2	18	8.5		0.0751***	0.023–0.249	0.000	0.075***	0.018–0.318	0.000
Symptoms reported												
Fever, headache, dizziness	Yes	168	68.6	172	81.1	0.001	2.021***	1.317–3.101	0.001	2.589***	1.501–4.465	0.000
	No (reference)	77	31.4	40	18.9		1.000			1.000		
Body aches, chills, convulsions	Yes	130	53.1	133	62.7	0.096	1.508*	0.929–2.448	0.096			
	No (reference)	115	46.9	79	37.3		1.000					
Weak, fatigue, no appetite	Yes	120	49.0	134	63.2	0.011	1.813**	1.144–2.872	0.011	1.951**	1.043–3.649	0.036
	No (reference)	125	51.0	78	36.8		1.000			1.000		
Bitter taste in the mouth	Yes	29	11.8	33	15.6	0.241	1.381	0.806–2.367	0.240			
	No (reference)	216	88.2	179	84.4		1.000					
Congestion, shallow breathing	Yes	38	15.5	20	9.4	0.016	0.570**	0.361–0.902	0.016	0.619*	0.372–1.030	0.065
	No (reference)	207	84.5	192	90.6		1.000			1.000		
Vomiting, diarrhea	Yes	30	12.2	24	11.3	0.752	0.920	0.548–1.545	0.752			
	No (reference)	215	87.8	188	88.7		1.000					

Table 3. Cont.

		Pharmacy n=245	%	PPMV n=212	%	P-value	Bivariate OR[1]	95% CI	P-val	Multivariate OR[1]	95% CI	P-val
Other: blisters, dark urine, yellow eyes	Yes	15	6.1	48	22.6	0.000	4.515***	2.345–8.696	0.000	3.138***	1.381–7.128	0.0063
	No (reference)	230	93.9	164	77.4		1.000			1.000		
Number of days waited before seeking care[2]	<1 day (reference)	56	25.9	65	31.7	0.016	1.000			1.000		
	1 day	30	13.9	49	23.9		1.378	0.854–2.225	0.189	2.070***	1.256–3.411	0.004
	2 days	37	17.1	40	19.5		0.931	0.510–1.700	0.817	1.624	0.890–2.962	0.114
	3–5 days	66	30.6	37	18.0		0.483*	0.220–1.058	0.069	0.659	0.289–1.504	0.322
	6 days or more	27	12.5	14	6.8		0.447*	0.181–1.100	0.080	0.431	0.137–1.355	0.150
Source of diagnosis	Myself/family/friend (reference)	213	86.9	205	96.7	0.011	1.000			1.000		
	Hospital/clinic/lab	19	7.8	1	0.5		0.055***	0.008–0.393	0.004	0.022**	0.001–0.412	0.011
	Pharmacy/PPMV	13	5.3	6	2.8		0.482	0.149–1.557	0.222	0.424	0.137–1.311	0.136
Observations							457			420		

[1]Odds ratios reported.
[2]Pharmacy (n=212), PPMV (n=205), Total (n=417).
Standard errors are clustered at the shop level;
***p<0.01,
**p<0.05,
*p<0.1.

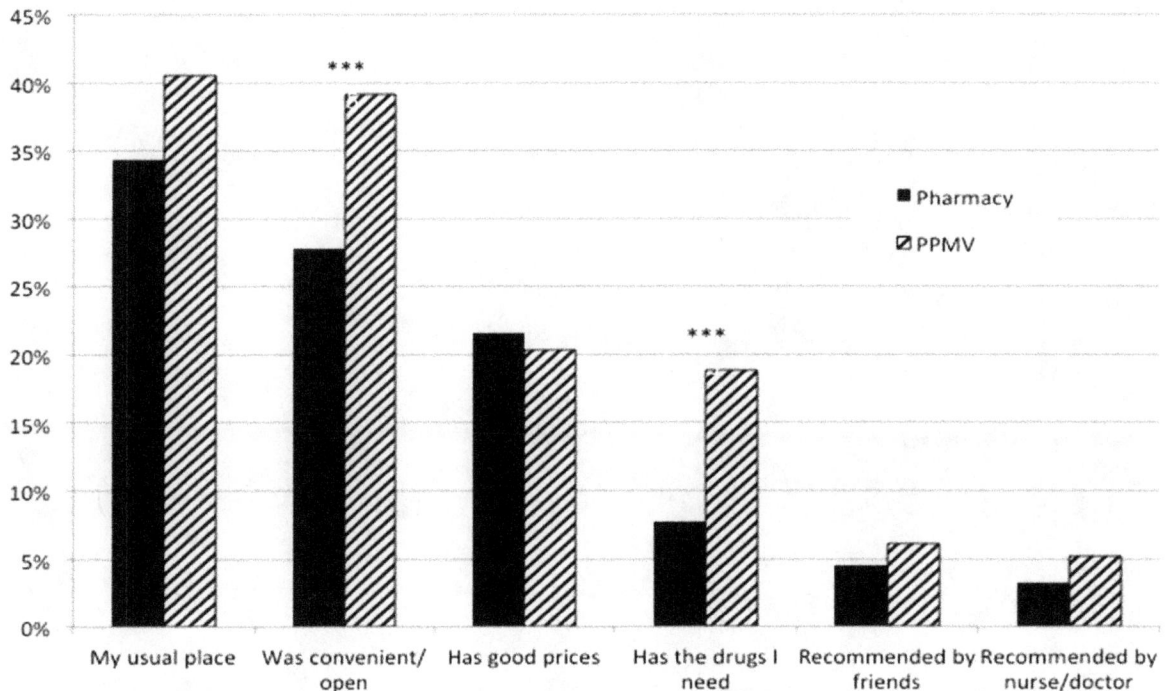

Figure 2. Reasons for choosing a drug shop (N = 457). When asked for reasons why they chose the particular drug shop, most respondents stated reasons of habit and convenience (see Figure 2). A significantly higher percentage of participants at PPMVs said that the shop was convenient and had the drugs that s/he needed. In similar percentages, both types of outlets were cited for their prices. Note: *** p<0.01, ** p<0.05, * p<0.1.

422) had sought additional care. For those who were RDT-positive (and for whom drug information is available), 68.8% (n = 11/16) reported taking an ACT; none took a non-ACT anti-malarial and all took some type of non-anti-malarial drug that they had also purchased (n = 12). Among RDT-negative participants, 28.9% still used some form of anti-malarial medication: 9.7% (n = 39/402) took an ACT and 19.2% (n = 77/402) took a non-ACT anti-malarial. For those who also purchased a non-anti-malarial, 76.5% (n = 189/247) took these drugs. When asked which places could be trusted to provide RDTs, 77.4% (n = 328/425) indicated hospitals or clinics and 17.5% (n = 74) named a diagnostic laboratory; only 4.2% stated pharmacies, 1.2% (n = 5) named PPMVs, and 3.5% (n = 15) indicated a family or friend could be trusted.

Discussion

Like elsewhere in sub-Saharan Africa [17,24–26], medicine retailers in Nigeria are an important source of treatment for uncomplicated malaria even though the quality of care and knowledge among these providers is poorer compared to other types of health professionals. This study sought to better characterize the practice of presumptive treatment at drug outlets in Nigeria. Recruited as they exited drug shops, nearly all study participants reported that they had self-diagnosed their condition and chose to patron the particular shop because it was either their usual place to buy drugs or was convenient. Individuals who went to PPMVs were typically younger, poorer, waited fewer days before seeking care, and had not gone to a hospital/clinic for diagnosis. These results suggest that relatively poorer populations, and potentially less-educated, are disproportionately serviced by PPMVs, potentially motivated by a variety of factors, including proximity and accessibility [27,28] and cost [29,30].

In this study, even though patrons of PPMVs spent less on their drug purchases on average, they were also more likely to purchase sub-standard, non-ACT anti-malarials. Going to a PPMV was the largest risk factor for not buying an ACT, indicating that PPMVs continue to sell non-recommended drugs for malaria. Studies show that receiving ACTs is highly associated with consumer demand [6], and that PPMVs in particular tend to sell what customers demand and avoid referring patients for confirmatory blood tests because they fear losing customers due to added inconvenience or cost [18]. Thus, consumer preferences for presumptive treatment and non-recommended drugs may drive individuals to patron PPMVs rather than pharmacies, even both types of outlets are generally perceived to provider lower quality services than hospitals or clinics [31]. Profit motives may further constrain proper dispensing behavior due to strong consumer demand for substandard drugs [26].

In addition to fever, many participants attributed a wide variety of symptoms to malaria, and those going to PPMVs were especially likely to name symptoms unrelated to malaria. Further, only 3.9% of sick adults seeking care for malaria were found to be positive for malaria using an RDT. This corroborates qualitative evidence that malaria is identified as the illness for a large swath of conditions in Nigeria [18], and that malaria is over-diagnosed and over-treated, similar to other urban areas of Nigeria [32] and elsewhere in sub-Saharan malaria-endemic countries [33–36]. There is also an entrenched perception that malaria is rampant and many people have been regaled with the need to treat malaria promptly by public health messages in the past aimed at increasing awareness. This highlights the importance of malaria behavior change messages that inform people that not all fever cases can be attributed to malaria and the need for individuals to seek out malaria diagnosis.

Table 4. Logistic regression of the likelihood of buying an ACT (versus other anti-malarial drugs).

		ACT		Other anti-malarial			Bivariate			Multivariate		
		n = 233	%	n = 184	%	P-value	OR¹	95% CI	P-val	OR¹	95% CI	P-val
Type of shop¹	PPMV	136	58.4	136	29.3	0.002	0.296***	0.135–0.650	0.002	0.371**	0.168–0.821	0.015
	Pharmacy	97	41.6	97	70.7		1.000			1.000		
Age of respondents	18–29 (reference)	70	30.0	70	22.3	0.541	1.000					
	30–39	64	27.5	64	29.3		1.441	0.800–2.595	0.224			
	40–49	52	22.3	52	23.9		1.445	0.775–2.694	0.247			
	50+	47	20.2	47	24.5		1.635	0.767–3.485	0.203			
Sex	Male	125	53.6	125	48.4	0.398	0.809	0.496–1.322	0.398			
	Female (reference)	108	46.4	108	51.6		1.000					
Education	No education (reference)	18	7.7	18	6.5	0.182	1.000					
	Primary education	36	15.5	36	9.8		0.750	0.300–1.873	0.538			
	Secondary education	96	41.2	96	39.1		1.125	0.513–2.466	0.769			
	Higher education	83	35.6	83	44.6		1.482	0.647–3.395	0.352			
Marital status	Not married (reference)	76	32.6	76	29.9	0.654	1.000					
	Married	157	67.4	157	70.1		1.135	0.652–1.978	0.654			
Employment status	Employed full time (reference)	59	25.3	59	34.2	0.105	1.000					
	Employed part time	6	2.6	6	2.7		0.780	0.174–3.499	0.746			
	Self-employed	136	58.4	136	46.2		0.585**	0.368–0.930	0.023			
	Unemployed	32	13.7	32	16.8		0.907	0.541–1.522	0.712			
Wealth quintile	Poorest (reference)	50	21.5	50	14.7	0.008	1.000			1.000		
	Second	59	25.3	59	14.1		0.816	0.454–1.466	0.497	0.652	0.357–1.192	0.165
	Third	48	20.6	48	17.4		1.235	0.610–2.500	0.558	0.875	0.412–1.861	0.730
	Fourth	44	18.9	44	23.9		1.852	0.870–3.943	0.110	1.234	0.615–2.477	0.554
	Richest	32	13.7	32	29.9		3.183***	1.499–6.758	0.003	1.931	0.880–4.236	0.101
Symptoms reported												
Fever, headache, dizziness	Yes	171	73.4	171	73.4	0.996	0.999	0.635–1.571	0.996			
	No (reference)	62	26.6	62	26.6		1.000					
Body aches, chills, convulsions	Yes	136	58.4	136	57.1	0.818	0.948	0.601–1.494	0.818			
	No (reference)	97	41.6	97	42.9		1.000					
Weak, fatigue, no appetite	Yes	138	59.2	138	54.3	0.387	0.820	0.522–1.287	0.387			
	No (reference)	95	40.8	95	45.7		1.000					
Bitter taste in the mouth	Yes	31	13.3	31	14.7	0.654	1.121	0.681–1.844	0.654			
	No (reference)	202	86.7	202	85.3		1.000					
Congestion, shallow breathing	Yes	24	10.3	24	16.3	0.110	1.696	0.887–3.244	0.110			
	No (reference)	209	89.7	209	83.7		1.000					

Table 4. Cont.

		ACT		Other anti-malarial		P-value	Bivariate			Multivariate		
		n = 233	%	n = 184	%		OR[1]	95% CI	P-val	OR[1]	95% CI	P-val
Vomiting, diarrhea	Yes	26	11.2	26	10.9	0.916	0.971	0.561–1.679	0.916			
	No (reference)	207	88.8	207	89.1		1.000					
Other: blisters, dark urine, yellow eyes	Yes	33	14.2	33	11.4	0.448	0.781	0.412–1.480	0.448			
	No (reference)	200	85.8	200	88.6		1.000					
Number of days waited before seeking care[1]	<1 day (reference)	68	30.8	68	24.8	0.140	1.000					
	1 day	46	20.8	46	15.5		0.924	0.455–1.875	0.827			
	2 days	42	19.0	42	18.6		1.214	0.691–2.135	0.500			
	3–5 days	45	20.4	45	29.2		1.776**	1.038–3.039	0.0362			
	6 days or more	20	9.0	20	11.8		1.615	0.798–3.269	0.183			
Source of diagnosis	Myself/family/friend (reference)	219	94.0	219	89.1	0.019	1.000			1.000		
	Hospital/clinic/lab	4	1.7	4	7.1		4.340**	1.323–14.24	0.0155	3.124*	0.987–9.894	0.053
	Pharmacy/PPMV	10	4.3	10	3.8		0.935	0.345–2.530	0.894	0.758	0.301–1.909	0.557
Observations							417			417		

[1]Odds ratios reported.
[2]Pharmacy (n = 221), PPMV (n = 161), Total (n = 382).
Standard errors are clustered at the shop level;
***p<0.01,
**p<0.05,
*p<0.1.

Table 5. RDT result and self-reported drug administration.

		n	N	%
RDT result	Positive	18	457	3.9
	Negative	439	457	96.1
Generally feeling better since baseline	Yes	415	424	97.9
	No	9	424	2.1
Drugs taken				
RDT-positive				
ACT	Yes	11	16	68.8
	No	5	16	31.3
Non-ACT anti-malarial	Yes	0	16	0
	No	0	16	0
Non-anti-malarial	Yes	12	12	100
	No	0	12	0
RDT-negative				
ACT	Yes	39	402	9.7
	No	363	402	90.3
Non-ACT anti-malarial	Yes	77	402	19.2
	No	325	402	80.8
Non-anti-malarial	Yes	189	247	76.5
	No	58	247	23.5
Sought additional care	Yes	25	422	5.9
	No	397	422	94.1
Places trusted to provide RDTs				
Hospital/clinic	Yes	328	424	77.4
	No	96	424	22.6
Diagnostic lab	Yes	74	424	17.5
	No	350	424	82.5
Pharmacy	Yes	18	424	4.2
	No	406	424	95.8
PPMV	Yes	5	424	1.2
	No	419	424	98.8
Community health worker	Yes	23	424	5.4
	No	401	424	94.6
Traditional healer	Yes	4	424	0.9
	No	420	424	99.1
Family/friend	Yes	15	424	3.5
	No	409	424	96.5
Felt well at follow up and RDT positive				
Took ACTs	Yes	9	16	56.3
	No	7	16	43.7
Took non- ACT anti-malarial	Yes	7	16	43.7
	No	9	16	56.7
Non- antimalarial	Yes	0	16	0
	No	16	16	100
Felt well at follow up and RDT negative				
Took ACTs	Yes	206	389	53.0
	No	183	389	47.0
Took non- ACT anti-malarial	Yes	181	389	46.5
	No	208	389	53.5
Non- antimalarial	Yes	2	389	0.5
	No	387	389	99.5

Although the study did not have a comparison control group, it is assumed that most sick individuals who purchased malaria drugs in this study were intending to take their purchased drugs to presumptively treatment him/herself. Over 44% of participants bought ACTs and the median amount spent on purchasing anti-malarial drugs was 240 Naira (~US$1.50). This level of overtreatment suggests that large quantities of ACTs may be wasted if reliable testing is not first carried out. It is therefore imperative to train all health workers as well as the populace on malaria symptoms and the need for a diagnostic test has become vital in health communications and education. Since PPMVs and pharmacies serve the majority of the population seeking treatment for malaria, standard diagnostic testing prior to treatment should be considered as part of a concerted strategy for malaria control. Some countries, including Tanzania, Senegal, and Zambia have successfully implemented RDTs in the public health sector and provider acceptability has improved over time, resulting in sizable cost-savings [7–10]. Further, this is the first study to assess patient adherence to test results (rather than provider prescription behavior) showing that simply providing diagnostic information to sick individuals can result in high rates of appropriate treatment behavior [22].

In addition, this also underscores the need to provide alternative means of management of non-malaria febrile illness. There is currently not a good understanding of the etiology of non-malaria febrile illnesses and only a handful of studies have documented the variety of causes of pediatric illnesses in select countries [33,37]. Such information is vital for developing more comprehensive treatment guidelines for childhood illnesses that are country-relevant and should be the focus of future studies.

Limitations of the study

Populations in Southwest Nigeria are likely to be from higher socioeconomic status than populations in other areas of the country and consequently likely to be healthier overall [14]. A sample of adults as carried out in the study may not necessarily be representative of children under five who are yet to develop immunity to malaria. Further studies will be needed to look at the incidence of malaria in this group as well as in other parts of Nigeria to determine if this picture is consistent nationwide. Characteristics of the shop and its workers may also be important determinants of shop patronage and buying drugs which the current study was not able to capture, but which future studies will aim to include in the assessment of care-seeking behavior for malaria.

The study could not look at counterfeit or substandard drugs purchased at the medicine shops. However, quality-assured ACTs were given free of charge in order to address the risk of participants taking substandard drugs. Although shop workers did not participate in the recruitment or screening of customer participants, they may have altered their sales or prescriptive behavior in ways that we cannot account for.

Acknowledgments

The authors wish to acknowledge Exxon Mobil and the Global Fund to Fight AIDS, Tuberculosis and Malaria. Our appreciation also goes to the drug stores and PPMVs shops where the study was implemented, as well as the participants who agreed to receive an RDT and answer survey questions. Many thanks to Adetunji Ilori for excellent assistance in field work management and surveyor training, Tunde Ogunbenro for facilitating and supporting project management, and Alana Schwartz at San Francisco General Hospital for lab assistance. We are grateful for the comments and feedback from seminar participants at the UCSF Global Health Sciences and Infectious Diseases Group, the 6th MIM (Multilateral Initiative on Malaria) Pan-African Malaria Conference, the Population Association of America Annual Meeting, the International Health Economics Association Conference, Stanford School of Medicine's General Medical Disciplines Departmental Seminar, and the World Social Marketing Conference.

Author Contributions

Conceived and designed the experiments: ADLC SM JL DM. Performed the experiments: ADLC ES JL SM CI CU. Analyzed the data: CI JL. Contributed reagents/materials/analysis tools: ADLC SM JL DM ES JA EN CI CU. Wrote the paper: CI JA JL ES. Provided technical support: JA EN.

References

1. WHO World Malaria Report 2008. Available: http://www.who.int/malaria/publications/world_malaria_report_2008/en/index.html. Accessed 2014 Feb 20.
2. Okeke TA, Uzochukwu BSC, Okafor HU (2006) An in-depth study of patent medicine sellers' perspectives on malaria in a rural Nigerian community. Malaria Journal 2006 5: 97.
3. Onwujekwe O, Chima R, Okonkwo P (2000) Economic burden of malaria illness versus that of a combination of all other illnesses. A study in five malaria holo-endemic communities. Health Policy 54: 143–159.
4. WHO World Malaria Report 2010. Available: http://www.who.int/malaria/publications/atoz/9789241547925/en/index.html. Accessed 2014 Feb 20.
5. AMFm Independent Evaluation Team (2012) Independent Evaluation of Phase 1 of the Affordable Medicines Facility - malaria (AMFm), Multi-Country Independent Evaluation Report: Final Report. Calverton, Maryland and London: ICF International and London School of Hygiene and Tropical Medicine.
6. Mangham LJ, Cundill B, Ezeoke O, Nwala E, Uzochukwu BS, et al (2011) Treatment of uncomplicated malaria at public health facilities and medicine retailers in south-eastern Nigeria. Malar J 10(1): 155.
7. Hamer DH, Ndhlovu M, Zurovac D, Fox M, Yeboah-Antwi K, et al (2007) Improved diagnostic testing and malaria treatment practices in Zambia. JAMA: the journal of the American Medical Association 297(20): 2227–2231.
8. Masanja MI, McMorrow M, Kahigwa E, Kachur SP, McElroy PD (2010) Health workers' use of malaria rapid diagnostic tests (RDTs) to guide clinical decision making in rural dispensaries, Tanzania. The American journal of tropical medicine and hygiene 83(6): 1238.
9. Thiam S, Thior M, Faye B, Ndiop M, Diouf ML, et al (2011) Major reduction in anti-malarial drug consumption in Senegal after nation-wide introduction of malaria rapid diagnostic tests. PLOS One 6(4): 1–7.
10. Yukich J, D'Acremont V, Kahama J, Swai M, Lengeler C (2010) Cost savings with rapid diagnostic tests for malaria in low-transmission areas: evidence from Dar es Salaam, Tanzania. American Journal of Tropical Hygiene and Medicine 83(1): 61–68.
11. Cohen J, Fink G, Berg K, Aber F, Jordan M (2012) Feasibility of distributing rapid diagnostic tests for malaria in the retail sector Evidence from an implementation study in Uganda. PLOS One 7(11): 1–10.
12. Retail prices of ACTs co-paid by the AMFm and other antimalarial medicines: Ghana, Kenya, Madagascar, Nigeria, Tanzania and Uganda Report of price tracking surveys. August 2013. Available: http://www.google.com/url?sa=t&rct=j&q=&esrc=s&source=web&cd=4&ved=0CDcQFjAD&url=http%3A%2F%2Fwww.theglobalfund.org%2Fdocuments%2Famfm%2FAMFm_PriceTrackingByHAIAugust2013Survey_Report_en%2F&ei=ZdwDU9-eDJfYoASto4G4DQ&usg=AFQjCNHk61FW85C0QSf2L2qG8CEnvGc7Xw&bvm=bv.61535280, d.cGU&cad = rja. Accessed 2014 Feb 20.
13. Uzochukwu BSC, Onwujekwe E, Ezuma NN, Ezeoke OP, Ajuba MO, et al (2011) Improving rational treatment of malaria: perceptions and influence of RDTs on prescribing behaviour of health workers in southeast Nigeria. PLOS One 6: e14627.
14. National Population Commission (NPC), National Malaria Control Programme (NMCP), ICF International (2012) Nigeria Malaria Indicator Survey 2010. Abuja, Nigeria: NPC, NMCP, and ICF International.
15. Salako LA, Brieger WR, Afolabi BM, Umeh RE, Agomo PU, et al (2001) Treatment of childhood fevers and other illnesses in three rural Nigerian communities. Tropical Pediatrics 47: 38–46.
16. Oladepo O, Kabiru S, Adeoye BW, Oshiname F, Ofi B, et al. (2008) Malaria treatment in Nigeria: the role of patent medicine vendors. The Future Health Systems, Innovations and knowledge for future health systems for the poor. Policy Brief March. 2008. 01.
17. Goodman C, Brieger W, Unwin A, Mills A, Meek S, et al (2007) Medicine sellers and malaria treatment in sub-Saharan Africa: what do they do and how can their practice be improved? Am J Trop Med Hyg 77: 203–218.

18. De La Cruz A, Liu J, Schatzkin E, Modrek S, Oladepo O, et al. (2012) The Influence of policy, hierarcy, and competition on malaria case management among retail providers in Nigeria. Poster #342 presented at the American Society for Tropical Medicine and Hygiene 62nd Annual Meeting, Atlanta GA.

19. Ezeoke OP, Ezumah NN, Chandler CC, Mangham-Jefferies IJ, Onwujekwe OE, et al (2012) Exploring health providers' and community perceptions and experiences with malaria tests in South-East Nigeria: a critical step towards appropriate treatment. Malar J 11: 368.

20. Bastiaens GJH, Bousema T, Leslie T (2014) Scale-up of Malaria Rapid Diagnostic Tests and Artemisinin Based Combination Therapy: Challenges and Perspectives in Sub-Saharan Africa. PLOS Med 11(1): e1001590. doi:10.1371/journal.pmed.1001590.

21. Basu S, Modrek S, Bendavid E (2014) Comparing decisions for malaria testing and presumptive treatment: a net health benefit analysis. Med Decis Making. 2014 May 14. pii: 0272989X14533609. [Epub ahead of print]

22. Modrek S, Schatzkin E, De La Cruz A, Isiguzo C, Nwokolo E, et al (2014) Malaria Journal 2014, 13: 69.

23. Filmer D, Pritchett LH (2001). Estimating Wealth Effects without Expenditure Data—Or Tears: An Application to Educational Enrollments in States of India. Demography. Volume 38, Issue 1, 115–132.

24. Nshakira N, Kristensen M, Ssali F, Reynolds Whyte S (2002) Appropriate treatment of malaria? Use of antimalarial drugs for children's fevers in district medical units, drug shops and homes in eastern Uganda. Tropical Medicine & International Health 7(4): 309–316.

25. Hetzel MW, Dillip A, Lengeler C, Obrist B, Msechu JJ et al (2008). Malaria treatment in the retail sector: knowledge and practices of drug sellers in rural Tanzania. BMC public health 8(1): 157.

26. Wafula FN, Goodman CA (2010) Are interventions for improving the quality of services provided by specialized drug shops effective in sub-Saharan Africa? A systematic review of the literature. International Journal for Quality in Health Care 22(4): 316–323.

27. Snow RW, Peshu N, Forster D, Mwenesi H, Marsh K (1992) The role of shops in the treatment and prevention of childhood malaria on the coast of Kenya. Transactions of the Royal Society of Tropical Medicine and Hygiene 86(3): 237–239.

28. Van Der Geest S (1987) Self-care and the informal sale of drugs in South Cameroon. Social science & medicine 25(3): 293–305.

29. Amin AA, Marsh V, Noor AM, Ochola SA, Snow RW (2003) The use of formal and informal curative services in the management of paediatric fevers in four districts in Kenya. Tropical Medicine & International Health 8(12): 1143–1152.

30. Brieger WR, Sesay HR, Adesina H, Mosanya ME, Ogunlade PB, et al (2000) Urban malaria treatment behaviour in the context of low levels of malaria transmission in Lagos, Nigeria. African journal of medicine and medical sciences 30: 7–15.

31. Onwujekwe O, Onoka C, Uguru N, Nnenna T, Uzochukwu B, et al (2010) Preferences for benefit packages for community-based health insurance: an exploratory study in Nigeria BMC Health Services Research 10: 162.

32. Oyibo WA (2013) Overdiagnosis and Overtreatment of Malaria in Children That Presented with Fever in Lagos, Nigeria. ISRN Infectious Diseases, 2013.

33. Crump JA, Morrissey AB, Nicholson WL, Massung RF, Stoddard RA, et al (2013) Etiology of severe non-malaria febrile illness in northern Tanzania: a prospective cohort study. PLOS neglected tropical diseases 7(7): e2324.

34. Reyburn H, Mbatia R, Drakeley C, Carneiro I, Mwakasungula E, et al (2004) Overdiagnosis of malaria in patients with severe febrile illness in Tanzania: a prospective study. BMJ: British Medical Journal 329(7476): 1212.

35. Okebe JU, Walther B, Bojang K, Drammeh S, Schellenberg D, et al (2010) Prescribing practice for malaria following introduction of artemether-lumefantrine in an urban area with declining endemicity in West Africa. Malaria journal 9(1): 180.

36. Mangham IJ, Cundill B, Achonduh OA, Ambebila JN, Lele AK, et al (2012) Malaria prevalence and treatment of febrile patients at health facilities and medicine retailers in Cameroon. Tropical Medicine & International Health 17(3): 330–342.

37. Acestor N, Cooksey R, Newton PN, Menard D, Guerin PJ, et al. (2012) Mapping the aetiology of non-malarial febrile illness in Southeast Asia through a systematic review—terra incognita impairing treatment policies. PLOS one 7(9): e44269.

9

Tuberculosis Treatment Managed by Providers outside the Public Health Department: Lessons for the Affordable Care Act

Melissa Ehman[1,2]*, Jennifer Flood[1], Pennan M. Barry[1]

1 Tuberculosis Control Branch, Division of Communicable Disease Control, Center for Infectious Diseases, California Department of Public Health, Richmond, California, United States of America, 2 Institute of Global Health, Global Health Sciences, University of California San Francisco, San Francisco, California, United States of America

Abstract

Introduction: Tuberculosis (TB) requires at least six months of multidrug treatment and necessitates monitoring for response to treatment. Historically, public health departments (HDs) have cared for most TB patients in the United States. The Affordable Care Act (ACA) provides coverage for uninsured persons and may increase the proportion of TB patients cared for by private medical providers and other providers outside HDs (PMPs). We sought to determine whether there were differences in care provided by HDs and PMPs to inform public health planning under the ACA.

Methods: We conducted a retrospective, cross-sectional analysis of California TB registry data. We included adult TB patients with culture-positive, pulmonary TB reported in California during 2007–2011. We examined trends, described case characteristics, and created multivariate models measuring two standards of TB care in PMP- and HD-managed patients: documented culture conversion within 60 days, and use of directly observed therapy (DOT).

Results: The proportion of PMP-managed TB patients increased during 2007–2011 (p = 0.002). On univariable analysis (N = 4,606), older age, white, black or Asian/Pacific Islander race, and birth in the United States were significantly associated with PMP care (p<0.05). Younger age, Hispanic ethnicity, homelessness, drug or alcohol use, and cavitary and/or smear-positive TB disease, were associated with HD care. Multivariable analysis showed PMP care was associated with lack of documented culture conversion (adjusted relative risk [aRR] = 1.37, confidence interval [CI] 1.25–1.51) and lack of DOT (aRR = 8.56, CI 6.59–11.1).

Conclusion: While HDs cared for TB cases with more social and clinical complexities, patients under PMP care were less likely to receive DOT and have documented culture conversion. This indicates a need for close collaboration between PMPs and HDs to ensure that optimal care is provided to all TB patients and TB transmission is halted. Strategies to enhance collaboration between HDs and PMPs should be included in ACA implementation.

Editor: John Z. Metcalfe, University of California, San Francisco, United States of America

Funding: The authors have no support or funding to report.

Competing Interests: The authors have declared that no competing interests exist.

* Email: Melissa.Ehman@cdph.ca.gov

Introduction

Despite a decline in tuberculosis (TB) in the United States (U.S.) in the past two decades, TB remains a significant public health problem and is a challenging, resource-intensive disease to diagnose and treat. Treatment of active disease requires at least six months of a multidrug regimen and necessitates systematic monitoring for side effects and response to treatment. Because most TB patients have historically been managed by publicly funded local and state TB programs, [1] these programs have substantial expertise to successfully detect and treat TB disease in the U.S. However, the private sector plays an increasingly important role in diagnosing and treating TB. [2] As TB cases continue to decline in the U.S., [3] community health care providers may not see enough cases to build or maintain expertise in managing cases of TB. Regardless of the source of direct patient care, public health programs are responsible for oversight of TB patient treatment, to ensure that transmission is prevented. This need to protect the public from TB makes public-private collaboration crucial for effective management of TB. [2,4,5]

Effective management of TB should ensure timely conversion of sputum cultures to negative and prevent acquired drug resistance (ensure adherence to treatment). [6–8] Documenting prompt culture conversion also allows for the use of short-course TB therapy. [9] The practice of directly observed therapy (DOT) does not simply ensure treatment adherence, but also facilitates overall monitoring of treatment efficacy and provides patient support through structured contact with the health care system. [4,9]

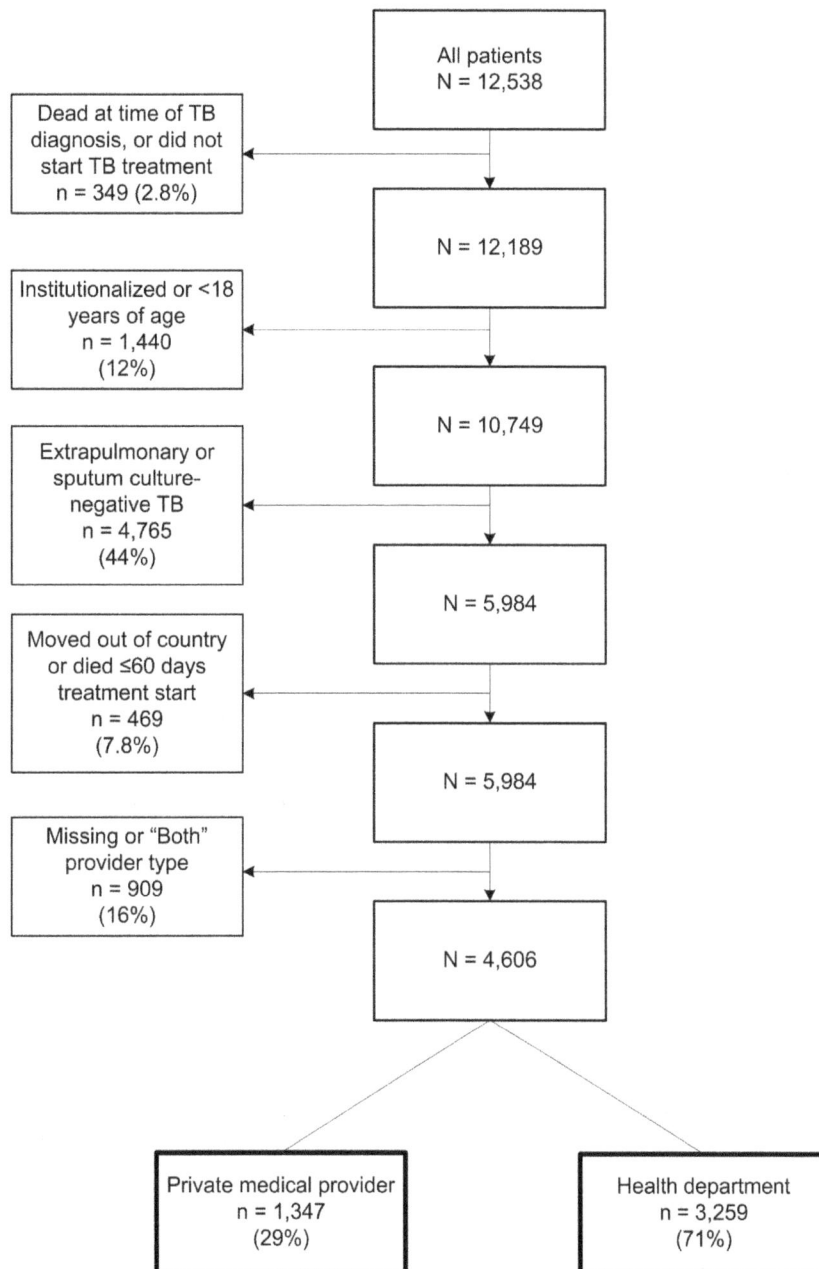

Figure 1. Analytic cohort, 2007–2011. TB = tuberculosis.

The Patient Protection and Affordable Care Act (ACA) [10] expands opportunities for patients to obtain health insurance and may increase health care provision in the private sector. In order to understand the potential impact of a shift in TB care from public TB programs to the private sector, we examined trends in providers caring for California TB patients over time, and examined differences in demographic and clinical characteristics of these two patient populations. We also sought to determine whether differences exist between care practices, including documenting that a patient has converted sputum cultures to negative and providing DOT to prevent acquisition of drug resistance.

Materials and Methods

Ethics statement

The California Department of Public Health (CDPH) routinely collects surveillance data, performs analyses and monitors trends for public health purposes. This analysis was determined to be a non-research public health analysis, and not subject to human subjects review. [11] All patient data were anonymized and de-identified prior to analysis.

Analytic design

We used TB surveillance data in a retrospective, cross-sectional analysis to model the relationships between the provider type for TB care – within the public health department or outside the health department (e.g. private and other providers) – and two measures of optimal TB management: documenting culture conversion to negative, and ensuring treatment adherence through DOT.

Data sources

TB surveillance data were captured through mandatory reporting by public health departments (HDs) of all TB cases to CDPH, using a standard report form containing demographic, clinical, and management information, including the type of clinical provider that managed the TB care. [12,13] On the TB reporting form, a case was classified as "Health Department," "Private/Other," or "Both." "Health Department" refers to patient care in a clinic directly managed by the public health department; for the vast majority of TB patients under HD care, this was a clinic devoted solely to TB diagnosis and treatment. "Private/Other" (hereafter private medical provider, or PMP) designates any other type of provider outside the public health department, including health maintenance organizations (HMOs), and county hospitals and clinics not directly managed by the HD. "Both" means that the patient received both HD and PMP care. Human immunodeficiency virus (HIV) infection status was determined by matching TB case records with the CDPH HIV/ acquired immune deficiency syndrome registry.

Inclusion criteria

For analysis of TB management, TB cases reported to CDPH during 2007–2011 among persons 18 years and older with a sputum culture positive for *M. tuberculosis* and no extrapulmonary disease were selected (Figure 1). The study population inclusion criteria were designed to create a cohort of cases for which TB case management standards are best defined: culture-positive pulmonary TB in adults. [9] Patients who did not start TB treatment, died within 60 days of starting treatment, moved out of the U.S. during treatment, or were diagnosed in an institutional setting, i.e., a correctional or long-term care facility, were excluded. Because exclusive management of patients by PMPs or HDs are the most clearly defined and consistently reported provider types across California, [14] we limited the analysis to PMP and HD provider types, and excluded those designated as Both.

Measures of optimal TB management

We examined two measures of TB management because of their importance for protecting the public's health: evidence of converting sputum culture from positive to negative during the initial treatment phase, and use of DOT. Calculations for these measures were based on indicators routinely used by CDPH [15] and the Centers for Disease Control and Prevention (CDC) [16] to monitor performance of TB control programs.

Culture conversion was defined as a report of a documented sputum culture-negative specimen which was collected within 60 days of the patient's treatment start date. We selected 60 days as the standard window used in clinical guidelines to assess treatment response and need for extension of therapy. [9] A patient was determined to have received DOT if therapy was reported to have been either totally directly observed, or both directly observed and self-administered.

Data analysis

We examined trends, stratified by type of provider for TB cases, using Joinpoint version 4.0.4. [17] We fit the regression lines to the counts of PMP and HD patients during 1993–2011, identified join points that best fit the data using a Monte Carlo permutation test, and compared the trends for TB patients managed by PMPs compared to HDs, using a permutation test for parallelism. [18]

For all other calculations, we used SAS version 9.3. [19] We tested trends for statistical significance with the Cochrane-Armitage test for trend, for the study cohort and also for a cohort that included patients reported as managed by both PMPs and HDs. We compared PMP-managed patients to HD-managed patients for a range of clinical and demographic factors, and tested associations using the Mantel-Haenszel chi square test, or Fisher's exact test where any expected cell count was less than five. We assessed correlation with phi coefficient less than 0.30 for multivariable models. We combined race and ethnicity into mutually exclusive categories, where Hispanic ethnicity was coded as Hispanic, regardless of race; and white, black, and Asian race categories each excluded persons of Hispanic ethnicity. In the multivariable models, we used birth in the U.S. instead of race/ ethnicity categories due to correlation of these two variables. Other correlated variables were combined into categories: smear-positive and cavitary TB disease, and homelessness and substance use (alcohol, injecting and non-injecting). We modeled the association of provider type with the two measures of TB management in univariable and multivariable analyses. We calculated crude and adjusted relative risk using modified Poisson regression with robust error variance. [20,21] Covariables associated with both provider type and measures of TB case management, and factors cited in the literature as possible confounders, were included *a priori* in each multivariable model. We compared models with additional covariables in different combinations using the QIC statistic (quasi-likelihood under the independence model criterion). [22] We selected the model with the lowest QIC as the final model. To assess the impact of excluding patients reported with a provider type of Both (PMP and HD), we analyzed a cohort that included patients managed by Both, and with all other study exclusions. We constructed multivariate models using this cohort in two ways: 1) PMP+Both vs. HD, and 2) PMP vs. HD+Both. We conducted a sensitivity analysis of the relationship between PMP care, DOT, and death during therapy, by excluding patients who died at varying times, to assess the robustness of the 60-day cut point for excluding deaths. We created two separate models to investigate documented culture conversion: documented culture conversion in greater than 60 days after starting treatment, and lack of documented culture conversion ever, to assess whether PMP care was associated with never having a culture conversion documented, or with culture conversion documented after 60 days of treatment. Because California guidelines prioritize key patient groups for DOT when resources do not allow for universal DOT, [23] such as homeless or those with drug-resistant disease, we conducted a subanalysis of predictors of DOT with a cohort restricted to patients with at least one indication for DOT.

Results

Among the 12,538 TB patients reported in California during 2007–2011, 4,606 were included in the analysis (Figure 1). While most patients were managed by the HD (3,259 or 71%), 29% (1,347) were privately managed.

The number of TB patients reported in California steadily declined during 1993–2011, [24] and TB cases meeting our study population criteria also declined during this time. Figure 2 shows the differences in TB incidence trends between public and private sectors. During 1993–2006, the incidence of HD TB patients declined 3.1% per year (95% confidence interval [CI] −3.6, −

2.7); whereas PMP patients declined 5.8% per year (CI −7.0, −4.7). During 2006–2011, however, the decline in PMP-managed TB cases leveled off (annual percent change [APC] = 1.9, CI −4.2, 8.3), whereas HD-managed patients continued to decline at the previous rate. This difference in the rate of incidence decline was statistically significant (p = 0.001).

In our analytic cohort, the proportion of cases with PMP care increased, rising from 25% in 2007 to 32% in 2011 (p = 0.002). In the modified study cohort that included patients with a provider type of Both, the proportion of patients categorized as Both declined from 18% in 2007 to 8.8% in 2011 (p<0.001).

Univariable analysis

Table 1 shows the characteristics of cases managed by PMPs compared with cases managed by HDs. Older patients, those of white, black or Asian/Pacific Islander race, or born in the U.S., were all significantly more likely to have PMP care. Patients cared for by HDs were more likely to be young, Hispanic, homeless, excess alcohol users, non-intravenous drug users, or have cavitary and/or smear-positive TB disease. No patients reported stopping treatment or having treatment extension beyond 12 months due to adverse reactions to TB medication. Documented culture conversion and DOT were observed less frequently among patients managed by PMPs.

Multivariable analysis

A total of 4,604 (99.9%) patients in the analytic cohort had complete information on culture conversion. The absence of documented culture conversion within 60 days of treatment start was significantly associated with privately managed care in multivariable analysis (adjusted relative risk [aRR] 1.37, CI 1.25–1.51). This model adjusted for ten covariables including age, cavitary and/or smear-positive TB disease, and drug resistance. In addition to private medical care, factors predicting lack of documented culture conversion in the adjusted model included:

cavitary and/or smear-positive TB disease, moving during treatment, no DOT, birth in the U.S., male sex, and any homelessness or drug use (Table 2). Privately managed care was a significant predictor of both never having culture conversion documented (aRR 3.34, CI 2.54–4.36) and of delayed culture conversion, documented later than 60 days (aRR 1.24, CI 1.12–1.39).

Nearly all patients (99.5%) had complete information on therapy administration method (DOT or self-administered therapy [SAT]). In the adjusted model, patients under private care were significantly more likely to have received SAT during the course of TB treatment, and PMP care was the strongest predictor of SAT among all covariables (aRR 8.56, CI 6.59–11.1). Lack of documented culture conversion within 60 days was also associated with SAT. Patient characteristics associated with receipt of DOT included homelessness or drug use, cavitary and/or smear-positive TB, a history of TB disease, resistance to any first-line drug used to treat TB, and age 65 years old or greater (Table 3). Similar results were found when excluding patients who died during therapy at 30 or 90 days. Among patients who received DOT, 85% received at least 21 weeks of DOT, and 94% received at least 10 weeks of DOT.

In a subanalysis, limited to patient groups prioritized for DOT under California guidelines, PMP care also had the greatest association with lack of DOT (aRR 6.46, CI 4.61–9.06). Patient groups for whom DOT is a priority in California include the homeless, drug or alcohol users, HIV infected, and patients with drug-resistant TB, smear-positive TB, delayed culture conversion, or prior history of TB.

Multivariable models using the modified study cohort including Both HD and PMP patients showed similar results for each study outcome, with no change in the direction nor significance of association for any covariable.

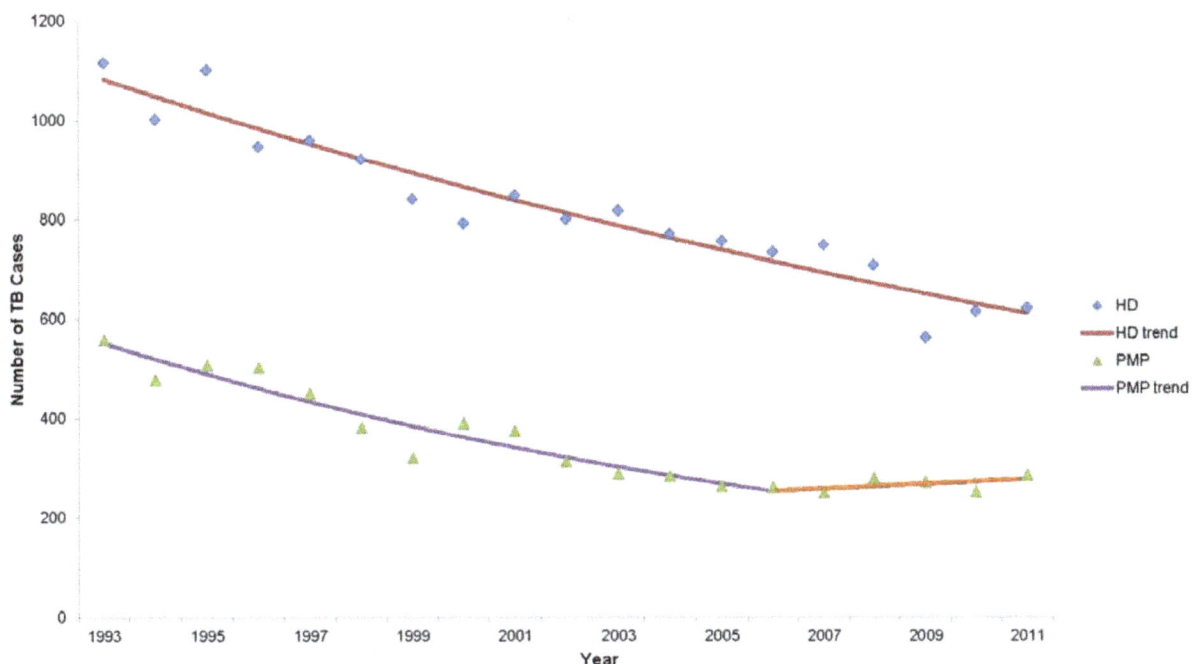

Figure 2. Tuberculosis case count trend, by provider type, California 1993–2011. HD = health department, PMP = private medical provider. Annual percent change (APC): HD 1993–2011 = −3.13, PMP 1993–2006 = −5.83, PMP 2006–2011 = +1.85.

Table 1. Characteristics of TB Patients by Provider Type, Reported in California, 2007–2011 (n = 4606).

Characteristic	All patients[a] n (col %)	PMP (n = 1347) n (col %)	HD (n = 3259) n (col %)	PMP vs. HD P value[b]
Male	2893 (63)	819 (61)	2074 (64)	0.070
18–24 years old	456 (9.9)	100 (7.4)	356 (11)	<0.001
25–44 years old	1421 (31)	366 (27)	1055 (32)	<0.001
45–64 years old	1611 (35)	423 (31)	1188 (36)	0.001
Age ≥65 years old	1118 (24)	458 (34)	660 (20)	<0.001
White	369 (8.0)	147 (11)	222 (6.8)	<0.001
Black	283 (6.2)	110 (8.2)	173 (5.3)	<0.001
Hispanic	1586 (34)	293 (22)	1293 (37)	<0.001
Asian/Pacific Islander	2359 (51)	797 (59)	1562 (48)	<0.001
American Indian/Alaskan Native	8 (0.2)	0 (0)	8 (100)	0.114
Born in United States	792 (17)	297 (22)	495 (15)	<0.001
Moved ever during treatment	234 (5.1)	72 (5.4)	162 (5.0)	0.599
Homeless	273 (5.9)	53 (3.9)	220 (6.8)	<0.001
Excessive alcohol use	431 (9.4)	98 (7.3)	333 (10)	0.002
Intravenous drug use	40 (0.9)	11 (0.8)	29 (0.9)	0.804
Nonintravenous drug use	250 (5.4)	51 (3.8)	199 (6.2)	0.002
Homelessness, alcohol or drug use	682 (15)	143 (11)	539 (17)	<0.001
History of TB disease	286 (6.3)	89 (6.7)	197 (6.1)	0.448
HIV-positive[c]	143 (3.1)	47 (3.4)	96 (3.0)	0.333
Cavitary and/or smear-positive TB disease	3183 (70)	881 (66)	2302 (71)	<0.001
Resistance to any first-line TB drug	651 (14)	183 (14)	468 (14)	0.506
No documented culture conversion ≤60 days	1469 (32)	533 (40)	936 (29)	<0.001
No directly observed therapy	342 (7.4)	270 (20)	72 (2.2)	<0.001

[a]alive at diagnosis and starting treatment, pulmonary only, culture-positive TB, age ≥18 years old; excluding missing or Both provider type, moved out of United States, deaths ≤60 days after treatment start.
[b]for Mantel-Haenszel chi-square, or Fisher's Exact Test where any expected cell count is <5.
[c]vs. HIV-negative or unknown status.
TB = tuberculosis, PMP = private medical provider, HD = health department, HIV = human immunodeficiency virus.

Discussion

We found that during 2007–2011, before implementation of the ACA, an increasing proportion of TB cases in California were exclusively managed by PMPs. We also found that patients managed by PMPs were less likely to have received optimal management of their pulmonary TB even after adjusting for possible confounding clinical and social factors. These findings may have implications for TB care under the ACA, when a more dramatic shift of TB care to the private sector is expected. If PMP patients are less likely to receive optimal management, then shifting toward PMP care without a concomitant increase in HD partnership with PMPs could be a threat to TB control.

Our findings are consistent with evidence showing that patients in public health TB clinics are more likely to receive care recommended in TB control guidelines. [25–31] Similar findings have been published in which clinicians and clinics with the most experience and volume provide care resulting in better outcomes to patients for other diagnoses such as HIV [32] and *Staphylococcus aureus* bacteremia. [33–35] The results also highlight the concept that public health TB clinics and programs warrant consideration as expert, specialty referral clinics, and not simply government sector safety net providers. In fact, specialty TB care has been established across the U.S. since the early 1900s, and has

been intentionally centered in public health TB clinics since the 1960s. [1] These TB specialty clinics provide patient-centered clinical care, case management, and monitoring for persons with complex health issues over months of treatment. However, TB control programs are charged with "ensuring the quality and completeness" [4] of care for all patients and these findings also point out that there should be close collaboration between PMPs and TB control programs to ensure that patients managed exclusively by PMPs receive the same optimal care that patients managed exclusively by the HD do.

Further highlighting the important role of HD TB care, we found that HDs care for a disproportionate burden of complex patients, such as homeless or drug users, who may be more difficult to treat. HDs also will remain critical "safety net" providers for populations uncovered by ACA, such as undocumented immigrants, who comprise an estimated 23% of persons with active TB disease in the United States. [36] Regardless of where TB patients access care, any lack of optimal care that results in increased transmission would increase the risk of TB in the community, and require heightened response from HDs in California, because they will retain responsibility for outbreak management and contact investigations. Shifting patients from HD to PMP care may therefore increase the need for HD resources, rather than lessen it. Studies have shown that increased

Table 2. No Documented Culture Conversion within 60 Days of TB Treatment Start, TB Cases Reported in California, 2007–2011 (n = 4604).

Characteristic	All patients[a] (col %)	No CC (n = 1469) (col %)	CC (n = 3135) (col %)	Univariable RR	CI	Multivariable aRR	CI
Private provider/other	1346 (29)	533 (36)	813 (26)	1.38	1.27–1.50	1.37	1.25–1.51
Male	2893 (63)	994 (68)	1899 (61)	1.24	1.13–1.36	1.19	1.08–1.31
Age ≥65 years old	1118 (24)	341 (23)	777 (25)	0.94	0.85–1.04	0.95	0.86–1.06
Born in United States	792 (17)	313 (21)	479 (15)	1.31	1.19–1.44	1.18	1.06–1.31
Moved ever during treatment	234 (5.1)	94 (6.4)	140 (4.4)	1.28	1.09–1.50	1.23	1.04–1.46
Homelessness, alcohol or drug use	692 (15)	269 (18)	413 (13)	1.29	1.16–1.43	1.16	1.04–1.30
History of TB disease	286 (6.3)	97 (6.7)	189 (6.1)	1.07	0.91–1.27	1.09	0.92–1.29
HIV-positive[b]	143 (3.1)	41 (2.8)	102 (3.3)	0.90	0.69–1.16	0.82	0.63–1.08
Cavitary and/or smear-positive TB	3181 (70)	1168 (80)	2013 (65)	1.73	1.54–1.93	1.80	1.61–2.02
Resistance to any first-line TB drug	651 (14)	182 (13)	469 (15)	0.86	0.76–0.98	0.91	0.80–1.04
No directly observed therapy	342 (7.4)	138 (9.4)	204 (6.5)	1.30	1.13–1.48	1.24	1.07–1.45

[a] alive at diagnosis and starting treatment, pulmonary only, culture-positive TB, age ≥18 years old; excluding missing or Both provider type, moved out of United States, deaths ≤60 days after treatment start.
[b] vs. HIV-negative or unknown status.
TB = tuberculosis, CC = culture conversion, RR = relative risk, CI = 95% confidence interval, aRR = adjusted relative risk, HIV = human immunodeficiency virus.

Table 3. No Directly Observed Therapy throughout TB Treatment, TB Cases Reported in California, 2007–2011 (n = 4585).

Characteristic	All patients[a] (col %)	No DOT (n = 342) (col %)	DOT (n = 4226) (col %)	Univariable RR	CI	Multivariable aRR	CI
Private provider/other	1335 (29)	270 (79)	1065 (25)	9.13	7.10–11.7	8.56	6.59–11.1
Male	2880 (63)	196 (57)	2684 (63)	0.79	0.64–0.98	NA	NA
Age ≥65 years old	1108 (24)	97 (28)	1011 (24)	1.24	0.99–1.56	0.79	0.64–0.99
Born in United States	791 (17)	68 (20)	723 (17)	1.20	0.93–1.54	NA	NA
Moved ever during treatment	228 (5.0)	23 (6.7)	205 (4.8)	1.38	0.92–2.06	NA	NA
Homelessness, alcohol or drug use	682 (15)	16 (4.7)	666 (16)	0.28	0.17–0.46	0.39	0.24–0.66
History of TB disease	284 (6.3)	14 (4.1)	270 (6.4)	0.64	0.39–1.09	0.53	0.30–0.94
HIV-positive[b]	143 (3.1)	5 (1.4)	138 (3.3)	0.46	0.19–1.10	0.51	0.21–1.22
Cavitary and/or smear-positive TB disease	3168 (70)	150 (45)	3018 (72)	0.35	0.29–0.43	0.41	0.33–0.49
Resistance to any first-line TB drug	648 (14)	31 (9.2)	617 (15)	0.61	0.43–0.88	0.64	0.46–0.91
No documented culture conversion ≤60 days	1459 (32)	138 (40)	1321 (31)	1.44	1.18–1.78	1.23	1.01–1.49

[a]alive at diagnosis and starting treatment, pulmonary only, culture-positive TB, age ≥18 years old; excluding missing or Both provider type, moved out of United States, deaths ≤60 days after treatment start.
[b]vs. HIV-negative or unknown status.
TB = tuberculosis, DOT = directly observed therapy, RR = relative risk, CI = 95% confidence interval, aRR = adjusted relative risk, NA = not in final multivariate model, HIV = human immunodeficiency virus.

funding is associated with better public health performance, [37] specifically for infectious disease morbidity. [38]

Our analysis assessed two aspects of clinical TB care that are modifiable and important. Documenting sputum culture conversion to negative during the initiation phase of treatment is a key clinical measure of treatment efficacy, and allows determination of appropriate length of therapy. [9] Directly observed therapy is a strategy widely used throughout the world to ensure treatment adherence. [9,39] Providing DOT has been shown to reduce rates of acquired drug resistance. [6]

There are many reasons PMPs may not provide DOT or collect sputum cultures for TB patients, including 1) financial resources, 2) a lack of knowledge of how to provide DOT and sputum induction, and 3) lack of understanding of the value of DOT and need to document sputum culture results during treatment. There is also a tradition of HDs providing DOT for patients. [1] However, HDs with limited resources may not be able to provide DOT or sputum induction to PMP patients, or may have policies preventing this. In California, sputum induction and HD-provided DOT are reimbursable procedures under Medicaid, [40] but capacity and agreements to bill private insurance for services provided by the health department are not in place in many HDs. Encouragement under the ACA for accountable care organizations to include HD TB specialists in their group of providers might promote HD-PMP collaboration in a way that is reimbursable for the HD. Ensuring that HDs have policies and procedures in place to facilitate access to sputum induction and DOT for PMP patients is an important first step.

With an anticipated increase in private care, and a history of uneven assurance of private TB care by HDs, how will TB care be strengthened for privately-managed patients? Despite barriers, improvement is possible and has been demonstrated by California TB control programs that systematically and routinely review PMP-managed patients during case conferences. [41] Health departments have reported success in working with PMPs on TB prevention when HDs have administrative support, have a toolkit of educational information, protocols and forms, and work to develop relationships with PMPs in the community. Alerts generated by electronic health records that could trigger PMP action such as collecting sputum or notifying the HD may also contribute to success. These lessons from TB prevention could be applied to HD-PMP partnership for active TB treatment as well. [42] These interventions can be replicated in HDs undergoing fiscal cuts. The HD staff time needed to put oversight, tracking and collaborative measures in place can save time downstream as follow-up and patient care issues are averted.

Two additional points deserve comment. First, the measures of patient care analyzed in this paper are interrelated. Lack of documented culture conversion and not receiving DOT were each far more likely among PMP patients, and each also predicted the other in multivariable models. This was expected because DOT and monitoring culture conversion are case management activities overseen by the HD for both privately and publicly managed patients. These activities are likely to occur together as part of routine monitoring. We adjusted for each practice in the multivariable models to account for confounding. Second, several groups of patients were found to be more likely to receive DOT, including those with previous TB, cavitary or smear-positive TB, drug resistance, or social factors complicating treatment. This was not surprising because in California, patients with these factors are prioritized for DOT. In both the main analysis, and the

subanalysis which included only patients with at least one indication for DOT in California, PMP care remained the strongest independent predictor of not receiving DOT.

Our analysis is subject to some limitations. First, our exclusion criteria were constructed to focus on adults with culture-positive, pulmonary TB, and as a result may not be generalizable to extrapulmonary, pediatric, or culture-negative TB cases. However, the relationship between PMPs and the measures of interest held even among excluded groups of cases where sample sizes were sufficient and analysis was possible, e.g., we could not assess culture conversion among culture-negative cases. Second, information on provider type in TB surveillance data may be subject to misclassification because HDs may not apply a uniform definition. [14] Patients reported as managed by Both HD and PMP may be co-managed, or sequentially managed, depending on local policies and procedures or individual situation; these distinctions would affect the interpretation of results for this category of patients. However, we restricted our analytic cohort to cases managed solely by either private or public health providers, types for which the definitions are clearest. We also showed that the proportion of patients reported as Both HD and PMP was small and declining, and that grouping these patients with either HD or PMP patients did not affect the overall results. Third, we were unable to distinguish between types of private medical provider settings (e.g., HMOs, private medical practices, non-profit clinics, and private or non-HD public hospitals). Aggregating disparate provider groups in our analysis may have masked important findings specific to one type of private provider. Stratified analysis by these private provider types, or even by specific large provider groups, would be an important next step in determining tailored interventions. Last, the TB report form was unable to distinguish whether a recorded delay in culture conversion was due to a delay in sputum collection, or persistent culture-positive sputum. Therefore, it may be that PMPs are equally able to render patients culture negative but PMP patients are less likely to have this documented in the public health record in a consistent and timely way. However, PMP care predicted both delayed culture conversion and never documented conversion in our analysis. Regardless of the reason for delayed culture conversion, our findings show the need for increasing PMP education and collaboration between HDs and PMPs.

In conclusion, our findings point to an opportunity for improvement in clinical care provided to TB patients managed exclusively in the private sector. Implementation of the ACA should take into account the TB expertise found in public sector TB programs, reinforce the role of public health departments to ensure optimal treatment of persons with TB disease, and make resources for key TB management practices available and accessible to all patients, regardless of where care is received.

Acknowledgments

The authors wish to acknowledge Alex Golden, for assistance with manuscript preparation; Lisa Pascopella, for statistical methodology consultation; Cathy Miller, Peter Oh, Jan Young, and Stephanie Spencer for key reference materials; and the California Tuberculosis Control Branch Registry, for data quality assurance and database preparation.

Author Contributions

Conceived and designed the experiments: ME JF PMB. Analyzed the data: ME. Wrote the paper: ME JF PMB.

References

1. Sbarbaro JA (1970) The public health tuberculosis clinic: its place in comprehensive health care. Am Rev Respir Dis 101: 463–465.
2. Binkin NJ, Vernon AA, Simone PM, McCray E, Miller BI, et al. (1999) Tuberculosis prevention and control activities in the United States: an overview of the organization of tuberculosis services. Int J Tuberc Lung Dis 3: 663–674.
3. Centers for Disease Control and Prevention (2012) Reported Tuberculosis in the United States, 2011. Available at: http://www.cdc.gov/tb/statistics/reports/2011. Accessed on October 31, 2013.
4. Taylor Z, Nolan CM, Blumberg HM (2005) Controlling tuberculosis in the United States. Recommendations from the American Thoracic Society, CDC, and the Infectious Diseases Society of America. MMWR Recomm Rep 54: 1–81. rr5412a1 [pii].
5. Institute of Medicine (2000) Ending Neglect: The Elimination of Tuberculosis in the United States. Washington, D.C.: National Academy Press.
6. Porco TC, Oh P, Flood JM (2013) Antituberculosis drug resistance acquired during treatment: an analysis of cases reported in California, 1994–2006. Clin Infect Dis 56: 761–769. cis989 [pii]; 10.1093/cid/cis989 [doi].
7. Moonan PK, Quitugua TN, Pogoda JM, Woo G, Drewyer G, et al. (2011) Does directly observed therapy (DOT) reduce drug resistant tuberculosis? BMC Public Health 11: 19, . 1471-2458-11-19 [pii]; 10.1186/1471-2458-11-19 [doi].
8. Weis SE, Slocum PC, Blais FX, King B, Nunn M, et al. (1994) The effect of directly observed therapy on the rates of drug resistance and relapse in tuberculosis. N Engl J Med 330: 1179–1184. 10.1056/NEJM199404283301702 [doi].
9. American Thoracic Society, Centers for Disease Control and Prevention, Infectious Diseases Society of America (2003) Treatment of tuberculosis. MMWR Recomm Rep 52: 1–77.
10. US Government Printing Office (2012) Public Law 111–148: Patient Protection and Affordable Care Act.
11. U.S. Department of Health and Human Services (2009) U.S. Code of Federal Regulations, 45 CFR 46.101.
12. Centers for Disease Control and Prevention (2003) Report of Verified Case of Tuberculosis (RVCT). CDC 72.9A.
13. Centers for Disease Control and Prevention (2009) Report of Verified Case of Tuberculosis (RVCT). CDC 72.9A.
14. Sprinson JE, Lawton ES, Porco TC, Flood JM, Westenhouse JL (2006) Assessing the validity of tuberculosis surveillance data in California. BMC Public Health 6: 217.
15. Ehman M, Shaw T, Cass A, Lawton E, Westenhouse J, et al. (2013) Developing and Using Performance Measures Based on Surveillance Data for Program Improvement in Tuberculosis Control. J Public Health Manag Pract 19: E29–E37. 10.1097/PHH.0b013e3182751d6f [doi].
16. Centers for Disease Control and Prevention (2010) Monitoring tuberculosis programs - National Tuberculosis Indicator Project, United States, 2002–2008. MMWR Morb Mortal Wkly Rep 59: 295–298. mm5910a3 [pii].
17. National Cancer Institute (2013) Joinpoint Regression Program, Version 4.0.4. Available at: http://srab.cancer.gov/joinpoint. Accessed on October 31, 2013.
18. Kim HJ, Fay MP, Feuer EJ, Midthune DN (2000) Permutation tests for joinpoint regression with applications to cancer rates. Stat Med 19: 335–351. 10.1002/(SICI)1097-0258(20000215)19:3<335::AID-SIM336>3.0.CO; 2-Z [pii].
19. SAS Institute Inc. (2012) SAS, version 9.3 [Software].
20. McNutt LA, Wu C, Xue X, Hafner JP (2003) Estimating the relative risk in cohort studies and clinical trials of common outcomes. Am J Epidemiol 157: 940–943.
21. Zou G (2004) A modified poisson regression approach to prospective studies with binary data. Am J Epidemiol 159: 702–706.
22. Pan W (2001) Akaike's information criterion in generalized estimating equations. Biometrics 57: 120–125.
23. California Department of Public Health, California Tuberculosis Controller's Association (2011) Guidelines for Directly Observed Therapy Program Protocols in California. http://www.ctca.org/fileLibrary/file_347_pdf.
24. Tuberculosis Control Branch (2013) Report on Tuberculosis in California, 2012. http://www.cdph.ca.gov/data/statistics/Pages/TuberculosisDiseaseData_aspx.
25. Golub JE, Bur S, Cronin WA, Gange S, Baruch N, et al. (2005) Patient and health care system delays in pulmonary tuberculosis diagnosis in a low-incidence state. Int J Tuberc Lung Dis 9: 992–998.
26. Liu Z, Shilkret KL, Finelli L (1998) Initial drug regimens for the treatment of tuberculosis: evaluation of physician prescribing practices in New Jersey, 1994 to 1995. Chest 113: 1446–1451.
27. Liu Z, Shilkret KL, Ellis HM (1999) Predictors of sputum culture conversion among patients with tuberculosis in the era of tuberculosis resurgence. Arch Intern Med 159: 1110–1116.
28. Rao SN, Mookerjee AL, Obasanjo OO, Chaisson RE (2000) Errors in the treatment of tuberculosis in Baltimore. Chest 117: 734–737.
29. Richardson NL (2000) Evaluating provider prescribing practices for the treatment of tuberculosis in Virginia, 1995 to 1998: an assessment of educational need. J Contin Educ Health Prof 20: 146–155. 10.1002/chp.1340200303 [doi].
30. Silin M, Laraque F, Munsiff SS, Crossa A, Harris TG (2010) The impact of monitoring tuberculosis reporting delays in New York City. J Public Health Manag Pract 16: E09–E17. 10.1097/PHH.0b013e3181c87ae5 [doi]; 00124784-201009000-00018 [pii].
31. Kong DG, Watt JP, Marks S, Flood J (2013) HIV status determination among tuberculosis patients from California during 2008. J Public Health Manag Pract 19: 169–177. 10.1097/PHH.0b013e3182550a83 [doi]; 00124784-201303000-00010 [pii].
32. Handford CD, Rackal JM, Tynan AM, Rzeznikiewiz D, Glazier RH (2012) The association of hospital, clinic and provider volume with HIV/AIDS care and mortality: systematic review and meta-analysis. AIDS Care 24: 267–282. 10.1080/09540121.2011.608419 [doi].
33. Honda H, Krauss MJ, Jones JC, Olsen MA, Warren DK (2010) The value of infectious diseases consultation in Staphylococcus aureus bacteremia. Am J Med 123: 631–637. S0002-9343(10)00128-2 [pii]; 10.1016/j.amjmed.2010.01.015 [doi].
34. Jenkins TC, Price CS, Sabel AL, Mehler PS, Burman WJ (2008) Impact of routine infectious diseases service consultation on the evaluation, management, and outcomes of Staphylococcus aureus bacteremia. Clin Infect Dis 46: 1000–1008. 10.1086/529190 [doi].
35. Schmitt S, McQuillen DP, Nahass R, Martinelli L, Rubin M, et al. (2013) Infectious Diseases Specialty Intervention is Associated with Decreased Mortality and Lower Healthcare Costs. Clin Infect Dis. cit610 [pii]; 10.1093/cid/cit610 [doi].
36. Davidow AL, Katz D, Reves R, Bethel J, Ngong L (2009) The challenge of multisite epidemiologic studies in diverse populations: design and implementation of a 22-site study of tuberculosis in foreign-born people. Public Health Rep 124: 391–399.
37. Mays GP, McHugh MC, Shim K, Lenaway D, Halverson PK, et al. (2004) Getting what you pay for: public health spending and the performance of essential public health services. J Public Health Manag Pract 10: 435–443.
38. Erwin PC, Greene SB, Mays GP, Ricketts TC, Davis MV (2011) The association of changes in local health department resources with changes in state-level health outcomes. Am J Public Health 101: 609–615. AJPH.2009.177451 [pii]; 10.2105/AJPH.2009.177451 [doi].
39. World Health Organization (2010) Treatment of tuberculosis: guidelines. Geneva: WHO Press.
40. California Department of Health Services (CDHS) (2013) Medi-Cal Rates. Available at: http://files.medi-cal.ca.gov/pubsdoco/rates/rateshome.asp. Accessed on October 31, 2013.
41. Cass A, Shaw T, Ehman M, Young J, Flood JM, et al. (2013) Improved Outcomes Found After Implementing a Systematic Evaluation and Program Improvement Process for Tuberculosis. Public Health Rep 128: 367–376.
42. Curry International Tuberculosis Center (2012) Engaging the Private Sector in TB Prevention. Available at: http://www.nationaltbcenter.ucsf.edu/training/webarchive/private/arch_private.cfm. Accessed on October 31, 2013.

10

Factors Predict Prolonged Wait Time and Longer Duration of Radiotherapy in Patients with Nasopharyngeal Carcinoma: A Multilevel Analysis

Po-Chun Chen[1], Ching-Chieh Yang[2], Cheng-Jung Wu[3], Wen-Shan Liu[4], Wei-Lun Huang[4], Ching-Chih Lee[5,6,7]*

1 Department of Radiation Oncology, Pingtung Christian Hospital, Pingtung, Taiwan, 2 Department of Radiation Oncology, Chi-Mei Medical Center, Tainan, Taiwan, 3 Department of Otolaryngology, Kaohsiung Veterans General Hospital, Kaohsiung, Taiwan, 4 Department of Radiation Oncology, Kaohsiung Veterans General Hospital, Kaohsiung, Taiwan, 5 Department of Otolarygology, Dalin Tzu Chi Hospital, Buddhist Tzu Chi Medical Foundation, Chiayi, Taiwan, 6 Cancer Center, Dalin Tzu Chi Hospital, Buddhist Tzu Chi Medical Foundation, Chiayi, Taiwan, 7 School of Medicine, Tzu Chi University, Hualin, Taiwan

Abstract

Purpose: Radiotherapy with or without chemotherapy is the primary treatment for patients with nasopharyngeal carcinoma (NPC). It wastes time from diagnosis to treatment. Treatment time of radiotherapy generally takes at least seven weeks. The current study aimed to evaluate factors associated with prolonged wait time and longer duration of radiotherapy in NPC patients.

Methods and Materials: From Taiwan's National Health Insurance research database, we identified 3,605 NPC patients treated with radiotherapy between 2008 and 2011. Wait time was calculated from the date of diagnosis to the start of radiotherapy. The impact of each variable on wait time and duration of radiotherapy was examined by multilevel analysis using a random-intercept model.

Results: The mean wait time and duration of radiotherapy were 1.78±3.33 and 9.72±7.27 weeks, respectively. Multilevel analysis revealed prolonged wait time in patients aged 45–65 years, those receiving radiotherapy alone, those with more comorbidities, those with low SES, and those living in eastern Taiwan. A prolonged duration of radiotherapy was associated with receipt of concurrent chemoradiotherapy, more comorbidities, and moderate SES.

Conclusions: Understanding the factors associated with longer wait times and duration of radiotherapy in patients with NPC may help healthcare providers better assist both these patients and potentially those with other head-and-neck cancers.

Editor: Bart O. Williams, Van Andel Institute, United States of America

Funding: These authors have no support or funding to report.

Competing Interests: The authors have declared that no competing interests exist.

* Email: hematcd2@hotmail.com

Introduction

Nasopharyngeal carcinoma (NPC) is endemic in Southeast Asia, with an annual incidence of 6.17 per 100,000 in Taiwan; its annual incidence in Western countries, by contrast, is <1 per 100,000 [1]. Radiotherapy with or without chemotherpy, which has long been the primary treatment for NPC, varies slightly in treatment modalities [2,3]. Although NPC is highly radiosensive, a high failure rate is noted in patients with advanced stage. Treatment stratigies and some time factors, such as wait time or length of treatment, have yet to be optimized [4–5].

The impact of time delay on disease control has been investigated in patients with head-and-neck cancers [6]. Moreover, a previous report showed that a treatment delay of >40 days was significantly associated with poorer survival rates in early-stage head-and-neck cancer patients [7]. A longer course of radiother-apy may result in poor disease control in early-stage NPC patients (>12 weeks) or early-stage head-and-neck cancer patients (>7 weeks) [8,9]. It is important to raise awareness of time delay and prolonged treatment time for decision makers in clinical practice. At present, it remains unclear which factors are associated with time delay and a prolonged duration of radiotherapy in NPC.

We used the nationwide claims data from Taiwan's National Health Insurance (NHI) research database to analyze NPC patients who received radiotherapy between 2008 and 2011. This database provides basic demographic data as well as hospital characteristics, patient characteristics and treatment modality. We sought to identify key factors associated with prolonged wait time and a longer duration of radiotherapy in NPC patients. In terms of improving treatment effects, we hope these information may help to improve future public health stategies and welfare policies.

Patients and Methods

Ethical consideration

This study was approved by the Institutional Review Board of Buddhist Dalin Tzu Chi General Hospital, Taiwan. Review board requirements for written informed consent were waived because all personal identifying information was removed from the dataset prior to analysis.

Study population

We inspected 5,026 NPC patients who received radiotherapy from Taiwan's NHI research database between 2008 to 2011. Taiwan's NHI program covered 99% of the population after 2003, with chart reviews and patient interviews used to verify the accuracy of diagnosis and treatment coding. Patients who received induction or systemic chemotherapy as the initial treatment were excluded except those who received chemotherapy within 14 days prior to radiotherapy. We also excluded patients who were treated for second irradiation. This left 3,605 patients who matched the inclusion criteria for this study. Basic data collected included wait time, duration of radiotherapy, hospital characteristics, gender, age, treatment modality, Charlson Comorbidity Index Score (CCIS), and patient socioeconomic status (SES).

Treatment modality

Concurrent chemotherapy regimen mostly used in Taiwan is cisplatin 100 mg/m^2 every 3 weeks for 3 cycles or weekly cisplatin 40 mg/m^2, followed by adjuvant cisplatin-based chemotherapy (cisplatin 80 mg/m^2 D1, 5-FU 1000 mg/m^2 D1-4, repeat cycle every 4 weeks for 1–3 cycles). External beam irradiation of 66–78 Gy was delivered in 33–39 fractions daily using three-dimensional conformal radiotherapy or intensity-modulated radiotherapy.

Wait time and duration of radiotherapy

Wait time was calculated from the date of diagnosis to the start of radiotherapy. We used the cutpoint of >4 weeks to define prolonged wait time. Duration of radiotherapy was calculated from the start of radiotherapy to the end of radiotherapy. We used the cutpoint of >10 weeks to define longer duration of radiotherapy.

Other covariates

SES and urbanization of residence were taken from insurance premiums, using income in Taiwan and urbanization variables previously described [10]. Patients were classified into 3 subgroups: high SES (civil servants, full-time or regular paid personnel with a government affiliation or employees of privately owned institutions), moderate SES (self-employed individuals, other employees, and members of the farmers' or fishermen's associations), and low SES (veterans, low-income families, and substitute service draftees). Severity of comorbidity was based on the modified CCIS as recorded before the diagnosis of NPC. The CCIS is a widely accepted scale used for risk adjustment in administrative claims data sets [11]. Different level of hospitals may have inequalities in treatment delay and clinical management during radiotherapy. The hospitals were categorized by hospital teaching level (medical center, regional hospital, or district hospital) or hospital ownership (porfit, non-profit, or public). The geographic regions were recorded as northern, central, southern, and eastern Taiwan.

Statistical analysis

The key dependent variables of interest were wait time and duration of radiotherapy. The distribution of diseases was described and compared using chi-squared testing. The continuous variables were compared with one-way ANOVA test. Patient characteristics (age, gender, individual SES, CCIS, urbanization and region of patient residence) and hospital characteristics (including ownership and teaching level) were included in the regression model. In this series, the herarchical linear regression method was used due to the potential clustering effect within a hospital. A hospital-level random effect might account for possible correlations between the wait time and duration of radiotherapy within a hospital's panel. A two-tailed value of p<0.05 was considered significant. All statistical operations were performed using SPSS (version 15, SPSS Inc., Chicago, IL).

Results

A total of 3,605 NPC patients in Taiwan received radiotherapy from 2008 to 2011. Table 1 summarizes the basic demographic characteristics of these patients. In all, 317 patients (8.8%) had wait times greater than 4 weeks. There were 1404 patients (38.9%) who had longer duration of radiotherapy. The mean duration of radiotherapy is 7.68 weeks and 10.16 weeks in patients who received radiotherapy alone and concurrent chemoradiotherapy (CCRT), respectively. Most patients (87.5%) were younger than 65 years. More than half of patients (59.1%) were treated at a medical center. Most, or 2,970 patients (82.4%), received CCRT. Approximately 15.9% of all patients had low SES. Most patients (72%) had lower CCIS. The mean wait time and duration of radiotherapy were 1.78±3.33 and 9.72±7.27 weeks, respectively (Table 2).

Wait time

Univariate analysis revealed that wait times were prolonged in patients older than 45 years, those who received radiotherapy alone, those with higher CCIS, those with low to moderate SES, and those who did not live in northern Taiwan.

After adjusting for patient and hospital characteristics, the herarchical linear regression revealed significant factors assoicated with wait time as the followings: for those age 45–65 years was 0.25 week longer than those age less than 45 years (p = 0.03); for those with RT alone was 1.78 week longer than those with CCRT (p<0.001); for those with higher morbidities was 0.72 week longer than those with lower comorbidities (p<0.001); for those with low SES was 0.34 week longer than those with high SES (p = 0.029) and those in eastern area was 1.29 week longer than the northern area (Table 3).

Duration of radiotherapy

Univariate analysis revealed a longer duration of radiotherapy in patients who received CCRT, with a mean of 10.16 weeks; in those with higher CCIS, with a mean of 10.62 weeks; and in those with low or moderate SES, with a mean of 10.04 weeks.

After adjusting for patient and hospital characteristics, the herarchical linear regression revealed significant factors assoicated with duration of radiotherapy as the followings: for those with RT alone was 2.42 week shorter than those with CCRT (p<0.001); for those with higher morbidities was 1.08 week longer than those with lower comorbidities (p<0.001); for those with moderate SES was 0.65 week longer than those with high SES (p = 0.021) (Table 3).

Table 1. Demographic characteristics for nasopharyngeal cancer patients from 2008 to 2011 (n = 3,605).

Characteristics	Wait time					Duration of radiotherapy				
	Less than 4 weeks (n = 3288)		More than 4 weeks (n = 317)		P value	Less than 10 weeks (n = 2201)		More than 10 weeks (n = 1404)		P value
	No.	%	No.	%		No.	%	No.	%	
Hospital characteristics										
Ownership					0.008					<0.001
For Profit (n = 1,915)	1,770	53.8	145	45.7		1,114	50.6	801	57.1	
Non-profit (n = 563)	498	15.1	65	20.5		396	18.0	167	11.9	
Public (n = 1,127)	1,020	31.1	107	33.8		691	31.4	436	31.1	
Teaching level					0.442					0.006
Medical center (n = 2,332)	2,131	64.8	201	63.4		1,394	63.3	938	66.8	
Regional (n = 1,121)	1,015	30.9	106	33.4		724	32.9	397	28.3	
District (n = 152)	142	4.3	10	3.2		83	3.8	69	4.9	
Gender					0.498					0.151
Male (n = 2,711)	2,472	75.2	239	75.4		1,637	74.4	1,074	76.5	
Female (n = 894)	816	24.8	78	24.6		564	25.6	330	23.5	
Age group					<0.001					0.185
0–44.99 years (n = 1,239)	1,166	35.5	73	23.0		733	33.3	506	36.0	
45–64.99 years (n = 1,916)	1,739	52.9	177	55.8		1,182	53.7	734	52.3	
Older than 65 years (n = 450)	383	11.6	67	21.1		286	13.0	164	11.7	
Treatment					<0.001					<0.001
CCRT[†] (n = 2,970)	2,789	84.8	181	57.1		1,705	77.5	1,265	90.1	
RT[‡] alone (n = 635)	499	15.2	136	42.9		496	22.5	139	9.9	
Charlson Comorbidity Index Score					<0.001					0.053
Lower than mean (n = 2,597)	2,411	73.3	186	58.7		1,611	73.2	986	70.2	
Higher than mean (n = 1,008)	877	26.7	131	41.3		590	26.8	418	29.8	
Socioeconomic status (SES)					0.031					0.050
High SES (n = 1,857)	1,709	52.0	148	46.7		1,169	53.2	688	49.0	
Moderate SES (n = 1,176)	1,073	32.6	103	32.5		690	31.3	486	34.6	

Table 1, continued

Characteristics	Wait time					Duration of radiotherapy				
	Less than 4 weeks (n = 3288)		More than 4 weeks (n = 317)		P value	Less than 10 weeks (n = 2201)		More than 10 weeks (n = 1404)		P value
	No.	%	No.	%		No.	%	No.	%	
Low SES (n = 572)	506	15.4	66	20.8		342	15.5	230	16.4	
Urbanization					0.045					0.728

Table 1. Cont.

Characteristics	Wait time					Duration of radiotherapy					
	Less than 4 weeks (n=3288)		More than 4 weeks (n=317)		P value	Less than 10 weeks (n=2201)		More than 10 weeks (n=1404)		P value
	No.	%	No.	%		No.	%	No.	%	
Urban (n=1,149)	1,056	32.1	93	29.3		692	31.4	457	32.5	
Suburban (n=1,508)	1,386	42.2	122	38.5		922	41.9	586	41.7	
Rural (n=948)	846	25.7	102	32.2		587	26.7	361	25.8	
Geographic Region					<0.001					0.021
Northern (n=1,745)	1,745	53.1	133	42.0		1,122	51.0	756	53.8	
Central (n=502)	502	15.3	53	16.7		370	16.8	185	13.2	
Southern (n=946)	946	28.8	113	35.6		636	28.9	423	30.1	
Eastern (n=95)	95	2.9	18	5.7		73	3.3	40	2.8	

†CCRT, Concurrent chemoradiotherapy.
‡RT, Radiotherapy.

Discussion

Our study demonstrated that higher CCIS was an independent factor for both prolonged wait time and longer duration of radiotherapy in NPC patients. Lower SES was an independent factor for time delay but not for duration of radiotherapy. CCRT was associated with the greatest duration of radiotherapy, prolonging treatment 2.42 weeks more than radiotherapy alone.

The strengths of our study include the endemic nature of NPC in Taiwan, allowing for the collection of a large sample size to make valid estimates and compare treatment modalities. Moreover, the NHI research database captures complete follow-up information, provides comprehensive health care benefits with a moderate cost sharing, and records all treatments. Ongoing validation of the NHI research database is conducted via comparison of chart-based and claims-based records [12]. To avoid causes of delay not identified in our study, we excluded patients with an interval of more than 120 days between diagnosis and start of radiotherapy. To our knowledge, this is the first study investigating the association between time factors and hospital characteristics, patient characteristics, and treatment modality in NPC patients.

As cancer incidence has increased in various parts of the world, so has the demand for radiotherapy for each type and stage of cancer [13,14]. Radiotherapy facilities are available worldwide, but are often inadequate to the population demands placed on them. In Taiwan, the nearly 60 radiotherapy facilities provide medical care for more than 20 million people. Taiwan's NHI program has provided for the medical needs of Taiwan for 20 years. Nevertheless, treatment delays are common. Similarly, Round et al. [13] compared predictive models for radiotherapy demand. The Methus model estimated a 13.1% increase in need for radiotherapy between 2011 and 2016. In general, treatment delays may result from health policy, patients themselves, or hospital characteristics. In our study, we did not find any significant difference in wait time between medical centers and other types of hospitals. Furthermore, alternating radiotherapy helps to relieve the burden on the system and shorten the wait time. However, such treatment is not indicated for certain cancers.

A literature review reported a negative impact of comorbidity on incidence of treatment complication, quality of life, increased cost of treatment and survival [15]. Assessment of comorbid diseases should be an important part in clinical practice. Moreover, the impact of comorbid diseases on therapeutic decision-making in head and neck cancer has been reported [16]. Comorbidity was assessed with Adult Comorbidity Evaluation (ACE-27) and Charlson Comorbidity Index (CCI). Results showed moderate to strong positive correlation between comorbidity and change in therapeutic decision-making. In our study, higher CCIS is an independent factor for both prolonged wait time and longer duration of radiotherapy in NPC patients. It is important to correct any underlying comorbid diseases prior to and during radiotherapy. Moreover, radiotherapy is a local treatment. The most common treatment-related side effects which lead to unplanned treatment interruptions are severe mucositis and skin reaction. The recovery time depends on the degree of the injury. Some comorbid conditions are associated with delayed wound healing, especially poor nutritional status, vascular disease, and diabetes mellitus [17]. Since the exact cause of treatment interruptions in our study is unknown, possible causes have been discussed using Charlson Comorbidity Index Score instead of a specific comorbid disease. A recently published study has developed a revised comorbidity index for head and neck cancer

Table 2. Distribution of wait time and duration of radiotherapy for nasopharyngeal cancer patients from 2008 to 2011 by univariate analysis (n = 3,605).

Characteristics	Wait time			Duration of radiotherapy		
	Mean	± SD	P value	Mean	± SD	P value
	1.78	3.33		9.72	7.27	
Hospital characteristics						
Ownership			0.092			0.064
Profit organization (n = 1,915)	1.71	3.45		9.92	7.88	
Non-profit organization (n = 563)	2.06	3.44		9.10	6.19	
Public (n = 1,127)	1.77	3.05		9.69	6.65	
Teaching level			0.226			0.171
Medical center (n = 2,332)	1.72	3.21		9.81	7.34	
Regional (n = 1,121)	1.93	3.54		9.43	7.21	
District (n = 152)	1.77	3.47		10.43	6.55	
Gender			0.803			0.811
Male (n = 2,711)	1.79	3.35		9.70	7.32	
Female (n = 894)	1.76	3.27		9.77	7.11	
Age group			<0.001			0.407
0–44.99 years (n = 1,239)	1.44	2.71		9.90	6.83	
45–64.99 years (n = 1,916)	1.90	3.54		9.68	6.98	
Older than 65 years (n = 450)	2.23	3.85		9.39	9.37	
Treatment			<0.001			<0.001
CCRT[†] (n = 2,970)	1.47	2.60		10.16	7.49	
RT[‡] alone (n = 635)	3.27	5.36		7.68	5.71	
Charlson Comorbidity Index Score			<0.001			<0.001
Lower than mean (n = 2,597)	1.58	2.80		9.37	6.50	
Higher than mean (n = 1,008)	2.30	4.37		10.62	8.90	
Socioeconomic status (SES)			0.008			0.036
High SES (n = 1,857)	1.66	2.99		9.42	6.37	
Moderate SES (n = 1,176)	1.81	3.42		10.04	8.37	
Low SES (n = 572)	2.15	4.08		10.04	7.53	
Table 2, continued						
Characteristics	**Wait time**			**Duration of radiotherapy**		
	Mean	±SD	P value	Mean	±SD	P value
Urbanization			0.348			0.482
Urban (n = 1,149)	1.73	3.30		9.61	7.53	
Suburban (n = 1,508)	1.74	3.29		9.89	7.53	
Rural (n = 948)	1.92	3.42		9.58	6.45	
Geographic Region			<0.001			0.698
Northern (n = 1,745)	1.58	3.06		9.68	7.28	
Central (n = 502)	1.87	3.22		9.50	6.40	
Southern (n = 946)	1.99	3.54		9.92	7.81	
Eastern (n = 95)	2.76	5.32		9.55	5.78	

[†]CCRT, Concurrent chemoradiotherapy.
[‡]RT, Radiotherapy.
SD, standard deviation;

patients [18]. It is worth investigating this revised comorbidity index in NPC patients in future studies.

In fact, patients with low SES have inequalities in health. They have delays in diagnosis, are offered different treatment modalities than those with higher income, and experience inferior outcomes to those of patients with higher SES, mostly shown in research on breast cancer [10,12,19]. A systemic review shows that patients from lower social classes receive significantly less positive socio-emotional utterances, a more directive and a less participatory consulting style, characterized by by significantly less information

Table 3. Distribution of wait time and duration of radiotherapy for nasopharyngeal cancer patients from 2008 to 2011 by multivariate analysis using a random-intercept model (n = 3605).

Characteristics	Wait time			Duration of radiotherapy		
	Estimate	95% CI*	p value	Estimate	95% CI*	p value
Intercept	0.97	(0.53–1.41)	<0.001	9.74	(8.77–10.71)	<0.001
Hospital characteristics						
Ownership						
Profit organization	Reference			Reference		
Non-profit organization	0.13	(−0.41–0.68)	0.628	−0.27	(−1.48–0.93)	0.648
Public	0.09	(−0.37–0.55)	0.690	−0.08	(−1.10–0.93)	0.865
Teaching level						
Medical center	Reference			Reference		
Regional	0.20	(−0.21–0.62)	0.336	−0.33	(−1.25–0.59)	0.475
District	−0.07	(−0.74–0.60)	0.831	0.81	(−0.68–2.30)	0.285
Gender						
Male	Reference			Reference		
Female	−0.030	(−0.27–0.21)	0.806	0.08	(−0.45–0.62)	0.312
Age group						
0–44.99 years	Reference			Reference		
45–64.99 years	0.25	(0.02–0.49)	0.030	−0.23	(−0.75–0.28)	0.377
Older than 65 years	−0.03	(−0.41–0.33)	0.840	−0.20	(−1.04–0.62)	0.622
Treatment						
CCRT[†]	Reference			Reference		
RT[‡] alone	1.78	(1.49–2.07)	<0.001	−2.42	(−3.06–−1.77)	<0.001
Charlson Comorbidity Index Score						
Lower than mean	Reference			Reference		
Higher than mean	0.72	(0.48–0.96)	<0.001	1.08	(0.56–1.61)	<0.001
Socioeconomic status (SES)						
High SES	Reference			Reference		
Low SES	0.34	(0.03–0.64)	0.029	0.65	(−0.02–1.33)	0.059
Moderate SES	−0.01	(−0.26–0.23)	0.920	0.65	(0.09–1.20)	0.021
Table 3, continued						
Characteristics	**Wait time**			**Duration of radiotherapy**		
	Estimate	95% CI*	p value	Estimate	95% CI*	p value
Urbanization						
Urban	Reference			Reference		
Suburban	−0.18	(−0.45–0.07)	0.159	0.31	(−0.27–0.90)	0.291
Rural	−0.28	(−0.61–0.03)	0.081	−0.09	(−0.81–0.62)	0.796
Geographic Region						
Northern	Reference			Reference		
Central	0.17	(−0.25–0.60)	0.426	0.01	(−0.94–0.95)	0.992
Southern	0.29	(−0.06–0.66)	0.111	0.04	(−0.76–0.85)	0.909
Eastern	1.29	(0.51–2.08)	0.01	−0.21	(−1.94–1.51)	0.805

[†]CCRT, Concurrent chemoradiotherapy.
[‡]RT, Radiotherapy.
CI, confidence interval.

giving, less directions and less socio-emotional and partnership building utterances from their doctor [20]. In Taiwan, SES does not affect the medical care patients receive, as all receive universal health insurance which reimburses hospitals directly for care. Even so, patients in our study who had low SES had significantly prolonged wait times over others. Thorough communication between doctors and patients is crucial so that mutual understanding can be achieved to improve patients' compliance, thereby reduce prolonged wait times, especially in low SES patients.

An early report from Hong Kong confirmed that interruptions in and prolongation of treatment adversely affect outcomes in radiotherapy for NPC [21]. Other studies have also demonstrated the impact of a longer duration of radiation treatment on local failure risk and overall survival in patients with NPC and other types of head-and-neck cancers [8,9,22]. However, there is little evidence to suggest which factors are associated with prolonged duration of radiotherapy. To find a possible correlation, we looked in this study for factors associated with prolonged radiation treatment time. CCRT was associated with the greatest duration of radiotherapy in this study. In general, acute toxicity caused by radiation and chemotherapy is responsible for this. Concurrent chemotherapy would increase acute toxicity over that of radiotherapy alone. Supportive medications to improve symptoms such as odynophagia and severe skin reaction should be provided as early as possible. Kim et al. [23] reported a prescription of a 3-week cycle of 100 mg/m^2 cisplatin prolonged treatment 1.8 weeks more than weekly cisplatin 30 mg/m^2. Current evidence suggested no difference in survival between the two chemotherapy groups. In our study, concurrent chemotherapy regimen mostly used is either cisplatin 100 mg/m^2 every 3 weeks for 3 cycles or weekly cisplatin 40 mg/m^2. Weekly Cisplatin that causes less complications may be effectively used to avoid treatment interruptions, thereby shorten the radiation treatment period.

This study has three potential limitations. Firstly, cancer stage was not obtained. However, we excluded patients who had potentially distant metastases by capturing information on the interval between initial chemotherapy and radiotherapy. In fact, the association between cancer stage and time factos has not yet to be identified from previous literatures. Secondly, the diagnosis of NPC and the record of comorbid conditions are dependent on ICD codes. Different coding quality between different levels of hospitals may result in bias. Finally, the assoicaiton of time factors

ad NPC outcomes were not explored in this series, and we will lanuch a new study in the furure. However, the NHI program in Taiwan reviews selected charts to verify the accuracy of diagnosis and treatment coding.

Conclusion

Radiotherapy is a multi-step, time-consuming treatment. It is difficult to determine whether the time delay related to health policy, patient factors, hospital characteristics, or some combination of these. With available administrative data, we found significant factors associated with prolonged wait time and longer duration of radiotherapy in patients with NPC. Our study may help healthcare providers and those responsible for health policy better understand this patient population and even apply these results to those with other head-and-neck cancers so as to make informed decisions on how to reduce wait time and length of treatment in the future. The impact of both wait time and duration of radiotherapy on survival remains to be investigated.

Acknowledgments

This study is based on data from the National Health Insurance Research Database provided by the Bureau of National Health Insurance, Department of Health, Taiwan, and managed by the National Health Research Institute. The interpretations and conclusions contained herein do not represent those of the Bureau of National Health Insurance, the Department of Health, or the National Health Research Institute.

Author Contributions

Conceived and designed the experiments: PCC CCL. Performed the experiments: PCC CCL. Analyzed the data: CCL. Contributed reagents/materials/analysis tools: PCC CCL. Wrote the paper: PCC CCY CJW WSL WLH CCL.

References

1. Taiwan Cancer Registry Annual Report, 2001. (2004) Department of Health, The Executive Yuan, Republic of China. Available: http://tcr.cph.ntu.edu.tw/main.php?Page=N2. Accessed 17 March 2014.
2. Wei WI, Sham JS (2005) Nasopharyngeal carcinoma. Lancet 365: 2041–2054.
3. Zhang L, Zhao C, Ghimire B, Hong MH, Liu Q, et al. (2010) The role of concurrent chemoradiotherapy in the treatment of locoregionally advanced nasopharyngeal carcinoma among endemic population: a meta-analysis of the phase III randomized trials. BMC Cancer 10: 558.
4. Lin JC, Jan JS, Hsu CY, Liang WM, Jiang RS, et al. (2003) Phase III study of concurrent chemoradiotherapy versus radiotherapy alone for advanced nasopharyngeal carcinoma: positive effect on overall and progression-free survival. J Clin Oncol 21: 631–637.
5. Chan AT, Teo PM, Ngan RK, Leung TW, Lau WH, et al. (2002) Concurrent chemotherapy-radiotherapy compared with radiotherapy alone in locoregionally advanced nasopharyngeal carcinoma: progression-free survival analysis of a phase III randomized trial. J Clin Oncol 20: 2038–2044.
6. Huang J, Barbera L, Brouwers M, Browman G, Mackillop WJ (2003) Does delay in starting treatment affect the outcomes of radiotherapy? A systematic review. J Clin Oncol 21: 555–563.
7. Fortin A, Bairati I, Albert M, Moore L, Allard J, et al. (2002) Effect of treatment delay on outcome of patients with early-stage head-and-neck carcinoma receiving radical radiotherapy. Int J Radiat Oncol Biol Phys 52: 929–936.
8. Cannon DM, Geye HM, Hartig GK, Traynor AM, Hoang T, et al. (2013) Increased local failure risk with prolonged radiation treatment time in head and neck cancer treated with concurrent chemotherapy. Head Neck 36: 1120–1125.
9. Chang JT, See LC, Liao CT, Chen LH, Leung WM, et al. (1998) Early stage nasopharyngeal carcinoma: radiotherapy dose and time factors in tumor control. Jpn J Clin Oncol 28: 207–213.
10. Chang TS, Chang CM, Hsu TW, Lin YS, Lai NS, et al. (2013) The combined effect of individual and neighborhood socioeconomic status on nasopharyngeal cancer survival. PLoS One 8:e73889.
11. Deyo RA, Cherkin DC, Ciol MA (1992) Adapting a clinical comorbidity index for use with ICD-9-CM administrative databases. J Clin Epidemiol 45: 613–619.
12. Cheng CL, Kao YH, Lin SJ, Lee CH, Lai ML (2011) Validation of the National Health Insurance Research Database with ischemic stroke cases in Taiwan. Pharmacoepidemiol Drug Saf 20: 236–242.
13. Round CE, Williams MV, Mee T, Kirkby NF, Cooper T, et al. (2013) Radiotherapy demand and activity in England 2006–2020. Clin Oncol (R Coll Radiol) 25: 522–530.
14. Abdel-Wahab M, Bourque JM, Pynda Y, Iżewska J, Van der Merwe D, et al. (2013) Status of radiotherapy resources in Africa: an International Atomic Energy Agency analysis. Lancet Oncol 14:e168–e175.
15. Paleri V, Wight RG, Silver CE, Haigentz M Jr, Takes RP, et al. (2010) Comorbidity in head and neck cancer: a critical appraisal and recommendations for practice. Oral Oncol 46: 712–719.
16. Baijal G, Gupta T, Hotwani C, Laskar SG, Budrukkar A, et al. (2012) Impact of comorbidity on therapeutic decision-making in head and neck cancer: audit from a comprehensive cancer center in India. Head Neck 34: 1251–1254.
17. Takahashi PY, Kiemele LJ, Chandra A, Cha SS, Targonski PV (2009) A retrospective cohort study of factors that affect healing in long-term care residents with chronic wounds. Ostomy Wound Manage 55: 32–37.
18. Bøje CR, Dalton SO, Primdahl H, Kristensen CA, Andersen E, et al. (2014) Evaluation of comorbidity in 9388 head and neck cancer patients: a national cohort study from the DAHANCA database. Radiother Oncol 110: 91–97.
19. Wu XC, Lund MJ, Kimmick GG, Richardson LC, Sabatino SA, et al. (2012) Influence of race, insurance, socioeconomic status, and hospital type on receipt of guideline-concordant adjuvant systemic therapy for locoregional breast cancers. J Clin Oncol 30: 142–150.
20. Willems S, De Maesschalck S, Deveugele M, Derese A, De Maeseneer J, et al. (2005) Socio-economic status of the patient and doctor-patient communication: does it make a difference? Patient Educ Couns 56: 139–146.
21. Kwong DL, Sham JS, Chua DT, Choy DT, Au GK, et al. (1997) The effect of interruptions and prolonged treatment time in radiotherapy for nasopharyngeal carcinoma. Int J Radiat Oncol Biol Phys 39: 703–710.
22. Sher DJ, Posner MR, Tishler RB, Sarlis NJ, Haddad RI, et al. (2011) Relationship between radiation treatment time and overall survival after induction chemotherapy for locally advanced head-and-neck carcinoma: a subset analysis of TAX 324. Int J Radiat Oncol Biol Phys 81:e813–e818.
23. Kim TH, Ko YH, Lee MA, Kim BS, Chung SR, et al. (2008) Treatment outcome of cisplatin-based concurrent chemoradiotherapy in the patients with locally advanced nasopharyngeal cancer. Cancer Res Treat 40: 62–70.

11

Osteopontin Upregulates the Expression of Glucose Transporters in Osteosarcoma Cells

I-Shan Hsieh[1], Rong-Sen Yang[2]*, Wen-Mei Fu[1]*

1 Department of Pharmacology, College of Medicine, National Taiwan University, Taipei, Taiwan, 2 Department of Orthopedic Surgery, National Taiwan University Hospital, Taipei, Taiwan

Abstract

Osteosarcoma is the most common primary malignancy of bone. Even after the traditional standard surgical therapy, metastasis still occurs in a high percentage of patients. Glucose is an important source of metabolic energy for tumor proliferation and survival. Tumors usually overexpress glucose transporters, especially hypoxia-responsive glucose transporter 1 and glucose transporter 3. Osteopontin, hypoxia-responsive glucose transporter 1, and glucose transporter 3 are overexpressed in many types of tumors and have been linked to tumorigenesis and metastasis. In this study, we investigated the regulation of glucose transporters by osteopontin in osteosarcoma. We observed that both glucose transporters and osteopontin were upregulated in hypoxic human osteosarcoma cells. Endogenously released osteopontin regulated the expression of glucose transporter 1 and glucose transporter 3 in osteosarcoma and enhanced glucose uptake into cells via the $\alpha v \beta 3$ integrin. Knockdown of osteopontin induced cell death in 20% of osteosarcoma cells. Phloretin, a glucose transporter inhibitor, also caused cell death by treatment alone. The phloretin-induced cell death was significantly enhanced in osteopontin knockdown osteosarcoma cells. Combination of a low dose of phloretin and chemotherapeutic drugs, such as daunomycin, 5-Fu, etoposide, and methotrexate, exhibited synergistic cytotoxic effects in three osteosarcoma cell lines. Inhibition of glucose transporters markedly potentiated the apoptotic sensitivity of chemotherapeutic drugs in osteosarcoma. These results indicate that the combination of a low dose of a glucose transporter inhibitor with cytotoxic drugs may be beneficial for treating osteosarcoma patients.

Editor: Effie C. Tsilibary, National Center for Scientific Research Demokritos, Greece

Funding: This study was financially supported by Ministry of Science and Technology (NSC 101-2325-B-002-070). The funders had no role in study design, data collection and analysis, decision to publish, or preparation of the manuscript.

Competing Interests: The authors have declared that no competing interests exist.

* Email: wenmei@ntu.edu.tw (WMF); rsyang@ntuh.gov.tw (RSY)

Introduction

Osteosarcoma is the most common type of bone cancer in teenagers and is highly metastatic [1,2]. Surgery and chemotherapy are the standard treatment options for high-grade osteosarcoma. However, approximately 20% of patients have lung metastases at initial diagnosis and 40% patients experience metastasis at a later stage. The 5-year survival rate for osteosarcoma patients with metastases is 20%, compared with 65% for patients with localized disease [3].

Glucose is a source of metabolic energy that maintains tumor cells' ability to proliferate and survive. Glucose transporters (GLUTs) move glucose into the cytosol to fuel aerobic glycolysis, also known as the Warburg effect [4–6]. GLUT1 and GLUT3 are class I glucose transporters that possess a high affinity for glucose and are hypoxia-responsive. Hypoxia is an important factor during tumor progression. Under hypoxic conditions, HIF-1 (hypoxia-inducible factor 1) regulates the expression of numerous genes, such as VEGF (vascular endothelial growth factor), iNOS, EPO, LDHA (lactate dehydrogenase A), PDK1 (pyruvate dehydrogenase kinase 1), GLUT1, and GLUT3 [7]. Expression of GLUT1 and GLUT3 is regulated by developmental stage and metabolic state. Upregulation of GLUT1 and GLUT3 are reported to be associated with poor prognosis in breast cancer [8]. Overexpression of GLUT1 also corresponds with poor survival in non-small cell lung cancer [9] and tumor aggressiveness in transitional cell carcinoma of the bladder [10]. Many cancers overexpress GLUTs because of the energy requirement associated with uncontrolled proliferation and metastasis [11]; however, few studies examine the relationship between osteosarcoma progression and GLUTs.

Osteopontin (OPN) is a noncollagenous bone matrix protein that earned its name from its discovery in osteoblasts [12,13]. OPN interacts with cells through many different integrins, including $\alpha v \beta 1$, $\alpha v \beta 3$, and $\alpha v \beta 5$, via the GRGDS. OPN also binds to the CD44 receptor on the cell membrane to regulate cytokine production, cell trafficking, cell proliferation, migration, and cell survival [14,15]. OPN expression is associated with the progression of several cancers, including breast, ovarian, prostate, renal, oral, colorectal, pancreatic, liver, lung, skin, and thyroid cancers, glioblastoma, and sarcomas. The interaction of OPN with various receptors, including several integrins and CD44, induces the activation of signal transduction pathways leading to cell migration and invasion. The level of OPN is also related to tumor stage and is a biomarker for cancer progression and prognosis in many cancers. The upregulation of OPN levels concomitant with cancer type-specific markers aids in early detection of many malignancies [16–18]. VEGF, THBS3 (thrombospondin 3), osteocalcin, osteonectin, VS38c, and S100 are specific markers for osteosarcoma [19]. Higher levels of these markers are detected in the peripheral blood of osteosarcoma patients [20]. Overexpression of OPN also occurs in many osteosarcoma samples [21]. Although osteopontin has multiple physiological functions, including the attachment of osteogenic cells to the bone matrix, control of mineralization, coupling of bone formation, and resorption [22], however, the role of OPN in osteosarcoma is still not clear. In this study, we found that GLUTs and OPN increased during hypoxic conditions in osteosarcoma. OPN upregulated GLUT1 and GLUT3 expression via $\alpha v \beta 3$ integrin and the AKT, JNK, and p38 pathways in osteosarcoma cells. Knockdown of OPN increased cell death in osteosarcoma cell lines. Chemotherapeutic drugs in combination with a low dose of glucose transporter inhibitor exerted synergistic cytotoxic action. Taken together, these data suggest a new therapeutic strategy for osteosarcoma.

Materials and Methods

Cell culture

The human osteosarcoma cell lines MG63, U-2OS, and 143B were purchased from the American Type Culture Collection (Rockville, MD). MG63 cells were cultured with DMEM (Gibco; Grand Island, NY), U-2OS cells were cultured with RPMI 1640, and 143B cells were cultured with MEM. All cell cultures were supplemented with 10% fetal bovine serum (FBS; Hyclone, Logan, UT) and maintained at 37°C in a humidified atmosphere with 5% CO_2.

RNA interference

An OPN-shRNA (short-hairpin RNA) conjugated to the pLKO.1 vector containing a puromycin-resistant region was provided by the National RNAi Core Facility at the Institute of Molecular Biology/Genomic Research Center in Taipei in Taiwan. The sequences as shown below:
OPN-shRNA #1:

CCGG**CTTCAGGGTTATGTCTATGTT**CTCGAGAACA-TAGACATAACCCTGAAGTTTTT
OPN-shRNA #2:
CCGG**CCACAAGCAGTCCAGATTATA**CTCGAGTA-TAATCTGGACTGCTTGTGGTTTTT
Control-shRNA:
CCGG**TCACAGAATCGTCGTATGCAG**CTCGAGCTG-CATACGACGATTCTGTGATTTTTG

shRNA plasmids and TurboFect Transfection Reagent (#R0531; Thermo Scientific) were premixed with Opti-MEM I (Gibco, Grand Island, NY) separately for 5 min, mixed with each other for 25 min, and then applied to MG63 and U-2OS cell cultures. The control shRNA (empty vector; ev) was used as a negative control. For transient transfection, cells were transfected with two different OPN-shRNA plasmids for 24 h.

Western blot

After washing with cold phosphate-buffered saline (PBS), cells were lysed with 50 μl radioimmunoprecipitation assay buffer [RIPA; 50 mM HEPES, 150 mM NaCl, 4 mM EDTA, 10 mM $Na_4P_2O_7$, 100 mM NaF, 2 mM Na_3VO_4, 1% Triton X-100, 0.25% sodium deoxycholate, 50 mM 4-(2-aminoethyl)-benzene sulfonylfluoride, 50 μg ml^{-1} leupeptin, 20 μg ml^{-1} aprotinin, pH 7.4] on ice for 30 min. Following centrifugation of lysates at 14,500 r.p.m. for 1 h, the supernatant was isolated and used for western blotting. Protein concentration was measured using a BCA assay kit (Pierce, Rockford, IL) with bovine serum albumin as a standard. Equal concentrations of protein were separated on 8% sodium dodecyl sulfate-polyacrylamide (SDS) gels and transferred to nitrocellulose membranes (Millipore, Bedford, MA, USA). The membranes were incubated for 1 h with 5% dry skim milk in PBS buffer to block nonspecific binding and then incubated overnight at 4°C with the following primary antibodies: rabbit anti-GLUT-1, 2, 3, and 4 (1:1,000; Millipore, Billerica, MA), anti-OPN (1:1,000; Abcam Inc., Cambridge, MA), and mouse anti-β-actin (1:10,000; Santa Cruz Biotechnology, Dallas, TX). After washing with phosphate buffered saline Tween (PBST), the membranes were then incubated with mouse anti-rabbit or goat anti-mouse peroxidase-conjugated secondary antibody (1:1,000; Santa Cruz

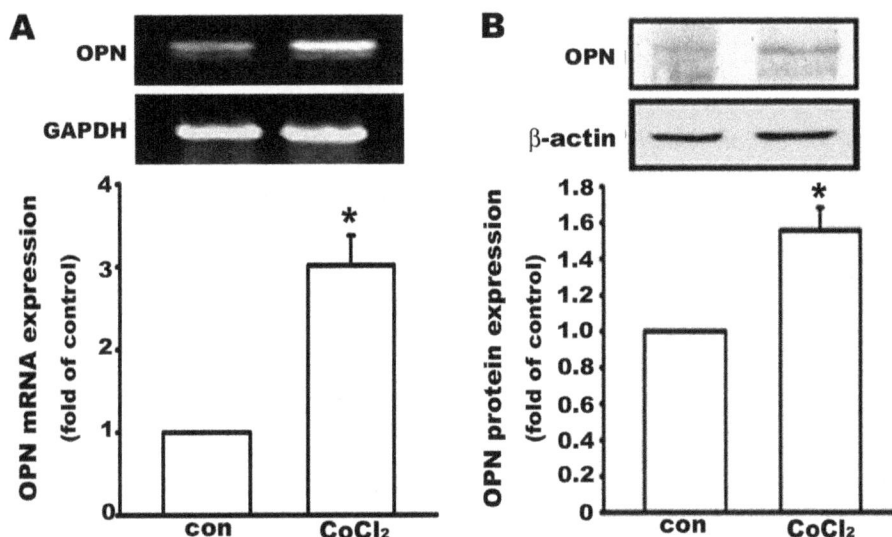

Figure 1. Hypoxia increases osteopontin expression in human osteosarcoma cells. MG63 osteosarcoma cells were treated with the chemical hypoxic agent $CoCl_2$ (100 μM). Osteopontin (OPN) mRNA (6 h) (A) and protein (24 h) (B) levels were increased by $CoCl_2$ treatment. Data are presented as the mean ± S.E.M. (n = 3), *p ≤ 0.05, as compared with the control (con).

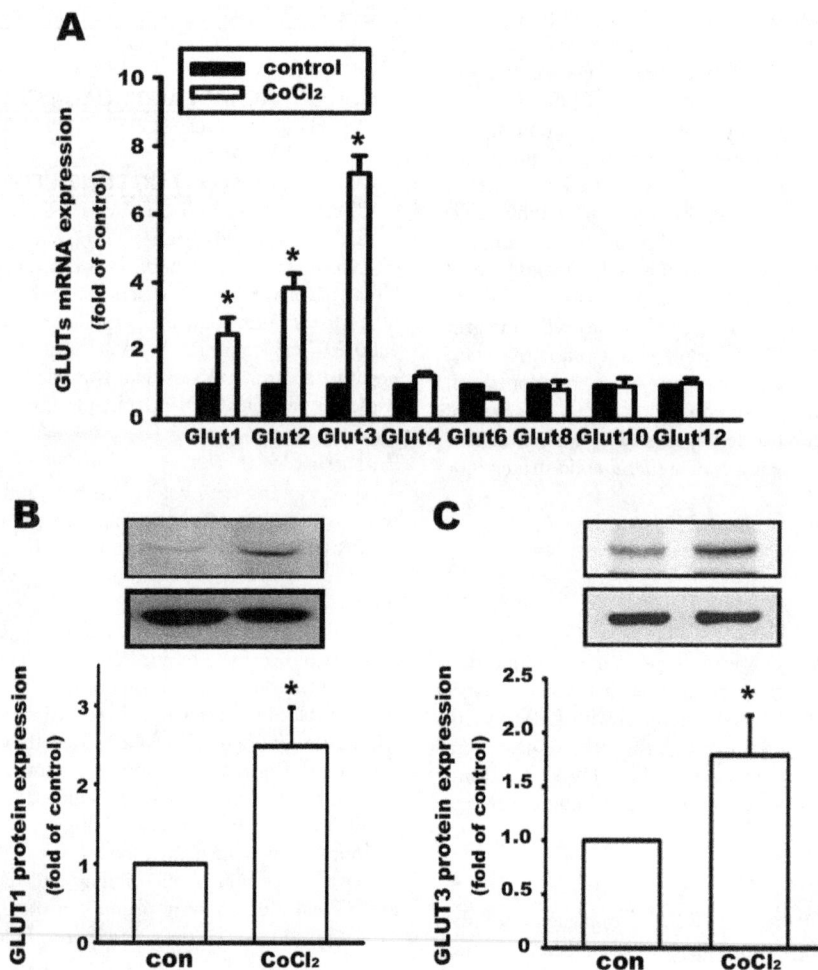

Figure 2. Hypoxia increases the expression of glucose transporters in human osteosarcoma cells. (A) The mRNA levels of glucose transporter (GLUT) 1, 2, 3, 4, 6, 8, 10, and 12 were evaluated using quantitative PCR. After treatment with $CoCl_2$ (100 μM, 6 h), GLUT 1, 2, and 3 mRNA levels were increased. $CoCl_2$ (100 μM, 24 h) also increased GLUT1 (B) and GLUT3 (C) protein levels in MG63 cells. Data are presented as the mean ± S.E.M. (n = 3), *p≤0.05, compared with the control group (con).

Biotechnology, Dallas, TX) for 1 h. The blots were visualized by enhanced chemiluminescence (ECL; Millipore, Billerica, MA) using a UVP imaging system (UVP, Upland, CA). For normalization purposes, each blot was also probed with mouse anti-β-actin (1:10,000; Santa Cruz Biotechnology, Dallas, TX).

Quantitative Real-Time PCR

Total RNA was extracted using a TRIzol kit (MDBio, Inc., Taipei, Taiwan). 2 μg RNA was used for reverse transcription that was performed with a commercial kit (Invitrogen, Carlsbad, CA). Quantitative real-time PCR was performed using a TaqMan/SYBR Master Mix (Thermo Scientific) and analyzed with a model StepOne plus System (Applied Biosystems; Foster City, CA). After pre-incubation at 50°C for 2 min and 95°C for 10 min, the PCR was performed at 40 cycles of 95°C for 15 sec and 60°C for 1 min. The threshold was set above the non-template control background and within the linear phase of target gene amplification to calculate the cycle number at which the transcript was detected (denoted as CT). The cDNA was amplified with gene specific primers as shown below:

GLUT1:
Forward: CCAGC TGCCA TTGCC GTT

Reverse: GACGT AGGGA CCACA CAGTT GC
GLUT2:
Forward: CACAC AAGAC CTGGA ATTGA CA
Reverse: CGGTC ATCCA GTGGA ACAC
GLUT3:
Forward: CAATG CTCCT GAGAA GATCA TAA
Reverse: AAAGC GGTTG ACGAA GAGT
GLUT4:
Forward: CTGGG CCTCA CAGTG CTAC
Reverse: GTCAG GCGCT TCAGA CTCTT
GLUT6:
Forward: GCCCG GACTA CGACA CCT
Reverse: AGCTG AAATT GCCGA GCAC
GLUT8:
Forward: TCATG GCCTT TCTCG TGAC
Reverse: TCCTT TAGTT TCAGG GACAC AG
GLUT10:
Forward: CTGTG GAGAT ACGAG GAAGA
Reverse: TCAGT CCGTA GAGCA GGA
GLUT12:
Forward: GGTAC CTGTT GAAAA CACCG
Reverse: GCAGT GACAG ATGAC AGGAA

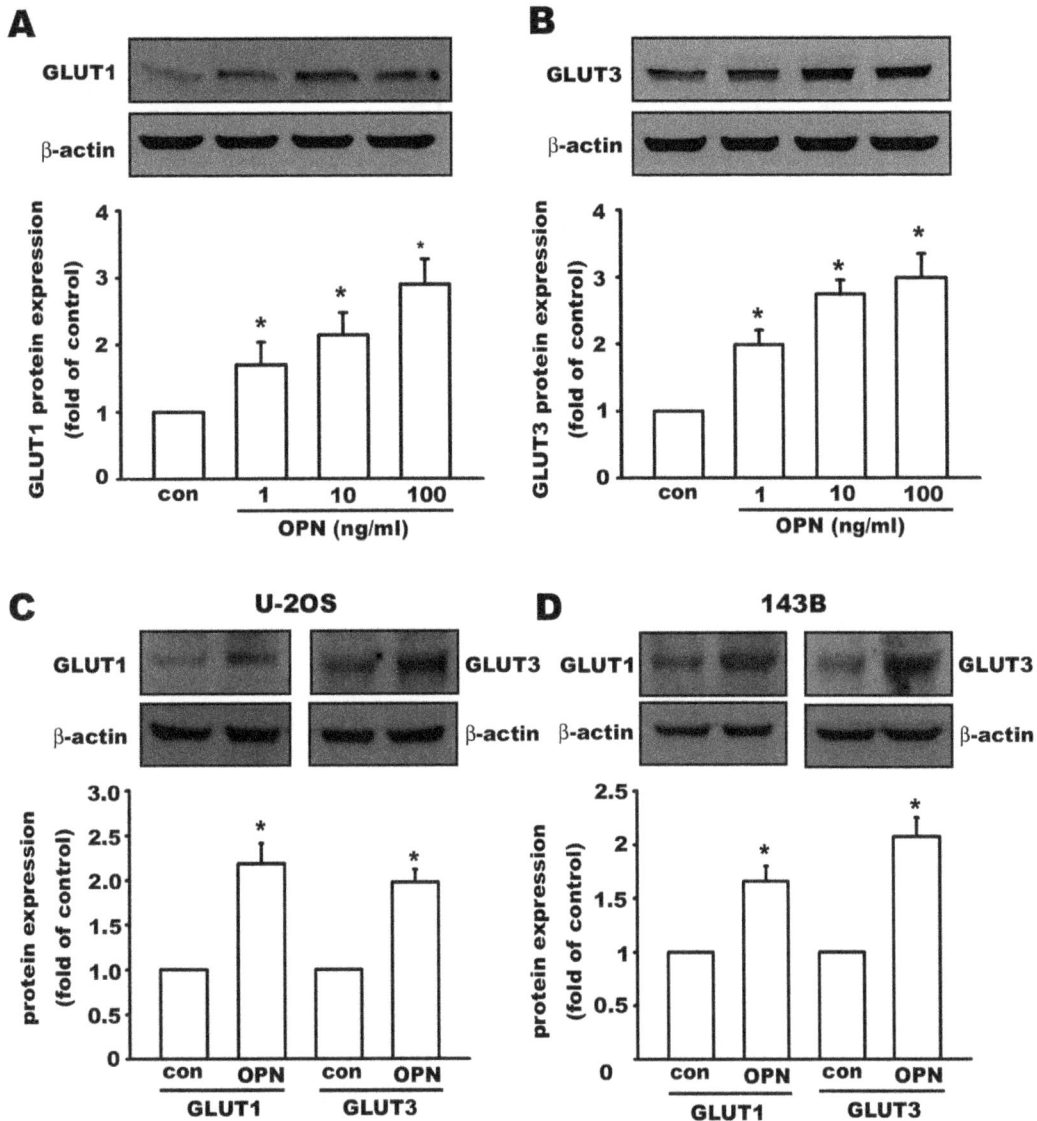

Figure 3. Osteopontin increases GLUT1 and GLUT3 expression in osteosarcoma cell lines. OPN (24 h) increased GLUT1 (A) and GLUT3 (B) protein levels in a concentration-dependent manner in MG63 osteosarcoma cells. OPN (10 ng/ml, 24 h) also increased GLUT1 and GLUT3 protein expression in U-2OS (C) and 143B (D) osteosarcoma cells. Data are presented as the mean ± S.E.M. (n = 4), *p≤0.05, as compared with the control group (con).

OPN:
Forward: CTGTG CCATA CCAGT TAA
Reverse: GATGT CAGGT CTGCG AAA
GAPDH:
Forward: CAGAA CATCA TCCCT GCCTC T
Reverse: GCTTG ACAAA GTGGT CGTTG AG
TagMan probes (Applied Biosystems; Foster City, CA)
SPP1 (OPN): Hs 00167093_ml
SLC2A1 (GLUT1): Hs 00892681_ml
SLC2A3 (GLUT3): Hs 00359840_ml
SLC2A4 (GLUT4): Hs 00168966_ml
GAPDH: Hs 99999905_ml

Cell viability assay

Cell viability was assessed by MTT [3-(4,5-dimethyl thiazol-2-yl)-2,5-diphenyl tetrazolium bromide] (Sigma-Aldrich, St. Louis, MO) assay. The culture medium was aspirated 24 h after drug treatment and MTT (0.5 mg/ml) was added to each well. The MTT was removed after 30 min and the cells were lysed using 100 μl dimethylsulfoxide (DMSO). The absorbance was measured at 550 nm and 630 nm using a microplate reader (Bio-Tek, Winooski, VT).

Glucose uptake assay

Glass coverslips were coated with poly-D-lysine for 1 h at room temperature and then rinsed with sterile d.d. H₂O (3 times/5 min). Cells were seeded onto coverslips for 24 h. They were then treated with OPN (100 ng/ml) for 24 h followed by 2-deoxy-D-glucose (2-NBDG) for 30 min at 37°C. After uptake of 2-NBDG, the cells were put on ice and fixed with 4% paraformaldehyde in PBS for 15 min at 4°C. Images were obtained from a fluorescent microscope using an excitation wavelength of 485 nm and an emission wavelength of 535 nm (model SP5 TCS; Leica, Heidelberg, Germany).

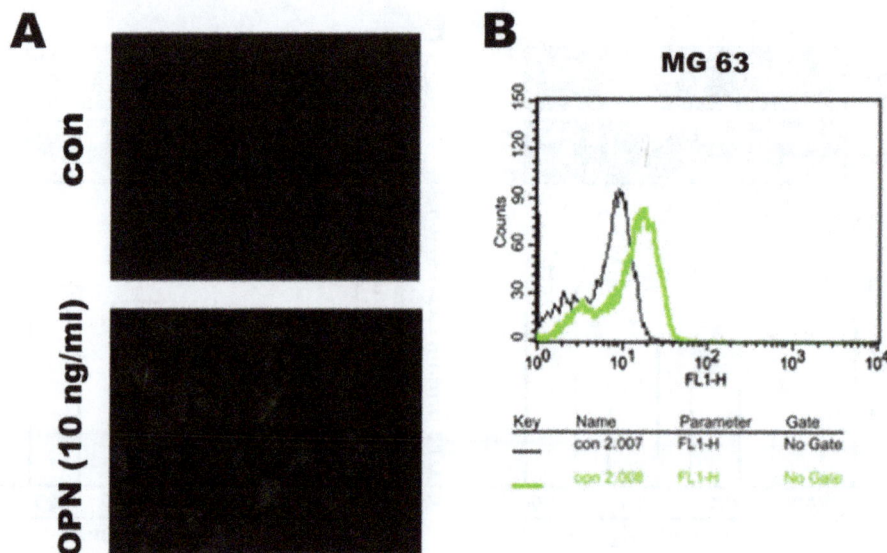

Figure 4. Osteopontin increases glucose uptake in MG63 osteosarcoma cells. 2-NBDG, a fluorescent D-glucose analog, was used as an indicator of glucose uptake. Note that treatment with OPN (100 ng/ml) for 24 h enhanced 2-NBDG uptake into MG63 cells, as shown by confocal microscopy (A) and flow cytometric analysis (B).

Flow cytometry

The effect of OPN on the cellular uptake of 2-NBDG was also measured by flow cytometry. Briefly, 5×10^5 cells were incubated in 6-well plates for 24 h. The cells were treated with OPN (100 ng/ml) at 37°C for 24 h. The cells were then detached by trypsin and 2-NBDG was added and incubated at 37°C for another 0.5 h. The cells were collected and washed twice with ice-cold PBS buffer. Finally, the cells were resuspended in cold PBS buffer for flow cytometric analysis. The relative values of 2-NBDG staining intensity were obtained by dividing the fluorescence intensity of each measurement by that of control cells.

Statistics

Values are expressed as the mean ± S.E.M from at least three experiments. Results were analyzed with one-way analysis of variance (ANOVA), followed by Student's t-test. Significance was defined as $p < 0.05$.

Results

Hypoxia increases osteopontin expression in human osteosarcoma cells

Hypoxia is a major regulator of tumor development and aggressiveness [23]. Osteopontin levels are also known to be upregulated in a variety of cancers. A dose of 100 μM cobalt chloride (CoCl₂), a hypoxia-mimetic agent that induces HIF1α expression, stabilization, and activation, was used to mimic the hypoxia seen during tumor development. We observed that osteopontin mRNA (6 h, Figure 1A) and protein (24 h, Figure 1B) levels were markedly increased in MG63 human osteosarcoma cells after treatment with CoCl₂, indicating that osteopontin may play a role in osteosarcoma progression.

Hypoxia increases the expression of glucose transporters in human osteosarcoma cells

Glucose transporters are another common regulator of tumor growth [5,24]. Tumor cells turn on the hypoxia-inducible

transcription factor oxygen-sensing system and regulate the downstream genes, such as VEGF, iNOS, EPO, GLUT1, and GLUT3, to adapt to hypoxia and increase tissue oxygenation [7,25–27]. In MG63 human osteosarcoma cells, the mRNA levels of GLUT1, GLUT2, and GLUT3, but not GLUT 4, 6, 8, 10, or 12, were increased after a 6-h treatment of CoCl₂ (100 μM) (Figure 2A). Because GLUT1 and GLUT3 possess a high affinity for glucose, we then measured the protein expression of GLUT1 and GLUT3. We observed that protein levels of GLUT1 and GLUT3 were upregulated after treatment of CoCl₂ (100 μM, 24 h) (Figures 2B and 2C).

Osteopontin increases GLUT1 and GLUT3 expression in osteosarcoma cells

Because osteopontin is one of the hypoxia-inducible genes and a cancer progression marker, we performed further investigations of the effect of OPN on the regulation of glucose transporters. We observed that treatment with OPN for 24 h increased GLUT1 (Figure 3A) and GLUT3 (Figure 3B) protein expression in a concentration-dependent manner in MG63 osteosarcoma cells. GLUT1 and GLUT3 are also upregulated by OPN (10 ng/ml) treatment in two other osteosarcoma cell lines, U-2OS (Figure 3C) and 143B (Figure 3D). These results demonstrate that OPN can regulate glucose transporter expression in osteosarcoma.

Increase of glucose uptake by OPN in osteosarcoma cells

Because of the fact that OPN can upregulate the expression of glucose transporters in osteosarcoma cells, we further examined the effect of OPN on glucose uptake in MG63 cells. 2-NBDG, a fluorescent D-glucose analog for direct measurement of glucose uptake, was used to examine the effect of OPN on glucose uptake. Immunofluorescence showed that 2-NBDG uptake was increased following treatment with OPN (100 ng/ml, 24 h) (Figure 4A). Flow cytometric analysis showed that the fluorescence of 2-NBDG was right-shifted by treatment with OPN (100 ng/ml, 24 h) (Figure 4B). These results indicate that exogenous OPN can further increase glucose uptake into hypoxic osteosarcoma cells.

A

B

C

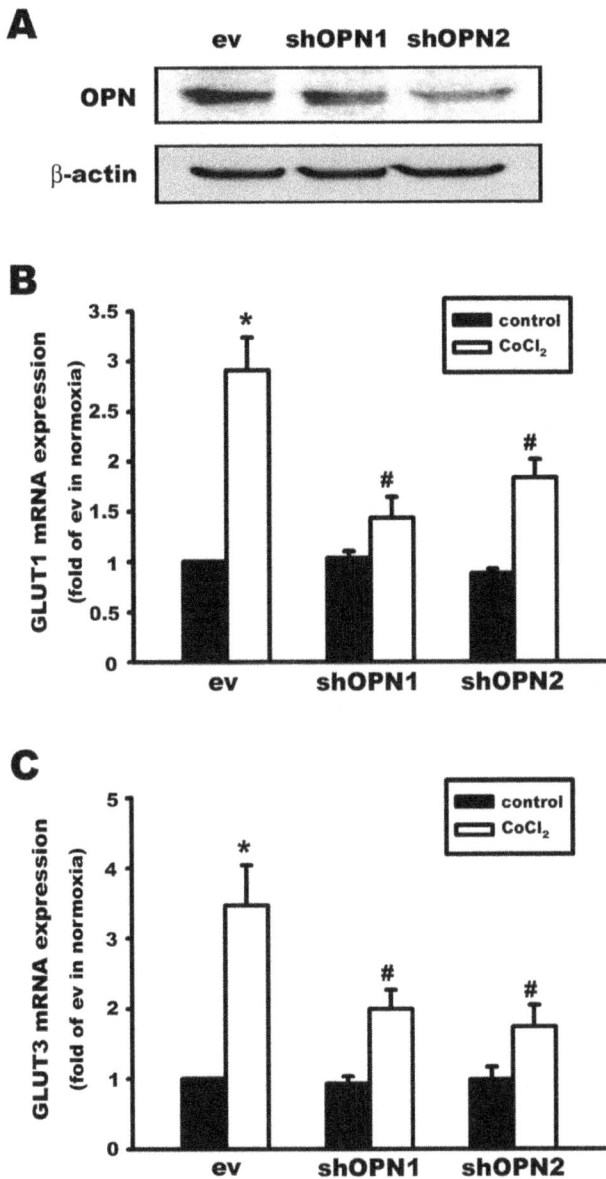

Figure 5. Knockdown of osteopontin decreases glucose transporters expression in a hypoxic osteosarcoma cell line. (A) Two OPN-shRNA plasmids (shOPN1 and shOPN2) and one empty vector (ev) plasmid were transiently transfected (24 h) in MG63 cells. OPN protein expression was downregulated by both shOPN1 and shOPN2. After treatment with the chemical hypoxia agent CoCl$_2$ (100 μM, 6 h), GLUT1 (B) and GLUT3 (C) mRNA expression was markedly upregulated in the empty vector (ev) group. This effect was significantly antagonized by OPN knockdown (shOPN1 and shOPN2) in MG63 cells. Data are presented as the mean ± S.E.M. (n=4), *p≤0.05, compared with the empty vector group (ev) in the control group, #p≤0.05, compared with the empty vector group (ev) in the CoCl$_2$ treatment group.

A

B

Figure 6. Knockdown of osteopontin enhances glucose transporter inhibitor phloretin-induced cell death in osteosarcoma cell lines. Knockdown of OPN expression by transient transfection of OPN-shRNA (shOPN1 and shOPN2) induced approximately 20% cell death in MG63 (A) and U-2OS (B) cells. Inhibition of glucose transporter activity by phloretin (500 μM, 24 h) also caused cell death in the empty vector (ev) group. The cytotoxic effect of phloretin was enhanced by OPN knockdown in both MG63 (A) and U-2OS (B) cells. Cell viability was measured by MTT assay. Data are presented as the mean ± S.E.M. (n=4), *p≤0.05, compared with the control group (con), #p≤0.05, compared with respective vehicle-treated group.

with empty vector (ev) (Figure 5A). CoCl$_2$ treatment (100 μM, 6 h) upregulated GLUT1 (Figure 5B) and GLUT3 (Figure 5C) mRNA expression in MG63 cells, which was antagonized by OPN shRNA transfection, indicating that endogenously released OPN is involved in hypoxia-induced GLUT1 and GLUT3 expression.

In addition, OPN knockdown for 48 h decreased cell viability in both MG63 (Figure 6A) and U-2OS (Figure 6B) osteosarcoma cells. Treatment with phloretin (500 μM), a glucose transporter inhibitor, for 24 h also decreased cell viability in MG63 (Figure 6A) and U-2OS (Figure 6B) osteosarcoma cells. The apoptotic effect of phloretin was further enhanced in OPN knockdown cells. These results indicate that endogenously released OPN plays an important role in regulating GLUTs expression and cell survival in osteosarcoma cells.

The αvβ3 integrin and MAPK pathways are involved in osteopontin-induced glucose transporter upregulation in osteosarcoma cells

Osteopontin, a secreted adhesive glycoprotein with a functional RGD cell-binding domain, interacts primarily with the αvβ3 integrin. As shown in Figure 7A, the OPN-induced increase of GLUT1 and GLUT3 protein expression was significantly antagonized by a αvβ3 monoclonal antibody (2 μg/ml) and

Knockdown of osteopontin decreases the expression of glucose transporters and cell viability in osteosarcoma cells

The role of endogenously released OPN was investigated by OPN knockdown in osteosarcoma cells using shRNA transfection. Transfection with two sequences of OPN-specific shRNA (sh1 and sh2) for 24 h downregulated OPN protein expression compared

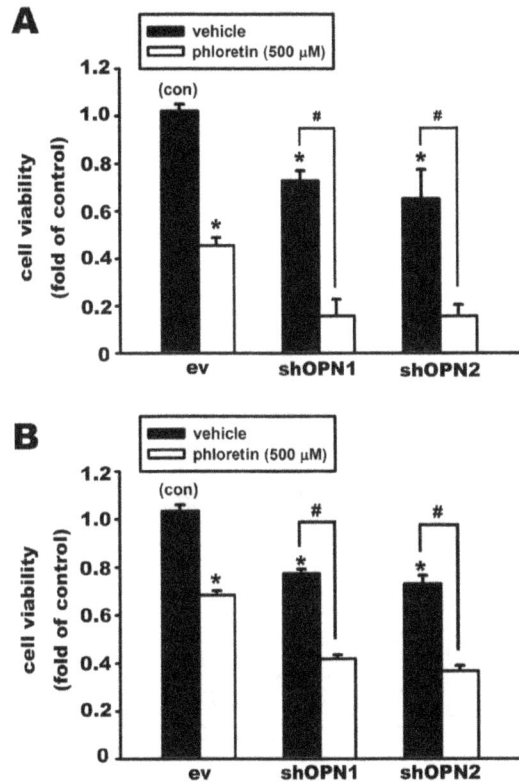

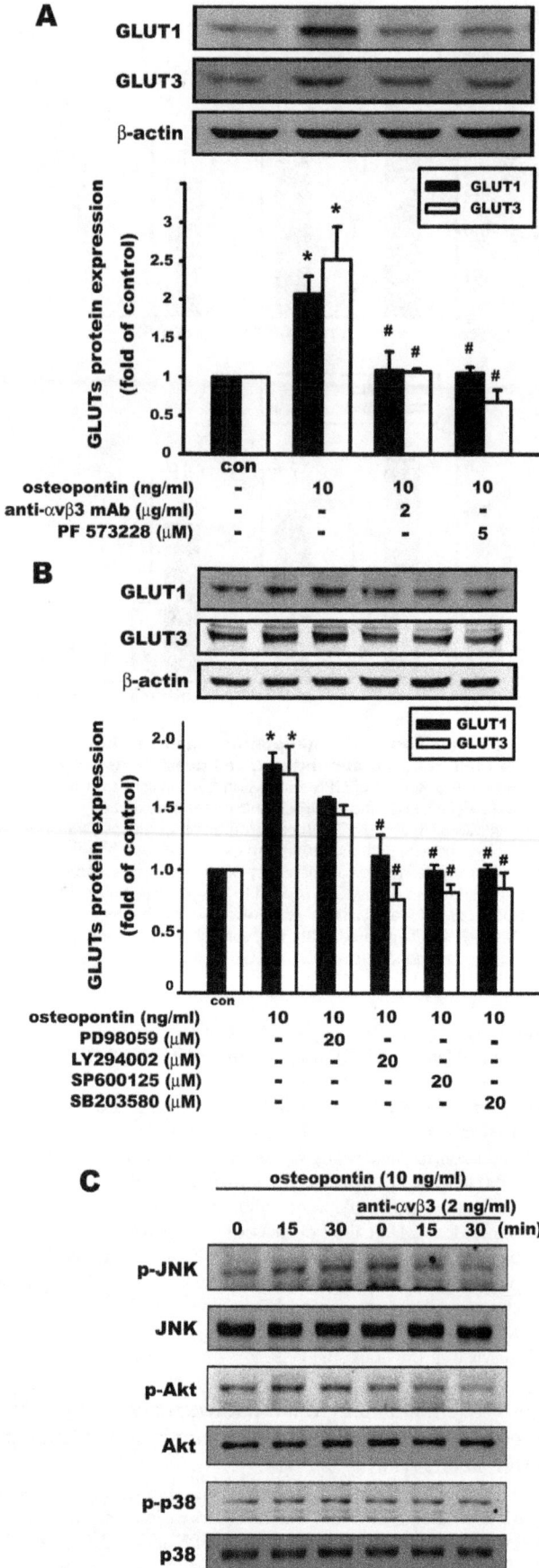

A

B

C

Figure 7. Osteopontin regulates GLUT1 and GLUT3 expression via the αvβ3 integrin and MAPK pathways in osteosarcoma cells. OPN (10 ng/ml) increased GLUT1 and GLUT3 protein expression in MG63 cells. This effect was significantly antagonized by pretreatment with an anti-αvβ3 mAb (2 µg/ml) and PF573228 (5 µM, FAK inhibitor) (A). (B) MG63 cells were pretreated with PD98059 (20 µM), LY294002 (20 µM), SP600125 (20 µM), and SB203580 (20 µM) for 30 min and then stimulated with OPN (10 ng/ml, 24 h). OPN-induced increase of GLUT1 and GLUT3 protein expression was significantly antagonized by LY294002, SP600125, and SB203580. (C) OPN (10 ng/ml) increased the phosphorylation of AKT, JNK, and p38 in a time-dependent manner, and pretreatment with an anti-αvβ3 mAb (2 µg/ml) inhibited OPN-induced AKT, JNK, and p38 phosphorylation. Data are presented as the mean ± S.E.M. (n = 3). *p ≤ 0.05, compared with the control group (con), #p ≤ 0.05, compared with OPN treatment alone.

PF573228 (focal adhesion kinase (FAK) inhibitor, 5 µM) in MG63 cells, indicating that OPN increased GLUT1 and GLUT3 expression via αvβ3 integrin and caused the activation of the downstream protein kinase FAK. OPN-induced increase of GLUT1 and GLUT3 protein expression was also markedly inhibited by the PI3K inhibitor LY294002 (20 µM), the JNK inhibitor SP600125 (20 µM), and the p38 inhibitor SB203580 (20 µM), whereas the ERK inhibitor PD98059 (20 µM) did not affect the OPN-induced expression of GLUT1 and GLUT3 (Figure 7B). It was also found that OPN time-dependently phosphorylated phosphoinositide-3 kinase (PI3K/AKT), Jun-amino-terminal kinase (JNK), and the p38 pathway, which were antagonized by an αvβ3 integrin monoclonal antibody (Figure 7C). These results indicate that several kinases, including PI3K/AKT, JNK, and p38, are involved in the regulation of glucose transporters by OPN via αvβ3 integrin.

The synergistic cytotoxic effect of chemotherapy drugs in combination with a GLUT inhibitor in osteosarcoma cells

Phloretin is a competitive inhibitor of glucose transporters that has potent antioxidant activity, as well as anti-proliferative and apoptotic effects in cancer cells, such as hepatocellular carcinoma (HepG2) [28], colon cancer (HT-29) [29], melanoma (B16) [30], and breast cancer (MCF10A). Here we used a low concentration of phloretin (100 µM) in combination with chemotherapeutic drugs, such as daunomyacin (1 µM), 5-Fu (10 µM), etoposide (10 µM), and methotrexate (10 µM), in the osteosarcoma cell lines MG63, U-2OS, and 143B. Treatment with phloretin (100 µM), daunomyacin (1 µM), 5-Fu (10 µM), etoposide (10 µM), or methotrexate (10 µM) alone for 24 h caused only 20% cell death. However, the combination of phloretin with these chemotherapeutic drugs markedly increased cell death (>50%) in all three osteosarcoma cell lines (Figure 8A). Representative images of phloretin in combination with chemotherapeutic drugs are shown in Figure 8B. These results indicate that the addition of a low dose of glucose transporter inhibitor with chemotherapeutic drugs can enhance cytotoxicity in osteosarcoma cells.

Discussion

In this study we demonstrate that both osteopontin and glucose transporters are crucial factors in osteosarcoma. Endogenously released OPN regulated GLUTs expression in hypoxia, which was reversed by knockdown of OPN. Inhibition of the function of OPN and GLUTs induced cell death in osteosarcoma cell lines. Combination of a GLUT inhibitor and chemotherapy drugs exerted a synergistic apoptotic effect in osteosarcoma.

Cobalt chloride (CoCl$_2$), a hypoxia-mimetic agent, has been demonstrated to inhibit the prolyl hydroxylase domain-containing

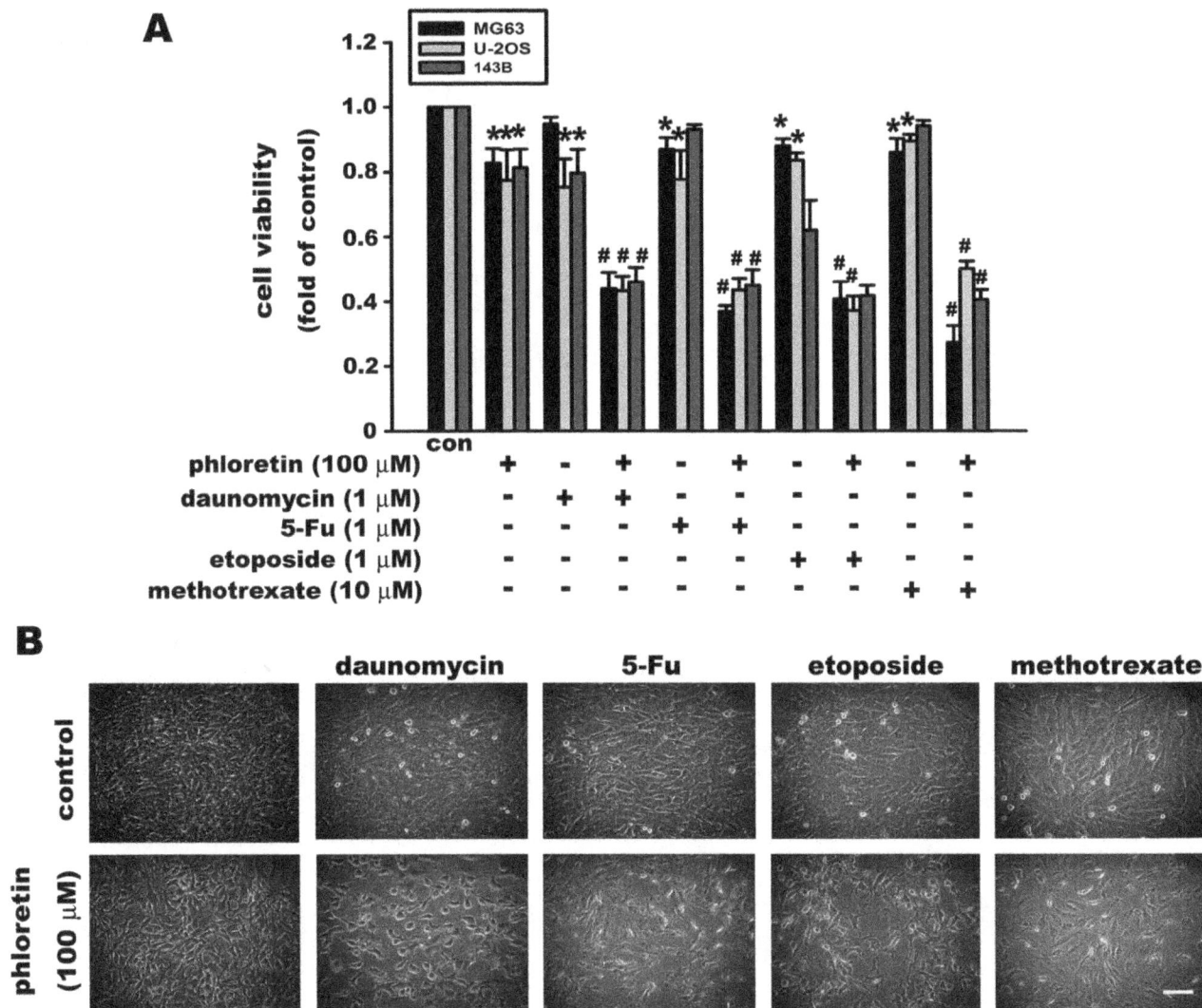

Figure 8. The cytotoxic effect of chemotherapeutic drugs is enhanced by combination with a glucose transporter inhibitor. (A) Treatment of MG63 cells with phloretin (100 μM), daunomycin (1 μM), 5-Fu (10 μM), etoposide 10 μM, or methotrexate (10 μM) alone for 24 h induced a low level of cell death. However, the combination of phloretin with chemotherapeutic drugs (daunomycin, 5-Fu, etoposide, and methotrexate) markedly increased cell death in three osteosarcoma cell lines: MG63, U-2OS, and 143B. Representative photographs are shown in panel B. Data are presented as the mean ± S.E.M. (n = 4). *p≤0.05, compared with the control (con), #p≤0.05, compared with the respective treatment of the chemotherapeutic drug alone.

enzymes (PHDs) [31], which plays a key role in oxygen-dependent degradation of the transcription factor, to activate hypoxia-mediated signaling by stabilizing hypoxia-inducible transcription factor-1α (HIF-1α) [32–34]. Here we used $CoCl_2$ to mimic the hypoxic condition, an inevitable cellular stress experienced during tumor progression and solid tumor development [35,36]. During hypoxia, HIF-1α degradation is inhibited and its activity is increased. Increase of HIF-1α activity is mediated through the PI3K-Akt and MAPK signaling pathways [37,38]. OPN is a bone-associated extracellular matrix protein that is produced by numerous cell types, such as osteoblasts, osteoclasts, T lymphocytes, NK cells, and epithelial cells. OPN influences normal physiological processes, including bone resorption, wound healing, tissue remodeling, and vascularization [39]. OPN has also been shown to be involved in all stages of cancer progression; for instance, tumor invasion, angiogenesis, and metastasis [40–42]. Here, we found that $CoCl_2$-induced hypoxia upregulated OPN

mRNA and protein expression in osteosarcoma cells. The overexpression of GLUTs is requisite for cell proliferation, like that seen in cancer, in order to increase the energy supply. We also demonstrated that GLUTs can be upregulated by both $CoCl_2$ and OPN.

Because GLUTs were upregulated by OPN, glucose uptake was evaluated using a fluorescent D-glucose analog, 2-NBDG, in MG63 osteosarcoma cells with confocal microscopy and flow cytometry [43,44]. The intracellular fluorescence intensity of 2-NBDG was enhanced by treatment with OPN in MG63, indicating that OPN increases nutrient availability to osteosarcoma cells. This effect was mediated by αvβ3 integrin, FAK phosphorylation, and the AKT, JNK, and p38 MAPK pathways.

Knockdown of OPN expression was performed in the osteosarcoma cell lines MG63 and U-2OS using two different shRNA plasmids. Cell survival was decreased by approximately 20% in OPN knockdown cells. Hypoxia-induced expression of

GLUTs was also inhibited by OPN knockdown. These results indicate that endogenously released OPN can regulate GLUTs expression, glucose uptake, and the survival of osteosarcoma cells.

Phloretin, a natural product, exists in the fruit trees in glucosidic form, namely phloridzin. Both of phloretin and phloridizin are present in apple and pulp [45]. Phloretin amounts to 12.5 μg/mL in apple juice and 219 μg/mL in carrot juice. Phloretin has a marked effect on the survival of colon cancer cells at concentrations as low as 50 μmol/L [46]. It has been demonstrated that phloretin, isoliquiritigenin and other hydroxylated chalcones had cytotoxic activity by inducing collapse of mitochondrial membrane potential and increasing oxygen uptake [47]. Phloretin (the aglucon of phlorizin) is reported to induce human liver cancer cell apoptosis and exert significant anti-tumor effects in HepG2 xenograft animal model by administering phloretin (10 mg/kg) intraperitoneally [28]. Although phlorizin makes the tumor cells impermeable to glucose, it also makes all other cells all over the body impermeable to glucose cells. However, phlorizin derivatives can sensitize the cancer cells for treatment with heat and other modalities in patients [48]. Here we used phloretin in osteosarcoma. Inhibition of GLUTs by 500 μM phloretin induced approximately 50% cell death in osteosarcoma cell lines. OPN knockdown enhanced the cell death induced by phloretin to 80%, indicating that phloretin-induced cell death was more sensitive in OPN knockdown osteosarcoma cells. This apoptosis enhancing effect also appeared at low dose of phloretin (100 μM, 6 h) in both MG63 (Figure S1A) and U-2OS (Figure S1B) osteosarcoma cells, indicating that OPN knockdown sensitized the tumor cells to phloretin-induced apoptosis. Both glucose and OPN are important to osteosarcoma cell survival. Glucose uptake is related to cancer cell survival and drug sensitivity. For instance, the decrease in glucose uptake at an early time point after a high dose of cisplatin reflects cisplatin chemosensitivity in ovarian cancer cells [49]. Phloretin also sensitizes cancer cells to daunorubicin and overcomes drug resistance in hypoxia [50]. Chemotherapy is used in the treatment of osteosarcoma. As shown above, osteosarcoma

is sensitive to the glucose transporter inhibitor phloretin. Moreover, combination of a low dose of glucose transporter inhibitor with chemotherapy drugs markedly enhanced cell death in osteosarcoma cell lines. These results indicate that a combination therapy of a low dose of a GLUTs inhibitor and a cytotoxic drug may offer a new therapeutic option to osteosarcoma patients.

In conclusion, endogenously released OPN is important for the regulation of GLUT1 and GLUT3 expression in osteosarcoma. Inhibition of glucose uptake by a transporter inhibitor can induce cell death in osteosarcoma. Furthermore, the combination of a low dose of phloretin with chemotherapeutic drugs markedly enhanced cell death in osteosarcoma cells.

Supporting Information

Figure S1 Low dose of phloretin enhances cell death of osteosarcoma in osteopontin knockdown cells. Knockdown of OPN expression (24 h) by transient transfection of OPN-shRNA (shOPN1 and shOPN2) induced approximately 10% cell death in MG63 (A) and U-2OS (B) cells. Inhibition of glucose transporter activity by phloretin (100 μM, 6 h) caused cell death in the empty vector (ev) group. The cytotoxic effect of phloretin was enhanced by OPN knockdown in both MG63 (A) and U-2OS (B) cells after short duration of 6 h treatment. Cell viability was measured by MTT assay. Data are presented as the mean ± S.E.M. (n = 4). *p≤0.05, compared with control group (con); #p≤ 0.05, compared with respective vehicle-treated group.

Author Contributions

Conceived and designed the experiments: WMF RSY. Performed the experiments: ISH. Analyzed the data: ISH. Contributed reagents/materials/analysis tools: ISH. Contributed to the writing of the manuscript: ISH. Preparation of the first draft of manuscript: ISH. Interpretation of the results and draft revision: WMF. Scientific guidance and draft revision: RSY.

References

1. Clark JC, Dass CR, Choong PF (2008) A review of clinical and molecular prognostic factors in osteosarcoma. J Cancer Res Clin Oncol 134: 281–297. doi: 10.1007/s00432-007-0330-x.
2. Wittig JC, Bickels J, Priebat D, Jelinek J, Kellar-Graney K, et al. (2002) Osteosarcoma: a multidisciplinary approach to diagnosis and treatment. Am Fam Physician 65: 1123–1132.
3. Schwab JH, Springfield DS, Raskin KA, Mankin HJ, Hornicek FJ (2012) What's new in primary bone tumors. J Bone Joint Surg Am 94: 1913–1919. doi: 10.2106/JBJS.L.00955.
4. Macheda ML, Rogers S, Best JD (2005) Molecular and cellular regulation of glucose transporter (GLUT) proteins in cancer. J Cell Physiol 202: 654–662. doi: 10.1002/jcp.20166.
5. Medina RA, Owen GI (2002) Glucose transporters: expression, regulation and cancer. Biol Res 35: 9–26.
6. Vander Heiden MG, Cantley LC, Thompson CB (2009) Understanding the Warburg effect: the metabolic requirements of cell proliferation. Science 324: 1029–1033. doi: 10.1126/science.1160809.
7. Semenza GL (2010) HIF-1: upstream and downstream of cancer metabolism. Curr Opin Genet Dev 20: 51–56. doi: 10.1016/j.gde.2009.10.009.
8. Meneses AM, Medina RA, Kato S, Pinto M, Jaque MP, et al. (2008) Regulation of GLUT3 and glucose uptake by the cAMP signalling pathway in the breast cancer cell line ZR-75. J Cell Physiol 214: 110–116. doi: 10.1002/jcp.21166.
9. Younes M, Brown RW, Stephenson M, Gondo M, Cagle PT (1997) Overexpression of Glut1 and Glut3 in stage I nonsmall cell lung carcinoma is associated with poor survival. Cancer 80: 1046–1051.
10. Younes M, Juarez D, Lechago LV, Lerner SP (2001) Glut 1 expression in transitional cell carcinoma of the urinary bladder is associated with poor patient survival. Anticancer Res 21: 575–578.
11. Airley R, Loncaster J, Davidson S, Bromley M, Roberts S, et al. (2001) Glucose transporter glut-1 expression correlates with tumor hypoxia and predicts metastasis-free survival in advanced carcinoma of the cervix. Clin Cancer Res 7: 928–934.
12. Denhardt DT, Guo X (1993) Osteopontin: a protein with diverse functions. FASEB J 7: 1475–1482.
13. Denhardt DT, Noda M (1998) Osteopontin expression and function: role in bone remodeling. J Cell Biochem Suppl 30–31: 92–102.
14. Yamamoto N, Sakai F, Kon S, Morimoto J, Kimura C, et al. (2003) Essential role of the cryptic epitope SLAYGLR within osteopontin in a murine model of rheumatoid arthritis. J Clin Invest 112: 181–188. doi: 10.1172/JCI17778.
15. Denhardt DT, Giachelli CM, Rittling SR (2001) Role of osteopontin in cellular signaling and toxicant injury. Annu Rev Pharmacol Toxicol 41: 723–749. doi: 10.1146/annurev.pharmtox.41.1.723.
16. Tilli TM, Franco VF, Robbs BK, Wanderley JL, da Silva FR, et al. (2011) Osteopontin-c splicing isoform contributes to ovarian cancer progression. Mol Cancer Res 9: 280–293. doi: 10.1158/1541-7786.MCR-10-0463.
17. Weber GF, Lett GS, Haubein NC (2010) Osteopontin is a marker for cancer aggressiveness and patient survival. Br J Cancer 103: 861–869. doi: 10.1038/sj.bjc.6605834.
18. Weber GF (2011) The cancer biomarker osteopontin: combination with other markers. Cancer Genomics Proteomics 8: 263–288.
19. Carlos-Bregni R, Contreras E, Hiraki KR, Vargas PA, Leon JE, et al. (2008) Epithelioid osteosarcoma of the mandible: a rare case with unusual immunoprofile. Oral Surg Oral Med Oral Pathol Oral Radiol Endod 105: e47-52. doi: 10.1016/j.tripleo.2007.09.003.
20. Savitskaya YA, Rico-Martinez G, Linares-Gonzalez LM, Delgado-Cedillo EA, Tellez-Gastelum R, et al. (2012) Serum tumor markers in pediatric osteosarcoma: a summary review. Clin Sarcoma Res 2: 9. doi: 10.1186/2045-3329-2-9.
21. Dalla-Torre CA, Yoshimoto M, Lee CH, Joshua AM, de Toledo SR, et al. (2006) Effects of THBS3, SPARC and SPP1 expression on biological behavior and survival in patients with osteosarcoma. BMC Cancer 6: 237. doi: 10.1186/1471-2407-6-237.
22. Giachelli CM, Steitz S (2000) Osteopontin: a versatile regulator of inflammation and biomineralization. Matrix Biol 19: 615–622.

23. Rankin EB, Giaccia AJ (2008) The role of hypoxia-inducible factors in tumorigenesis. Cell Death Differ 15: 678–685. doi: 10.1038/cdd.2008.21.

24. Adekola K, Rosen ST, Shanmugam M (2012) Glucose transporters in cancer metabolism. Curr Opin Oncol 24: 650–654. doi: 10.1097/CCO.0-b013e328356da72.

25. Airley RE, Mobasheri A (2007) Hypoxic regulation of glucose transport, anaerobic metabolism and angiogenesis in cancer: novel pathways and targets for anticancer therapeutics. Chemotherapy 53: 233–256. doi: 10.1159/000104457.

26. Denko NC (2008) Hypoxia, HIF1 and glucose metabolism in the solid tumour. Nat Rev Cancer 8: 705–713. doi: 10.1038/nrc2468.

27. Rey S, Semenza GL (2010) Hypoxia-inducible factor-1-dependent mechanisms of vascularization and vascular remodelling. Cardiovasc Res 86: 236–242. doi: 10.1093/cvr/cvq045.

28. Wu CH, Ho YS, Tsai CY, Wang YJ, Tseng H, et al. (2009) In vitro and in vivo study of phloretin-induced apoptosis in human liver cancer cells involving inhibition of type II glucose transporter. Int J Cancer 124: 2210–2219. doi: 10.1002/ijc.24189.

29. Park SY, Kim EJ, Shin HK, Kwon DY, Kim MS, et al. (2007) Induction of apoptosis in HT-29 colon cancer cells by phloretin. J Med Food 10: 581–586. doi: 10.1089/jmf.2007.116.

30. Kobori M, Shinmoto H, Tsushida T, Shinohara K (1997) Phloretin-induced apoptosis in B16 melanoma 4A5 cells by inhibition of glucose transmembrane transport. Cancer Lett 119: 207–212.

31. Epstein AC, Gleadle JM, McNeill LA, Hewitson KS, O'Rourke J, et al. (2001) C. elegans EGL-9 and mammalian homologs define a family of dioxygenases that regulate HIF by prolyl hydroxylation. Cell 107: 43–54.

32. Wang GL, Semenza GL (1993) Desferrioxamine induces erythropoietin gene expression and hypoxia-inducible factor 1 DNA-binding activity: implications for models of hypoxia signal transduction. Blood 82: 3610–3615.

33. Ho VT, Bunn HF (1996) Effects of transition metals on the expression of the erythropoietin gene: further evidence that the oxygen sensor is a heme protein. Biochem Biophys Res Commun 223: 175–180. doi: 10.1006/bbrc.1996.0865.

34. Vengellur A, LaPres JJ (2004) The role of hypoxia inducible factor 1alpha in cobalt chloride induced cell death in mouse embryonic fibroblasts. Toxicol Sci 82: 638–646. doi: 10.1093/toxsci/kfh278.

35. Wang GL, Jiang BH, Rue EA, Semenza GL (1995) Hypoxia-inducible factor 1 is a basic-helix-loop-helix-PAS heterodimer regulated by cellular O2 tension. Proc Natl Acad Sci U S A 92: 5510–5514.

36. Harris AL (2002) Hypoxia–a key regulatory factor in tumour growth. Nat Rev Cancer 2: 38–47. doi: 10.1038/nrc704.

37. Dimova EY, Kietzmann T (2006) The MAPK pathway and HIF-1 are involved in the induction of the human PAI-1 gene expression by insulin in the human hepatoma cell line HepG2. Ann N Y Acad Sci 1090: 355–367. doi: 10.1196/annals.1378.039.

38. Zhong H, Chiles K, Feldser D, Laughner E, Hanrahan C, et al. (2000) Modulation of hypoxia-inducible factor 1alpha expression by the epidermal growth factor/phosphatidylinositol 3-kinase/PTEN/AKT/FRAP pathway in human prostate cancer cells: implications for tumor angiogenesis and therapeutics. Cancer Res 60: 1541–1545.

39. Denhardt DT, Noda M, O'Regan AW, Pavlin D, Berman JS (2001) Osteopontin as a means to cope with environmental insults: regulation of inflammation, tissue remodeling, and cell survival. J Clin Invest 107: 1055–1061. doi: 10.1172/JCI12980.

40. Ahmed M, Behera R, Chakraborty G, Jain S, Kumar V, et al. (2011) Osteopontin: a potentially important therapeutic target in cancer. Expert Opin Ther Targets 15: 1113–1126. doi: 10.1517/14728222.2011.594438.

41. Jain S, Chakraborty G, Bulbule A, Kaur R, Kundu GC (2007) Osteopontin: an emerging therapeutic target for anticancer therapy. Expert Opin Ther Targets 11: 81–90. doi: 10.1517/14728222.11.1.81.

42. Wai PY, Kuo PC (2008) Osteopontin: regulation in tumor metastasis. Cancer Metastasis Rev 27: 103–118. doi: 10.1007/s10555-007-9104-9.

43. O'Neil RG, Wu L, Mullani N (2005) Uptake of a fluorescent deoxyglucose analog (2-NBDG) in tumor cells. Mol Imaging Biol 7: 388–392. doi: 10.1007/s11307-005-0011-6.

44. Zou C, Wang Y, Shen Z (2005) 2-NBDG as a fluorescent indicator for direct glucose uptake measurement. J Biochem Biophys Methods 64: 207–215. doi: 10.1016/j.jbbm.2005.08.001.

45. Tsao R, Yang R, Young JC, Zhu H (2003) Polyphenolic profiles in eight apple cultivars using high-performance liquid chromatography (HPLC). J Agric Food Chem 51: 6347–6353. doi: 10.1021/jf0346298.

46. Katarzyna Przybylska RNB, Krystyna Kromer, Jennifer M Gee (2007) Assessment of the antiproliferative activity of carrot and apple extracts. Pol J Food Nutr Sci 57: 307–314.

47. Sabzevari O, Galati G, Moridani MY, Siraki A, O'Brien PJ (2004) Molecular cytotoxic mechanisms of anticancer hydroxychalcones. Chem Biol Interact 148: 57–67. doi: 10.1016/j.cbi.2004.04.004.

48. Leveen, Harry H, Leveen, Robert F, Leveen, etal. (1989) Treatment of cancer with phlorizin and its derivatives. C07G003/00;C07G011/00;C07H015/00;C07H017/00;A01N043/04;A61K031/70;C07H015/24;A61K036/00;C07K001/00;C07K014/00;C07K014/37;C07K016/00;C07K017/00;C07H015/06 ed. Us.

49. Egawa-Takata T, Endo H, Fujita M, Ueda Y, Miyatake T, et al. (2010) Early reduction of glucose uptake after cisplatin treatment is a marker of cisplatin sensitivity in ovarian cancer. Cancer Sci 101: 2171–2178. doi: 10.1111/j.1349-7006.2010.01670.x.

50. Cao X, Fang L, Gibbs S, Huang Y, Dai Z, et al. (2007) Glucose uptake inhibitor sensitizes cancer cells to daunorubicin and overcomes drug resistance in hypoxia. Cancer Chemother Pharmacol 59: 495–505. doi: 10.1007/s00280-006-0291-9.

12

The Prevalence of HIV-1 Drug Resistance among Antiretroviral Treatment Naïve Individuals in Mainland China

Yingying Su[1], Fujie Zhang[1], Huixin Liu[1], M. Kumi Smith[2], Lin Zhu[1], Jing Wu[1], Ning Wang[1]*

1 National Center for AIDS/STD Control and Prevention, Chinese Center for Disease Control and Prevention, Beijing, China, 2 Department of Epidemiology, University of North Carolina, Chapel Hill, North Carolina, United States of America

Abstract

Background: Surveillance of drug resistance in antiretroviral treatment-naïve patients in China is needed to ensure optimal treatment outcomes and control of the human immunodeficiency virus (HIV) epidemic.

Methods: A systematic literature search was conducted in English and Chinese through PubMed (English), China National Knowledge Infrastructure (Chinese), Chinese Biomedical Literature Database (Chinese), and Wanfang (Chinese). Random effects models were used to calculate the pooled prevalence of transmitted drug resistance and subgroup analyses examined prevalence estimates across time periods, study locations, and study populations.

Results: Analysis of data from 71 studies (47 in Chinese and 24 in English) yielded a pooled prevalence of transmitted HIV drug resistance to any antiretroviral drug class of 3.64% (95% confidence interval [CI]: 3.00%–4.32%). Rates were significantly high at initial stage of free ART program from 2003 to 2005 (5.18%, 95%CI: 3.13%–7.63%), and were much lower among studies conducted in 2006–2008 (3.02%, 95%CI: 2.03%–4.16%). A slight increase was observed again in the most recent study period from 2009 to 2012 (3.68%, 95%CI: 2.78%–4.69%). Subgroup analysis revealed highest prevalence levels of transmitted drug resistance in Beijing city, and Henan and Hubei provinces (above 5%), and although differences in prevalence rates among risk groups were negligible, men who have sex with men were unique in their relatively large portion of protease inhibitor resistance, a second-line drug of limited availability in China.

Conclusions: Overall prevalence of transmitted HIV drug resistance in China is classified as "low" by the World Health Organization. However regional and temporal variability suggest a more complex epidemic for which closer HIV drug resistance surveillance is needed. A nationwide HIV drug resistance surveillance system to monitor both treatment-experienced and treatment-naïve patients will be a cornerstone to ensure the effectiveness of treatment scale-up, particularly as China seeks to expand a national policy of antiretroviral treatment as prevention.

Editor: Xia Jin, University of Rochester, United States of America

Funding: This work was supported by funding from the Mega-projects of national science research for the 12th Five-Year Plan (2012ZX10001-001) of China. The funders had no role in study design, data collection and analysis, decision to publish, or preparation of the manuscript.

Competing Interests: The authors have declared that no competing interests exist.

* Email: wangnbj@163.com

Introduction

China has one of the largest populations of persons infected with human immunodeficiency virus type-1(HIV-1). As of 2011 an estimated 780,000 people living with HIV/AIDS and among them 154,000 living with AIDS in China [1]. The HIV epidemic is largely concentrated in injecting drug users (IDU), as well as in groups with higher risk sexual exposures including female sex workers and men who have sex with men (MSM) [2]. As of 2007, however, data from the national case report system has suggested that heterosexual transmission (HST) has become the primary mode of transmission in China, signaling a potential transmission to a more generalized epidemic [1].Of the about 70,000 new HIV diagnoses from January to September in 2013, those believe to be acquired through unprotected sex accounted for 89.9% (heterosexual transmission for 69.1%, homosexual transmission for 20.8%) [3].

To combat the spread of HIV through the general population, the Chinese Center for Disease Control has launched a policy initiative to harness suppressive antiretroviral therapy (ART) to slow the spread of HIV in China. The existing national free ART program established in 2003, is expected to provide a strong foundation for such an effort. Initially started as a pilot program for patients who were former plasma donors (FPD), the program has undergone rapid scale up [4,5]. And by the end of September 2013, the national free ART program has treated about 260,000 cumulative patients [3], and has reduced AIDS associated mortality from 39.3 to 14.2 deaths per 100 persons from 2002 to 2009 [6].

Rapid scale up of ART access has been accompanied by a concomitant rise in drug resistance among treated HIV patients. This has been largely attributed to the limited selection of antiviral agents through the national ART program on which most patients rely, and the lack of critical disease monitoring tools like CD4 or viral load testing in most treatment settings [5,7,8]. Though the relationship between poor treatment outcomes, insufficient viral suppression, and emerge of drug resistance is well understood [9,10], little is known about onward transmission of resistant strains in Chinese settings. Primary infection with drug resistant strains severely limits new patients' treatment options and shortens time to treatment failure. The prevalence of transmitted drug resistance (TDR) in wider circulation could also undermine program efficacy of the national treatment efforts [11]. A better understanding of the prevalence of drug resistance in treatment naïve HIV/AIDS patients in China will provide insight critical for both clinical management and for broader disease control efforts [12].

The goal of this systematic review is to provide an overview and pooled prevalence estimate of HIV drug resistance among treatment-naïve patients in China. We also provide a simple analysis of several trends and distributions available from the data in order to provide more insight into better treatment and control of HIV in China.

Methods

Search strategy

We conducted a systematic literature in English and Chinese using the following four databases: PubMed, China National Knowledge Infrastructure (CNKI), Chinese Biomedical Literature Database (CBM), and Wanfang, from January 1, 1990 through February 28, 2014. Search terms included ("HIV" OR "AIDS" OR "human immunodeficiency virus" OR "acquired immuno-deficiency syndrome") AND ("drug resistance" or "drug resistant") AND ("China"). Details on search strategy can be found in the Appendix S1. We further reviewed the reference lists for other relevant articles not captured in our initial search.

Selection Criteria

Investigators YYS and HXL independently assessed eligibility of articles and performed the data extraction. Discrepancies between the two investigators were resolved by consulting the other authors (NW and MKS). Eligible articles all met the following inclusion criteria: (1) inclusion of data on HIV-1-infected and treatment-naïve individuals; (2) availability of basic demographic information for study subjects such as age, sex, or most likely HIV transmission route; (3) availability of information on study design, location, and period; and (4) HIV drug resistance patterns were interpreted using the WHO recommended Stanford HIV Drug Resistance Database (http://hivdb.stanford.edu). Articles that restricted study subjects to HIV patients of a single subtype were excluded, as were those without information on patient treatment status or that pooled results of treated and untreated patients. Studies based outside of mainland China such as Taiwan, Hong Kong and Macao were excluded due to the fact that these regions maintain autonomous and separate HIV/AIDS treatment programs. Articles based on the same or overlapping study populations were included only once to avoid duplication, with preference given to the article with more detailed information about the population, or, all else equal, with the larger sample size.

Data extraction

A standardized form was used to assess article eligibility and to extract data including author names, year of publication, study period, language of article, study location, age range and sex of participants, most likely routes of primary HIV infection, time of infection(chronic or new diagnose), study design (cohort vs. cross section), recruitment method, system of HIV drug resistance typing, portion of tested samples whose HIV RNA was successfully amplified and sequenced, and characteristics of the sequences genotype including number of mutations with at least low-level resistance 1) to any antiretroviral agent, 2) to nucleoside reverse transcriptase inhibitor(NRTI), 3) to non-nucleoside reverse transcriptase inhibitor(NNRTI), 4) to protease inhibitor(PI).

Statistical analysis

The proportion of TDR was defined as number of samples exhibiting at least a lower-level resistance to any antiretroviral agent, divided by the total number of samples successfully amplified and sequenced [13]. This definition of TDR prevalence is consistent with that used for the WHO TDR surveillance mutation list [14]. The Freeman-Tukey Double arcsine transformation of proportions was used to calculate an overall proportion. Model choice (fixed versus random effects models) was based on heterogeneity assessment by examining the Cochran Q statistic (p-value of <0.1 was considered a statistically significant) [15] and the I^2 statistic (values of 25%, 50% and 75% are considered to represent low, medium and high heterogeneity respectively) [16]. The DerSimonian-Laird estimate was used in case of random effects. Subgroup analyses were conducted according to study period, study location and study population to assess the heterogeneity between studies. Publication bias was assessed with the funnel plot and Egger's test, which found no evidence of bias (Figure S1). Analyses were carried out using R EpiTools package [17] and SAS(version 9.3, SAS Institute).

Results

Study selection and characteristics

Of the 4964 articles (4656 in Chinese, 308 in English) initially identified, of which 1934 were excluded as duplicates, another 2858 were removed for relevance based on a title and abstract screening. Following a closer full text review of the remaining 172 articles we identified 71 studies for inclusion in the final analysis, of which 47 were in Chinese, 24 in English (Figure 1). Seventeen of these employed the WHO HIV drug resistance survey method which recommends use of truncated sequential sampling (TSS) to classify levels of transmitted drug resistance for each drug class in resource poor settings [18]. Among the remainder, 54 were cross-sectional studies. Details on resistance to specific classes of antiretroviral drug were available in 68 studies (Table S1).

Transmitted drug resistance prevalence rates

The 71 studies included in this analysis represented results from a collective total of 11,633 HIV-1 treatment naïve individuals, among whom 9,167 HIV RNA sequences were successfully amplified and analyzed. The random effects estimate for overall pooled prevalence of HIV-1 TDR to any antiretroviral drug was 3.64% (95% confidence interval [CI]: 3.00%–4.32%). The pooled prevalence of mutations resistant to NRTI's, NNRTI's, and PI's was 0.91% (95%CI: 0.60%–1.27%), 1.14% (95%CI: 0.75%–1.59%), 0.68% (95%CI: 0.41%–1.01%), respectively.

TDR prevalence was further explored within identifiable subgroups in studies where relevant information was provided (Table 1). Figure 2 shows temporal trends in TDR prevalence

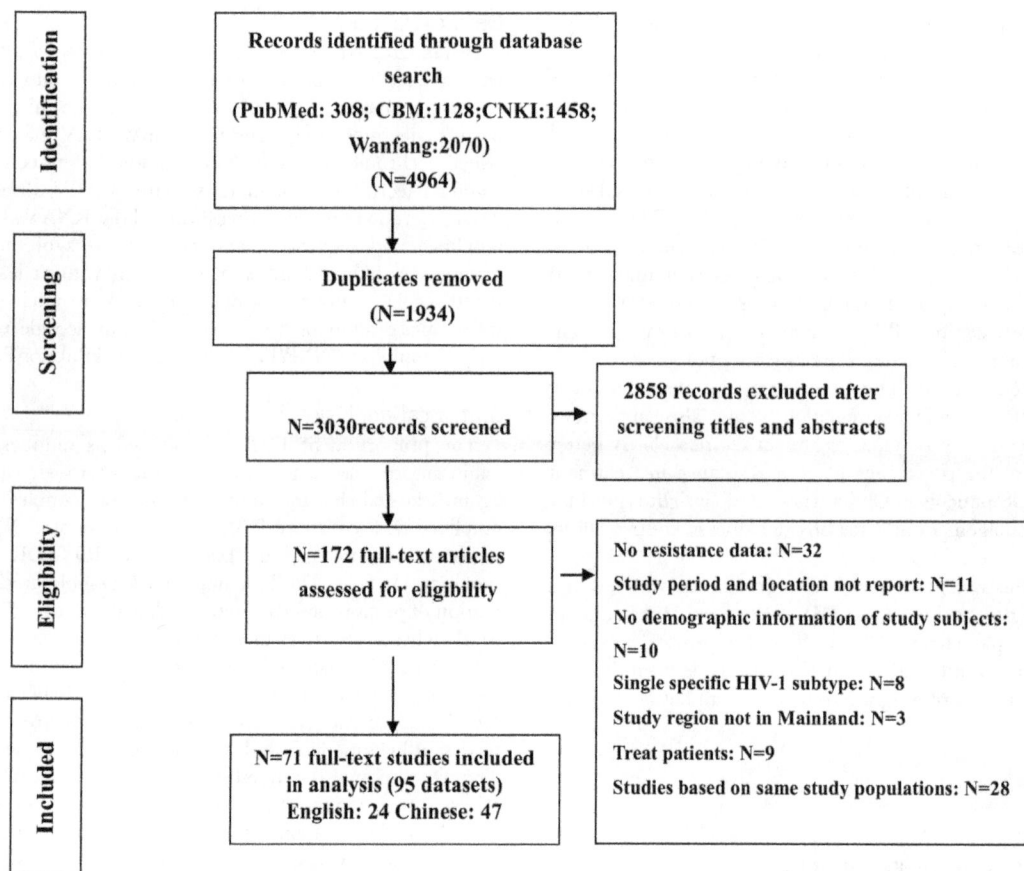

Figure 1. Flow chart of the process of studies selection.

according to the midpoint of the year in which study participants were recruited. A slightly upward trend can be detected in the composite time trend, though the trend was not statistically significant. We further categorized study times into four time periods roughly corresponding to the following phases of the national free ART program: pilot (before 2003), initiation (2003 to 2005), scale-up (2006 to 2008), and introduction of second line therapy (2009–2012) [5,8]. Results of the analyses showed that the overall TDR prevalence for any antiretroviral drug class was significantly high at initial stage of free ART program (5.18%, 95%CI: 3.13%–7.63%), but much lower during the scale-up phase (3.02%, 95%CI: 2.03%–4.16%). TDR prevalence rose again slightly after 2008 (3.68%, 95%CI: 2.78%–4.69%). Geographic subgroup analyses excluded studies in which the study represented the sole report on TDR from a given province [19–23] or in which results were reported as pooled prevalence of patients from multiple provinces [24–32]. Stratified analyses showed that TDR prevalence rates in the city of Beijing and the provinces of Henan and Hubei were all above 5%, but the rest were below this threshold. Finally, where information on most likely routes of HIV infection was provided, we estimated TDR prevalence for the following groups: FPD (5 articles), MSM (17 articles), IDU (5 articles), and those otherwise described as heterosexual individuals (3 articles). Pooled prevalence of TDR in these four risk groups were highest among MSM (4.03%, 95%CI:2.81%–5.43%), and slightly lower among FPD (3.78%, 95% CI: 2.48%–5.31%) and heterosexuals (3.73%, 95% CI: 1.85%–6.20%). Rates were lowest

among IDU (2.78%, 95% CI: 1.04%–5.12%), but substantial overlap of the 95% confidence intervals suggests no significant difference in TDR rates among these groups. Figure 3 shows the prevalence of TDR to specific classes of antiretroviral drug within each subgroup, in which a disproportionately large prevalence of PIs resistance can be seen in MSM.

Discussion

Our meta-analysis showed that estimated prevalence of TDR in ART-naïve patients in China was 3.64% (95%CI: 3.00%–4.32%). Such a pooled prevalence rate of primary drug resistance is similar to those from other developing country settings such as Thailand (0.5%, 95% CI: 0.1%–1.4%) and India (2.7%, 95% CI: 1.1%–4.7%) [33], but lower than those estimated in Europe (8.4%, 95%CI: 7.4%–9.5%) [34] and the United States (14.6%, 95% CI: 12.9%–16.0%) [35]. The far lower rates of TDR in Chinese HIV patients as compared to those in western countries may be due to differences in sampling strategies, but may also reflect real differences in the prevalence of circulating strains of drug resistance HIV in the two settings. China's HIV epidemic is at a relatively earlier phase compared to those in Africa and the west, as has a shorter history of population level exposure to ART, leading to less drug resistance in the population.

Changes in estimated TDR prevalence across populations sampled over distinct time periods likely reflect population level response to the antiretroviral drug used most widely by beneficiaries of China's free ART program at each phase. Higher

Table 1. Result of stratified meta-analysis based on time period, study region and risk group.

Category	Number of estimates	Pooled prevalence (%)	95%CI (%)	Heterogeneity p-value[a]
Time period[b]				
before 2003	3	2.65	0.89–5.17	0.15
2003–2005	5	5.18	3.13–7.63	0.01
2006–2008	20	3.02	2.03–4.16	0.18
2009–2012	53	3.68	2.78–4.69	<0.0001
Region[c]				
Hubei	3	7.37	4.61–10.65	0.42
Henan	7	7.11	4.10–10.80	0.00
Beijing	5	6.52	4.35–9.05	0.27
Shanghai	3	4.91	2.25–8.38	0.87
Tianjin	2	4.90	1.25–10.31	0.65
Zhejiang	2	4.76	2.35–7.86	0.51
Liaoning	2	4.40	2.26–7.15	0.95
Guangdong	7	3.43	2.17–4.91	0.70
Guangxi	6	2.72	1.70–3.94	0.14
Hunan	2	2.69	0.91–5.22	0.83
Yunnan	11	2.44	1.14–4.11	0.08
Guizhou	2	2.25	0.00–14.08	0.04
Anhui	3	1.89	0.02–5.51	0.60
Shandong	2	1.56	0.07–4.24	0.67
Sichuan	3	0.49	0.00–2.16	0.24
Risk group[d]				
MSM	17	4.03	2.81–5.43	0.05
FPD	5	3.78	2.48–5.31	0.19
HST	3	3.73	1.85–6.20	0.05
IDU	5	2.78	1.04–5.12	0.22

Note: [a]Heterogeneity p value was calculated by examining the Cochran Q statistic (p-value of <0.1 was considered a statistically significant); [b]For time period subgroup analysis, 81 HIV TDR prevalence estimates from 71 articles were used; [c]For study region subgroup analysis, 60 HIV TDR prevalence estimates from 58 articles were used; [d]For risk group subgroup analysis, 30 HIV TDR prevalence estimates from 28 articles were used. MSM: men who have sex with men; FPD: former plasma donors; HST: Heterosexual transmission; IDU: Injecting drug users.

TDR prevalence estimates in the earliest phase of the national free ART program may be due to the widespread use of generic agents including zidovudine, didanosine, and nevirapine [5]. Subsequent survey work as shown a strong association between didanosine use and virological failure in the earliest participants of the free ART program, suggesting high drug resistance rates due to antiretroviral drug choice [36,37]. In addition, ART dispensation in the early phase of the epidemic relied on village clinics where clinicians who often lacked formal medical training and who worked without the benefit of routine laboratory monitoring to aid their patient management [5,7,38]. After 2005, routinization of ART practices [39] and availability of branded drugs including lamivudine and efavirenz may have led to lower population level prevalence of drug resistant strains [4]. Slightly higher rates of TDR following 2008 may be due to broad expansion of ART access during this phase [8,40] or due to a cumulative increase in the prevalence of drug strains in HIV infected person on therapy [41]. However the lack of a statistically significant difference in pooled prevalence of TDR in these two periods may reflect a spurious difference.

Geographic sub-analyses showed that pooled estimates of TDR were highest in Beijing (a provincial-level city) and Henan and Hubei provinces. Higher rates of TDR in Beijing may be due to the fact that three out of the five studies based in Beijing were of MSM [42–44]. Past reports of TDR in MSM in Beijing have been high [42]—as compared to rates among MSM recruited in Guangzhou city [45], Liaoning province [46] and Yunnan province [47]—but for reasons that are still poorly understood. Higher rates in Henan province likely reflect the fact that it has the largest concentration of treated HIV patients in China with the earliest access to ART due to the piloting of the national treatment program in this population [4]. Finally, the three articles conducted in Hubei province were carried out in the early phase of the free ART program, a possible explanation for the higher prevalence of TDR.

Though drug resistance patterns did not vary significantly across risk populations, one noteworthy finding was the elevated prevalence of PI-specific TDR among MSM. The fact that PI's were not available through China's free ART program until 2008 [48] and its limited use even today [25] may suggest acquisition of PI-specific TDR from individuals treated outside of

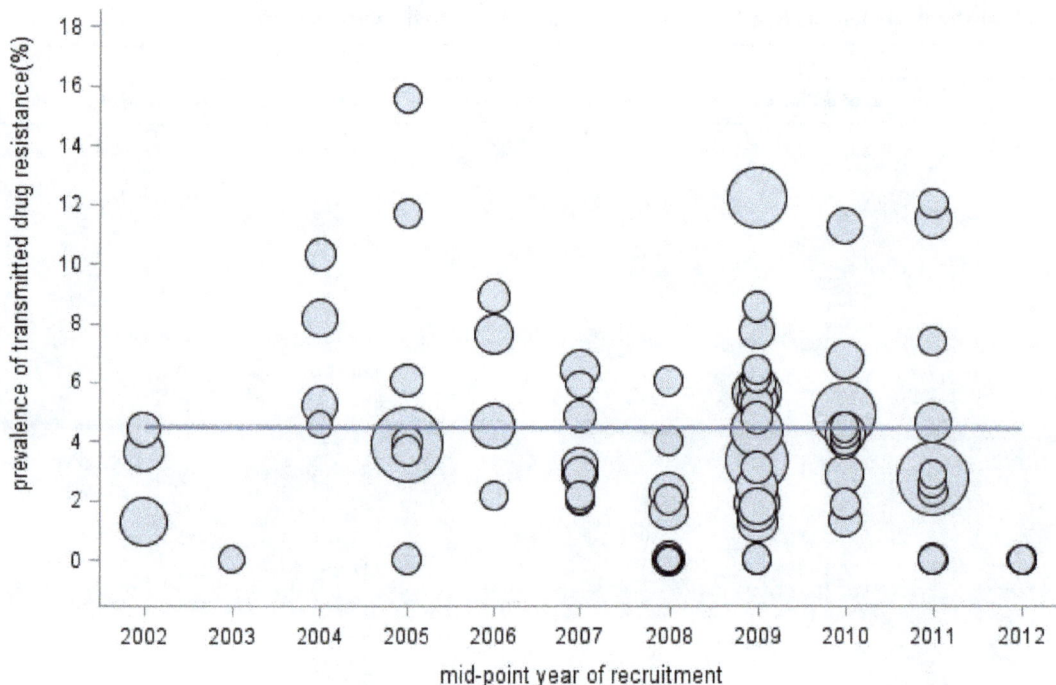

Figure 2. Temporal trends of prevalence of drug resistance in HIV ART-naïve patients in China. The size of circle correspond to sample size of every study, 81 estimates from 71 articles were used in this subgroup analysis.

the free ART program or foreign nationals treated abroad. Mixing between foreign-born and Chinese men in MSM sexual networks, and the relative affluence of MSM (or the subset captured in epidemiological studies) which allows for increased international travel [25] may be partial explanations for this phenomenon.

Our analysis faces several important limitations. Convenience sampling was the most common recruitment method for most studies included in this analysis which limits representativeness of findings. Selection bias may also have led to oversampling of studies in regions with high levels of ART penetration such as Guangdong, Beijing, Yunnan, Henan and Guangxi.

Despite these limitations, findings from this study represent the first comprehensive investigation of HIV TDR in treatment naïve individuals in China. Though estimated rates are lower than many western settings, the relative infancy of the Chinese ART program underscores the importance of consistent monitoring of onward transmission of drug resistant HIV at the population level. Beyond the clinical considerations of limited therapeutic options for TDR in treatment naïve patients, China's focus on treatment as prevention as part of its newly articulated HIV control strategy in the 12th Five-Year Action Plan [12] underscores the HIV prevention tradeoffs of expanded ART access.

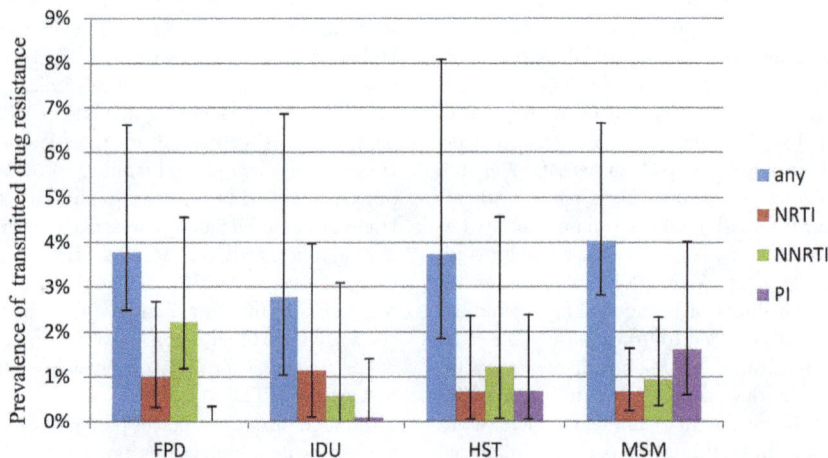

Figure 3. Prevalence of transmitted drug resistance in difference risk groups. Note: MSM: men who have sex with men; HST: Heterosexual transmission; FPD: former plasma donors; IDU: Injecting drug users; NRTI: nucleoside reverse transcriptase inhibitor; NNRTI: non-nucleoside reverse transcriptase inhibitor; PI: protease inhibitor.

Supporting Information

Figure S1   Funnel plot.

Table S1   Characteristics of included studies.

Checklist S1   PRISMA checklist.

References

1. Ministry of Health, People's Republic of China, Joint United Nations Programme on HIV/AIDS, World Health Organization (2011) 2011 Estimates for the HIV/AIDS Epidemic in China. Beijing, China.
2. Zhang L, Chow EP, Jing J, Zhuang X, Li X, et al. (2013) HIV prevalence in China: integration of surveillance data and a systematic review. Lancet Infect Dis 13: 955–963.
3. National Health and Family Planning Commission of the People's Republic of China (2013) Background of HIV/AIDS prevention and control in China. Available: http://www.nhfpc.gov.cn/jkj/s3586/201312/2b871ccd2ef446eb9542875d3d68bbca.shtml. Accessed March 31, 2014.
4. Dou Z, Chen RY, Xu J, Ma Y, Jiao JH, et al. (2010) Changing baseline characteristics among patients in the China National Free Antiretroviral Treatment Program, 2002-09. Int J Epidemiol 39 Suppl 2: ii56–64.
5. Zhang F, Haberer JE, Wang Y, Zhao Y, Ma Y, et al. (2007) The Chinese free antiretroviral treatment program: challenges and responses. AIDS 21 Suppl 8: S143–148.
6. Zhang F, Dou Z, Ma Y, Zhang Y, Zhao Y, et al. (2011) Effect of earlier initiation of antiretroviral treatment and increased treatment coverage on HIV-related mortality in China: a national observational cohort study. Lancet Infect Dis 11: 516–524.
7. Zhang FJ, Pan J, Yu L, Wen Y, Zhao Y (2005) Current progress of China's free ART program. Cell Res 15: 877–882.
8. Zhao DC, Wen Y, Ma Y, Zhao Y, Zhang Y, et al. (2012) Expansion of China's free antiretroviral treatment program. Chin Med J (Engl) 125: 3514–3521.
9. Little SJ (2000) Transmission and prevalence of HIV resistance among treatment-naive subjects. Antivir Ther 5: 33–40.
10. Bennett DE, Bertagnolio S, Sutherland D, Gilks CF (2008) The World Health Organization's global strategy for prevention and assessment of HIV drug resistance. Antivir Ther 13 Suppl 2: 1–13.
11. Wittkop L, Gunthard HF, de Wolf F, Dunn D, Cozzi-Lepri A, et al. (2011) Effect of transmitted drug resistance on virological and immunological response to initial combination antiretroviral therapy for HIV (EuroCoord-CHAIN joint project): a European multicohort study. Lancet Infect Dis 11: 363–371.
12. Zhao Y, Poundstone KE, Montaner J, Wu ZY (2012) New policies and strategies to tackle HIV/AIDS in China. Chin Med J (Engl) 125: 1331–1337.
13. Avila-Rios S, Garcia-Morales C, Garrido-Rodriguez D, Ormsby CE, Hernandez-Juan R, et al. (2011) National prevalence and trends of HIV transmitted drug resistance in Mexico. PLoS One 6: e27812.
14. Bennett DE, Camacho RJ, Otelea D, Kuritzkes DR, Fleury H, et al. (2009) Drug resistance mutations for surveillance of transmitted HIV-1 drug-resistance: 2009 update. PLoS One 4: e4724.
15. Higgins J, Thompson SG (2002) Quantifying heterogeneity in a meta-analysis. Statistics in medicine 21: 1539–1558.
16. Huedo-Medina TB, Sanchez-Meca J, Marin-Martinez F, Botella J (2006) Assessing heterogeneity in meta-analysis: Q statistic or I2 index? Psychol Methods 11: 193–206.
17. R Core Team (2013) R: A language and environment for statistical computing. R Foundation for Statistical Computing, Vienna, Austria. Available: http://www.R-project.org/. Accessed April 7, 2014.
18. Bennett DE, Myatt M, Bertagnolio S, Sutherland D, Gilks CF (2008) Recommendations for surveillance of transmitted HIV drug resistance in countries scaling up antiretroviral treatment. Antivir Ther 13 Suppl 2: 25–36.
19. Qiu LJ, Wu SL, Liu XH, Xie MR, Yan PP, et al. (2013) Study on drug resistant mutations for HIV-1 strains in Fujian Province. Chin J AIDS STD 19: 6–9.
20. Li L, Lu X, Li H, Chen L, Wang Z, et al. (2011) High genetic diversity of HIV-1 was found in men who have sex with men in Shijiazhuang, China. Infect Genet Evol 11: 1487–1492.
21. Li WJ, Li H, Wang FX, Li YG (2012) Drug resistance mutations in HIV-1 strains of treatment-naive patients in Harbin, China. Chin J Viral Dis 2: 40–45.
22. Yang HT, Xiao ZP, Huang XP, Hu HY, Xu XQ, et al. (2012) Threshold survey of transmitted HIV-1 drug resistance in Jiangsu province. Acta Universitatis Medicinalis Nanjing (Natural Science) 2012: 1–5.
23. Han XX, Zhao B, Sun F, An MM, Yin LL, et al. (2012) Primary HIV-1drug resistance among injecting drug users in Xinjiang. Chin J Public Health 28: 810–811.
24. Liao L, Xing H, Li X, Ruan Y, Zhang Y, et al. (2007) Genotypic analysis of the protease and reverse transcriptase of HIV type 1 isolates from recently infected injecting drug users in western China. AIDS Res Hum Retroviruses 23: 1062–1065.
25. Yang J, Xing H, Niu J, Liao L, Ruan Y, et al. (2013) The emergence of HIV-1 primary drug resistance genotypes among treatment-naive men who have sex with men in high-prevalence areas in China. Arch Virol 158: 839–844.
26. Kuang JQ (2007) Genotypic HIV-1 Drug Resistance and Factors associated with the effect of Antiretroviral therapy Among Chinese HIV/AIDS Patients: Peking Union Medical College.
27. Liao L, Xing H, Shang H, Li J, Zhong P, et al. (2010) The prevalence of transmitted antiretroviral drug resistance in treatment-naive HIV-infected individuals in China. J Acquir Immune Defic Syndr 53 Suppl 1: S10–14.
28. Wang X, He C, Xing H, Liao L, Xu X, et al. (2012) Short communication: emerging transmitted HIV type 1 drug resistance mutations among patients prior to start of first-line antiretroviral therapy in middle and low prevalence sites in China. AIDS Res Hum Retroviruses 28: 1637–1639.
29. Li L, Sun G, Liang S, Li J, Li T, et al. (2013) Different Distribution of HIV-1 Subtype and Drug Resistance Were Found among Treatment Naive Individuals in Henan, Guangxi, and Yunnan Province of China. PLoS One 8: e75777.
30. Si XF, Huang HL, Wei M, Guan Q, Song YH, et al. (2004) Prevalence of drug resistance mutations among antiretroviral drug-naive HIV-1-infected patients in China. Chinese J Exp Chin Virol 18: 308–311.
31. Zeng P, Wang J, Huang Y, Guo X, Li J, et al. (2012) The human immunodeficiency virus-1 genotype diversity and drug resistance mutations profile of volunteer blood donors from Chinese blood centers. Transfusion 52: 1041–1049.
32. Yin CY, Lu HZ, Huang XX, Li XO, Lou GQ, et al. (2011) HIV-1 drug-resistance mutations in treatment-naive patients in China. Chin J Clin Infect Dis 4: 201–205.
33. Gupta RK, Jordan MR, Sultan BJ, Hill A, Davis DH, et al. (2012) Global trends in antiretroviral resistance in treatment-naive individuals with HIV after rollout of antiretroviral treatment in resource-limited settings: a global collaborative study and meta-regression analysis. Lancet 380: 1250–1258.
34. Vercauteren J, Wensing AM, van de Vijver DA, Albert J, Balotta C, et al. (2009) Transmission of drug-resistant HIV-1 is stabilizing in Europe. J Infect Dis 200: 1503–1508.
35. Wheeler WH, Ziebell RA, Zabina H, Pieniazek D, Prejean J, et al. (2010) Prevalence of transmitted drug resistance associated mutations and HIV-1 subtypes in new HIV-1 diagnoses, U.S.-2006. AIDS 24: 1203–1212.
36. Li T, Dai Y, Kuang J, Jiang J, Han Y, et al. (2008) Three generic nevirapine-based antiretroviral treatments in Chinese HIV/AIDS patients: multicentric observation cohort. PLoS One 3: e3918.
37. Xing H, Wang X, Liao L, Ma Y, Su B, et al. (2013) Incidence and associated factors of HIV drug resistance in Chinese HIV-infected patients receiving antiretroviral treatment. PLoS One 8: e62408.
38. Zhang FJ, Maria A, Haberer J, Zhao Y (2006) Overview of HIV drug resistance and its implications for China. Chin Med J (Engl) 119: 1999–2004.
39. Manual for National free HIV antiretroviral drug treatment: first edition (2005) Beijing: People's Medical Publishing House.
40. World Health Organization (WHO) (2012) WHO HIV drug resistance report 2012. Available: http://www.who.int/hiv/pub/drugresistance/report2012/en/. Accessed January 31, 2014.
41. Liao L, Xing H, Su B, Wang Z, Ruan Y, et al. (2013) Impact of HIV drug resistance on virologic and immunologic failure and mortality in a cohort of patients on antiretroviral therapy in China. AIDS 27: 1815–1824.
42. Zhang X, Li S, Li X, Li X, Xu J, et al. (2007) Characterization of HIV-1 subtypes and viral antiretroviral drug resistance in men who have sex with men in Beijing, China. AIDS 21 Suppl 8: S59–65.
43. Wu YS, Zhang T, Wei FL, Li DM, Zhang WW, et al. (2011) Study on transmitted drug resistance in new recently or recently infected persons. Chinese Medical Association-Fifth national academic conferences of HIV/AIDS, viral hepatitis C and tropical diseases. Wu Han, Hubei.
44. Li L, Han N, Lu J, Li T, Zhong X, et al. (2013) Genetic characterization and transmitted drug resistance of the HIV type 1 epidemic in men who have sex with men in Beijing, China. AIDS Res Hum Retroviruses 29: 633–637.
45. Zhao GL, Feng TJ, Hong FC, Wang F, Cai YM, et al. (2009) Study on drug-resistant gene mutation in HIV-1 infected MSM population in Shenzhen. Chin J AIDS STD 15: 589–591.

Appendix S1   Detailed search strategy.

Author Contributions

Conceived and designed the experiments: YYS NW. Performed the experiments: YYS HXL LZ MKS. Analyzed the data: YYS. Contributed reagents/materials/analysis tools: FJZ MKS LZ JW. Wrote the paper: YYS FJZ HXL MKS LZ JW NW.

46. Zhao B, Han X, Dai D, Liu J, Ding H, et al. (2011) New trends of primary drug resistance among HIV type 1-infected men who have sex with men in Liaoning Province, China. AIDS Res Hum Retroviruses 27: 1047–1053.

47. Chen M, Ma Y, Su Y, Yang L, Zhang R, et al. (2014) HIV-1 Genetic Characteristics and Transmitted Drug Resistance among Men Who Have Sex with Men in Kunming, China. PLoS One 9: e87033.

48. Manual for National free HIV antiretroviral drug treatment: second edition (2008) Beijing: People's Medical Publishing House.

13

High-Dose Cytarabine in Acute Myeloid Leukemia Treatment

Wei Li[1], Xiaoyuan Gong[1], Mingyuan Sun[1], Xingli Zhao[1], Benfa Gong[1], Hui Wei[1], Yingchang Mi[1], Jianxiang Wang[1,2]*

1 Leukemia Diagnosis and Treatment Center, Institute of Hematology and Blood Disease Hospital, Chinese Academy of Medical Sciences and Peking Union of Medical College, Tianjin, China, 2 State Key Laboratory of Experimental Hematology, Institute of Hematology and Blood Disease Hospital, Chinese Academy of Medical Sciences and Peking Union of Medical College, Tianjin, China

Abstract

The optimal dose, scheme, and clinical setting for Ara-C in acute myeloid leukemia (AML) treatment remain uncertain. In this study, we performed a meta-analysis to systematically assess the impact of high-dose cytarabine (HDAC) on AML therapy during the induction and consolidation stages. Twenty-two trials with a total of 5,945 de novo AML patients were included in the meta-analysis. Only patients less than 60 year-old were included in the study. Using HDAC in induction therapy was beneficial for RFS (HR = 0.57; 95% CI, 0.35–0.93; $P = 0.02$) but not so for CR rate (HR = 1.01; 95% CI, 0.93–1.09; $P = 0.88$) and OS (HR = 0.83; 95% CI, 0.66–1.03; $P = 0.1$). In consolidation therapy, HDAC showed significant RFS benefits (HR = 0.67; 95% CI, 0.49–0.9; $P = 0.008$) especially for the favorable-risk group (HR = 0.38; 95% CI, 0.21–0.69; $P = 0.001$) compared with SDAC (standard dose cytarabine), although no OS advantage was observed (HR = 0.84; 95% CI, 0.55–1.27; $P = 0.41$). HDAC treatment seemed less effective than auto-BMT/allo-BMT treatment (HR = 1.66, 95% CI, 1.3–2.14; $P<0.0001$) with similar OS. HDAC treatment led to lower relapse rate in induction and consolidation therapy than SDAC treatment, especially for the favorable-risk group. Auto-BMT/allo-BMT was more beneficial in prolonging RFS than HDAC.

Editor: Wilbur Lam, Emory University/Georgia Institute of Technology, United States of America

Funding: This study was supported by National Natural Science Foundation (81270635), National Public Health Grand Research Foundation (201202017), National Science & Technology Major Projects (201 1ZX09302-007-04) of China and Tianjin Major Science and Technology Project (12ZCDZSY17500). The funders had no role in study design, data collection and analysis, decision to publish, or preparation of the manuscript.

Competing Interests: In this article we declared that Jianxiang Wang acts as consultant of Novartis and Bristol Myers Squibb. ALL authors have no conflict of interest to declare.

* Email: wangjx@ihcams.ac.cn

Introduction

Cytarabine (Ara-C) has been a major drug for acute myeloid leukemia (AML) treatment for more than three decades. Initially, the drug was used at 100–200 mg/m^2 for 7–10 days for standard treatment [1]. In recent years, multiple cycles of high-dose cytarabine (HDAC) therapy (at 3.0 g/m^2 every 12 hours) have been commonly used as the consolidation therapy in multicenter trials; it was observed to maximize Ara-C's anti-leukemia effect in AML patients, leading to improve disease- free-survival (DFS) [2,3]. After that, HDAC instead of standard-dose cytarabine multiagent chemotherapy has become a common practice in the treatment of AML, especially in patients younger than 60 years of age, either for remission induction or consolidation, based on the guidelines of the National Comprehensive Cancer Network (VI. 2013). However, recent randomized controlled trials with 781 patients have challenged the benefits of HDAC [4]. HDAC failed to show significant improvement in five-year relapse-free survival and five-year overall survival as compared with SDAC regimen in AML treatments, especially in the consolidation therapy. After these new studies, the dose and effect of HDAC during AML induction and consolidation therapies are open for new evaluation [5]. Therefore, a systematic analysis needs to be performed to clarify these issues, which is the focus of this meta-analytical review. Specifically, this review study compared the effectiveness of HDAC versus SDAC as AML therapy in adult patients during the induction and consolidation phases, in order to shed lights on defining the optimal dose and scheme of Ara-C treatment with minimum possible toxicity. On the other hand, we assessed the effectiveness of HDAC compared with bone marrow transplantation (BMT) in order to explore the best therapy in the consolidation phase.

Methods

Literature Search

Independent reviewers (L.W and G. XY) systematically searched PubMed for relevant research papers published in English between January 1990 and March 2013 using the following query terms: acute myeloid leukemia, high-dose, and cytarabine. The titles and abstracts of the identified studies were reviewed to determine potential eligibility for meta-analysis. Relevant review and meta-analysis articles were included to identify additional studies that met the inclusion criteria. Further studies were referred by means of manual search of secondary

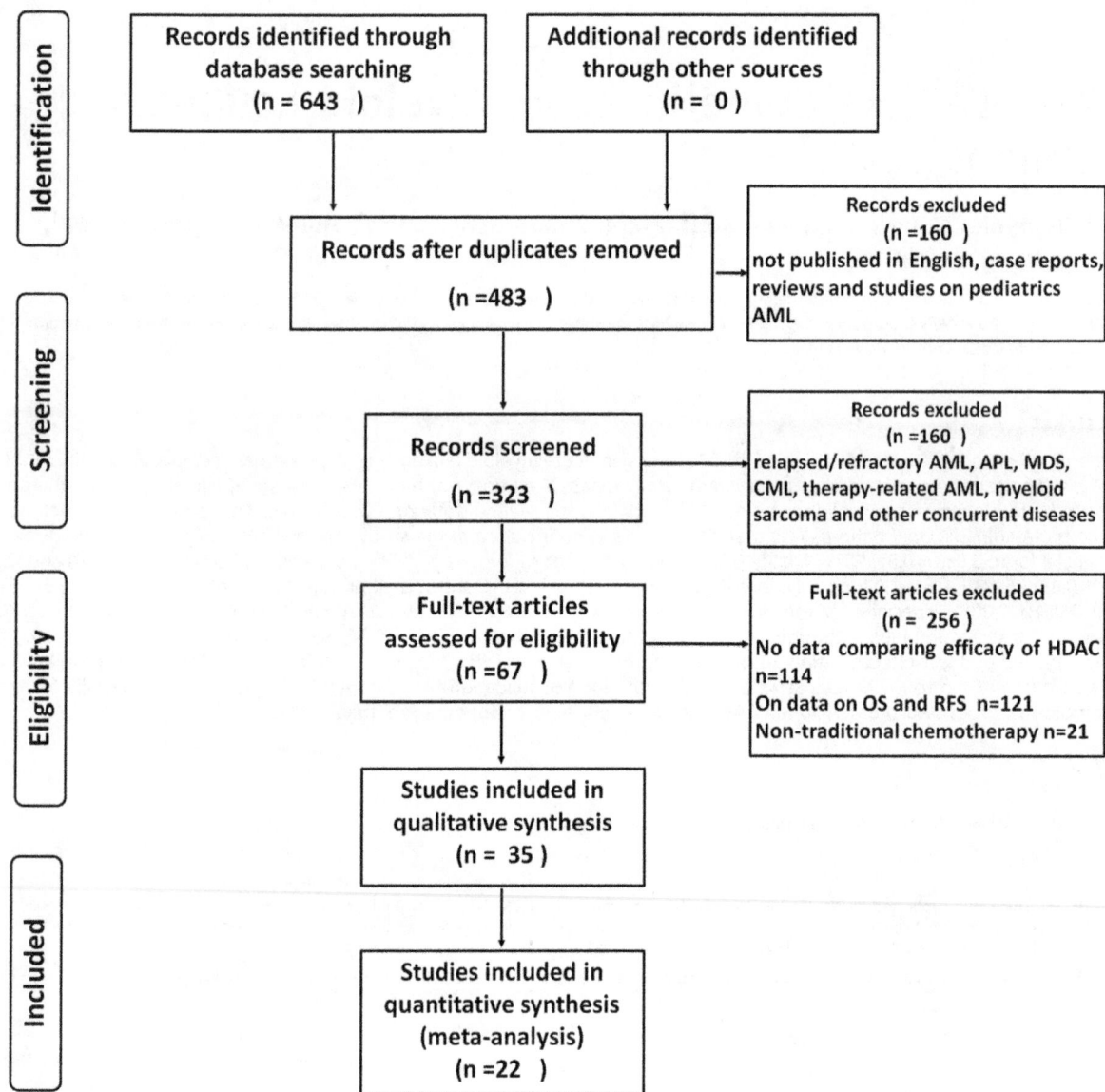

Figure 1. Flow chart explaining the selection of eligible studies included in the meta-analysis.

sources. Divergences among the reviewers must be resolved to reach a consensus after further discussion.

Inclusion and Exclusion Criteria

Identified articles were independently appraised according to the inclusion criteria by the same two reviewers (L.W and G. XY). All patients were required to have untreated acute myeloid leukemia, de novo AML, and patients with acute promyelocytic leukemia and translocation t(15;17) did not included this study. The included trials described the comparsion of HDAC (2.0–3.0 g/m^2) and standard-dose cytarabine (SDAC, ≤200 mg/m^2) in induction and consolidation therapy, or bone marrow transplantion (BMT) in consolidation therapy. new medicine research and phase II/III clinical trials were excluded. Studies reported hazard ratios (HRs) and 95% confidence intervals (CIs) for overall survival (OS)/relapse free survival (RFS) benefit, or those provided data to estimate HR by the method of Parmar *et al* [6]. If multiple articles were identified to report on the same study, the most recent one

was analyzed. Only randomized controlled trials (RCT) were included in the comparison of HDAC and SDAC, but observed study met the inclusion criteria for the study of BMT vs HDAC, because it was difficult to ensure that each patient had donor and even more difficult to complete RCT.

Data Extraction. Data were extracted in the standardized format by two independent reviewers. Data collected for each study included study name, name of first author, year of publication, period of enrollment, total number of subjects allocated to therapies, median patient age (years), chemotherapy regimens, number of events (death, relapse) in each group, and study end points of overall survival benefit, RFS benefit, or both. We used overall survival (OS) and relapse free survival (RFS) of individual studies. Discrepancies in data extraction were resolved by identifying consensus, referring back to the original article, or contacting study authors if necessary. When missing data were encountered, the authors were contacted to complete data analysis.

Table 1. Characteristics of included Studies for induction therapy.

Source	Study ID	Enrollment Period	Multi-center	No. of patients	RCTs	Study entry criteria	Induction therapy
J.P. Matthews et al, 2001 [7]	ALSG	1987–1991	Yes	248	Yes	de novo AML median age: 42 years	DEA (DNR+VP-16+Ara-c 100 mg/m^2/d×7d) DEA (DNR+VP-16+Ara-c 3 g/m^2 q12 h d1,3,5,7d)
JK. Weick et al, 1996 [8]	SWOG	1986–1991	Yes	723	Yes	de novo or secondary AML M/F: 397/326 age range: 15–64 years WBC range: 0.4–416×10^9/L	DA (DNR+Ara-c 200 mg/m^2/d×7d) DA (DNR+Ara-c 3 g/m^2 q12 h×6d)
T. Büchner et al, 2006 [9]▲	—	1999–2005	Yes	1770	Yes	de novo or secondary AML, age range: 16~85 years※	Double induction TAD (6-TG+DNR+Ara-c 100 mg/m^2/d×8d) + HAM (MTZ+Ara-c 3 g/m^2 q12 h×3d) HAM+HAM (MTZ+Ara-c 3 g/m^2 q12 h×3d)
T. Büchner et al, 1999 [10]	CAMLCG	1985–1992	Yes	725	Yes	de novo AML, M/F: 336/389 median age: 44 (16–60) years WBC range: 0.1–405×10^9/L	Double induction TAD+TAD (6-TG+DNR+Ara-c100 mg/m^2/d×8d) TAD (6-TG+DNR+Ara-c 100 mg/m^2/d×8d) + HAM (MTZ+Ara-c 3 g/m^2 q12 h×3d)
T. Büchner et al, 2009 [11]▲	CAMLCG	1993–2005	Yes	1284	Yes	de novo AML, years range: 16~85 years※ WBC range: 0.05–1017×10^9/L	Double induction TAD (6-TG+DNR+Ara-c 100 mg/m^2/d×8d) + HAM (MTZ+Ara-c 3 g/m^2 q12 h×3d) HAM+HAM (MTZ+Ara-c 3 g/m^2 q12 h×3d)

Note: ▲ T. Büchner et al, 2009 repeated the same trial of T. Büchner et al, 2006.
※analyze <60 years patients in each trial.
Abbreviations: NR, not reported; IDA, idarubicin; Ara-c, cytarabin; VP-16, etoposide; DNR, daunorubicin.

A

Study or Subgroup	Experimental Events	Total	Control Events	Total	Weight	Risk Ratio M-H. Random. 95% CI
J.P. Matt hews(ALSG)2001	91	124	88	124	17.3%	1.03 [0.89, 1.21]
JK. Weick(SWOG) 1996	275	493	120	230	18.7%	1.07 [0.92, 1.24]
T. Bu¨chner(CAMLCG) 2006	336	473	307	451	34.4%	1.04 [0.96, 1.14]
T. Bu¨chner(CAMLCG)1999	234	360	260	365	29.6%	0.91 [0.83, 1.01]
Total (95% CI)		**1450**		**1170**	**100.0%**	**1.01 [0.93, 1.09]**
Total events	936		775			

Heterogeneity: Tau² = 0.00; Chi² = 5.15, df = 3 (P = 0.16); I² = 42%
Test for overall effect: Z = 0.15 (P = 0.88)

B

Study or Subgroup	log[Risk Ratio]	SE	Weight	Risk Ratio IV. Fixed. 95% CI
J.P. Matt hews(ALSG)2001	-0.78	0.33	11.8%	0.46 [0.24, 0.88]
JK. Weick(SWOG) 1996	-0.39	0.76	2.2%	0.68 [0.15, 3.00]
T. Bu¨chner(CAMLCG)1999	-0.09	0.16	50.3%	0.91 [0.67, 1.25]
T.Bu¨chner (CAMLCG)2009	-0.12	0.19	35.7%	0.89 [0.61, 1.29]
Total (95% CI)			**100.0%**	**0.83 [0.66, 1.03]**

Heterogeneity: Chi² = 3.79, df = 3 (P = 0.28); I² = 21%
Test for overall effect: Z = 1.67 (P = 0.10)

C

Study or Subgroup	log[Risk Ratio]	SE	Weight	Risk Ratio IV. Random. 95% CI
J.P. Matt hews(ALSG)2001	-1.39	0.34	20.8%	0.25 [0.13, 0.48]
JK. Weick(SWOG) 1996	-0.71	0.26	24.7%	0.49 [0.30, 0.82]
T. Bu¨chner(CAMLCG)1999	-0.27	0.19	28.3%	0.76 [0.53, 1.11]
T.Bu¨chner (CAMLCG)2009	-0.08	0.23	26.3%	0.92 [0.59, 1.45]
Total (95% CI)			**100.0%**	**0.57 [0.35, 0.93]**

Heterogeneity: Tau² = 0.18; Chi² = 12.13, df = 3 (P = 0.007); I² = 75%
Test for overall effect: Z = 2.25 (P = 0.02)

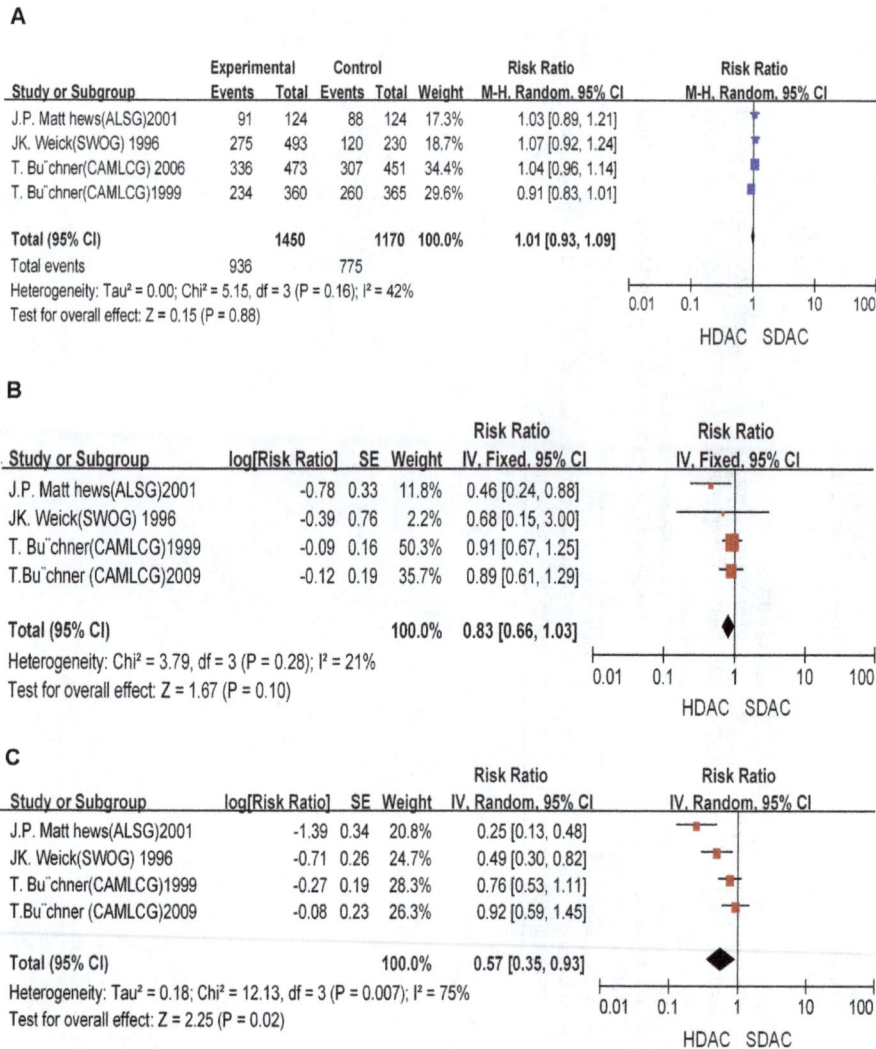

Figure 2. Effect of HDAC versus SDAC in induction therapy. A: Effect of HDAC versus SDAC in induction therapy on CR rate. **B**: Overall survival benefit of HDAC in induction therapy. **C**: Relapse free survival benefit of HDAC in induction therapy.

Assessment of methodological quality. Two reviewers assessed the methodological quality of each trial. The risk of bias in each trial was assessed according to Cochrane methodology by using the following criteria: considering random sequence generation, allocation concealment, the blinding of patients and personnel, incomplete outcome data, selective reporting, and Begg's funnel plots and Egger's test were used to reveal possible publication bias. Heterogeneity was assessed by forest plots and with a standard Chi² test and an inconsistency (I^2) statistic. Both the fixed-effect model and the random-effect model were initially used to calculate total HRs, and finally selected with regards to heterogeneity in the survival analyses. If the heterogeneity ($I^2 >$ 75%) was too great for a summary estimate to be calculated, subgroup analysis was needed.

Data synthesis. Data were synthesized using the Cochrane Statistics package RevMan (version 4.0.4). The threshold of significance was $P \leq 0.05$. A forest plot with combined HRs (with 95% CIs) for OS and RFS benefit of SDAC vs. HDAC, or HDAC vs. auto-BMT/allo-BMT was constructed using random-effects meta-analysis. We also performed additional analysis that stratified treatment options by cytogenetic characteristics. In such analysis,

patients were stratified into poor-, intermediate-, and favorable-risk groups by cytogenetic characteristics. OS and RFS benefits of HDAC for different cytogenetic risk groups were analyzed.

Results

Studies selected for meta-analysis

The initial search on MEDLINE (PubMed) database and the abstract review identified 643 articles. After the screening of titles and abstracts (by two reviewers L.W and G. XY), 160 non-relevant articles were excluded, which were those that were published in languages other than English, case reports, reviews, and studies on pediatrics AML. For the secondary search, the reference lists of review articles were manually examined to identify additional studies. The 483 selected articles were retrieved for further reviews in a structured format. As a result, 160 more articles were excluded, because those studies involved relapsed/refractory AML, APL, high-risk MDS, CML, therapy-related AML, myeloid sarcoma, or other concurrent diseases (including status of other concurrent tumors, definite MDS history) of AML that conflicted with the inclusion criteria. For the remaining 323

Table 2. Characteristics of Included Studies for consolidation therapy.

Source	Study ID	Enrollment Period	RCT	Multicenter	No. of patients	Median age/age range (years)	Consolidation therapy	follow-up (years)
JK. Weick et al. 1996 [8]	SWOG	1986–1991	Yes	Yes	287	45 (15–64)	DA (DNR+Ara-C 200 mg/m²/d×7) continuous 2 courses DA (DNR+Ara-C 3 g/m² q12 h×6) 1 course	4.3
K.F. Bradstock et al, 2005 [12]	ALLG	1995–2000	Yes	Yes	202	43 (15–60)	ICE (IDA+VP-16+Ara-c 100 mg/m²/d×5) continuous 2 courses ICE (IDA+VP-16+Ara-c 3 g/m² q12 h d1,3,5,7) 1 course	4
M. Fopp et al, 1997 [13]	SAKK	1985–1992	Yes	Yes	137	16–64	DA (DNR+Ara-C 100 mg/m²/d×7) 1 courses DA (DNR+Ara-C 3 g/m² q12 h×3) 1 course	6
PA. Cassileth et al, 1992 [14]	ECOG	1984–1988	Yes	Yes	170	15~65	TA (6-TG+Ara-c 60 mg/m²/d×5) AA (Amsa+Ara-c 3 g/m² q12 h×3) (no courses in detail)	4
R.J.Mayer et al, 1994 [15]	CALGB	1985–1990	Yes	Yes	389	16–86★	SDAC (Ara-c 100 mg/m²/d×5) continuous 4 courses HDAC (Ara-c 3 g/m² q12 h×3) continuous 4 courses (no detail therapy)	4.3
S. Miyawaki et al, 2011b [4]▲	JALSG	2001–2005	Yes	Yes	781	15–64	DA, MA, AA, VEA (DNR, MTZ, ACl-a, VP-16, VCR+Ara-C200 mg/m²/dx5) continuous 4 courses HDAC (2 g/m² q12 h×5) continuous 3 courses	4
S, Ohtake et al, 2011a [16]▲	JALSG	2001–2005	Yes	Yes	781	15–64	DA, MA, AA, VEA (DNR, MTZ, ACl-a, VP-16, VCR+Ara-C200 mg/m²/dx5) continuous 4 courses HDAC (2 g/m² q12 h×5) continuous 3 courses	4
T. Büchner et al, 2003 [17]	CAMLCG	1992–1999	Yes	Yes	576	16–82★	TAD (6-TG, DNR, Ara-C200 mg/m²/dx5) continuous several courses HAM (MTZ+Ara-c 2 g/m² q12 h d1,2,8,9)	NR
CD. Bloomfield et al, 1998 [19]	CALGB	1985–1990	Yes	No	186	>16	Ara-C 100 mg/m²/dx5 continuous 4 courses Ara-c 3.0 g/m² q12 h d1,3,5 continuous 4 courses (no detail therapy)	5
X. Thomas et al, 2011 [20]	ALFA	1999–2006	Yes	Yes	237	15–50	AA (Amsa+Ara-C), TSC (MTZ+VP-16+Ara-C500 mg/m²/dx d8–10) continuous 2 course Ara-c 3.0 g/m² q12 h d1,3,5 continuous 4 courses	10
AM. Tsimberidu et al, 2003 [21]	HCG	1996–2000	No	No	120	15–60	Ara-c 3.0 g/m² q12 h d1,3,5 continuous 2 courses preparative regimen: BU+VP-16+CTX Allo-BMT/auto- SCT	5.3
JL. Harousseau et al, 1997 [22]	GOELAM	1987–1994	No	No	517	15–60	ICC (IDR+Ara-c 3.0 g/m² q12 h d1–4) continuous 2 courses preparative regimen: BU+CTX/TBI+CTX Allo-BMT/auto-SCT	8.5
PA. Cassileth et al, 1998 [23]	No	1990–1997	Yes	Yes※	808	16–55	Ara-c 3.0 g/m² q12 h d1–3 preparative regimen: CTX+BU Allo-BMT/auto-SCT	4
RA. Zittoun et al, 1995 [24]	GIMEMA	1986–1993	Yes	Yes※	623	33 (10–59)	AA (Amsa+Ara-c 2.0 g/m² d1–6) continuous 2 courses preparative regimen: CTX+TBI+/–BU Allo-BMT/auto-SCT	8
S. Brunet et al, 2004 [25]	Spain	1994–1999	No	No	200	15–60	Ara-c 3.0 g/m² q12 h d1–3 continuous 2 courses preparative regimen: CTX+TBI+/–BU Allo-BMT/auto-SCT	7
R. Bassan et al, 1998 [26]	Italy	1987–1993	No	No	108	15–60	Ara-c 2.0 g/m²/d d1–6 preparative regimen: Dox+TBI Allo-BMT/auto-SCT	>5
PA. Cassileth et al, 1992 [14]	ECOG	—	No	Yes※	534	44 (15–65)	Ara-c 3.0 g/m² q12 h d1–6 1 course preparative regimen: CTX+TBI Allo-BMT	6

Table 2. Cont.

Source	Study ID	Enrollment Period	RCT	Multicenter	No. of patients	Median age/age range (years)	Consolidation therapy	follow-up (years)
GJ. Schiller et al, 1992 [27]	—	1982–1990	No	No	103	16–45	MA, DA (MTZ, DNR+Ara-c 2.0–3.0 g/m² q12 h d1–4) 2–3 course preparative regimen: TBI+CTX/MTX/Ara-C Allo-BMT	8
JL. Harousseau et al, 1991 [28]		1984–1987	No	Yes※	115	44 (13–65)	ICC (Amsa+Ara-c 3.0 g/m² q12 h d1–4) 2 course no preparative regimen Allo-BMT	7

Note: ▲ S. Miyawaki et al, 2011 repeated the same trial of S, Ohtake et al, 2011.
※BMT randomized trials were defined that if the patients didn't have donors, they were randomized into auto-BMT and high-dosed Ara-C groups.
★analyze analyze <60 years the patients in each trial.
Abbreviations: NR, not reported; IDA, idarubicin; Ara-c, cytarabin; VP-16, etoposide; DNR, daunorubicin MCT, multiagent chemotherapy;
CTX, cyclophosphamide; MTZ, mitoxantrone; AZQ, diaziquone; 6-TG, thioguanine; AMS, amsacrine.

articles, full texts were further reviewed. A total of 256 articles were further excluded: 114 articles did not report data comparing the efficacy of HDAC on the OS and RFS of adult AML patients; 121 articles did not provide prospective data on OS and RFS outcome; and 21 articles used non-traditional chemotherapy regimens. The remaining 67 articles met the inclusion criteria. However, 22 articles were further excluded by experts, because the induction or consolidation therapy used in these studies were not consistent, along with confusing risk groups in some articles; 10 more articles were also excluded because only HDAC was used thus no comparison data available; and 4 articles were reporting the same trials [2,9,18,4]. As a result, a total of 22 articles passed through all examinations and were finally used for the meta-analysis in this study [Figure 1].

Quality Assessment

According to Cochrane methodology, the risk of bias of total RCT articles were assessed by Cochrane factors. The studies at low risk of bias had values (a quantitative index of the risk of bias, range 0–100%) of 64.3%, 64.3%, 0, 92.9%, 50%, 42.9%. (Figure S1).

HDAC versus SDAC in induction therapy

Four randomized controlled trials compared HDAC with SDAC in induction therapy [Table1]. In all 4 trials, the end points of CR, OS, and RFS were reported. Initial baseline characteristics between the treatment group and the control group were quite balanced. A total of 2,980 de novo AML patients enrolled from 1985 to 2005 were included. In the CAMLCG2009 and CAMLCG 2006 trials, the inclusion criteria for patient age were different from those of the rest of trials. Patients younger than 60 year-old were analyzed in the majority of trials. No significant differences in CR between patients received HDAC and those received SDAC [Figure 2] (HR = 1.01; 95% CI, 0.93–1.09; $P = 0.88$). The OS and RFS results were overall heterogeneous. In the trial ALSG 1996, OS and RFS were much longer in the HDAC group than those in the SDAC group. On the other hand, a larger number of patients receiving HDAC treatment showed shorter OS in the CAMLCG trial. Overall, no significant differences in OS were observed between HDAC and SDAC in the induction phase (HR = 0.83; 95% CI, 0.66–1.03; $P = 0.1$) [Figure 2]. Patients in the HDAC group showed similar OS as that of the SDAC group. However, a statistically significant difference in RFS was observed between HDAC and SDAC in the induction phase (HR = 0.57; 95% CI, 0.35–0.93; $P = 0.02$) [Figure 2]. Therefore, HDAC used in the induction therapy clearly improved RFS but not OS in AML patients.

HDAC versus SDAC in consolidation therapy

Nine trials were identified to contain the comparison of HDAC and SDAC in consolidation therapy [Table 2]. All 9 trials were randomized controlled studies, and 7 of them were multicenter trials. A total of 2,965 de novo AML patients enrolled from 1978 to 2005 were included, and the longest follow-up period of each trial was 10 years. Only patients younger than 60 year-old were analyzed. The initial baseline characteristics (age, sex, race, FAB classification, and cytogenetics) between two groups were similar, although detailed information about initial baseline characteristics in the ECOG1992 trial was not shown. In addition, only 1 course of HDAC was used in the SWOG1996 and SAKK1997 trials, different from all other trials. In 5 trials, HDAC was used concomitantly with other drugs, while 4 other trials only used single dose of Ara-C (2–3 g/m²), which may lead to heterogeneity among different trials. All the 9 trials reported end points of 4-year

A

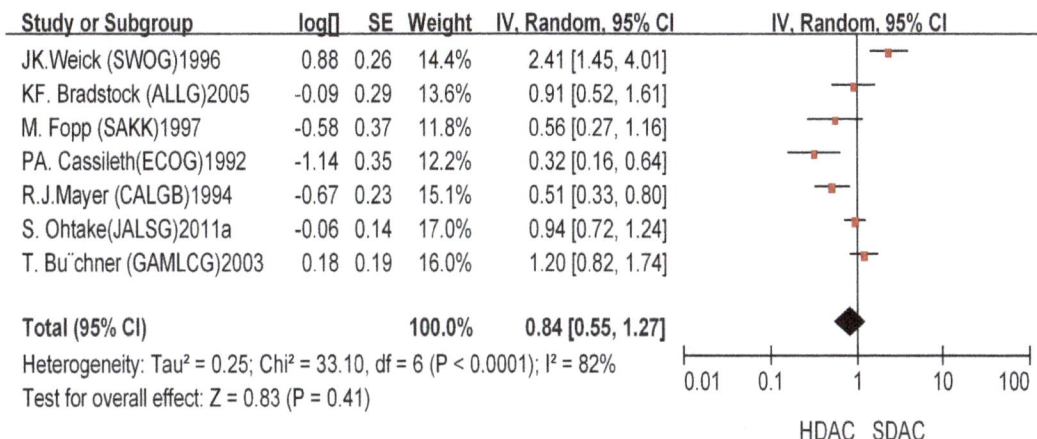

Study or Subgroup	log[]	SE	Weight	IV, Random, 95% CI
JK.Weick (SWOG)1996	0.88	0.26	14.4%	2.41 [1.45, 4.01]
KF. Bradstock (ALLG)2005	-0.09	0.29	13.6%	0.91 [0.52, 1.61]
M. Fopp (SAKK)1997	-0.58	0.37	11.8%	0.56 [0.27, 1.16]
PA. Cassileth(ECOG)1992	-1.14	0.35	12.2%	0.32 [0.16, 0.64]
R.J.Mayer (CALGB)1994	-0.67	0.23	15.1%	0.51 [0.33, 0.80]
S. Ohtake(JALSG)2011a	-0.06	0.14	17.0%	0.94 [0.72, 1.24]
T. Bu¨chner (GAMLCG)2003	0.18	0.19	16.0%	1.20 [0.82, 1.74]
Total (95% CI)			**100.0%**	**0.84 [0.55, 1.27]**

Heterogeneity: Tau² = 0.25; Chi² = 33.10, df = 6 (P < 0.0001); I² = 82%
Test for overall effect: Z = 0.83 (P = 0.41)

B

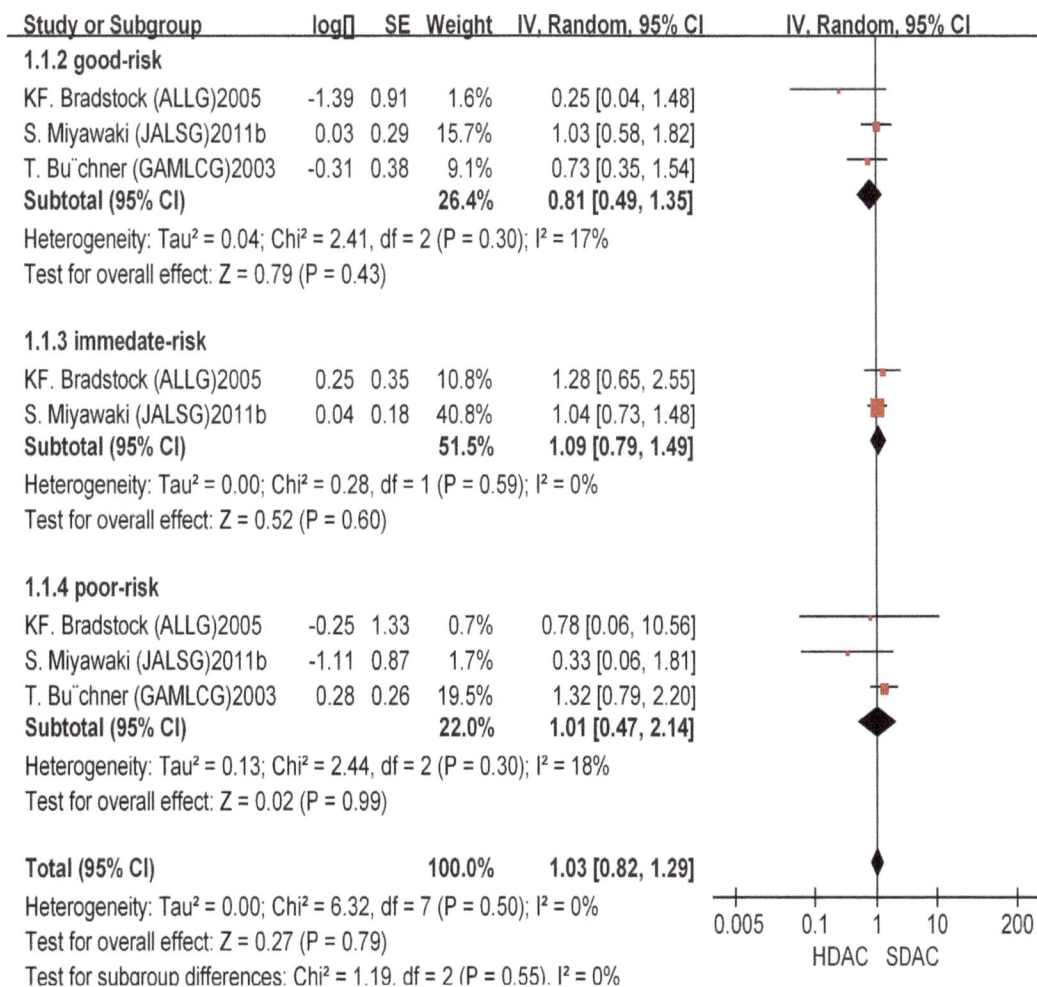

Study or Subgroup	log[]	SE	Weight	IV, Random, 95% CI
1.1.2 good-risk				
KF. Bradstock (ALLG)2005	-1.39	0.91	1.6%	0.25 [0.04, 1.48]
S. Miyawaki (JALSG)2011b	0.03	0.29	15.7%	1.03 [0.58, 1.82]
T. Bu¨chner (GAMLCG)2003	-0.31	0.38	9.1%	0.73 [0.35, 1.54]
Subtotal (95% CI)			**26.4%**	**0.81 [0.49, 1.35]**

Heterogeneity: Tau² = 0.04; Chi² = 2.41, df = 2 (P = 0.30); I² = 17%
Test for overall effect: Z = 0.79 (P = 0.43)

1.1.3 immedate-risk				
KF. Bradstock (ALLG)2005	0.25	0.35	10.8%	1.28 [0.65, 2.55]
S. Miyawaki (JALSG)2011b	0.04	0.18	40.8%	1.04 [0.73, 1.48]
Subtotal (95% CI)			**51.5%**	**1.09 [0.79, 1.49]**

Heterogeneity: Tau² = 0.00; Chi² = 0.28, df = 1 (P = 0.59); I² = 0%
Test for overall effect: Z = 0.52 (P = 0.60)

1.1.4 poor-risk				
KF. Bradstock (ALLG)2005	-0.25	1.33	0.7%	0.78 [0.06, 10.56]
S. Miyawaki (JALSG)2011b	-1.11	0.87	1.7%	0.33 [0.06, 1.81]
T. Bu¨chner (GAMLCG)2003	0.28	0.26	19.5%	1.32 [0.79, 2.20]
Subtotal (95% CI)			**22.0%**	**1.01 [0.47, 2.14]**

Heterogeneity: Tau² = 0.13; Chi² = 2.44, df = 2 (P = 0.30); I² = 18%
Test for overall effect: Z = 0.02 (P = 0.99)

Total (95% CI)			**100.0%**	**1.03 [0.82, 1.29]**

Heterogeneity: Tau² = 0.00; Chi² = 6.32, df = 7 (P = 0.50); I² = 0%
Test for overall effect: Z = 0.27 (P = 0.79)
Test for subgroup differences: Chi² = 1.19, df = 2 (P = 0.55), I² = 0%

Figure 3. Overall survival benefit of HDAC in consolidation therapy. A: Total overall survival benefit of HDAC in consolidation therapy. **B**: Overall survival benefit of different subgroups of HDAC in consolidation therapy.

A

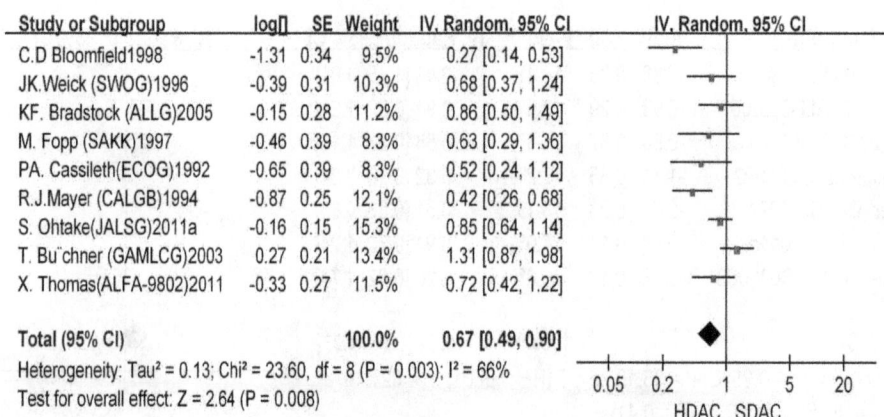

B

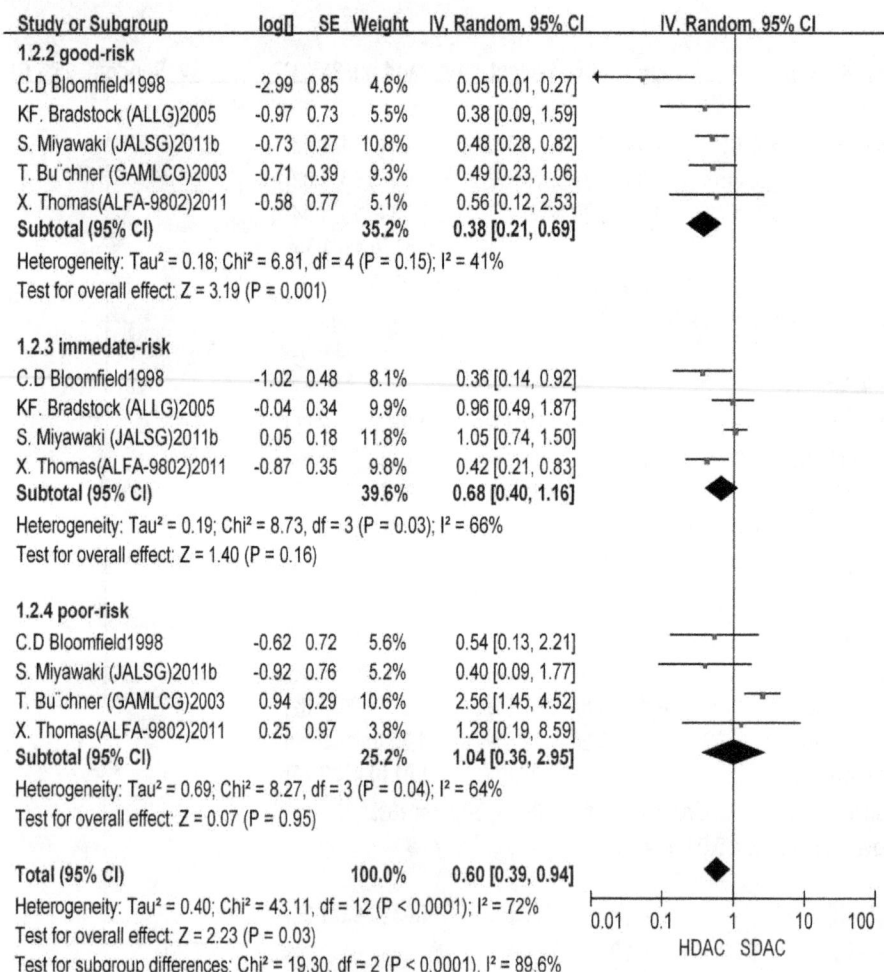

Figure 4. Relapse free survival benefit of HDAC in consolidation therapy. A: Total relapse free survival benefit of HDAC in consolidation therapy. **B**: Relapse free survival benefit of different subgroups of HDAC in consolidation therapy.

OS and RFS. The 4-year OS rate in the HDAC group ranged from 32%–71%. No significant differences in OS were observed between the HDAC and SDAC groups (HR = 0.84; 95% CI, 0.55–1.27; P = 0.41) [Figure 3]. However, patients that used

HDAC in consolidation therapy showed longer RFS than those used SDAC (HR = 0.67; 95% CI, 0.49–0.9; P = 0.008) [Figure 4]. Therefore, HDAC improved RFS but did not affect OS in consolidation therapy.

Study or Subgroup	log[Risk Ratio]	SE	Weight	Risk Ratio IV, Fixed, 95% CI	Risk Ratio IV, Fixed, 95% CI
4.1.1 HDAC/auto-BMT					
A.M.Tsimberidu2003	0.45	0.69	1.9%	1.57 [0.41, 6.06]	
JL. Harousseau 1997	-0.21	0.31	9.5%	0.81 [0.44, 1.49]	
PA. Cassileth 1998	-0.33	0.26	13.6%	0.72 [0.43, 1.20]	
RA.Zittoun(GIMEMA)1995	0.25	0.26	13.6%	1.28 [0.77, 2.14]	
S. Brunet 2004	-0.65	0.47	4.1%	0.52 [0.21, 1.31]	
Subtotal (95% CI)			**42.7%**	**0.89 [0.67, 1.19]**	
Heterogeneity: Chi² = 4.71, df = 4 (P = 0.32); I² = 15%					
Test for overall effect: Z = 0.79 (P = 0.43)					
4.1.2 HDAC/allo-BMT					
A.M.Tsimberidu2003	1.14	0.78	1.5%	3.13 [0.68, 14.42]	
GJ. Schiller1992	-0.29	0.47	4.1%	0.75 [0.30, 1.88]	
JL. Harousseau 1997	0.02	0.28	11.7%	1.02 [0.59, 1.77]	
PA. Cassileth 1998	-0.25	0.26	13.6%	0.78 [0.47, 1.30]	
PA. Cassileth(ECOG)1992	0	0.35	7.5%	1.00 [0.50, 1.99]	
RA.Zittoun(GIMEMA)1995	0.37	0.24	15.9%	1.45 [0.90, 2.32]	
S. Brunet 2004	-0.82	0.55	3.0%	0.44 [0.15, 1.29]	
Subtotal (95% CI)			**57.3%**	**1.01 [0.79, 1.30]**	
Heterogeneity: Chi² = 8.03, df = 6 (P = 0.24); I² = 25%					
Test for overall effect: Z = 0.11 (P = 0.92)					
Total (95% CI)			**100.0%**	**0.96 [0.80, 1.16]**	
Heterogeneity: Chi² = 13.19, df = 11 (P = 0.28); I² = 17%					
Test for overall effect: Z = 0.43 (P = 0.66)					
Test for subgroup differences: Chi² = 0.44, df = 1 (P = 0.51), I² = 0%					

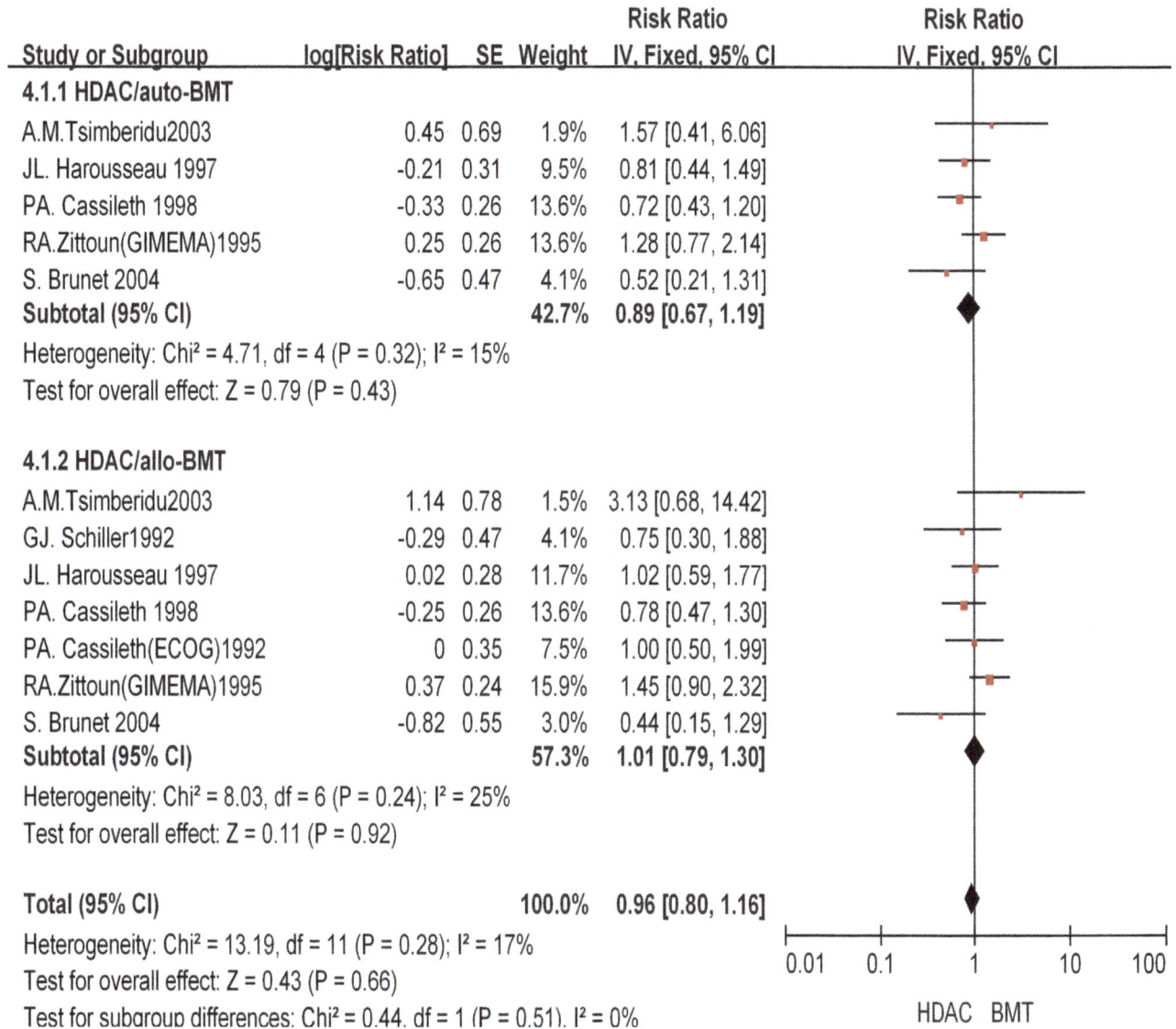

Figure 5. Effect of HDAC versus BMT on overall survival.

We further performed stratified analysis for different subgroups. We restricted the stratification for cytogenetic risk (SWOG/ECOG, NCCN, and MRC) (Table S1). Five trials were included in the stratified analysis. A significant RFS benefit was observed with HDAC treatment (HR = 0.38; 95% CI, 0.21–0.69; P = 0.001) in the favorable-risk group [Figure 4]. However, no significant RFS benefit was shown with HDAC treatment in the immediate-risk and poor-risk groups (HR = 0.68; 95% CI, 0.4–1.16; P = 0.16; HR = 1.04; 95% CI, 0.36–2.95; P = 0.95). On the contrary, HDAC did not show any significant effects on OS as compared to SDAC. The OS with HDAC was not significantly different from that with SDAC treatment in all 3 stratified risk groups (HR = 0.81; 95% CI, 0.49–1.35; P = 0.43; HR = 1.09; 95% CI, 0.79–1.49; P = 0.6; HR = 1.01; 95% CI, 0.47–2.14; P = 0.99) [Figure 3].

HDAC versus BMT in consolidation therapy

Nine trials containing the comparison of the effect of HDAC treatment with that of auto-SCT/all-BMT were included in the analysis. They included 5 randomized trials and 4 observational trials. Randomized trials were defined as those in which patients who did not have donors would be randomly allocated into the HDAC and auto-SCT groups. Only 2 trials were multicentre trials. End points of OS and RFS were reported across all cytogenetic risk groups in all 9 trials, so we were not able to perform stratified analysis for different cytogenetic risk groups when evaluating OS and RFS outcomes. A total of 3,128 *de novo* AML patients enrolled from 1986 to 2000 were included. The longest follow-up period of each trial was 8.5 years [Table 2]. Of them, 29.8% patients received auto-SCT; 30.8% received allo-BMT; and 39.4% received HDAC. No imbalance in preparative regimen was observed between trials. The data were highly homogeneous in different studies concerning RFS endpoint (I² = 0%). Only patients younger than 65 year-old were enrolled in the analysis considering the risk of transplantation.

This analysis revealed that the combined HR was 0.89 (95% CI, 0.67–1.19; P = 0.43), 1.01 (95% CI, 0.79–1.3; P = 0.92), and that patients received HDAC had an OS similar to that of patients received auto-SCT/allo-BMT in consolidation therapy [Figure 5].

Study or Subgroup	log[Risk Ratio]	SE	Weight	Risk Ratio IV, Random, 95% CI	Risk Ratio IV, Random, 95% CI
5.2.1 HDAC/auto-BMT					
A.M.Tsimberidu2003	0.37	0.72	2.7%	1.45 [0.35, 5.94]	
JL. Harousseau 1997	0.18	0.32	8.8%	1.20 [0.64, 2.24]	
PA. Cassileth 1998	0.5	0.27	10.5%	1.65 [0.97, 2.80]	
R.Bassan 1998	-0.02	0.51	4.8%	0.98 [0.36, 2.66]	
RA.Zittoun(GIMEMA)1995	0.59	0.26	10.9%	1.80 [1.08, 3.00]	
S. Brunet 2004	-0.29	0.47	5.4%	0.75 [0.30, 1.88]	
Subtotal (95% CI)			**43.1%**	**1.41 [1.06, 1.87]**	

Heterogeneity: Tau² = 0.00; Chi² = 3.82, df = 5 (P = 0.58); I² = 0%
Test for overall effect: Z = 2.39 (P = 0.02)

5.2.2 HDAC/allo-BMT					
A.M.Tsimberidu2003	1.7	0.8	2.2%	5.47 [1.14, 26.26]	
GJ. Schiller1992	0.31	0.47	5.4%	1.36 [0.54, 3.43]	
J.L. Harousseau 1991	0.03	0.57	4.0%	1.03 [0.34, 3.15]	
JL. Harousseau 1997	0.22	0.28	10.2%	1.25 [0.72, 2.16]	
PA. Cassileth 1998	1.32	0.28	10.2%	3.74 [2.16, 6.48]	
PA. Cassileth(ECOG)1992	0.55	0.36	7.7%	1.73 [0.86, 3.51]	
R.Bassan 1998	1.63	1.15	1.2%	5.10 [0.54, 48.62]	
RA.Zittoun(GIMEMA)1995	0.92	0.24	11.7%	2.51 [1.57, 4.02]	
S. Brunet 2004	0.03	0.54	4.4%	1.03 [0.36, 2.97]	
Subtotal (95% CI)			**56.9%**	**1.95 [1.35, 2.81]**	

Heterogeneity: Tau² = 0.13; Chi² = 14.68, df = 8 (P = 0.07); I² = 45%
Test for overall effect: Z = 3.56 (P = 0.0004)

Total (95% CI)			**100.0%**	**1.66 [1.30, 2.14]**	

Heterogeneity: Tau² = 0.08; Chi² = 22.20, df = 14 (P = 0.07); I² = 37%
Test for overall effect: Z = 4.00 (P < 0.0001)
Test for subgroup differences: Chi² = 3.70, df = 1 (P = 0.05), I² = 73.0%

0.01   0.1   1   10   100

HDAC   BMT

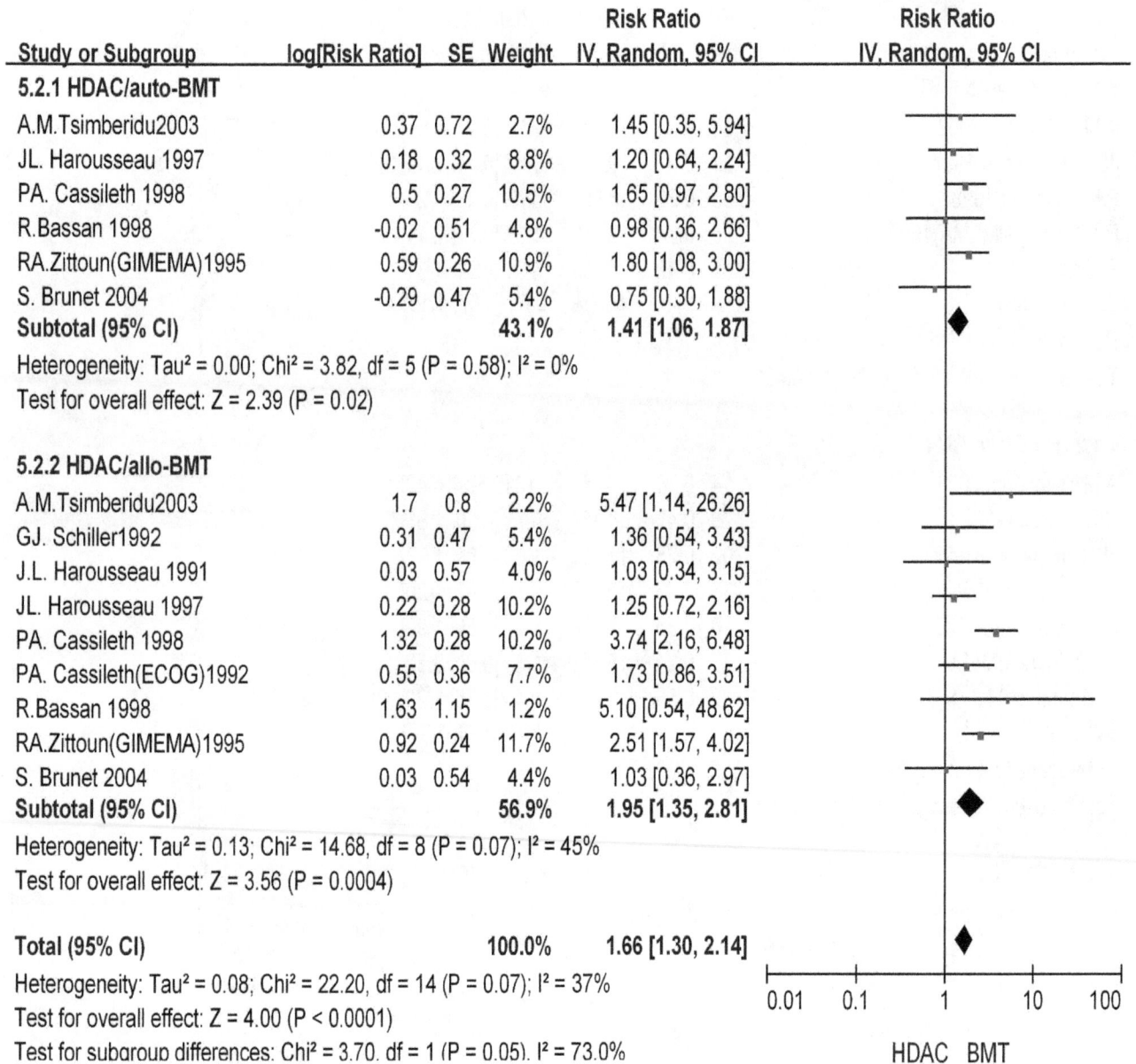

Figure 6. Effect of HDAC versus BMT on relapse free survival.

On the other hand, the RFS was significantly different between the auto-SCT/allo-BMT group and the HDAC group [Figure 6]. Auto-SCT had a combined HR of 1.41 (95% CI, 1.06–1.87; $P = 0.02$), while allo-BMT had a combined HR of 1.95 (95% CI, 1.35–2.81; $P = 0.0004$), indicating a significant RFS benefit of auto-SCT/allo-BMT over HDAC. Overall, the results indicated that auto-SCT/allo-BMT significantly reduced the hazard rate of relapse but failed to improve overall survival.

Discussion

In the past 20 years, Ara-C has been widely used in the induction and consolidation therapy for AML. Multiple prospective studies on Ara-C have been reported, and the application of HDAC has been tested extensively beyond first-line therapy and is considered a standard therapy. However, HDAC started to be questioned in recent studies with larger patient numbers. In this study, we performed a meta-analysis to address whether HDAC application in the induction and consolidation therapy prolongs RFS and decreases AML recurrence comparing with SDAC.

In a recent meta-analysis, 3 trials were analyzed, which discovered no differences in CR rates between HDAC and SDAC treatments. HDAC in induction therapy improved long-term disease control and OS in adults <60 years of age with *de novo* AML [29]. However, the effect of HDAC remains unclear in consolidation therapy, especially that for patients younger than 60 years. Therefore, we systematically collected all trials that used HDAC in both induction therapy and consolidation therapy from Jan. 1990 to Mar. 2013. The regimen of induction and consolidation therapy was restricted, which led to the exclusion of 20 articles containing different regimens of induction and consolidation therapy in HDAC and SDAC groups. All trials we identified were reported on an intent-to-treat basis and included a complete description of withdrawals and drop-outs. Some degrees of heterogeneity still existed in the age inclusion criterion. In one article, patients older than 60 years of age were not analyzed separately from patients younger than 60 years. However, this article was still included because the proportion of patients older than 60 years was very low. Based on the current data, we cannot conclude whether HDAC has the same effects on older patients. The dose of HDAC has also been questioned. In HOVON/SAKK study [30], Ara-C was used at 1.0 g/m^2 q12 h×6 days. In this meta-analysis, we limited HDAC at the dose level of 2.0–3.0 g/m^2 q12 h×3–5 days for the majority of trials.

Overall, endpoint heterogeneity within trials was limited. No evidence was found to support the notion that HDAC improves CR rate as compared to SDAC in induction therapy. However, our analysis revealed that HDAC had a clear benefit on RFS in induction therapy, consistent to the findings from ALSG and CAMLCG [8,10]. A retrospective analysis of CALGB and ECOG studies [14,15,31] discovered a survival advantage of HDAC in consolidation therapy over SDAC. However, our analysis failed to reach this conclusion. Data from the risk group stratified analysis demonstrated that HDAC significantly improved RFS in the favorable-risk group but no significant benefits in the intermediate and poor-risk groups. We also discussed the advantage of using BMT in consolidation therapy and discovered that auto-BMT/allo-BMT improved RFS, but not OS, as compared to HDAC.

In conclusion, this meta-analysis demonstrated that HDAC improved RFS in induction therapy while reducing the relapse rate in consolidation therapy, as compared with SDAC, especially for the favorable-risk group. Auto-BMT/Allo-BMT had a more beneficial effect in prolonging RFS as compared with HDAC. The analysis also posed some challenges to previous trial results. Overall, treatment with HDAC regimen did show some advantages for some outcome endpoints, especially in certain risk groups. However, it failed to show predominant advantages in all cases. Considering its high toxicity, caution should be taken when HDAC treatment regimen is chosen for patients. We also discovered varied degrees of heterogeneity within trials in our meta-analysis, which may interfere with the interpretation of results and limit the validity of the findings. In the future, more comprehensive clinical trails with improved study designs are needed to help elucidate the advantages and drawbacks of each treatment regimen in order to identify the optimal dose and treatment schedule for AML patients.

Supporting Information

Checklist S1 PRISMA Checklist.

Figure S1 Risk of bias graphs of Randomized Control Trials.

Table S1 Risk status based on validated cytogenetics.

Acknowledgments

We thank Professor Taixiang Wu (Head of Chinese Clinical Trial Registry; Head of Research Manager. e-mail: txwutx@hotmail.com) for his technical support and careful reading.

Author Contributions

Conceived and designed the experiments: JW. Performed the experiments: WL XG. Analyzed the data: MS XZ. Contributed reagents/materials/analysis tools: BG. Contributed to the writing of the manuscript: YM HW.

References

1. Löwenberg B, Downing JR, Burnett A (1999) Acute myeloid leukemia. N Engl J Med. 341(14): 1051–1062.
2. Bishop JF, Matthews JP, Young GA, Szer J, Gillett A, et al. (1996) A randomized study of high-dose cytarabine in induction in acute myeloid leukemia. Blood. 87: 1710–1717.
3. Moore JO, George SL, Dodge RK, Amrein PC, Powell BL, et al. (2005) Sequential multiagent chemo- therapy is not superior to high-dose cytarabine alone as postremission intensification therapy for acute myeloid leukemia in adults under 60 years of age: Cancer and Leukemia Group B Study 9222. Blood. 105(9): 3420–7.
4. Miyawaki S, Ohtake S, Fujisawa S, Kivoi H, Shinaqawak K, et al. (2011) A randomized comparison of 4 courses of standard-dose multiagent chemotherapy versus 3 courses of high-dose cytarabine alone in post remission therapy for acute myeloid leukemia in adults: the JALSG AML201 Study. Blood. 117(8): 2366–72.
5. Löwenberg B (2013) Sense and nonsense of high-dose cytarabine for acute myeloid leukemia. Blood. 121(1): 26–28.
6. Parmar MK, Torri V, Stewart L (1998) Extracting summary statistics to perform meta-analyses of the published literature for survival endpoints. Stat Med. 17(24): 2815–2834.
7. Matthews JP, Bishop JF, Young GA, Juneia SK, Lowenthal RM, et al. (2001) Patterns of failure with increasing intensification of induction chemotherapy for acute myeloid leukaemia. Br J Haematol. 113(3): 727–36.
8. Weick JK, Kopecky KJ, Appelbaum FR, Head DR, Kingsbury LL, et al. (1996) A randomized investig- ation of high-dose versus standard-dose cytosine arabinoside with daunorubicin inpatients with previously untreated acute myeloid leukemia: a Southwest Oncology Group study. Blood. 88(8): 2841–51.
9. Büchner T, Berdel WE, Schoch C, Haferlach T, Serve HL, et al. (2006) Double induction containing either two courses or one course of high–dose cytarabine plus mitoxantrone and post remission therapy by either autologous stem-cell transplantation or by prolonged maintenance for acute myeloid leukemia. J Clin Oncol. 24(16): 2480–9.
10. Büchner T, Hiddemann W, Wörmann B, Löffler H, Gassmann W, et al. (1999) Double induction strategy for acute myeloid leukemia: the effect of high-dose cytarabine with mitoxantrone instead of standard-dose cytarabine with daunorubicin and 6-thioguanine: a randomized trial by the German AML Cooperative Group. Blood. 15; 93(12): 4116–24.
11. Büchner T, Berdel WE, Haferlach C, Haferlach T, Schnittger S, et al. (2009) Age-related risk profile and chemotherapy dose response in acute myeloid leukemia: a study by the German Acute Mye- loid Leukemia Coo-perative Group. J Clin Oncol. 27(1): 61–9.
12. Bradstock KF, Matthews JP, Lowenthal RM, Baxter H, Catalano J, et al. (2005) A randomized trial of high-versus conventional-dose cytarabine in consolidation chemotherapy for adult de novo acute myeloid leukemia in first remission after induction therapy containing high-dose cytarabine. Blood. 105(2): 481–8.
13. Fopp M, Fey MF, Bacchi M, Cavalli F, Gmuer J, et al. (1997) Post-remission therapy of adult acute myeloid leukaemia: one cycle of high-dose versus standard-dose cytarabine. Leukaemia Project Group of the Swiss Group for Clinical Cancer Research (SAKK). Ann Oncol. 8(3): 251–7.
14. Cassileth PA, Lynch E, Hines JD, Oken MM, Mazza JJ, et al. (1992) Varying intensity of post- remission therapy in acute myeloid leukemia. Blood. 79(8): 1924–30.
15. Mayer RJ, Davis RB, Schiffer CA, Berq DT, Powell BL, et al. (1994) Intensive postremission chemotherapy in adults with acute myeloid leukemia. Cancer and Leukemia Group B. N Engl J Med. 331(14): 896–903.
16. Ohtake S, Miyawaki S, Fujita H, Kiyoi H, Shinaqawa K, et al. (2011) Randomized study of induction therapy comparing standard-dose idarubicin with high-dose daunorubin in adult patients with previously untreated acute myeloid leukemia: the JALSG AML201 Study. Blood. 117(8): 2358–65.
17. Büchner T, Hiddemann W, Berdel WE, Wörmann B, Schoch C, et al. (2003) 6-Thioguanine, cytarabine, and daunorubicin (TAD) and high–dose cytarabine and mitoxantrone (HAM) for induction, TAD for consolidation, and either prolonged maintenance by reduced monthly TAD or TAD-HAM-TAD and one course of intensive consolidation by sequential HAM in adult patients at all ages with de novo acute myeloid leukemia (AML): a randomized trial of the German AML Cooperative Group. J Clin Oncol. 21(24): 4496–504.
18. Schoch C, Haferlach T, Haase D, Fonatsch C, Löffler H, et al. (2001) Patients with de novo acute myeloid leukaemia and complex karyotype aberrations show a poor prognosis despite intensive treatment: a study of 90 patients. Br J Haematol. 112(1): 118–26.
19. Bloomfield CD, Lawrence D, Byrd JC, Carroll A, Pettenati MJ, et al. (1998) frequency of prolonged remission duration after high-dose cytarabine intensi- fication in acute myeloid leukemia varies by cytogenetic subtype. Cancer Res. Sep 15; 58(18): 4173–9.
20. Thomas X, Elhamri M, Raffoux E, Renneville A, Pautas C, et al. (2011) Comparison of high-dose cytarabine and timed-sequential chemotherapy as consolidation for younger adults with AML in first remission: the ALFA-9802 study. Blood. 118(7): 1754–1762.

21. Tsimberidu AM, Stavroyianni N, Viniou N, Papaioannou M, Tiniakou M, et al. (2003) Comparison of Allogeneic Stem Cell Transplantation, High-Dose Cytarabine, and Autologous Peripheral Stem Cell Transplantation as Post-remission Treatment in Patients with De Novo Acute Myelogenous Leukemia. Cancer. 97(7): 1721–1731.

22. Harousseau JL, Cahn JY, Pignon B, Witz F, Milpied N, et al. (1997) Chemotherapy as Postremission Therapy in Adult Acute Myeloid Leukemia Comparison of Autologous Bone Marrow Transplant- ation and Intensive. Blood. 90(8): 2978–2986.

23. Cassileth PA, Arington DP, Appelbaum FR, Lazarus HM, Rowe JM, et al. (1998) Chemotherapy compared with autologous or allogeneic bone marrow transplantation in the management of acute myeloid leukemia in first remission. N Engl J Med. 339: 1649–56.

24. Zittoun RA, Mandelli F, Willemze R, de Witte T, Labar B, et al. (1995) autologous or allogeneic bone marrow transplantion compared with intensive chemotherapy in acute myelogenous leukemia. N Engl J Med. 332: 217–23.

25. Brunet S, Esteve J, Berlanga J, Ribera JM, Bueno J, et al. (2004) Treatment of primary acute myeloid leukemia: results of a prospective multicenter trial including high-dose cytarabine or stem cell transplantation as post-remission strategy. Haematologica. 89: 940–949.

26. Bassan R, Raimondi R, Lerede T, D'emilio A, Buelli M, et al. (1998) Outcome assessment of age group-specific (±50 years) post-remission consolidation with high-dose cytarabine or bone marrow autograft for adult acute myelogenous leukemia. Haematologica. 83: 627–635.

27. Schiller GJ, Nimer SD, Territo MC, Ho WG, Champlin RE, et al. (1992) Bone Marrow Transplant- ation Versus High-Dose Cytarabine-based consolidation chemotherapy for acute myelogenous leukemia in First Remission. J Clin Oncol. 10(1): 41–46.

28. Harousseau JL, Milpied N, Briere J, Desablens B, Leprise PY, et al. (1991) Double Intensive Consolid -ation Chemotherapy in Adult Acute Myeloid Leukemia. J Clin Oncol. 9: 1432–1437.

29. Kern W, Estey EH (2006) High-dose cytosine arabinoside in the treatment of acute myeloid leukemia. Cancer. 107: 116–24.

30. Löwenberg B, Pabst T, Vellenga E, van Putten W, Schouten HC, et al. (2011) Cytarabine dose for acute myeloid leukemia. N Engl J Med. 364: 1027–1036.

31. Farag SS, Ruppert AS, Mrózek K, Mayer RJ, Stone RM, et al. (2005) Outcome of induction and postremission therapy in younger adults with acute myeloid leukemia with normal karyotype: a cancer and leukemia group B study. J Clin Oncol. 23(3): 482–93.

14

Lifespan Based Pharmacokinetic-Pharmacodynamic Model of Tumor Growth Inhibition by Anticancer Therapeutics

Gary Mo[1,2], Frank Gibbons[2], Patricia Schroeder[2], Wojciech Krzyzanski[1]*

1 Department of Pharmaceutical Sciences, University at Buffalo, Buffalo, New York, United States of America, 2 DMPK Modeling and Simulation, Oncology, iMED, AstraZeneca, Waltham, Massachusetts, United States of America

Abstract

Accurate prediction of tumor growth is critical in modeling the effects of anti-tumor agents. Popular models of tumor growth inhibition (TGI) generally offer empirical description of tumor growth. We propose a lifespan-based tumor growth inhibition (LS TGI) model that describes tumor growth in a xenograft mouse model, on the basis of cellular lifespan T. At the end of the lifespan, cells divide, and to account for tumor burden on growth, we introduce a cell division efficiency function that is negatively affected by tumor size. The LS TGI model capability to describe dynamic growth characteristics is similar to many empirical TGI models. Our model describes anti-cancer drug effect as a dose-dependent shift of proliferating tumor cells into a non-proliferating population that die after an altered lifespan T_A. Sensitivity analysis indicated that all model parameters are identifiable. The model was validated through case studies of xenograft mouse tumor growth. Data from paclitaxel mediated tumor inhibition was well described by the LS TGI model, and model parameters were estimated with high precision. A study involving a protein casein kinase 2 inhibitor, AZ968, contained tumor growth data that only exhibited linear growth kinetics. The LS TGI model accurately described the linear growth data and estimated the potency of AZ968 that was very similar to the estimate from an established TGI model. In the case study of AZD1208, a pan-Pim inhibitor, the doubling time was not estimable from the control data. By fixing the parameter to the reported *in vitro* value of the tumor cell doubling time, the model was still able to fit the data well and estimated the remaining parameters with high precision. We have developed a mechanistic model that describes tumor growth based on cell division and has the flexibility to describe tumor data with diverse growth kinetics.

Editor: Aamir Ahmad, Wayne State University School of Medicine, United States of America

Funding: This work is supported by a fellowship from AstraZeneca MBDDx Predictive Science Programme and National Institutes of Health grant GM57980. The funders had no role in study design, data collection and analysis, decision to publish, or preparation of the manuscript.

* Email: wk@buffalo.edu

Introduction

The integration of pharmacokinetic and pharmacodynamic (PK/PD) modeling in drug development has greatly improved the efficacy and safety of anti-cancer treatments. PK/PD models have allowed for better dose selection and optimized clinical trial designs. Recent efforts have demonstrated the benefits of applying PK/PD modeling in early stages of drug development. Advancement in PK/PD modeling, specifically the progression of PK/PD modeling from empirical to more mechanistic approaches have greatly increased the predictive power of models [1].

Empirical models are attractive because of their simplicity and parsimony, and for early compound screening based on specific criteria, they are very practical. The major drawback of empirical models is their reliance on drug-specific, rather than system-specific, parameters. Translation to higher species is expected to be challenging without knowledge of the biological system, since one would not know which parameters would change in a novel species. At the opposite end of the spectrum are mechanistic models of tumor growth, which combine drug-specific parameters with system-specific parameters for numerous molecular species. Although mechanistic models offer superior prediction accuracy, they often require rich datasets on numerous biomarkers in order to identify the parameters.

All tumor-growth inhibition (TGI) models have to be able to describe two hallmark characteristics of tumor growth and growth inhibition. Because tumor growth is a dynamic process, which can have profound effects on treatment success, accurate quantitative description of tumor growth is critical [2]. The unrestricted growth of solid tumors have been described using various mathematical functions (see [3,4] for review). The onset of chemotherapeutic effect, namely inhibition of growth or reduction of tumor size, is often delayed [5–7]. This disconnect between the drug pharmacokinetics and the efficacy time course has been addressed in several TGI models [8–11]. Many mechanistic TGI models based on the integration of biological systems, both in tumor growth and anti-cancer treatment, have been developed [12–14]. These complex models offer great predictive potential, but all require additional biomarkers beside just tumor growth data.

The model developed by Simeoni and colleagues is described as a semi-mechanistic approach for modeling TGI [11]. The model is widely used in preclinical development due to its simplicity and features relevant to the biology of anti-cancer treatment. The model is able to capture both the complex growth kinetics and the temporal delay in tumor growth inhibition. However, the model still relies on empirical description of tumor growth, and offers no relevance to biological mechanisms that mediate growth of tumor cells.

The aim of this study is to develop a mechanistic TGI model that describes tumor growth through the process of cell division using the lifespan approach. Lifespan models are ideal for describing systems that have a finite duration, such as population of cells [15]. Drug-induced perturbation of biological systems is also well described using lifespan models [16,17]. In our lifespan TGI model, the use of delay differential equations, which are developed to characterize delays in dynamic systems, offer a natural way of describing the delay in anti-cancer effect of drug treatment as have been previously reported [9]. Furthermore, using the lifespan approach to account for cellular division allows us to describe cell-cycle specific chemotherapeutics in a novel way.

In the following sections, we first review data collection, both *in vivo* and from literature. We introduce the lifespan concept, along with a cell-division efficiency parameter p, which will be central to our analysis. We describe a model of unperturbed tumor growth that is dependent on tumor size. We then extend this to perturbed tumor growth, with different drug mechanism of action, specifically non-cycle-specific drug effect model, and a cycle-specific model. After conducting sensitivity analysis on the models, we then apply them to three case studies of tumor growth inhibition by paclitaxel, AZ968 and AZD1208. We conclude the paper with a discussion of the results. We establish that this lifespan-based model has the versatility to describe TGI for anticancer drugs having various modes of action, and the robustness to estimate the required parameters from experimental data typical of a preclinical development program.

Materials and Methods

Literature Data Acquisition

Data used in Case Study 1 was obtained from mouse xenograft study reported by Simeoni and colleague [11]. To briefly summarize the study, mice bearing tumors derived from the HCT116 human colon carcinoma cell line were given intravenous (i.v.) injections of paclitaxel at 30 mg/kg every 4 days starting from day 8 after tumor inoculation. Data from the study was digitized using Graph Digitizer 2.0 (Nick's Production). Pharmacokinetics of paclitaxel was described using a two-compartment model outlined in the original report [11] and model parameters were fixed to $V = 0.81$ L/kg, $k_{el} = 0.868$/h, $k_{12} = 0.006$/h and $k_{21} = 0.0838$/h.

Animal Data

For Case Study 2 and 3, raw data from previous studies [18,19] were obtained from the investigators. In brief, female NCr and CD1 mice (5–6 week old) were treated with AZ968, an anti-cancer agent that was synthesized by AstraZeneca R&D (Waltham, MA). HCT116 tumor cells (6×10^6) were implanted by s.c. injection into the left flank of NCr mice. This is a human colon carcinoma line, commonly used in xenograft studies [20,21]. Animals with established tumor xenografts, determined by tumor size reaching ~150–200 mm³, were randomized and treated once daily with either vehicle (0.5% HPMC) or AZ968 by intraperitoneal (i.p.) injection with 10 to 15 mice per treatment group. Tumor volume

was measured with calipers and calculated as tumor volume = (length × width²) ×0.5. Female NCr and CD1 mice.

For pharmacodynamic studies, mice with tumors of 150–200 mm³ were treated with either vehicle or AZ968, with three mice per dose. AZ968 or vehicle was administered once per week for three weeks, and AZ968 were administered at 10, 20 or 30 mg/kg. Tumor volume was assessed three times a week for three weeks with measurements taken on the day of treatment, 48 h and 120 h after treatment. For AZ968 treatment groups, an additional measurement was taken on 216 h after the last dose administration.

For pharmacokinetic study of AZ968, CD1 mice were given single i.p. injection of AZ968 at 10, 20 or 30 mg/kg with 3 mice per dose group. Blood samples were collected via cardiac puncture. Total plasma concentrations of AZ968 were determined by LC/MS/MS method. Same procedure was used for the pharmacokinetic study of AZD1208, except AZD1208 was administered orally (p.o.) at 3, 10 or 30 mg/kg doses as outlined in the original study [18].

Model Development

Unperturbed tumor growth model. The schematic of the unperturbed tumor growth model is presented in Figure 1A. Lifespan models are similar to the widely used indirect response model [22] in that changes in the biological response of interest are governed by production and elimination [23]. In developing a lifespan formulation of tumor growth, we made the following assumptions: 1) Tumor size is controlled by two processes: production and elimination. 2) Each tumor cell has a lifespan T. When this time has elapsed, the cell divides in two, thus T is the tumor doubling time. 3) For simplicity, we assume all cells are at the same point of their lifespan. 4) Production of new tumor cells is exclusively due to division of existing cells. Under assumption (1), the net change in size is described by the following differential equation:

$$\frac{dw}{dt} = k_{in}(t) - k_{out}(t) \tag{eq.1}$$

where $k_{in}(t)$ and $k_{out}(t)$ are production and elimination rates, respectively. Under assumptions (2) and (3), the daughter cells produced from cell division become tumor cells and contribute to the growth of the tumor. Combined, these assumptions indicate that the lifespan of the tumor cells can be used to determine the elimination rate $k_{out}(t)$ from the production rate $k_{in}(t)$ using the following relationship [15]:

$$k_{out}(t) = k_{in}(t - T) \tag{eq.2}$$

We assume that the production of new tumor cells is exclusively due to division of the cells. This allows us to propose the concept that changes in tumor growth rate with increasing tumor size is a result of changes in cell division efficiency, which results from a decrease in accessible nutrients as previously suggested [24]. In our model we incorporate division efficiency using the relationship:

$$k_{in}(t) = p \cdot k_{out}(t) \tag{eq.3}$$

The dimensionless parameter p is the efficiency of cell division i.e., the number of cells that actually become new tumor cells. To

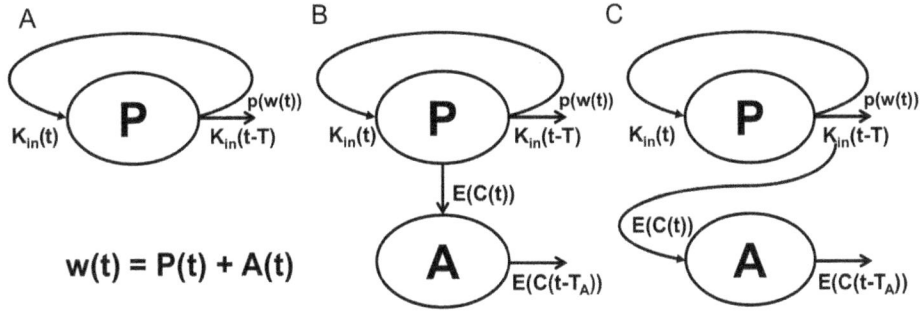

Figure 1. Model Schematics. A) Unperturbed tumor growth, B) Non-cycle-specific perturbed tumor growth, and C) Cycle-specific perturbed tumor growth. The meanings of the symbols and variables are explained in the model development section.

ensure the tumor continues to grow p should not be less than 1, and under normal cytokinesis it cannot be greater than 2. Therefore, the division efficiency parameter is constrained by $1 \leq p \leq 2$. This division efficiency parameter is central to our analysis and facilitates our theory that the tumor size impacts the efficiency of the division, and that tumor size limits growth by decreasing the efficiency of division of the tumor cells. Consequently, p must be a function that decreases with respect to tumor weight, w:

$$p = p(w) \qquad \text{(eq.4)}$$

Finally, we assume that the model (eq. 1) applies for times $t>0$, where time $t = 0$ can be arbitrarily chosen to mark the beginning of the experiment, data collection, or treatment initiation. Since the full description of $k_{out}(t)$ requires knowledge of $k_{in}(t)$ for times $-T < t \leq 0$, we assume that the doubling time T is relatively small compared to the duration of the experiment design, and consequently the tumor production rate is relatively constant over the $-T < t \leq 0$ time interval:

$$k_{in}(t) = k_{in0},$$
$$\text{for } -T < t \leq 0 \qquad \text{(eq.5)}$$

Based on the relationships outlined by eq. 2 and eq. 4, it is necessary to describe $k_{in}(t)$ using a recursive definition:

$$k_{in}(t) = p(w(t)) \cdot k_{in}(t - T) \qquad \text{(eq.6)}$$

The derivation of the recursive form of $k_{in}(t)$ is discussed in Appendix S1, and $k_{in}(t)$ can now be presented as:

$$k_{in}(t) = k_{in0} \cdot \prod_{i=0}^{INT(t/T)} p(w(t - iT)) \qquad \text{(eq.7)}$$

where $INT(x)$ denotes the biggest integer such that $INT(x) \leq x$. Please note that according to eq. 7, the number of delays is determined by the ratio $INT(t_{last}/T)$, where t_{last} is the last observation point or end of the time interval where the model

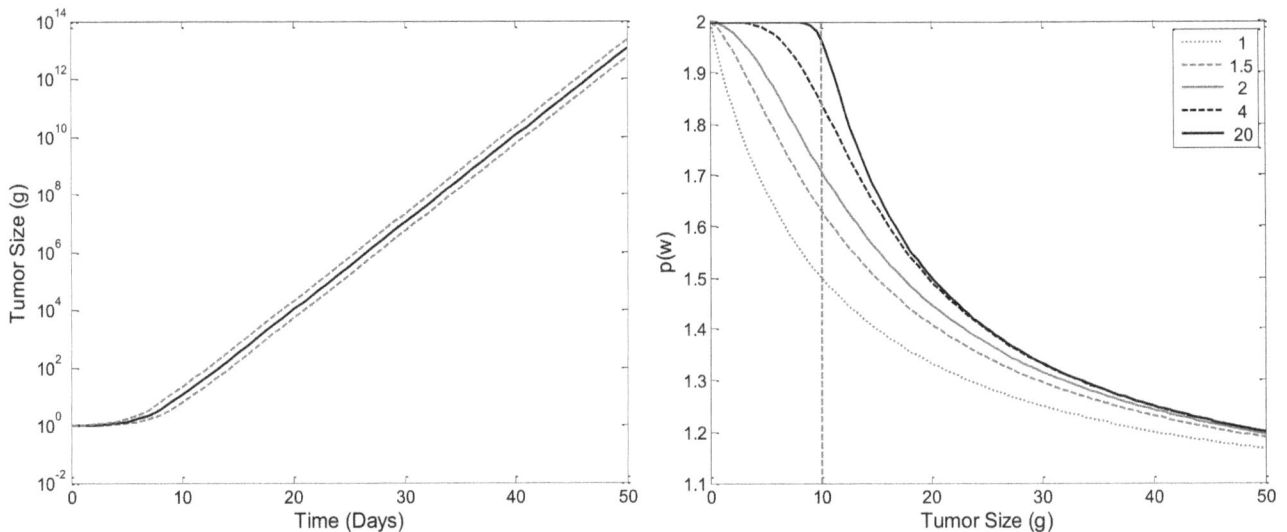

Figure 2. Simulated Effect of Division Efficiency on Tumor Growth. A) Semi-log plot of tumor growth with constant division efficiency of $p_0 = 2$. Upper and lower dashed lines indicate upper and lower bound described by eq. 12. B) Simulation of cell division efficiency function, $p(w)$, vs tumor weight, w, for different values of ψ. The threshold, w_{th}, was set to 10 g, and initial efficiency, p_0 is set to 2.

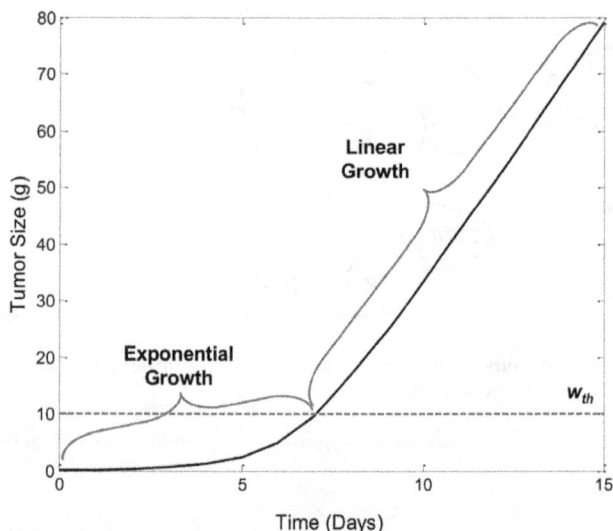

Figure 3. Simulation Tumor Growth Profile of TGI Lifespan Model. Plot of tumor weight vs. time. The threshold, w_{th}, which is set to 10 g, is indicated by the dashed line. Doubling time of the tumor cells, T, was set to 1 day, k_{in0} was set to 0.05 g/day and p_0 is set to 2.

applies. By combining the relationship outlined by eq. 7, eq. 2, and eq. 1 our model for unrestricted tumor growth can now be presented as:

$$\frac{dw}{dt} = \frac{k_{in0}(p(w(t))-1)}{p(w(t))} \cdot \prod_{i=0}^{INT(t/T)} p(w(t-iT)), \quad (eq.8)$$

for $t>0$

To solve this equation uniquely, an initial condition is required, for which we choose:

$$w(0) = w_0 \quad (eq.9)$$

where w_0 is the tumor size at time $t=0$ i.e., the start of the experiment.

Constant efficiency p. Since this is a novel mathematical recasting of the problem, we examine some simplistic scenarios, to confirm that it behaves as one would expect. First let us take the case in which cell division efficiency is *not* affected by the tumor size. Under the assumption of constant division efficiency (p(w) ≡ p_0) eq. 8 simplifies to:

$$\frac{dw}{dt} = k_{in0} \cdot (p_0-1) p_0^{INT(t/T)}, \quad (eq.10)$$

for t > 0

which can be solved explicitly (see Appendix S2):

$$w(t) = w_0 + k_{in0} \cdot T \cdot$$

$$\left(p_0^{INT(t/T)} - 1 + (p_0-1) \cdot p_0^{INT(t/T)} \cdot (t/T - INT(t/T)) \right), \quad (eq.11)$$

for t > 0

Since $0 \le t/T - INT(t/T) < 1$ one can obtain the lower and upper bounds for the solution that control the asymptotic behavior for large times:

$$w_0 + k_{in0} \cdot T \cdot (p_0^{t/T-1}-1) \le w(t) \le w_0 + k_{in0} \cdot T \cdot p_0^{t/T+1} \quad (eq.12)$$

It should be noted that because of the discontinuity of the function $INT(x)$, the exact asymptotic of $w(t)$ for large t values might be difficult to obtain. However, for small lifespan T values the relationship (12) essentially says that $w(t)$ grows exponentially with time as $p_0^{t/T}$ which reinforces the interpretation of T as the time necessary to increase the tumor size by the factor p_0. In the case of constant maximum division efficiency ($p_0 = 2$), then T becomes the exact doubling time of the tumor size. Figure 2A shows an example of the tumor growth curve described by eq. 11 with the upper and lower bounds (eq. 12).

Tumor size dependent efficiency. The data on growth of tumor xenograft in mouse models suggest an inverse relationship between the tumor size and the growth rate [25]. Numerous mathematical models have been developed to account for tumor size restriction of tumor growth rate using size-dependent inhibitory functions in model equations [11,26,27]. As outlined above, our approach is based on the assumption that the major impact of tumor size on its growth is on decreasing the efficiency of cell division. Therefore the function $p(w)$ should decrease with increasing tumor weight, w. According to eq. 8, if for a specific tumor size $p(w_{ss}) = 1$, then tumor growth is stopped and w_{ss} becomes the steady state solution. Alternatively, one can consider $p(w)$ decreasing to 1 as w approaches infinity, then the steady sate is never reached which is a necessary condition of unlimited tumor growth. By design, most mouse xenograft experiments do not reach steady tumor volume, so we will focus on the later scenario. Another feature of xenograft tumor growth time course is a biphasic profile with an initial exponential growth followed by a slower linear phase [28]. The model by Simeoni and colleagues [11] addressed this phenomenon by introducing a threshold tumor size below which the tumor growth is exponential and above which it becomes linear. Similarly, we propose the following relationship between tumor size and efficiency of cell proliferation:

$$p(w) = 1 + \frac{p_0-1}{\left(1 + \left(\frac{w}{w_{th}}\right)^\psi\right)^{\frac{1}{\psi}}} \quad (eq.13)$$

where p_0 is the cell division efficiency for tumor sizes below the threshold w_{th}. The power coefficient ψ serves as a continuous representation of a switch between exponential and non-exponential tumor growth phases. As $\psi \to \infty$, then:

$$p(w) \to \begin{cases} p_0, & w < w_{th} \\ 1 + \frac{p_0-1}{w/w_{th}}, & w > w_{th} \end{cases} \quad (eq.14)$$

Simulations of $p(w)$ vs. w for a number of ψ values shown in Figure 2B demonstrate that for $\psi = 20$ the $p(w)$ function exhibits a natural switch property (eq. 14).

In Appendix S3 we show that $w(t)$ is an increasing function of time that approaches infinity as $t \to \infty$. Simulations of $w(t)$ vs. t curves imply that for $w(t)>w_{th}$, change in $w(t)$ becomes linear (Figure 3). The calculation of the slope of this line is difficult.

However, if we assume that T is small compared to other model time scales, then:

$$\frac{dw}{dt} \to \frac{(p_0 - 1) \cdot w_{th}}{T},$$

$$\text{as } t \to \infty \qquad \text{(eq.15)}$$

eq. 15 implies that the slope of the linear growth phase is proportional to p_0-1, w_{th}, and inversely proportional to T, but does not depend on k_{in0} or w_0.

If the tumor growth data exhibit only linear rate of tumor growth, we can assume that the measurements of tumor weight are taken after the tumor size has surpassed the threshold, such that the w observed are larger than the threshold value. Under such a scenario the $p(w)$ function can be simplified to:

$$p(w) = 1 + \frac{(p_0 - 1) \cdot w_{th}}{w} \qquad \text{(eq.16)}$$

which is derived from eq. 14. For the simplified form of the $p(w)$ function (eq. 16), the parameters p_0 and w_{th} are not individually identifiable, but the product $(p_0 - 1) \cdot w_{th}$ can be consider as an identifiable model parameter, p_{wth}, thus replacing the need to estimate p_0 and w_{th}.

Perturbed tumor growth – non-cycle-specific drug effect model. The next phase of our model development is to introduce a model to account for anti-tumor drug induced tumor growth inhibition. We will first explore non-cycle-specific anti-cancer drugs that induce cell death (assumed to be apoptosis) in tumor during any stage of the tumor cell life cycle. The schematic representation of the non-cycle-specific drug effect model is presented in Figure 1B. Mathematical models of cytotoxic effect of anticancer agents relate drug plasma concentration $C(t)$ to the rate of cell removal as second-order or saturable processes [10,29,30]. Because these anti-cancer drugs can affect the tumor cells at any time, the drug effects can be modeled simply as a dose-dependent removal of a portion of tumor cells from the replicating population. We assign such tumor cells to a non-proliferating population that will die of apoptosis. This requires the tumor to be separated into two populations of cells: a proliferating population $M(t)$ and an apoptotic population $A(t)$, and sum of which makes up the tumor size:

$$w(t) = M(t) + A(t) \qquad \text{(eq.17)}$$

The process of removing the proliferating cells can be described as:

$$E(C(t)) \cdot M(t) = k_2 \cdot C(t) \cdot M(t) \qquad \text{(eq.18)}$$

which assumes a linear relationship between drug concentration, $C(t)$, and drug effect $E(C(t))$. The relationship is characterized by a second-order drug potency constant k_2.

The killing of tumor cells affects proliferation in that only cells which survive the cytotoxic effects of the anti-cancer drug can divide at the end of their lifespan T. Consequently, the cell removal rate, $k_{out}(t)$ in our model is now presented as [16]:

$$k_{out}(t) = k_{in}(t-T) \cdot e^{-\int_{t-T}^{t} E(C(z))dz} - E(C(t)) \cdot M(t) \qquad \text{(eq.19)}$$

where the integral multiplying $k_{in}(t\text{-}T)$ denotes the fraction of surviving cells. Given that only the surviving cells can divide with the efficiency $p(w(t))$, $k_{in}(t)$ is now presented as:

$$k_{in}(t) = p(w(t)) \cdot e^{-\int_{t-T}^{t} E(C(z))dz} \cdot k_{in}(t-T) \qquad \text{(eq.20)}$$

Using the same recursive derivation presented in the Appendix S2, we can present $k_{in}(t)$ in the closed form:

$$k_{in}(t) = k_{in0} \cdot e^{-\int_{0}^{t} E(C(z))dz} \cdot \prod_{i=0}^{INT(t/T)} p(w(t-iT)) \qquad \text{(eq.21)}$$

By combining eq. 19 and eq. 21 into eq. 1, the perturbed tumor growth by non-cycle-specific anti-cancer drugs can be expressed as:

$$\frac{dM}{dt} =$$

$$\frac{k_{in0}(p(w(t)) - 1)}{p(w(t))} \cdot e^{-\int_{0}^{t} E(C(z))dz} \cdot \prod_{i=0}^{INT(t/T)} p(W(t-iT)) - E(C(t)) \cdot M(t), \qquad \text{(eq.22)}$$

$$\text{for } t > 0$$

The initial condition for the proliferation population is:

$$M(0) = w_0 \qquad \text{(eq.23)}$$

A hallmark feature of anti-cancer treatment is a significant time delay between plasma drug concentration and reduction of tumor size or inhibition of tumor growth [5–7,9,10], which have been addressed by various models using transit compartments [10,11]. Similarly to the approach by Simeoni and colleagues [11], we assume that the cells affected by the drug are not killed instantaneously, but rather undergo programmed cell death (apoptosis) that takes a period of time T_A to complete. If $A(t)$ denotes the size of the apoptotic tumor cells due to a chemotherapeutic effect at time t, then according to the basic lifespan model [9,15]:

$$\frac{dA}{dt} = E(C(t)) \cdot M(T) - E(C(t-T_A)) \cdot M(t-T_A), \qquad \text{(eq.24)}$$

$$\text{for } t > 0$$

If no drugs were given prior to start of experiments then there is an absence of any non-proliferating tumor cells that are generated by anti-cancer drugs:

$$A(0) = 0 \qquad \text{(eq.25)}$$

The perturbed tumor growth model described by eq. 22 and eq. 24 accounts for non-cycle-specific drug effects since the tumor cells are susceptible to drug-induced killing at any stage of their development at the rate specified by eq. 18. An example of the MATLAB implementation of the non-cycle-specific drug effect model is provided in Material S1–S3.

Perturbed tumor growth - cycle specific drug effect model. For this section we will address cycle-specific anti-cancer compounds that inhibit tumor growth by inducing apoptosis at a specific point of the tumor cell life cycle. The concepts for the cycle-specific drug effect model are generalized in the model schematic in Figure 1C. Since the turnover of tumor cells in our model is determined by their lifespan T, according to eq. 2, we will utilize another mechanism of drug action on tumor cells where the drug affects the lifespan distribution of the affected tumor cells [17].

$$\ell(t,\tau) = E(C(t)) \cdot \delta(\tau) + (1 - E(C(t))) \cdot \delta(\tau - T) \qquad (eq.26)$$

Here $\ell(t,\tau)$ is the probability density function for the distribution of the cell lifespan τ at time t. The terms $\delta(\tau)$ and $\delta(\tau-T)$ are the point distributions (Dirac delta functions) centered at 0 and T, respectively, and the drug effect is described by the Emax model:

$$E(C) = \frac{E_{max} \cdot C}{EC_{50} + C} \qquad (eq.27)$$

with $0 \leq E_{max} \leq 1$ being the maximum effect, and EC_{50} representing the drug concentration eliciting 50% of the maximum effect. According to eq. 26, the chemotherapeutic effect shifts cells of lifespan T to a subpopulation of cells with lifespan of 0, and the partition between these populations is determined by the Emax model. Since a cell of lifespan $T = 0$ at a given time t must be immediately removed from the population, the drug effect results in instantaneous removal of portion of tumor cells from the population determined by the drug function $E(C(t))$. Based on concept [17], the cell elimination rate becomes:

$$k_{out}(t) = k_{in}(t) \cdot E(C(t)) + k_{in}(t - T) \cdot (1 - E(C(t-T)) \qquad (eq.28)$$

The cells which are not affected by the chemotherapy become new tumor cells with efficiency $p(w(t))$, since the tumor weight now consists of both the proliferating cells $w(t)$ and apoptotic cells $A(t)$. Thus, $k_{in}(t)$ must now be presented as:

$$k_{in}(t) = p(w(t)) \cdot (1 - E(C(t-T))) \cdot k_{in}(t-T) \qquad (eq.29)$$

The relationship described in eq. 29 provides a recursive definition of $k_{in}(t)$ which leads to the following:

$$k_{in}(t) = \frac{k_{in0}}{1 - E(C(t))} \cdot \prod_{i=0}^{INT(t/T)} (1 - E(C(t-iT))) \cdot p(w(t-iT)), \qquad (eq.30)$$

for $t > 0$

Consequently, as derived in Appendix S2, the perturbed tumor model becomes:

$$\frac{dM}{dt} = \frac{k_{in0} \cdot ((1 - E(C(t))) \cdot p(w(t)) - 1)}{(1 - E(C(t))) \cdot p(w(t))}$$

$$\cdot \prod_{i=0}^{INT(t/T)} (1 - E(C(t-iT))) \cdot p(w(t-iT)), \qquad (eq.31)$$

for $t > 0$

with the initial condition described by eq. 9.

Similar to the non-cycle-specific drug effect model, the apoptotic cell population is described by the lifespan model [15]:

$$\frac{dA}{dt} = k_{in}(t) \cdot (E(C(t)) - k_{in}(t - T_A) \cdot E(C(t - T_A)) \qquad (eq.32)$$

with the initial condition given by eq. 25:

The model outlined by eq. 31 and eq. 32 describes drug action that is cycle-specific because the drug can only affect cells that have reached the end of their lifespan T when they divide, and tumor cells at any other stage of their development are not affected by the drug, which is the fundamental definition of cycle-specific anti-cancer drug effect [31]. An example of the MATLAB implementation of the cycle-specific drug effect model is provided in Material S4–S6.

Data Analysis

All models in this report were implemented in MATLAB (R2012b, The MathWorks Inc.). Model parameter values were estimated using the function nlinfit, a nonlinear regression algorithm in MATLAB. The delay differential equations were solved using dde23 [32]. Unlike the other parameters, the lifespan TGI model is not a continuous function of T and T_A due to the use of the integer function in eq. 8, which causes jumps in the model output over continuous value of T. Therefore, a grid search method was performed to estimate T and T_A. Once the value of T and T_A are determined, they were fixed and the remaining model parameters were estimated using nlinfit. Due to higher number of model parameters in perturbed lifespan TGI models, a grid search with all the parameters was not feasible in terms of run time. Instead, values of T, p_0, k_{in0} and w_{th} were fixed to estimates obtained by fitting to the control group, T and T_A were determined using grid search, and finally, remaining parameters were refitted with nlinfit, having fixed the values of T and T_A.

For the comparison of the lifespan TGI model to the TGI model developed by Simeoni and colleagues [11], the tumor growth data from the AZ968 in vivo study outlined above were used. The data from that study only exhibit linear tumor growth, and are assumed to have surpassed the threshold size. Linear data can be accommodated in our lifespan TGI model using eq. 16 to describe division efficiency. For the reference TGI model, we have to make modification to the equation to only describe linear tumor growth data. The model equations are now presented as:

$$\frac{dx_1}{dt} = \frac{\lambda_1 \cdot x_1(t)}{w(t)} - k_2 \cdot C(t) \cdot x_1(t)$$

$$\frac{dx_2}{dt} = k_2 \cdot C(t) \cdot x_1(t) - k_1 \cdot x_2(t)$$

$$\frac{dx_3}{dt} = k_1 \cdot x_2(t) - k_1 \cdot x_3(t) \qquad (eq.33)$$

$$\frac{dx_4}{dt} = k_1 \cdot x_3(t) - k_1 \cdot x_4(t)$$

$$w(t) = x_1(t) + x_2(t) + x_3(t) + x_4(t)$$

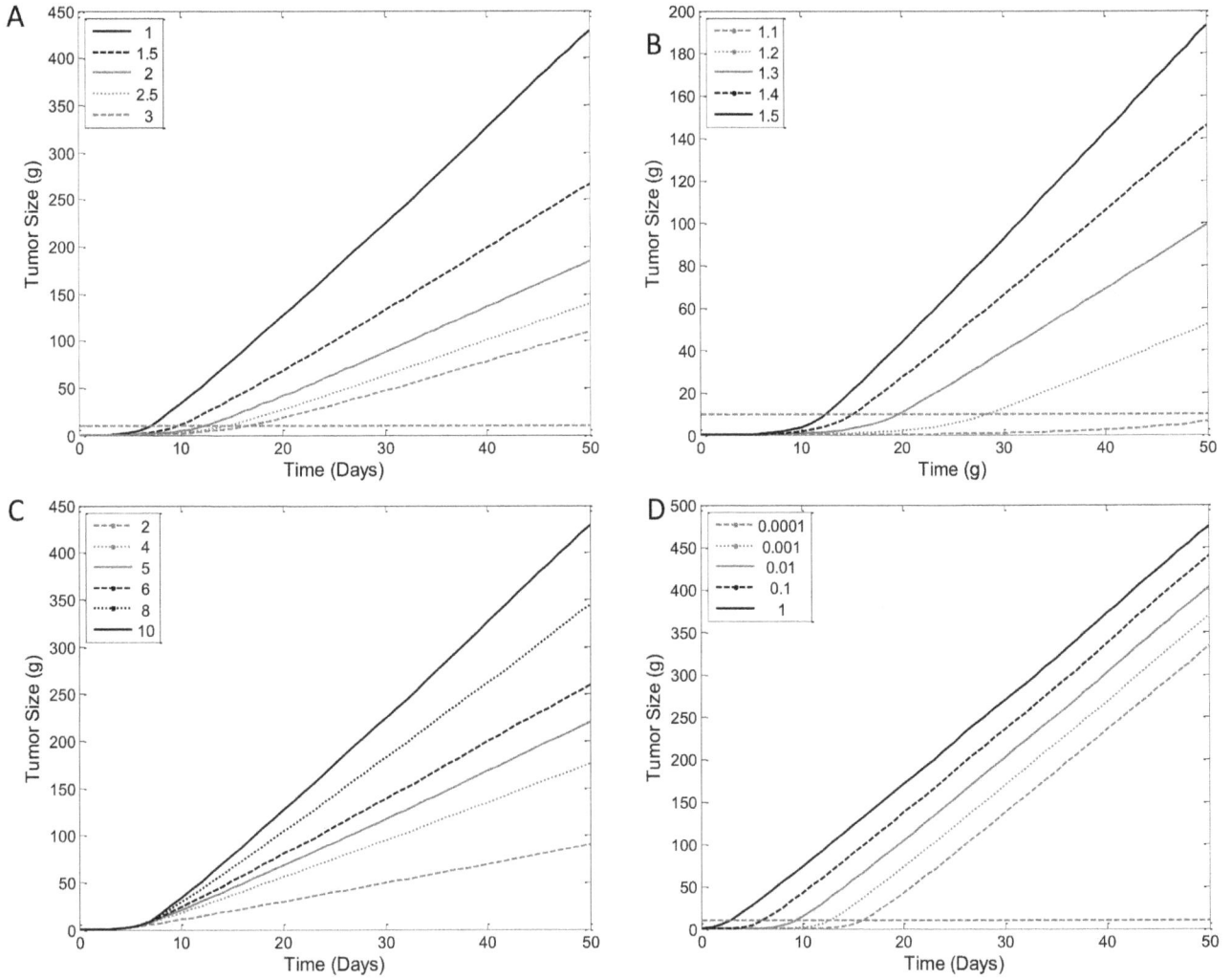

Figure 4. Sensitivity Analysis of Unperturbed Tumor Growth. Simulated model profiles of varying values of A) Tumor cell lifespan (T), B) Initial division efficiency (p_0), C) Tumor size threshold (w_{th}) for decrease in division efficiency, and D) Past tumor growth rate (k_{in0}). Simulation were carried with parameters values of $T = 1$ day, $p_0 = 2$, $k_{in0} = 0.05$ g/day and $w_{th} = 10$ g, unless otherwise specified for each figure. Dashed lines in panels A–C indicate the w_{th} value.

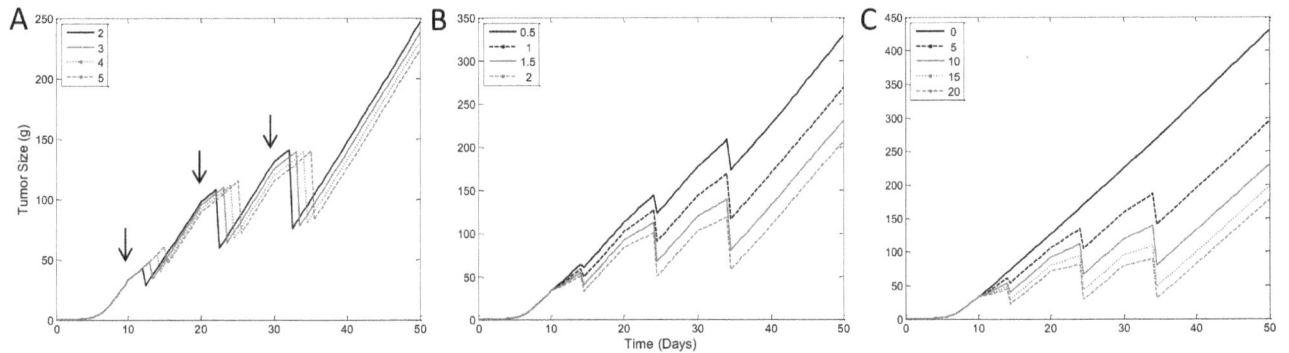

Figure 5. Sensitivity Analysis of Non-Cycle-Specific Drug Effect Model. Simulated model profiles with changes in A) Apoptosis duration, T_A, and B) Linear drug potency constant, k_2. C) Signature profile of cycle-specific drug mechanism model with dose escalation. Simulation were carried with parameters values of $T = 1$ day, $T_A = 4$ days, $p_0 = 2$, $k_{in0} = 0.05$, $w_{th} = 10$ g, and $k_2 = 1.5$ mL/ng, unless otherwise indicated. Arrows indicate dose administration on days 10, 20 and 30.

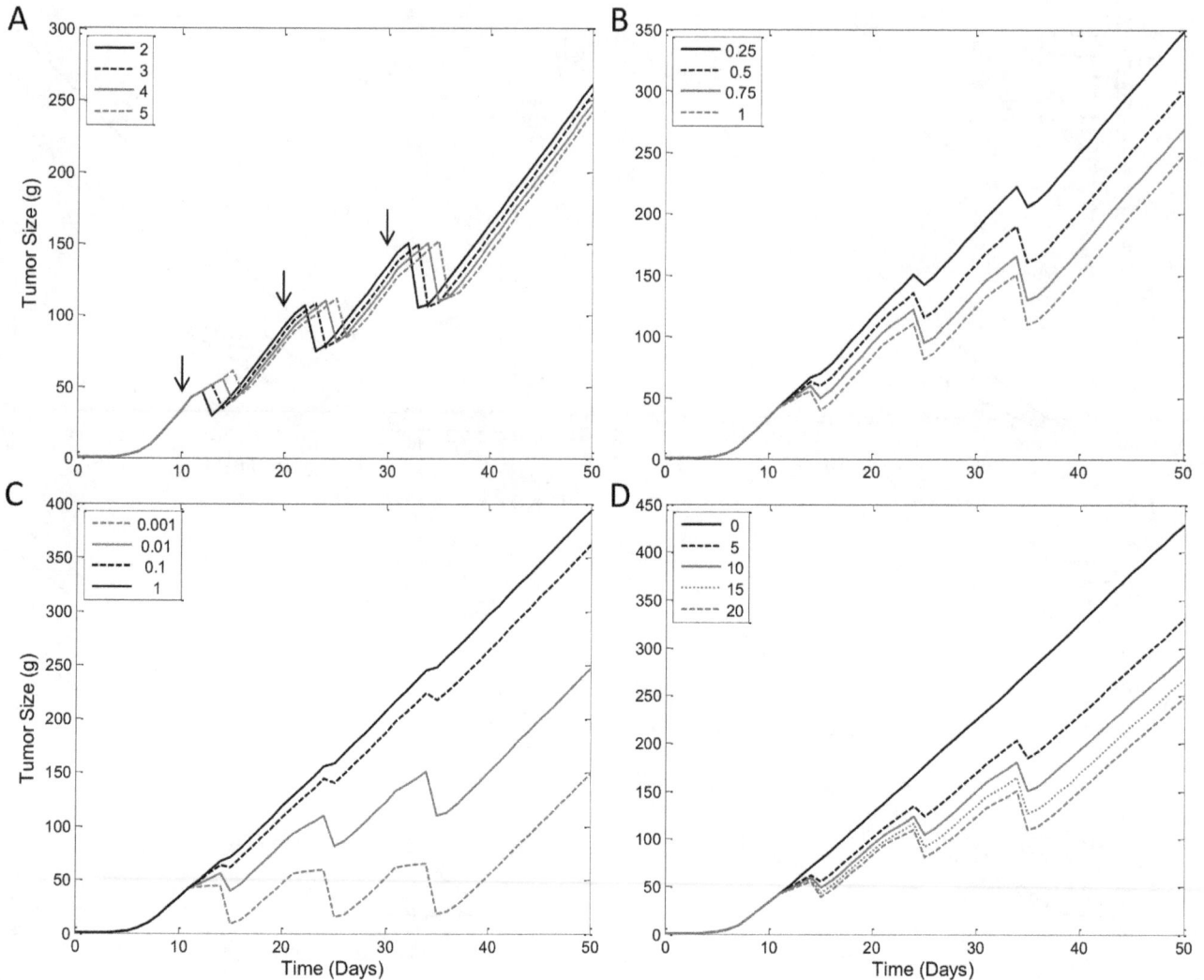

Figure 6. Sensitivity Analysis of Cycle-Specific Drug Effect Model. Simulated model profiles with changes in: A) Apoptosis duration, T_A, B) Maximum drug efficacy, E_{max}, and C) Drug potency, EC_{50}. D) Signature profile of cycle-specific drug mechanism model with dose escalation. Simulation were carried with parameters values of $T = 1$ day, $T_A = 4$ days, $p_0 = 2$, $k_{in0} = 0.05$ g/day, $w_{th} = 10$ g, $E_{max} = 1$ and $EC_{50} = 0.01$ concentration, unless otherwise indicated. Arrows indicate dose administration at days 10, 20 and 30.

where λ_1 is the linear growth rate, k_2 is the second order drug potency constant, k_1 is the transit rate constant, and $C(t)$ is the plasma drug concentration.

Results

Model Exploration – Unperturbed Tumor Growth

The lifespan model of tumor growth inhibition outlined in the model development section accounts for tumor growth through the process of cellular division of tumor cells, and is capable of describing non-cycle-specific anti-cancer drug effects and cycle-specific drug effects. Exploration of the characteristics of our model will begin with the unperturbed tumor growth model. The incorporation of a tumor size-dependent cell division efficiency factor, $p(w(t))$ as outlined by eq.13, allows the model to produce a bi-phasic growth kinetic with initial exponential growth rate and linear growth rate after a specific tumor size is reached (w_{th}), as indicated by the model profile in Figure 3.

Sensitivity Analysis – Unperturbed Tumor Growth

The model parameters that determine the aspects of the model profile, such as slope of linear growth phase, have been explored mathematically in the model development section. Here we will further examine the effects of the parameters. The sensitivity analysis demonstrates that each of the model parameters has different effects on model behavior (Figure 4). Increasing values of T resulted in slower growth kinetics. Both exponential growth rate and linear growth rate (slope of linear growth phase) are affected (Figure 4A). Decreasing values of p_0 had a similar effect as increasing value of T, except p_0 tends to affect exponential growth much more than the linear growth (Figure 4B). Increasing values of w_{th} does not have any effect on exponential growth, but does dictate the end of the exponential growth phase and more importantly the slope of the linear growth phase (Figure 4C). The effect of T, p_0, and w_{th} on linear growth as seen in the sensitivity analysis is in accordance to the relationship of these parameters in determining the slope of linear growth into later time points as outlined by eq.15. Unlike the other parameters, changes in k_{in0} do

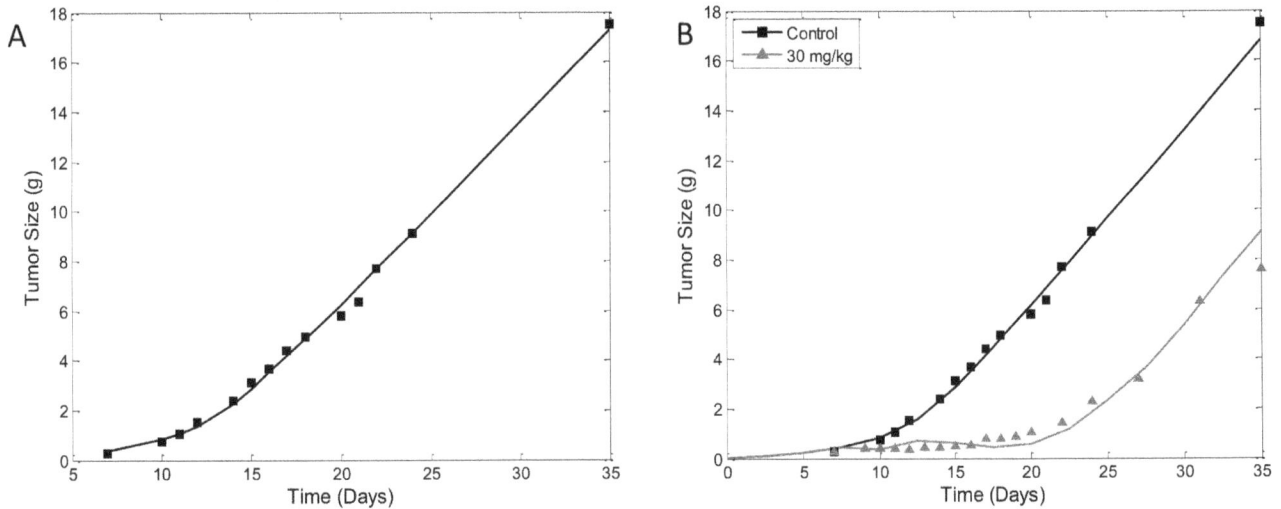

Figure 7. Modeling Tumor Growth Inhibition by Paclitaxel. A) Observed (black squares) and model fitted (black line) tumor weight during untreated tumor growth. Data was digitized from (Simeoni et al, 2004). Initial tumor volume was fixed at 0.033 g as estimated from original publication. B) Simultaneous fitting of unperturbed tumor growth data (black square) with model preduction (black line) and tumor growth inhibition data (grey triangle) and model prediction using the cycle-specific drug effect model (grey line) by 30 mg/kg of paclitaxel administered every 4 days for 3 rounds starting from day 8.

not seem to affect the kinetics of tumor growth in either phases, but rather determine when measureable level of growth begins (Figure 4 D). The results of the sensitivity analysis indicate that parameters in the unperturbed models are all identifiable. Confirmation of identifiability will be presented in the case studies with TGI data.

Sensitivity Analysis – Non-Cycle-Specific Drug Effect

Simulations for sensitivity analysis and model signature profiles were conducted with a two-compartment PK model with $k_{el} = 20$ day^{-1}, $k_{12} = 0.2$ day^{-1}, $k_{21} = 2$ day^{-1} and $V = 1$ mL. For sensitivity analysis, a dose of 10 units was administered at 10, 20 and 30 days (we take dose to be dimensionless). Simulations of changes in parameters for the non-cycle-specific drug effect model were performed and the resulting sensitivity analysis is shown in Figure 5. Simulation shows that changes in the duration-of-apoptosis parameter, T_A, have a direct effect on the length of delay of drug-induced tumor reduction after drug administration (Figure 5A). Changes in the linear drug potency constant, k_2, affect the degree of TGI and tumor size reduction, if any (Figure 5B). Signature profile of the non-cycle-specific drug effect model with increasing doses of anti-cancer drug is shown in Figure 5C, and as expected is very similar to the simulation of changing values of k_2.

Sensitivity analysis – cycle-specific drug effect. Although both the cycle-specific and non-cell cycle-specific drug effect models use the same tumor growth component as the non-cycle-specific drug effect model, there are significant differences between them, as outlined in the Model Development section. Furthermore, unlike the non-cycle-specific model, which uses a linear drug effect function, the cycle-specific model incorporates the Emax model for drug effect and different parameters are required. Similar to sensitivity analysis of the non-cycle-specific model, changes in T_A parameter exclusively affect the delay in anti-cancer drug effect (Figure 6A). The Emax drug effect requires both maximum efficacy, E_{max}, and drug potency, EC_{50}. Simulations show that changes in E_{max} and EC_{50} both affect the degree of anti-cancer drug induced tumor reduction (Figure 6B,C). Although similar, there are subtle differences in the effects of the two parameters that can be distinguished given the appropriate dose ranges in data. Notice the low EC_{50} values used for simulation in Figure 6B (Figure legend), when compared to the peak concentration of the drug in the system which is 10 units/mL. This is due to the nature of the equation for the cycle-specific drug effect model which only allows the drug to act on tumors cell the moment they reach the doubling time, T. This small window means the drug can only affect a fraction of the cells. The model has to adjust the potency of the drug to account for efficacy. For this reason a much lower EC_{50} value is required to account for the

Table 1. Parameter Estimates for Unperturbed Tumor Growth.

Parameter	Estimates	Units	CV%
T	1.46[a]	days	-
p_0	1.44	-	7.44
k_{ing}	3.86×10^{-2}	g/day	77.8
w_{th}	2.54	g	24.3

[a]Parameter was fixed.

Table 2. Parameter Estimates for Simultaneous Fitting of Unperturbed and Paclitaxel Inhibited Tumor Growth with Cycle-Specific Drug Effect.

Parameter	Estimates	Units	CV%
T	1.46^a	days	-
T_A	0.536^a	days	-
p_0	1.44	-	2.18×10^{-2}
k_{in0}	4.04×10^{-2}	g/day	0.149
w_{th}	2.48	g	2.24
E_{max}	1^a	-	-
EC_{50}	9.45	ng/mL	2.23

[a]Parameter was fixed.

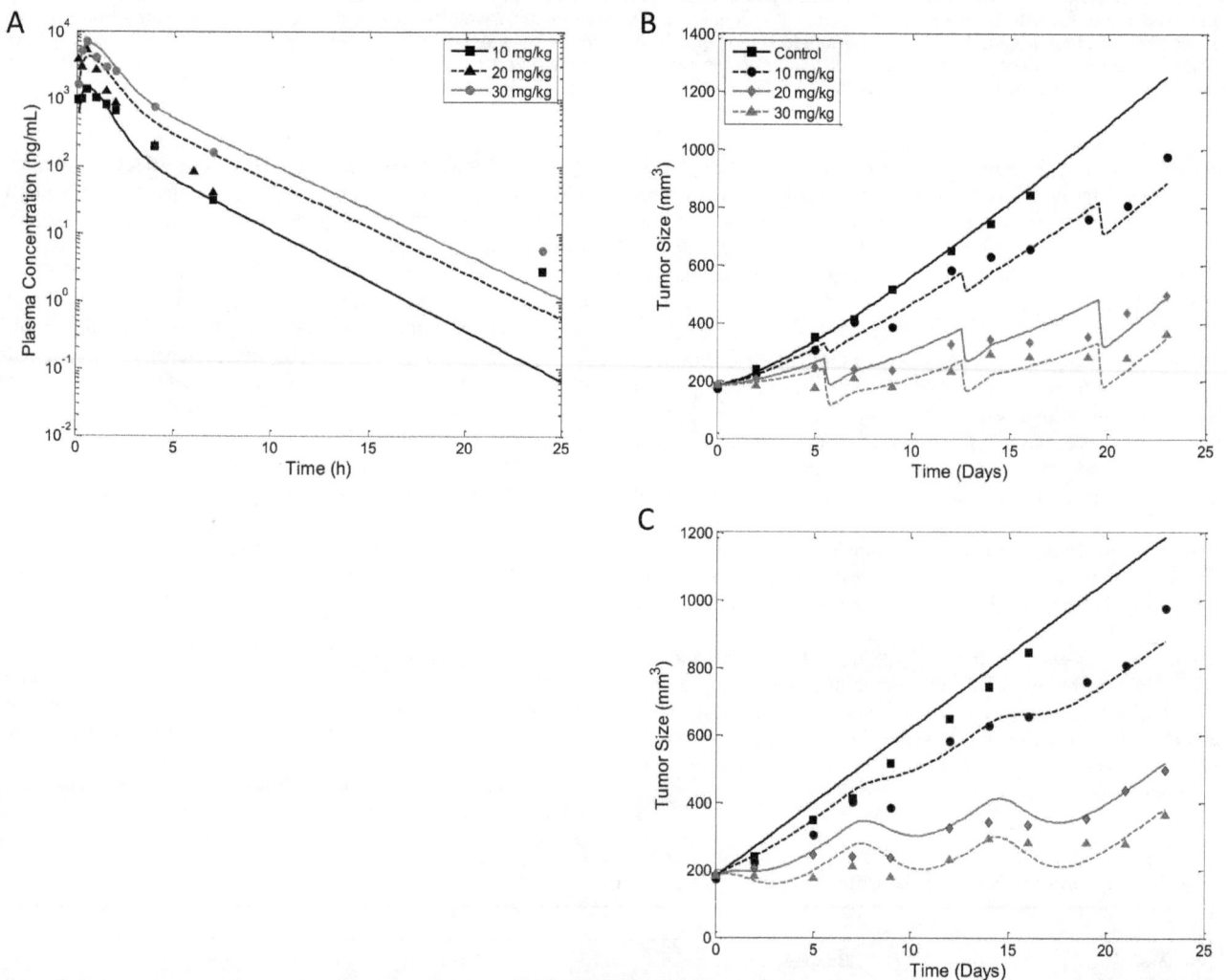

Figure 8. Model Comparison: Modeling Tumor Growth Inhibition by AZ968. A) Modeling of pharmacokinetic data after single i.p. dose of AZ968 at 10, 20 and 30 mg/kg. Data (symbols) was described with a 2 compartment model with dose-dependent elimination rate constant and central volume of distribution (model prediction in lines). B) Observed (symbols) and model predicted (lines) tumor volume using the lifespan model of tumor growth inhibition. Line style and color indicate unrestricted condition and oral treatment with AZ968 at 10, 20 and 30 mg/kg in mice xenograft. Symbols indicate control condition (black squares), 10 mg/kg AZ968 (black circles), 20 mg/kg (grey diamonds), and 30 mg/kg (grey triangles). Initial tumor volume was fixed at 180 mm^3 as estimated from initial data points. C) Fitting of same AZ968 data using the Simeoni model.

Table 3. Parameter Estimates for PK Fitting of AZ968.

Parameter	Estimates	Units	CV%
k_a	46.8[a]	1/day	-
k_{el} 10 mg/kg	33.9	1/day	1.40
k_{el} 20 mg/kg	26.0	1/day	1.40
k_{el} 30 mg/kg	24.7	1/day	1.40
k_{12}	8.74	1/day	3.44
k_{21}	11.2	1/day	0.801
V 10 mg/kg	2.70	L/kg	1.49
V 20 mg/kg	2.07	L/kg	1.49
V 30 mg/kg	1.97	L/kg	1.49

[a]Parameter was fixed.

observed drug effect on tumor size. The effect of this feature is seen in the signature profile of the cycle-specific drug effect model shown in Figure 6D. Note the low degree of dose-separation for the effect of drug on tumor size. A low EC_{50} value results in saturation of drug effect for all doses, prolonging the duration, but not the intensity, at higher doses. The effects of this model characteristic will be further evident in the following case study.

Case Study 1 - Tumor Growth Inhibition by Paclitaxel

Data for this case study was obtained from literature [11]. In this study paclitaxel was administered i.v. at 30 mg/kg every 4 days starting from day 8 after tumor inoculation. Tumor growth data and model prediction by our lifespan TGI are shown in Figure 7. We began by fitting the unperturbed growth data. Prediction from our lifespan TGI model overlapped well with the experimental data (Figure 7A). Examination of the parameter estimates shows biologically relevant values (Table 1). The doubling time, T, was estimated to be 1.46 days, initial division efficiency, p_0, estimated to be 1.44, past tumor production rate, k_{in0}, was estimated to be 0.0386 g·day^{-1}, and tumor threshold, w_{th}, to be 2.55 g. The precision of the parameter estimates are high for both p_0 and w_{th}, which had coefficient of variance (CV%) of 7.44% and 24.3%. The precision for the estimate of k_{in0} was not as high as the other two, but was still within acceptable levels of precision (CV% of 77.8%).

For the second part of this case study we fitted both unperturbed and paclitaxel inhibited tumor growth data. Because paclitaxel is considered a cycle-specific anti-cancer drug, we fitted the data using the cycle-specific drug effect model. Figure 7B shows the experimental data and lifespan TGI model predicted values, which overlap well. Examination of the model parameter estimates show that values from the simultaneous fit were very similar to the estimates from the unperturbed data (Table 2). Estimate for p_0 was 1.44, k_{in0} was 0.404 g day^{-1} and w_{th} was 2.461 g. The estimate of T was kept constant from the result of the grid search from the unperturbed data fitting. Parameters unique to the cycle-specific drug effect model are T_A, EC_{50} and E_{max}. EC_{50} was estimated to be 83.28 ng/mL, E_{max} was fixed to 1 due to lack of escalating doses, and T_A, which also has discontinuous property similar to T, was estimated to be 0.536 days. The advantage of the simultaneous fitting is the availability of more data points. As expected the precision of the model estimates was increased compared to fitting only unperturbed data. CV% value of p_0, k_{in0}, w_{th} and EC_{50} were 0.0744%, 0.0908%, 2.225% and 0.043%, respectively. This case study demonstrates that our model is fully

capable of fitting real experimental data from animal xenograft models. Interestingly, the estimated EC_{50} value is very low compared to the peak plasma concentration of paclitaxel, which can reach 37040 ng/mL (data not shown), according to the PK model. Similar to the sensitivity analysis of the cycle-specific drug effect model, this observation is due to the limited time that a fraction of the tumor cells will be affected by the drug. Implication of this model characteristic will be discussed further in the following section. Regardless of the unique characteristic of the model, the high precision of the parameter estimates confirms the identifiability of the model parameters in the unperturbed model of tumor growth and the cycle-specific drug effect model. However, interpretation of the model parameters must be done with care, and adjustments of the model may be required, which will be discussed in the following section.

Model Comparison – Tumor Growth Inhibition by AZ968

Now that we have demonstrated the flexibility of our lifespan TGI model, and confirm identifiability of the model parameters, we will explore the capability of our model to describe mouse xenograft data compared to the TGI model presented by Simeoni and colleagues [11]. We first modeled the PK profile of AZ968, using a two-compartment model. Model fitting is shown in Figure 8A. Estimates of model parameter values are listed in Table 3. Due to observed non-linear PK, dose-specific values of k_{el} and V were needed to fit PK data (Table 3). Unlike the paclitaxel datasets, data from this study show only linear growth kinetics. We will make the assumption that the tumor sizes at the first measurement have already surpassed the tumor threshold. The data will be modeled using the linear version of the lifespan TGI model (see eq. 16), and the linearized version of the Simeoni, et al., model of TGI (see eq. 33). AZ968 is a potent casein kinase 2 (CK2) inhibitor, which induces apoptosis of tumor cells. There is no known mechanism of AZ968 to suggest the compound is active only at specific cell cycles, therefore the non-cycle-specific drug effect model is used for this study. Model fitting of both the lifespan TGI model and the reference TGI model (eq. 33) are shown in Figure 8. Predictions from both models overlay well with the data points, and both models are able to capture the delayed onset of drug effect on tumor size. Parameter estimates for both model fittings are listed in Table 4. While the estimated value corresponding to 'time till cell death' ($T_A = 5.56$ days for our model, and mean transit time ($4/k_1$) = 2.68 days for Simeoni's) are not identical, they are comparable. The potency constant, k_2, from the two models is estimated to be very similar: the lifespan TGI

Table 4. Parameter Estimate for Model Fitting of Tumor Growth Inhibition by AZ968.

Lifespan TGI Model				Simeoni TGI Model			
Parameter	Estimates	Units	CV%	Parameter	Estimates	Units	CV%
T	1.28^a	days	-	λ_1	43.8	1/day	6.98×10^{-2}
T_A	5.56^a	days	-	k_1	1.12	1/day	4.27×10^{-2}
P_{wth}	80.8	mm^3	2.65	k_2	2.0×10^{-3}	mL/ng/day	0.101
k_{in0}	49.9	mm^3/day	4.46				
k_2	2.30×10^{-3}	mL/ng/day	3.69×10^{-2}				

^{a}Parameter was fixed.

model gives $k_2 = 0.0023$ ng^{-1} mL·day^{-1} and the Simeoni model $k_2 = 0.0020$ ng^{-1}·mL·day^{-1}. Examination of the precision of the model estimates demonstrates that both models were able to estimate the parameters with high precision (see Table 4). This comparative study demonstrates that the lifespan TGI model is fully capable of describing real experimental data with precision comparable to that of one of the most commonly used models of TGI.

Case Study 2 - Tumor Growth Inhibition by AZD1208

Data for this case study was provided by AstraZeneca [18]. For the purpose of this case study we will set time according to when the first dose of AZD1208 was administered, which we count as day 1. We began with a compartmental PK analysis after a single oral administration of AZD1208 at 3, 10 and 30 mg/kg and found it well described using a one-compartment PK model with first order absorption as shown in Figure 9A. Parameter values of $k_a = 5.52$ day^{-1} and $V/F = 4.86$ L/kg were estimated with high precision (Table 5), with the exception of the elimination rate constant, k_{el}, which was estimated to be same value as k_a and therefore we set k_{el} to equal k_a value in the final PK model.

After establishing the PK model, we fit the TGI data using the lifespan TGI model. Since AZD1208 is a pan-Pim kinase inhibitor that promotes apoptosis at any stages of cell cycle, the data were analyzed using the non-cycle-specific model. Model fitting of the AZD1208 TGI data is shown in Figure 9B. Interestingly, the tumor data in this study exhibited only exponential growth kinetics. In order to adapt the lifespan TGI model to account for only exponential growth we simply set the tumor threshold, w_{th}, to a very large value well beyond the observed values of tumor size. Another unique feature of this dataset is the inclusion of saturating doses. To accommodate the dose ranges we replaced the drug potency constant, k_2, in eq. 18 with the E_{max} model. The process of fitting was the same as for the previous studies, however, in this study the control data were very sparse and the doubling time, T, could not be estimated. In order to proceed with the analysis we set $T = 3$ days based on the doubling time reported by the commercial vendor of the MOLM-16 tumor cell used in the study, which was similar to the doubling reported the original study when the cells were initially collected [33]. Doubling times for mouse xenografts have been found to be in the range of 2–8 days, approximately [34]. The remaining parameters were estimated with high precision and are well within biologically feasible ranges (see Table 6). This case study demonstrates the flexibility of the lifespan model to accommodate different types of TGI data while maintaining parameter identifiability and precise estimates of parameter values.

Discussion

The lifespan model of TGI presented here is the first mechanistic model to describe tumor growth through the process of cellular division. By using division efficiency as the restriction factor due to tumor burden, the lifespan TGI model is able to account for multi-phasic growth patterns, a critical feature in many models of TGI [8,9,35–38]. Exploration of the model behavior through simulations, and data fitting capability through case studies have confirmed that our mechanistic approach to modeling TGI is fully capable of describing real experimental data in a biologically relevant context.

Major concerns for development of mechanistic models are the cost of increased number of parameters, and their identifiability. For comparative purposes, we will focus on a well-known TGI model developed by Simeoni and colleagues [11], which is one of

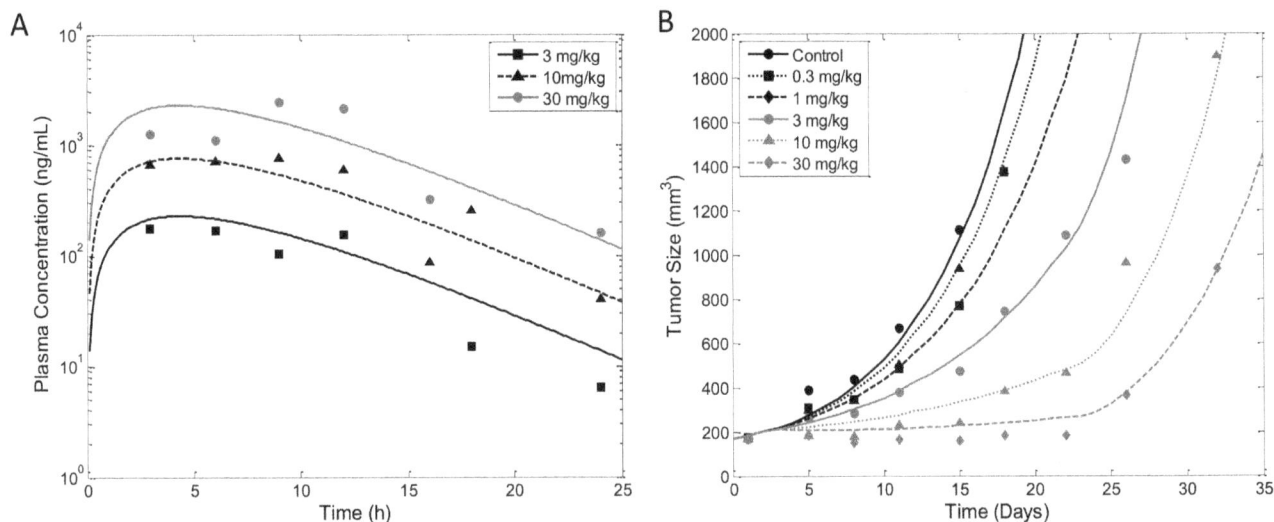

Figure 9. Tumor Growth Inhibition by AZD1208. A) Pharmacokinetic profile of AZD1208 was described using a 1 compartment model with equal values for absorption and elimination rate constants. PK data (symbols) were collected following a single oral administration of AZD1208 at 3, 10 and 30 mg/kg (model prediction in lines). B) Observed (symbol) and lifespan model predicted (lines) tumor growth and inhibition by AZD1208 at 0.3, 1, 3, 10 and 30 mg/kg given orally. Initial tumor volume was fixed to 170 mm³, which is the value of the first tumor size measurement.

the most popular models of TGI. The Simeoni model is a perfect example of modeling parsimony. Its flexibility and robustness allows the model to fully capture tumor growth and tumor growth inhibition data with very few parameters, making it an ideal model for rapid screening of drug libraries. However, the model describes tumor growth empirically through rate kinetics, and utilizes little information about physiological processes in its structural design. The foundation of our lifespan model is the biological mechanism of cancer growth: cell division. Although we introduce more parameters, (four parameters, compared to Simeoni et al.'s two parameters), the sensitivity analysis demonstrated that all the parameters are identifiable. Furthermore, the parameters we introduce have much greater biological relevance: T is the exact representation of the doubling time of tumor cells; p_0 is the division efficiency of the tumor cells at the first observation; and w_{th} is the tumor size at which the rate of tumor growth changes from exponential to linear. The biological relevance of these parameters can be valuable for inter-species translation, and increase the accuracy of our predictions to human patients. For instance, the doubling time T can be directly compared to the doubling time of tumor cells in cancer patients to evaluate any potential in predicting human efficacy of anti-cancer drugs. Appropriate clinical data is required to explore the predictive power of our lifespan TGI model.

The only parameter in the lifespan TGI model that is difficult to interpret is the k_{in0}, which is the tumor growth rate at the beginning of the experiment. A function describing the tumor growth in the past is necessary due to the use of delay differential equations in our model. By incorporating this parameter, we make

the assumption that tumor growth prior to start of the experiment (between t = −T to 0) is constant. This is a safe assumption since the doubling time is small in comparison to the duration of the experiment and any tumor growth during that period will be negligible compared to the tumor sizes that will be measured throughout the course of the experiment. It is theoretically feasible to describe the history as a function of time rather than a constant. However, other assumptions will still be necessary, and the implementation of the model becomes very complex and outside the scope of this report.

To incorporate anti-cancer drug mechanism into our lifespan model of TGI, specifically the non-cycle-specific drug effect, we introduced two additional parameters, the drug potency constant k_2 and duration of apoptosis, T_A. It should be noted that the drug effect can also be modeled using the Emax function or any other function, but for simplicity and model comparison purposes (reference model uses the same function) we used the simplest drug effect function possible. An additional cell population with a lifespan, T_A, was incorporated to account for the delay in onset of observable drug effect on tumor size, a well reported feature of anti-cancer drug treatment [5–7]. This population is generated as a result of anti-cancer drug effect and the lifespan of this population can be interpreted as the time for cell death via apoptosis. Many PKPD models use transit compartments to incorporate delays [9–11,39]. We used the lifespan model to describe the process of cell division, and since transit compartments are approximations of lifespan models, and are equivalent under certain conditions [40,41], it was natural for us to describe the dying tumor cells using a lifespan model as well.

Table 5. Parameter Estimates for PK Fitting of AZ968.

Parameter	Estimates	Units	CV%
k_a	5.52	1/day	7.48
V/F	4.86	L/kg	17.89

Table 6. Parameter Estimates for Lifespan Model fitting of Tumor Growth Inhibition by AZD1208.

Parameter	Estimates	Units	CV%
T	3^a	days	-
T_A	1.92^a	days	-
p_0	1.57	-	2.17
k_{in0}	27.8	mm^3/day	13.5
E_{max}	0.159	-	5.73
EC_{50}	182	ng/mL	2.29×10^{-2}

[a]Parameter was fixed.

The mechanistic nature of our lifespan TGI model also allows for incorporation of different anti-cancer drug mechanisms. Although many drugs exhibit the mechanism of action by inducing apoptosis at any stage of the tumor cell life cycle, there are numerous drugs that are cell-cycle-specific [31] and only target cells at specific points in their life cycle. Previous models relied on the time-dependent transition of tumor cells into different drug-sensitivity states [42]. More recent mechanistic models are describing the cell-cycle in more detail [29,43,44], however, these models are more complex and require rich data with numerous biomarkers. In our lifespan TGI model we can mechanistically describe a cycle-specific drug action because the model describes changes in tumor size after each round of cell division. After each division cycle, the effect of the drug can be imposed on the tumor cells. And since the time it takes for any cell-cycle stage to repeat itself is the doubling time, this model is applicable for drugs that target different stages of the cell cycle. The application of this cell-cycle-specific drug effect model was demonstrated in Case Study 1, where we examined the effect of paclitaxel on mice xenograft tumors. The model performed well and was able to estimate parameter values with high precision. Interestingly, the model predicted a very low EC_{50} relative to the plasma concentration. As discussed earlier, this is due to the model equation which only allows the drug to act for a short period of time, during which the drug can affect only a fraction of cells that are sensitive. In other models it is assumed that as soon as the tumor cells are exposed to the drug they are marked for death. The delay for cycle-specific drugs would include not only the time for apoptosis to occur, but also for the time it takes for the cells to become sensitive to the drug. This is not the case in our model, which only exposes the cells to the drug after the doubling time, but this, as demonstrated by the case study, has its drawbacks in the compensatory high estimate of potency. This suggests that cycle-specific drugs must have some means of accumulating in the system. Drug accumulation can be easily modeled using an effect compartment rather than linking the PD to plasma drug concentration. Tumor permeation and clearance can also cause disassociation of predicted drug effect based on plasma drug concentration. Modeling efforts are focused on addressing issues such as tumor vascularization, intra-tumor drug gradients, and tumor heterogeneity, which all can cause discrepancies between intra-tumor and plasma drug PK (see review [45]). However, such modeling efforts require additional data, such as intra-tumor drug PK measurements that we do not have access to. It would be very interesting to combine our lifespan TGI model with a more complex intra-tumor PK model, which would allow for more accurate prediction of efficacy than predictions made based on plasma PK. It should

be noted that although this model is able to describe the action of cycle-specific drugs, it is unable to identify the specific cell cycle phase at which the drug becomes active. Inclusion of cell cycle phases are required for cycle identification, and such model is outside the scope of this report.

Although all model parameters are identifiable, the estimation of the doubling time, T, and duration of apoptosis, T_A, cannot be accomplished using traditional minimization algorithms. As discussed earlier, this is due to a discontinuity of the model equation with respect to the two parameters. In order to have an estimate of the parameters, a grid search was performed. Although this method is capable of identifying the global minimum, its precision is limited by the run time and number of parameters to be estimated. Furthermore, there are no conventional statistical evaluations available for this approach. The other parameters were estimated using a minimization algorithm after values for T and T_A were determined by the grid search method and fixed. Although this is a limitation of the lifespan TGI model, there are options to overcome this issue. One solution is to fix the parameter to *in vitro* values as was done for Case Study 2 with AZD1208 induced TGI. The inclusion of a grid search process greatly adds to the computational time of this model, which can take several hours. This is in addition to the added computation time required for the delay differential equation solver in the algorithmic fitting process, which for the case study presented was more than ten times longer (179 s for lifespan TGI, and 12 s for Simeoni TGI model). Until we can resolve the requirement for a grid search, this model will continue to run much slower by comparison to conventional TGI models.

One of the biggest potential limitations of mechanistic models in general is the need for high resolution data due to their complexity and high number of parameters. The model comparison study showed that although we introduced two additional parameters in our lifespan TGI model compared to the reference TGI model [11], the parameters in our model were estimated with high precision, and that the model was able to describe the data well compared to the reference model. Furthermore, the estimated values of equivalent parameters between the two models were in very good concordance. This comparative study demonstrates that our model not only offers a mechanistic approach to describing tumor growth, it also has comparable robustness to the reference model when applied to real experimental data. Although the model comparison was done with real data, the cost of the extra parameters could become apparent with sparse data [46]. Even though our model is based on biological processes, some of the concepts we introduce are difficult if not impossible to confirm with current technologies. For instance the proliferation efficiency, described by the $p(w)$ function, cannot be confirmed as it is not feasible to track *in vivo* cell division in real time. Certain model parameters, such as the initial tumor growth rate, kin_0, the doubling time, T, and time for tumor death, T_A, are all values that cannot be confirmed *in vivo*. Therefore the accuracy of the model and its parameter estimates must be taken with caution. One of the greatest limitations of many TGI models is the oversimplification of the cellular composition of tumors. Tumor heterogeneity has been widely observed both clinically and experimentally [47–50]. However, in order to characterize heterogeneous cell populations, additional biomarkers are required. Although it is very feasible to quantify mixed cell populations through flow cytometry or histological techniques, such experiments are invasive and would disrupt accurate collection of continuous tumor growth data. Mixed cell population modeling would also require additional model parameters. In regards to model parsimony and given the nature of the available data, many established TGI models have relied on the simplification of the tumor cellular composition [8,10,11].

The lifespan TGI model presented in this report is a novel mechanistic approach to modeling tumor growth and tumor growth inhibition by anti-cancer drugs. We have demonstrated that the model has the versatility to address different tumor growth kinetics and different drug mechanisms of action, and the robustness to provide precise parameter estimates from experimental data. Most importantly, the mechanistic nature of the model and the parameters has biological relevance, which can have real implications in inter-species predictions.

Supporting Information

Appendix S1   Derivation of model equations.

Appendix S2   Explicit solution to the tumor growth model with constant cell division efficiency.

Appendix S3   Calculation of the slope of the tumor size vs. time curve.

Material S1   Non-cycle-specific model run script.

Material S2   Non-cycle-specific model file.

Material S3   Non-cycle-specific model history file.

Material S4   Cycle-specific model run script.

Material S5   Cycle-specific model file.

Material S6   Cycle-specific model history file.

Acknowledgments

We would like to acknowledge the contribution of Mike Grondine in carrying out the in-vivo studies for AZD1208. GM was supported in part by a postdoctoral fellowship through AstraZeneca Model-based Drug Discovery program.

Author Contributions

Conceived and designed the experiments: FG PS. Analyzed the data: GM WK. Wrote the paper: GM FG PS WK.

References

1. Danhof M, de Lange ECM, Della Pasqua OE, Ploeger BA, Voskuyl RA (2008) Mechanism-based pharmacokinetic-pharmacodynamic (PK-PD) modeling in translational drug research. Trends in Pharmacological Sciences 29: 186–191.

2. Schabel FM (1969) The Use of Tumor Growth Kinetics in Planning "Curative" Chemotherapy of Advanced Solid Tumors. Cancer Res 29: 2384–2389.

3. Bajzer Z, Marušić M, Vuk-Pavlović S (1996) Conceptual frameworks for mathematical modeling of tumor growth dynamics. Mathematical and Computer Modelling 23: 31–46.

4. Sachs RK, Hlatky LR, Hahnfeldt P (2001) Simple ODE models of tumor growth and anti-angiogenic or radiation treatment. Mathematical and Computer Modelling 33: 1297–1305.

5. Frei E 3rd, Bickers JN, Hewlett JS, Lane M, Leary WV, et al. (1969) Dose schedule and antitumor studies of arabinosyl cytosine (NSC 63878). Cancer Res 29: 1325–1332.

6. O'Dwyer PJ, Hudes GR, Walczak J, Schilder R, LaCreta F, et al. (1992) Phase I and pharmacokinetic study of the novel platinum analogue CI-973 on a 5-daily dose schedule. Cancer Res 52: 6746–6753.

7. Wiernik PH, Schwartz EL, Strauman JJ, Dutcher JP, Lipton RB, et al. (1987) Phase I clinical and pharmacokinetic study of taxol. Cancer Res 47: 2486–2493.

8. Jumbe NL, Xin Y, Leipold DD, Crocker L, Dugger D, et al. (2010) Modeling the efficacy of trastuzumab-DM1, an antibody drug conjugate, in mice. J Pharmacokinet Pharmacodyn 37: 221–242.

9. Koch G, Walz A, Lahu G, Schropp J (2009) Modeling of tumor growth and anticancer effects of combination therapy. J Pharmacokinet Pharmacodyn 36: 179–197.

10. Lobo ED, Balthasar JP (2002) Pharmacodynamic modeling of chemotherapeutic effects: application of a transit compartment model to characterize methotrexate effects in vitro. AAPS PharmSci 4: E42.

11. Simeoni M, Magni P, Cammia C, De Nicolao G, Croci V, et al. (2004) Predictive pharmacokinetic-pharmacodynamic modeling of tumor growth kinetics in xenograft models after administration of anticancer agents. Cancer Res 64: 1094–1101.

12. Bueno L, de Alwis DP, Pitou C, Yingling J, Lahn M, et al. (2008) Semi-mechanistic modelling of the tumour growth inhibitory effects of LY2157299, a new type I receptor TGF-beta kinase antagonist, in mice. Eur J Cancer 44: 142–150.

13. Ribeiro D, Pinto JM (2009) An integrated network-based mechanistic model for tumor growth dynamics under drug administration. Comput Biol Med 39: 368–384.

14. Tang L, Su J, Huang D-S, Lee DY, Li KC, et al. (2012) An Integrated Multiscale Mechanistic Model for Cancer Drug Therapy. ISRN Biomathematics 2012: 12.

15. Krzyzanski W, Ramakrishnan R, Jusko WJ (1999) Basic pharmacodynamic models for agents that alter production of natural cells. J Pharmacokinet Biopharm 27: 467–489.

16. Krzyzanski W, Jusko WJ (2002) Multiple-pool cell lifespan model of hematologic effects of anticancer agents. J Pharmacokinet Pharmacodyn 29: 311–337.

17. Krzyzanski W, Perez-Ruixo JJ, Vermeulen A (2008) Basic pharmacodynamic models for agents that alter the lifespan distribution of natural cells. J Pharmacokinet Pharmacodyn 35: 349–377.

18. Keeton EK, McEachern K, Dillman KS, Palakurthi S, Cao Y, et al. (2014) AZD1208, a potent and selective pan-Pim kinase inhibitor, demonstrates efficacy in preclinical models of acute myeloid leukemia. Blood 123: 905–913.

19. Schroeder P, Alimzhanov M, Bao L, Liu Z, Brassil PD, et al. (2012) PK/PD/Efficacy characterization of AZ968, a selective CK2 kinase inhibitor. Cancer Research 72.

20. Brattain MG, Fine WD, Khaled FM, Thompson J, Brattain DE (1981) Heterogeneity of malignant cells from a human colonic carcinoma. Cancer Res 41: 1751–1756.

21. Wei N, Chu E, Wipf P, Schmitz JC (2014) Protein kinase d as a potential chemotherapeutic target for colorectal cancer. Mol Cancer Ther 13: 1130–1141.

22. Dayneka NL, Garg V, Jusko WJ (1993) Comparison of four basic models of indirect pharmacodynamic responses. J Pharmacokinet Biopharm 21: 457–478.

23. Krzyzanski W, Perez Ruixo JJ (2012) Lifespan based indirect response models. J Pharmacokinet Pharmacodyn 39: 109–123.

24. Ribba B, Watkin E, Tod M, Girard P, Grenier E, et al. (2011) A model of vascular tumour growth in mice combining longitudinal tumour size data with histological biomarkers. Eur J Cancer 47: 479–490.

25. Creton G, Benassi M, Di Staso M, Ingrosso G, Giubilei C, et al. (2006) The time factor in oncology: consequences on tumour volume and therapeutic planning. J Exp Clin Cancer Res 25: 557–573.

26. Laird AK (1964) Dynamics of Tumor Growth. Br J Cancer 18: 490–502.

27. Panetta JC (1995) A logistic model of periodic chemotherapy. Applied Mathematics Letters 8: 83–86.

28. Wennerberg J, Willen R, Trope C (1988) Changes in histology and cell kinetics during the growth course of xenografted squamous cell carcinoma. Arch Otolaryngol Head Neck Surg 114: 781–787.

29. Hamed SS, Straubinger RM, Jusko WJ (2013) Pharmacodynamic modeling of cell cycle and apoptotic effects of gemcitabine on pancreatic adenocarcinoma cells. Cancer Chemother Pharmacol 72: 553–563.

30. Yang J, Mager DE, Straubinger RM (2010) Comparison of two pharmacodynamic transduction models for the analysis of tumor therapeutic responses in model systems. AAPS J 12: 1–10.

31. Parker WB (2009) Enzymology of purine and pyrimidine antimetabolites used in the treatment of cancer. Chem Rev 109: 2880–2893.

32. Shampine LF, Thompson S (2001) Solving DDEs in Matlab. Applied Numerical Mathematics 37: 441–458.

33. Matsuo Y, Drexler HG, Kaneda K, Kojima K, Ohtsuki Y, et al. (2003) Megakaryoblastic leukemia cell line MOLM-16 derived from minimally differentiated acute leukemia with myeloid/NK precursor phenotype. Leuk Res 27: 165–171.

34. Hlatky L, Olesiak M, Hahnfeldt P (1996) Measurement of potential doubling time for human tumor xenografts using the cytokinesis-block method. Cancer Res 56: 1660–1663.

35. Bassukas ID (1994) Comparative Gompertzian analysis of alterations of tumor growth patterns. Cancer Res 54: 4385–4392.

36. Brunton GF, Wheldon TE (1980) The Gompertz equation and the construction of tumour growth curves. Cell Tissue Kinet 13: 455–460.

37. Hart D, Shochat E, Agur Z (1998) The growth law of primary breast cancer as inferred from mammography screening trials data. Br J Cancer 78: 382–387.

38. Skehan P (1986) On the normality of growth dynamics of neoplasms in vivo: a data base analysis. Growth 50: 496–515.

39. Friberg LE, Karlsson MO (2003) Mechanistic models for myelosuppression. Invest New Drugs 21: 183–194.

40. Budha NR, Kovar A, Meibohm B (2011) Comparative performance of cell life span and cell transit models for describing erythropoietic drug effects. AAPS J 13: 650–661.

41. Koch G, Schropp J (2012) General relationship between transit compartments and lifespan models. J Pharmacokinet Pharmacodyn 39: 343–355.

42. Jusko W (1973) A pharmacodynamic model for cell-cycle-specific chemotherapeutic agents. J Pharmacokinet Biopharm 1: 175–200.

43. Kozusko F, Chen P, Grant SG, Day BW, Panetta JC (2001) A mathematical model of in vitro cancer cell growth and treatment with the antimitotic agent curacin A. Math Biosci 170: 1–16.

44. Panetta JC, Evans WE, Cheok MH (2006) Mechanistic mathematical modelling of mercaptopurine effects on cell cycle of human acute lymphoblastic leukaemia cells. Br J Cancer 94: 93–100.

45. Kim M, Gillies RJ, Rejniak KA (2013) Current advances in mathematical modeling of anti-cancer drug penetration into tumor tissues. Front Oncol 3: 278.

46. Shivva V, Korell J, Tucker IG, Duffull SB (2013) An approach for identifiability of population pharmacokinetic-pharmacodynamic models. CPT Pharmacometrics Syst Pharmacol 2: e49.

47. Campbell PJ, Pleasance ED, Stephens PJ, Dicks E, Rance R, et al. (2008) Subclonal phylogenetic structures in cancer revealed by ultra-deep sequencing. Proc Natl Acad Sci U S A 105: 13081–13086.

48. Dexter DL, Kowalski HM, Blazar BA, Fligiel Z, Vogel R, et al. (1978) Heterogeneity of tumor cells from a single mouse mammary tumor. Cancer Res 38: 3174–3181.

49. Inda MM, Bonavia R, Mukasa A, Narita Y, Sah DW, et al. (2010) Tumor heterogeneity is an active process maintained by a mutant EGFR-induced cytokine circuit in glioblastoma. Genes Dev 24: 1731–1745.

50. Macintosh CA, Stower M, Reid N, Maitland NJ (1998) Precise microdissection of human prostate cancers reveals genotypic heterogeneity. Cancer Res 58: 23–28.

15

Investigation of Cross-Species Translatability of Pharmacological MRI in Awake Nonhuman Primate - A Buprenorphine Challenge Study

Stephanie Seah[1,2]*, Abu Bakar Ali Asad[1,2], Richard Baumgartner[3], Dai Feng[3], Donald S. Williams[1], Elaine Manigbas[4], John D. Beaver[4¤a], Torsten Reese[2¤b], Brian Henry[2], Jeffrey L. Evelhoch[1], Chih-Liang Chin[1,2]

1 Imaging, Merck & Co. Inc., West Point, Pennsylvania, United States of America, 2 Translational Medicine Research Centre, MSD, Singapore, Singapore, 3 Biostatistics and Research Decision Sciences, Merck & Co. Inc., Rahway, New Jersey, United States of America, 4 Imaging, Maccine Pte Ltd, Singapore, Singapore

Abstract

Background: Pharmacological MRI (phMRI) is a neuroimaging technique where drug-induced hemodynamic responses can represent a pharmacodynamic biomarker to delineate underlying biological consequences of drug actions. In most preclinical studies, animals are anesthetized during image acquisition to minimize movement. However, it has been demonstrated anesthesia could attenuate basal neuronal activity, which can confound interpretation of drug-induced brain activation patterns. Significant efforts have been made to establish awake imaging in rodents and nonhuman primates (NHP). Whilst various platforms have been developed for imaging awake NHP, comparison and validation of phMRI data as translational biomarkers across species remain to be explored.

Methodology: We have established an awake NHP imaging model that encompasses comprehensive acclimation procedures with a dedicated animal restrainer. Using a cerebral blood volume (CBV)-based phMRI approach, we have determined differential responses of brain activation elicited by the systemic administration of buprenorphine (0.03 mg/kg i.v.), a partial μ-opioid receptor agonist, in the same animal under awake and anesthetized conditions. Additionally, region-of-interest analyses were performed to determine regional drug-induced CBV time-course data and corresponding area-under-curve (AUC) values from brain areas with high density of μ-opioid receptors.

Principal Findings: In awake NHPs, group-level analyses revealed buprenorphine significantly activated brain regions including, thalamus, striatum, frontal and cingulate cortices (paired *t*-test, versus saline vehicle, $p < 0.05$, $n = 4$). This observation is strikingly consistent with μ-opioid receptor distribution depicted by [6-O-[^{11}C]methyl]buprenorphine ([^{11}C]BPN) positron emission tomography imaging study in baboons. Furthermore, our findings are consistent with previous buprenorphine phMRI studies in humans and conscious rats which collectively demonstrate the cross-species translatability of awake imaging. Conversely, no significant change in activated brain regions was found in the same animals imaged under the anesthetized condition.

Conclusions: Our data highlight the utility and importance of awake NHP imaging as a translational imaging biomarker for drug research.

Editor: Alessandro Gozzi, Italian Institute of Technology, Italy

Funding: This research was funded by Merck & Co. The authors would like to declare that the following individuals are current or former employees of the funder - Stephanie Seah, Abu Bakar Ali Asad, Richard Baumgartner, Dai Feng, Don Williams, Torsten Reese, Brian Henry, Jeff Evelhoch and Chih-Liang Chin. Their roles include study design, data collection and analysis, decision to publish and preparation of the manuscript.

Competing Interests: Merck provided all funds for this work. As mentioned in the financial disclosures, some authors are current or former employees of Merck and may own stock or hold stock options in Merck. Co-authors Elaine Manigbas and John Beaver were employees of Maccine Pte. Ltd.

* Email: stephanie.seah@merck.com

¤a Current address: Translational Imaging, Global Pharmaceutical Research and Development, Abbott Park, Illonois, United States of America
¤b Current address: MR Imaging, CIC biomaGUNE, San Sebastlán, Gipuzkoa, Spain

Introduction

Pharmacological MRI (phMRI) is a neuroimaging technique that allows characterization of changes in neural activity following drug challenge. Drug-induced pharmacodynamic responses detected from alterations in blood oxygenation level dependence (BOLD) signals or relative cerebral blood volume/flow (rCBV/rCBF) can provide as imaging biomarkers to delineate the central effect of drug actions [1,2,3,4]. As a result, significant effort has been devoted to implement phMRI as a translational research tool to develop novel CNS compounds, considering that this *in vivo* imaging technique can be performed in both animals [5,6,7,8] and humans [9,10,11,12]. To date, phMRI has been adopted to interrogate several key neurotransmitter systems, and these findings collectively have highlighted the value of phMRI to elucidate neurobiological mechanisms of drug actions and to gain better understanding of human diseases. In most preclinical imaging studies, animals were anesthetized during image acquisition to minimize movements; however, several lines of evidence have shown that the use of anesthesia could attenuate basal neuronal activity and likely confound drug-induced brain activation patterns [13,14,15,16,17,18,19,20]. Therefore, it is critical to establish translational platforms that permit investigation of pharmacological responses of experimental therapeutics in preclinical species, healthy volunteers and eventually in patients. To this end, phMRI in awake animals has been extensively pursued across various species, such as rodents [19,21,22,23] and nonhuman primates (NHPs) [17,18,24,25,26,27,28].

Awake NHP models are particularly attractive for neuroscience research, in light of greater similarities with humans in clinical and pathological characteristics [29]. It has been demonstrated that NHP and human brains share features in neuronal cytoarchitecture [30] and functional connections [31]. Additionally, the activity and distribution of neurotransmitter systems [32,33], drug metabolism and pharmacokinetic responses [34] are more comparable to human in NHP than in rodent. Nonetheless, despite the improved cross-species translatability offered by awake NHP imaging, animal movements during image acquisition can pose as a major obstacle, since excessive motion can lead to image blurring or ghosting artifacts, and higher baseline signal fluctuations that could diminish sensitivity to detect changes of drug-induced phMRI signals. Furthermore, the level of resting state stability could vary significantly among imaging sessions, which can attribute to compromised test-retest reliability and hindrance to conducting longitudinal studies. To circumvent this challenge, several groups have attempted to develop awake NHP imaging paradigms, in which extensive acclimation procedures are often required [17,27,35,36,37]. Animals were trained to remain still and gradually habituate to the actual scanning environment while using a dedicated animal restrainer that affords better securing of the animal's head and/or body, such as a head-post model [35] or non-invasive helmet approaches [27,36]. In addition, improved data acquisition methods [37], use of contrast agent [38] and optimized data analysis strategies [39] have also been explored to enhance phMRI sensitivity. Nonetheless, it will be essential to establish a systematic approach to evaluate phMRI baseline signals attributable to animal movements and thus characterize the utility, or limitation, of these awake imaging platforms.

Buprenorphine is an opioid agonist that has a high affinity to various opioid receptors, such as μ, δ, κ subtypes [40], and it has been used clinically to treat opiate addiction or pain [41,42]. The clinical efficacy of buprenorphine for pain and opiate addiction is thought to be due to partial agonism at μ–opioid receptors and/or antagonism at κ–opioid receptors [41,42]. Previous studies performed by Upadhyay et al. have shown that buprenorphine elicited BOLD responses in humans correspond to brain regions with abundant μ–opioid receptors and modulate brain functional connectivity ascribed to pain-processing circuitry [43]. Interestingly, congruency in the spatial pattern of buprenorphine-induced brain activation between humans and conscious rats was also observed [21]. In light of these studies in both humans and awake rats, a phMRI study of buprenorphine in awake NHP can assess the congruency of imaging endpoints across species, and thereby determine the utility of an awake NHP imaging platform for translational research.

In this study, we sought to investigate differential responses in brain activity in NHP produced by the systemic administration of buprenorphine under awake and anesthetized conditions. We hypothesized that buprenorphine-induced brain activation pattern observed from awake NHP should highlight the known μ-opioid receptor distribution [44,45] and afford investigation of cross-species translatability of awake NHP imaging in conjunction with previous phMRI data obtained from humans and awake rats [21,43].

Toward this goal, we first constructed a dedicated animal restrainer based on a design previously reported by Andersen et al. [35] and then developed an awake NHP training protocol. Each animal received comprehensive training, including incremental sessions in a mock MRI scanner and acclimatization to the actual imaging environment. The effectiveness of training was evaluated via measured circulating cortisol levels and behavioral scores (e.g. rated by the trainer). Consequently, these criteria were used to select animals thought to be most habituated to the scanner environment for subsequent imaging studies. During the imaging phase, resting state BOLD signals were acquired under awake (both test and re-test) and anesthetized conditions to determine resting state baseline stability and reliability, which served as a measure of the effectiveness or limitation of our acclimation procedures. To assess the cross-species translatability of our awake NHP platform, we imaged brain activity induced by buprenorphine infusion (0.03 mg/kg i.v.) using a CBV-based phMRI approach, where an ultrasmall superparamagnetic iron oxide (USPIO) contrast agent was applied to increase sensitivity [46]. Imaging experiments were conducted following a within-subject study design to differentiate the central effect of buprenorphine and saline vehicle in NHPs imaged under both awake and isoflurane-anesthetized conditions. To characterize the regional specificity of drug effect, a group-level and region-of-interest (ROI) data analysis pipeline was implemented based on a standard monkey brain atlas [47], where drug-induced CBV-based signal change time-course data and corresponding area-under-curve (AUC) were derived from selected brain regions with high density of μ–opioid receptors.

Materials and Methods

Ethics Statement

The following experiments were conducted in accordance with the Institutional Animal Care and Use Committee at Merck & Co. The current study, in addition to its protocol, was approved by the Institutional Animal Care and Use Committee at Merck & Co (Permit Number: 11102130610016). No animals were sacrificed for the purpose of this experiment. Trained veterinarians and animal technicians were involved in the care of the animals as well as all the animal procedures performed during this study.

Animals

Adult female cynomolgus monkeys (Macaca fascicularis, PT Prestasi Fauna Nusantara, Indonesia; $n = 12$, age = 4 years - 6 years, body weight = 2 kg~4 kg) were allocated for this study. Animals were pair housed at the Maccine facility in temperature- (18 °C–26 °C) and humidity-controlled (30%–70%) rooms maintained on a 12:12 light/dark cycle with lights on at 7:00 AM. Mirrors were placed outside the home cage, and cage toys/manipulative enrichment, such as Kong toys, Flexi keys, were provided and rotated every week. Radios and televisions were also used as supplementary enrichments. Animals were fed with a diet of monkey chow free of animal protein, as well as a controlled amount of fruits or vegetables, offered twice daily. Aside from daily fruit rations, frozen homemade treats (i.e. fruits, raisins, cereals, etc.) were provided once a week. Tap water was offered ad libitum. Prior to the commencement of the study, a complete physical examination, including hematological/blood chemistry analysis, was performed and reviewed by the attending veterinarian.

Awake Training Protocol

Based on previous work done by Andersen et al. [35], a dedicated animal restrainer was constructed, and the animals were habituated to the restrainer and MRI scanner environment for awake imaging. To alleviate stress and minimize movement during awake imaging, each animal was blindfolded and trained in a phased manner, gradually habituated through different training procedures over several months (see Fig. 1; Phase 1a–c). As shown in Figure 1, our training protocol includes *restrainer training*, *mock scanner training* and *head-post surgery and head-restraint tethering training* phases. During each training session, animal's behavioral gestures (e.g. vocalization, excessive movement, head/body turn) were monitored and scored by a trainer. A low cumulative behavioral score at the end of the training was indicative of a well-behaved animal, suitable for the imaging study. Briefly, during Phase 1a: *restrainer training*, animals were trained to remain still in a primate restraining chair for a period of 30 minutes which was gradually prolonged to a steady state of 120 minutes. Upon achieving this requirement, animals were placed in a prone position in a confinement apparatus for 120 minutes to acclimatize to the restrainer environment. Next, animals were gradually exposed to an MRI-compatible restrainer and the duration of the training period increased by 15 minutes weekly until a steady state of 120 minutes was reached. Additionally, to assess the stress level associated with training procedures, cortisol concentrations were also measured using an electrochemiluminescence immunoassay toolkit (ECLIA, Roche Diagnostics, Singapore), in which blood samples (2 mL) were collected prior to placing the animals inside the restrainer tube and 90-minute-post training. Based on the measured cortisol levels and cumulative behavioral scores over the course of Phase 1a, eight

animals were selected and progressed to Phase 1b (*mock scanner training*).

In the *mock scanner training* phase, animals were placed in the restrainer in a mock scanner for a 2-hour time period every other day, in order to habituate them to the scanner environment. At the last training session of this phase, cortisol measurements were repeated (pre- and post-training, $n = 8$) to evaluate the effectiveness of acclimation, and the results were compared with a non-trained control cohort ($n = 6$). Finally, in the *head-post surgery and head-restraint tethering* phase for the selected animals, the head-post component of the restrainer was surgically attached to the skull of each subject [35]. Head tethering restraint training started after animals had fully recovered from the surgery and occurred twice a week until the actual imaging study.

Animal Preparation for the Imaging Study

Animals progressed from the training procedures to imaging studies (see Fig. 1), where they were imaged under both awake and anesthetized conditions for the stability and test-retest reliability study of resting state BOLD signal and subsequently the phMRI experiments. For the anesthetized imaging study, animals were sedated with ketamine (10 mg/kg IM) for induction, while ear plugs and eye lubricant were applied to all the animals, prior to bringing them into the scanner room. The animal was then placed on the patient bed of the MRI scanner in a prone position and ventilated by an MRI-compatible ventilator and bellows system (SurgiVet, Dublin, OH). Anesthesia was maintained through inhalation of a mixture of isoflurane (2%) in medical air. Physiological parameters of each animal, including heart rate, SpO_2, $EtCO_2$, and respiration rate were monitored and recorded throughout the imaging session using an MR-compatible Datex-Ohmeda physiological monitoring system (GE Healthcare, WI). The temperature of the animal was measured via a fiber-optic temperature sensor system (OpSens, Quebec, Canada) and recorded periodically throughout the experiment. For the awake imaging study, animals were blindfolded and placed in a sphinx position within the restrainer used during the training procedures.

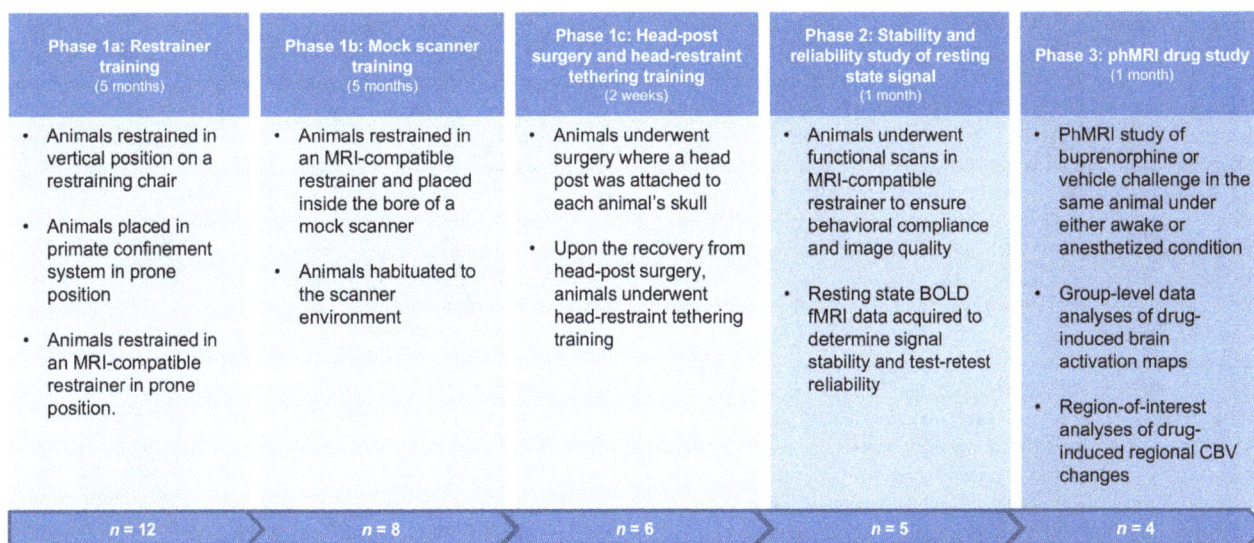

Phase 1a: Restrainer training (5 months)	Phase 1b: Mock scanner training (5 months)	Phase 1c: Head-post surgery and head-restraint tethering training (2 weeks)	Phase 2: Stability and reliability study of resting state signal (1 month)	Phase 3: phMRI drug study (1 month)
• Animals restrained in vertical position on a restraining chair • Animals placed in primate confinement system in prone position • Animals restrained in an MRI-compatible restrainer in prone position.	• Animals restrained in an MRI-compatible restrainer and placed inside the bore of a mock scanner • Animals habituated to the scanner environment	• Animals underwent surgery where a head post was attached to each animal's skull • Upon the recovery from head-post surgery, animals underwent head-restraint tethering training	• Animals underwent functional scans in MRI-compatible restrainer to ensure behavioral compliance and image quality • Resting state BOLD fMRI data acquired to determine signal stability and test-retest reliability	• PhMRI study of buprenorphine or vehicle challenge in the same animal under either awake or anesthetized condition • Group-level data analyses of drug-induced brain activation maps • Region-of-interest analyses of drug-induced regional CBV changes
$n = 12$	$n = 8$	$n = 6$	$n = 5$	$n = 4$

Figure 1. Study protocol of awake imaging in non-human primates. Initial Phase 1a–c focus on the training procedures to reduce animal movement/stress during awake imaging; Phase 2 was the assessment of the stability of resting state signal and its test-retest reliability; Phase 3 was the within-subject pharmacological challenge study, where buprenorphine (0.03 mg/kg i.v.) and vehicle were given to the same animals under awake and anesthetized conditions.

A customized head radiofrequency (RF) coil was securely attached to the head-post of the animal. Also, during each awake imaging session, at least one animal trainer would be assigned to visually monitor the animals.

Evaluation of the Effectiveness or Limitation of Awake Training Protocol

All imaging experiments were conducted on a 3 Tesla TIM Trio MRI scanner (Siemens Medical Solutions, Erlangen, Germany) using a dedicated 8-channel phased-array head coil (RAPID Biomedical GmbH, Germany). Resting state BOLD signal was collected by a single-shot gradient-echo EPI pulse sequence (TR/TE $= 3$ s/21 ms, in-plane pixel size $= 1$ mm $\times 1$ mm, slice thickness $= 2$ mm, and 24 slices with no gap), and 810 imaging volumes (40 minutes in total) were acquired. High resolution brain anatomical images (TR/TE $= 700$ ms/13 ms, in-plane pixel size $= 0.67$ mm $\times 0.67$ mm) of individual animals were also acquired in order to co-register with a standard monkey brain atlas [47] for further group-level and ROI analyses. Resting state BOLD signals were acquired from the same animals imaged under anesthetized and awake conditions separately ($n = 5$). Further, to examine the test-retest reliability of resting state BOLD signal during awake imaging, experiments were repeated on a different day. As a result, each animal was imaged three times in total.

Assessment of Cross-species Translatability of Awake NHP

For the phMRI study, selected animals ($n = 4$) underwent four separate sessions (1-week apart to ensure drug washout) on different days (16 scans in total), where a counterbalanced measures design was used to ensure each animal was imaged under different drug challenge (vehicle or buprenorphine) or imaging condition (awake or anesthetized). For each imaging experiment, brain anatomical image and functional datasets were acquired using the same imaging pulse sequences and parameters described above (see *Evaluation of the Effectiveness or Limitation of Awake Training Protocol* section).

To increase the sensitivity of phMRI signals [46], a CBV-based approach using a USPIO contrast agent, 7.5 mg/kg i.v. of Ferumoxytol (AMAG Pharmaceutical, Cambridge MA), was used. A tail vein line was cannulated for the administration of contrast agent and drug, while the indwelling catheter was attached to a saline-filled syringe placed on an infusion pump (Harvard Apparatus, Holliston, MA) located outside the scanner room. All animals were administered intravenously with either 0.03 mg/kg of buprenorphine (Reckitt Benckiser Pharmaceuticals, UK) or saline vehicle. Intramuscular injection of buprenorphine at 0.01 mg/kg or 0.03 mg/kg has been commonly used for analgesia in nonhuman primates [48] and we have adopted the higher dose in the current study. Notably, different doses of buprenorphine were selected in previous phMRI studies in rodent (0.04 mg/kg and 0.1 mg/kg i.v.) or human (0.2 mg/70 kg i.v.) [21,43]. The following imaging protocol was carried out: (i) 5-minute pre-contrast data acquisition, (ii) bolus injection of the contrast agent via the tail vein line (total injection volume $= 2$ mL), (iii) 10-minute pre-drug baseline acquisition (post-contrast), (iv) infusion of either buprenorphine at 0.03 mg/kg i.v. or saline vehicle (total injection volume $= 3$ mL) was split into three infusion periods (30 s each) separated by a 1.5-minute interval, in order to minimize potential respiratory suppression related to the buprenorphine injection [43]. Finally, (v) 20-minute period of post-drug imaging acquisition.

Data Analysis

Data analyses were conducted using the FMRIB Software Library (FSL) (http://www.fmrib.ox.au.ul/fls) and in-house Matlab (MathWorks, Natick, MA). First, voxels of the brain were extracted using a brain extraction tool (FSL BET). To characterize the fluctuation of resting state BOLD signals obtained from awake and anesthetized imaging experiments, time-course data of each voxel was derived and expressed as a percentage change relative to the average signal intensity over the entire imaging time period. Then, for each voxel the mean percentage change was calculated by averaging the absolute value of percentage change over time. Consequently, the mean value and standard deviation over the entire brain volume were calculated and reported. Finally, a Bland-Altman plot was used to assess test-retest reliability of awake resting state BOLD signal.

For the phMRI data analysis, FSL was used. Specifically, our data analysis pipeline included the following steps: motion correction (FSL MCFLIRT), brain extraction, spatial smoothing (FWHM $= 2$ mm) and co-registration to a standard monkey brain atlas [47]. To depict activated brain regions, time-course relative CBV change, $\Delta rCBV(t)$, was first calculated from the raw data using a known relationship [46,49],

$$\Delta rCBV(t) = \ln[S_{POST}/S(t)]/\ln[S_{PRE}/S_{POST}] \qquad (1)$$

where t is time after drug injection, $S(t)$ is the signal intensity after the drug infusion, S_{POST} is the mean pre-drug baseline signal intensity over the 10-minute period, post contrast agent administration, and S_{PRE} is the mean signal intensity over the 5-minute period, prior to the administration of contrast agent. Then, a general linear model (GLM) was used for the subject-level analysis, where a linear ramp model was used to mimic the infusion response, while the elimination of buprenorphine was based on the known plasma pharmacokinetic of buprenorphine in dogs (brain half-life ~4.5 hr) [50]. Due to the relatively long onset of the ramp function compared to the hemodynamic response function (HRF), the ramp stimulus function in our GLM was not convolved with HRF [43]. To perform unbiased univariate linear regression analysis, nuisance regressors were prepared that account for most of the confounding explanatory variables (EVs), where the mean time-course signals extracted from the ventricles and white matter were included to regress out additional confounds related to physiological noises and/or linear drifts. Further, an in-house Matlab script was written to identify excessive intensity changes (head movement) between imaging time-points, as a de-spiking in the EV. Spike detection was implemented using a median absolute residual variation (MARV) score-based approach [51], while imaging volumes with motion greater than half of a voxel were identified as spikes.

For the group-level and ROI analyses, functional data of each animal was first co-registered to the individual's anatomical images by rigid body translations and rotations and subsequently into a template monkey brain atlas [47] using 12 degrees of freedom affine transformation. These calculated transformation matrix parameters were then applied to the functional dataset and derived statistical maps. Group comparisons were conducted using a mixed-effects paired t-test (FSL FLAME) to determine the group means of the differential effect of vehicle and buprenorphine in both anesthetized and awake animals, threshold at p<0.05, in order to identify brain regions affected by the drug or vehicle challenge under awake and anesthetized imaging. In addition, to illustrate the temporal dynamics of rCBV change, time-course data for each imaging condition from selected brain regions were

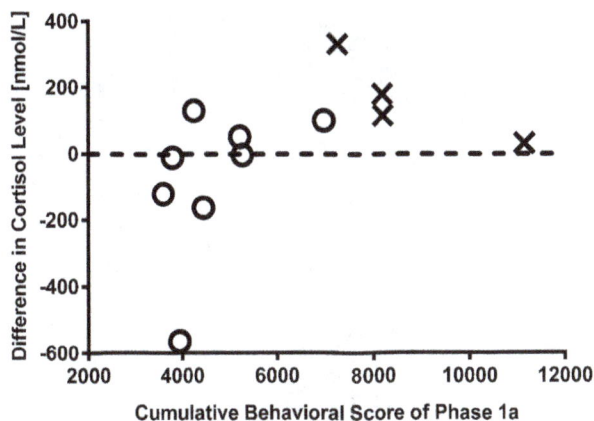

Figure 2. Differences in plasma cortisol concentration and cumulative behavioral scores during Phase 1a used to select animals for Phase 1b. Cumulative behavioral scores over the Phase 1a training obtained from all animals ($n = 12$), in which animals with lower behavioral scores ($n = 8$, 'O') were selected to transition into the Phase 1b study and ones with higher scores were deselected ($n = 4$, '×'). In addition, to assess the stress level during the awake training, plasma cortisol concentrations were measured from these animals at two separate time points (~ one month apart) during this phase, and results indicated that the reduction in cortical level is likely associated with better habituation (i.e. lower behavioral scores).

extracted, detrended and plotted. Regional time-course data was calculated by averaging the rCBV change over all the supra-threshold voxels within specific brain regions. Results obtained from the vehicle infusion were exploited to detrend buprenorphine data on a region-by-region basis. Also, ROI analyses of drug-induced ΔrCBV time-course data were performed, in which AUC were obtained from brain regions with high density of μ-opioid receptor such as putamen, caudate, thalamus, cingulate cortex and frontal cortex, where regional AUC values (mean ± SEM) were

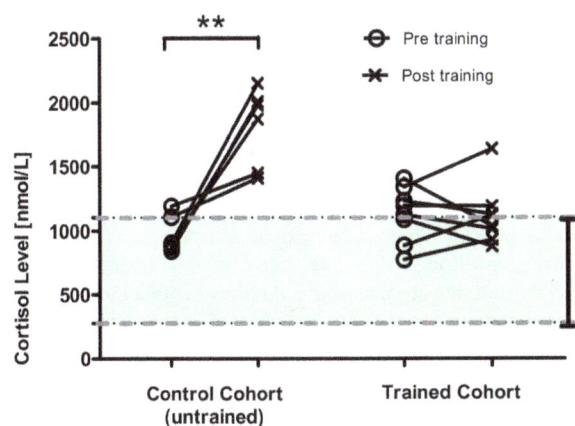

Figure 3. Awake training increased plasma cortisol concentrations in untrained animals, but not in trained animals. Plasma cortisol concentrations measured from the animals ($n = 8$) at prior- and post-90-minute training session during the Phase 1b period. Results indicate that, at the end of training session cortisol levels are significantly elevated in untrained/control animals ($n = 6$), while no significant change was observed in habituated animals (paired t-test, **$p < 0.01$). The dash lines highlight the range of normal cortisol concentration observed in cynomolgus monkeys (276 nmol/L to 1104 nmol/L) [52].

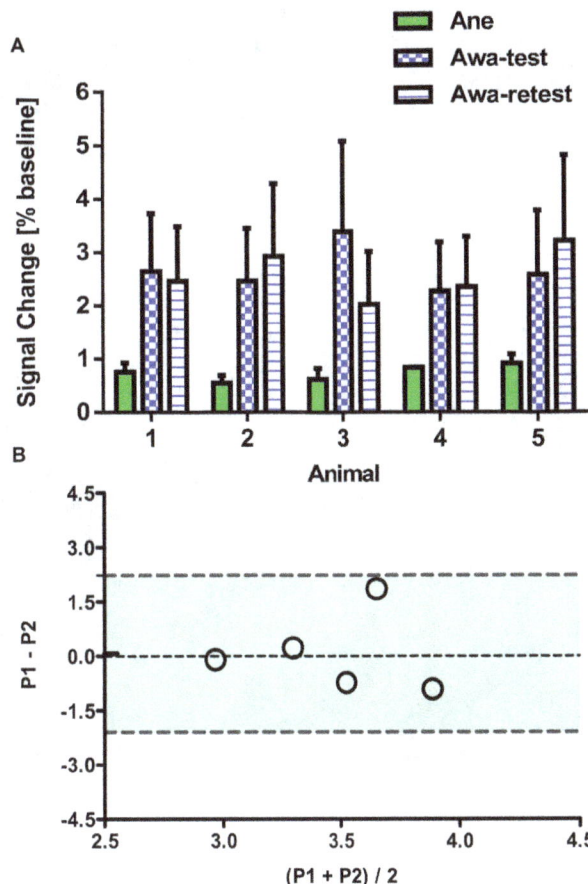

Figure 4. Comparison of resting state stability between anesthetized and awake imaging and test-retest reliability of awake baseline signal. (A) Resting state variation of BOLD signal (mean ± SD) obtained from each non-human primate (NHP) imaged under either awake (Awa, test and retest) or anesthetized (Ane) condition. (B) Bland-Altman plot for awake imaging data and the dash lines highlight the 95% limits of agreement (P1: represents the first test, P2 represents the retest).

calculated from all animals treated with either buprenorphine or vehicle and imaged under both anesthetized and awake conditions. Finally, calculated AUC data were subjected to a paired t-test (JMP 7.0.1, SAS Institute, Cary NC), with differences considered statistically significant at $p < 0.05$.

Results

Behavioral Scores and Cortisol Levels for Animal Selection

Cumulative behavioral scores obtained from all the animals ($n = 12$) over the entire Phase 1a period are plotted in Figure 2, in which animals with lower overall behavioral scores (better habituated) were selected to transition from Phase 1a to 1b ($n = 8$). These results demonstrate that levels of acclimation can vary within the training cohort, and thereby the selection of desired animals is essential. Within this phase, differences in the cortisol levels measured at two time points (separated by a month) are shown in Figure 2, indicating that elevated cortisol levels are likely observed from animals with higher behavioral scores. To assess the effect of training on stress levels, Figure 3 illustrates the cortisol concentrations obtained from untrained/control animals

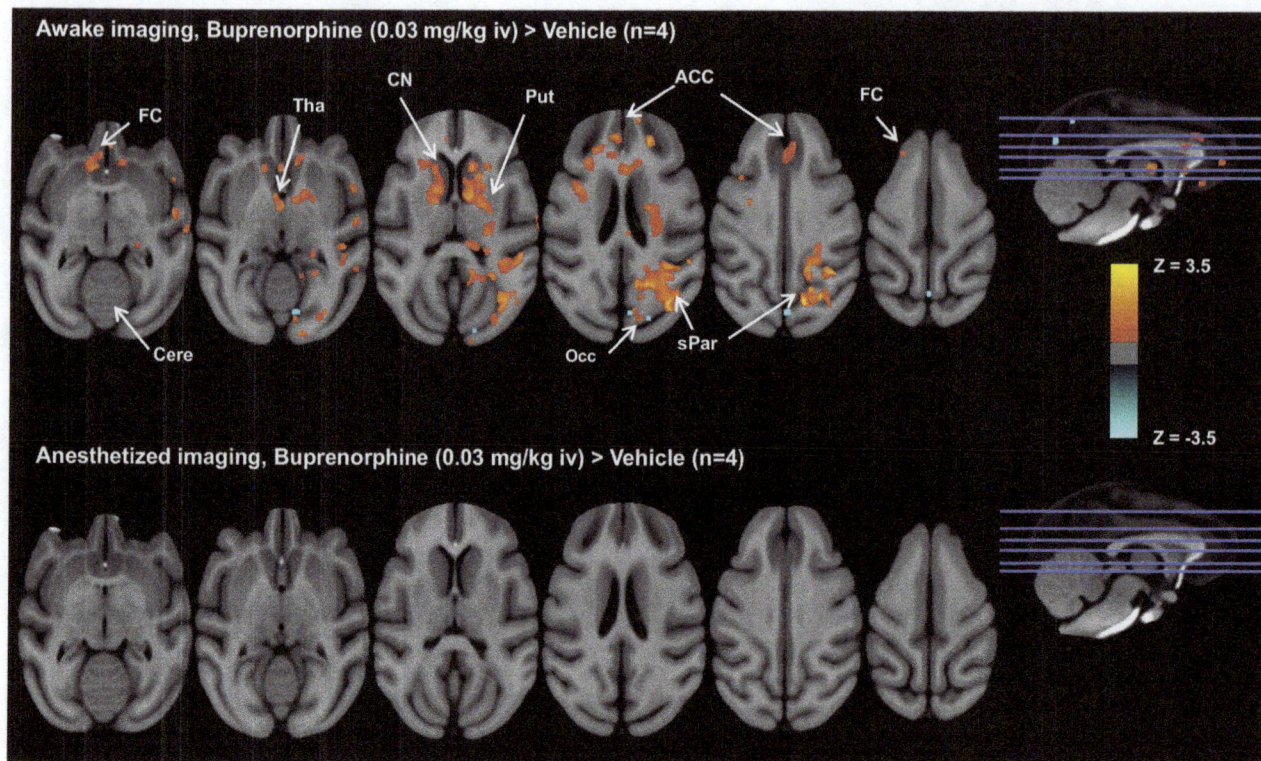

Figure 5. Group comparisons of brain activation patterns between buprenorphine and vehicle under awake and anesthetized imaging. Group comparisons of brain activation patterns showing significant effect of buprenorphine versus vehicle (paired *t*-test, p<0.05, *n* = 4) under awake and anesthetized imaging. In the awake study, buprenorphine activates brain regions with a high density of μ-opioid receptor, including frontal cortex (FC), thalamus (Tha), anterior cingulate cortices (ACC), caudate nucleus (CN), putamen (Put), and superior parietal lobule (sPar), and limited deactivation was found in occipital cortex (Occ). In contrast, no significant difference in brain activation between buprenorphine and vehicle infusion was observed in anesthetized animals.

($n = 6$) as well as our imaging cohort ($n = 8$) at pre- and 90-minute-post training session (Phase 1b). As shown, cortisol levels were significantly elevated in untrained animals after they underwent the training session (paired *t*-test, p<0.01), while no significant difference was observed in habituated animals. Further, only one from the trained imaging cohort had cortisol concentrations substantially above the previously reported normal range (between 276 nmol/L and 1104 nmol/L) [52]. The lower cortisol level found in the trained cohort implies reduced stress levels in these animals and effective habituation to the restrainer and MRI scanner environment. Finally, two animals were deselected from the cohort due to medical conditions (unrelated to the training), while the remaining six animals were moved forward to Phase 1c.

Effectiveness or Limitation of Awake Training Protocol

Figure 4A shows the percentage variation in resting state baseline signals within the whole brain volume (mean ± SD) from individual animals imaged under awake and anesthetized conditions. Our data indicate that compared to anesthetized imaging, the level of baseline variation was significantly higher (4~5 fold) under the awake condition (paired *t*-test, p<0.01). This observation is not unexpected, since there was some animal movement during awake imaging. These findings suggest that a larger change in drug-induced phMRI signals may be needed in order to achieve comparable sensitivity offered by imaging anesthetized animals (i.e. to offset the increased baseline noise). Reasonable test-retest reliability was found from the awake baseline data, considering all the data points were within 95%

limits of agreement of the Bland Altman plot (see Fig. 4b). Finally, two animals were deselected from the Phase 3 drug study, due to the increased body weight thus unable to fit into the animal restrainer or the need for repetitive head-post repairs.

Buprenorphine-induced phMRI response under awake and anaesthetized conditions

Figure 5 illustrates group comparisons of brain activation patterns showing significant effect of buprenorphine versus vehicle on rCBV changes (paired t-test, p<0.05, n = 4), while Table 1 lists the results of ROI analyses, including activated brain regions/coordinates, z-statistics, and total percentage activated volumes calculated from the awake study. As shown, under the awake imaging condition, buprenorphine activated brain regions with a high density of μ-opioid receptor including, frontal cortex, thalamus, cingulate cortex, caudate nucleus, putamen, occipital cortex, and superior parietal lobule. Notably, these findings are strikingly consistent with μ-opioid receptor distribution depicted by [6-O-[^{11}C]methyl]buprenorphine ([^{11}C]BPN) positron emission tomography (PET) study in baboons, where the highest [^{11}C]BPN uptakes was observed in striatum (caudate nucleus and putamen) followed by thalamus, cingulate, frontal, parietal, occipital cortices, and then cerebellum [44]. In accordance with the results obtained from the previous study in conscious rodent and human studies [21], similar region-specificity of activated brain structures are also observed in our awake NHP data. Conversely, no significant activation was observed from anesthetized animals (paired *t*-test, vs. vehicle treatment; see Fig. 5B), despite animal

Table 1. Activated brain regions and their volumes induced by buprenorphine infusion derived from the region-of-interest analysis.

Brain Region	Coordinates (X, Y, Z) [mm]	Z-statistics	Activated Volume (percentage) [mm³]
Cingulate cortex	29.7, 70.0, 25.2	2.52	182.52 (10.80%)
Gyrus rectus	29.5, 61.2, 21.0	2.61	44.39 (11.58%)
Orbital gyrus	26.0, 58.7, 19.5	2.39	2.83 (0.38%)
Caudate Nucleus	35.5, 57.2, 28.0	2.54	224.19 (28.51%)
Putamen	24.2, 57.2, 20.7	2.43	17.84 (2.02%)
Superior frontal gyrus	17.5, 54.5, 35.5	2.51	77.17 (1.46%)
Middle frontal gyrus	17.2, 54.7, 35.0	2.54	11.14 (0.86%)
Precentral gyrus	51.5, 50.5, 23.5	2.51	43.16 (0.79%)
Postcentral gyrus	53.0, 42.0, 25.7	2.66	34.48 (1.79%)
Globus pallidus	37.0, 50.2, 25.0	2.46	27.55 (13.42%)
Internal capsule	36.2, 49.7, 24.7	2.49	23.22 (10.56%)
Amygdala	40.5, 48.2, 12.7	2.50	13.94 (2.37%)
Thalamus	34.5, 48.2, 27.0	2.61	34.48 (3.18%)
Hippocampus	43.2, 43.0, 12.7	2.61	24.06 (4.84%)
Insular cortex	46.7, 42.7, 21.2	2.51	1.09 (0.28%)
Inferior temporal gyrus	48.0, 40.7, 9.5	2.33	0.25 (0.03%)
Superior temporal gyrus	50.2, 31.7, 29.5	2.53	213.33 (6.32%)
Middle temporal gyrus	50.5, 31.0, 29.7	2.61	43.61 (2.89%)
Midbrain	36.2, 39.7, 18.2	2.37	3.28 (0.34%)
Pulvinar nuclei	36.5, 36.2, 27.0	2.43	6.19 (6.14%)
Inferior parietal lobe	38.0, 24.5, 36.7	2.63	120.39 (4.32%)
Superior parietal lobe	36.2, 21.2, 34.5	2.61	72.75 (2.56%)
Superior occipital	37.7, 22.5, 35.0	2.61	87.05 (2.58%)
Lateral occipital	34.2, 12.0, 27.5	2.56	68.58 (3.16%)
Cerebellum	35.5, 19.0, 22.7	2.43	5.77 (0.08%)

Brain regions show differential responses of buprenorphine infusion (0.03 mg/kg i.v.) in awake imaging (vs vehicle, paired t-test, $z>2.3$, $n=4$). The z-statistic represents the maximum of each brain region with significant difference in rCBV changes between buprenorphine and vehicle treatments, while the coordinates correspond to the location of individual maxima in the standard monkey brain atlas space [47].

physiological parameters (mean $\pm$ SEM, $n = 4$) being maintained within normal ranges during these experiments (mean heart rate = (119.9 ± 5.1) beats/min, mean SpO_2 = $98.8\%\pm0.6\%$, mean $EtCO_2$ = $22.0\%\pm0.4\%$, and body temperature = 36.5 °C±0.1 °C). These results exemplify the undesired anesthetic-drug interactions embedded in the anesthetized animal experiments, while highlighting the need for awake imaging for phMRI studies.

Plots of time-course rCBV changes derived from our ROI analyses are shown in Figure 6, in which activated brain regions identified in the group-level brain activation maps (see Fig. 5) showed significant increases in rCBV following buprenorphine infusion. Buprenorphine produced significant increases in rCBV change (mean $\pm$ SD) at frontal cortex ($7.3\%\pm0.2\%$), thalamus ($6.5\%\pm0.2\%$), caudate nucleus ($6.2\%\pm0.2\%$), putamen ($5.8\%\pm0.2\%$), and cingulate cortex ($5.1\%\pm0.2\%$). Of note, it appears that rCBV reached the maximum value around 10-minute-post onset of drug infusion and then maintained at steady state that prolonged over the rest of the imaging period. Area-under-curve of the rCBV time-course data over the entire drug infusion period (AUC), or the above-mentioned steady state period (AUC_{ss}), were calculated and shown in Figure 7. Results depicted that both AUC and AUC_{ss} calculated from thalamus, caudate nucleus, and putamen are significantly higher in buprenorphine-

treated awake animals (paired t-test, p<0.05, vs vehicle), whilst no significant increases in AUC and AUC_{ss} were found in any brain region from the anesthetized study.

Discussion

Previous PET studies in baboons with the opioid receptor radioligand, [^{11}C]BPN revealed high binding activity in striatum, thalamus, cingulate gyrus, frontal cortex, parietal cortex, occipital cortex and cerebellum (in a descending order) [44] and these findings agree well with the known opioid receptor distribution in post-mortem human brain [53]. In this work, we found that buprenorphine infusion in awake, but not anesthetized, NHP produced significant and persistent increase in rCBV at specific brain regions including frontal and cingulate cortices, caudate nucleus, putamen, thalamus, parietal cortex and occipital cortices (see Fig. 5). These activated brain regions are consistent with the binding sites of μ–opioid receptors highlighted in the PET study [44], reflecting the underlying drug actions and subsequent biological responses. Recently, Becerra et al. demonstrated that brain regions activated by buprenorphine in awake rats paralleled that observed in humans, in which buprenorphine elicited BOLD signals in somatosensory and cingulate cortices, insula, striatum,

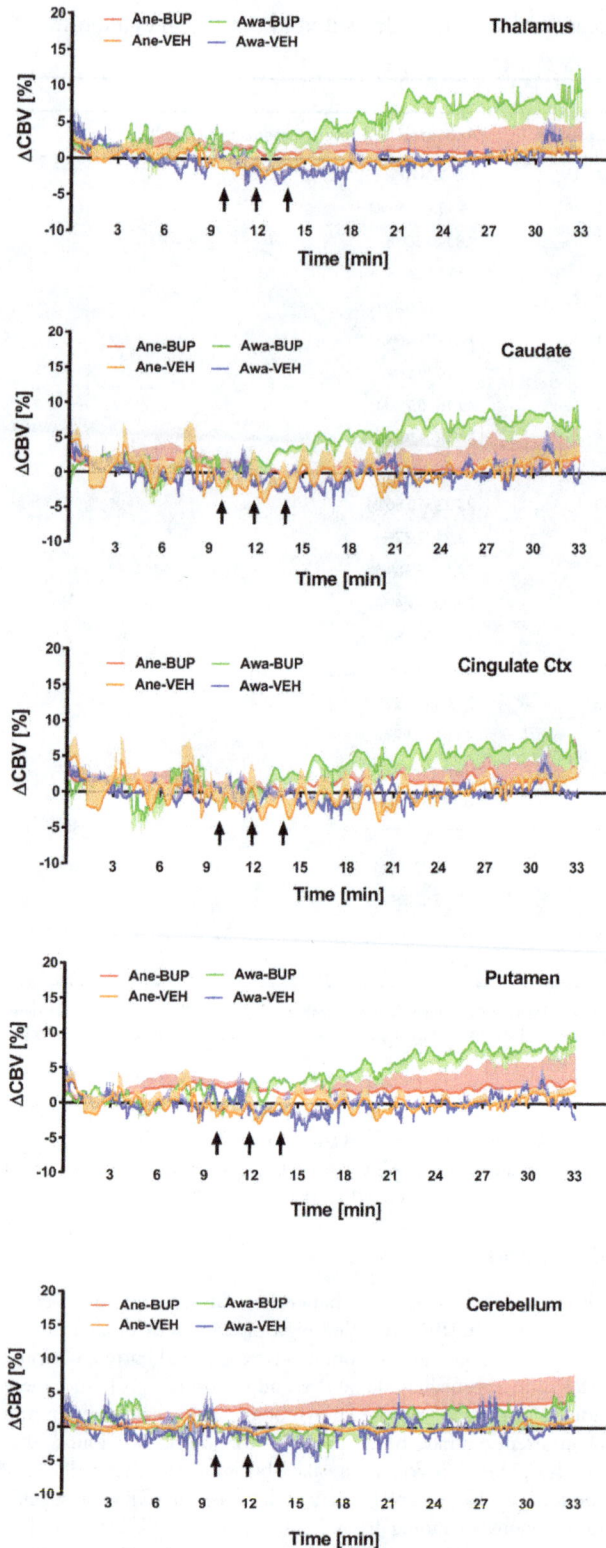

Figure 6. Regional time-course rCBV changes derived from the region-of-interest analysis. Plots of regional time-course rCBV change (mean ± SEM) derived from region-of-interest (ROI) analyses of the imaging cohort (*n* = 4) treated with either buprenorphine (BUP at 0.03 mg/kg i.v.) or vehicle (VEH) and imaged under awake (Awa) or anesthetized (Ane) conditions. The black arrows indicate the three individual dosing time periods (30 s drug infusion separated by 1.5-minute intervals), starting at 10-minute after the contrast agent

administration. Results indicated that in awake NHP, buprenorphine infusion produces significant increases in rCBV at brain regions with high density of μ-opioid receptors, but not the area with low concentration of μ-opioid receptors (i.e. cerebellum).

thalamus, periaqueductal gray (PAG), and cerebellum in a dose-dependent manner [21]. Further, in contrast to human data, negative BOLD signals were observed in several brain regions in awake rats and this discrepancy was reconciled with the difference in opioid receptor subtypes and binding affinities between these two species [21]. To examine the congruency of phMRI data across rodent, NHP and humans, it appears that the brain activation patterns obtained from our awake NHP study show greater similarity to human data. For example, very limited deactivation, or decreased rCBV, was found in occipital cortex (see Fig. 5). Also, with the exception of activation in the cerebellum, brain regions activated by buprenorphine in awake NHP are depicted in human data. We attributed inconsistency in cerebellar activation to the difference in drug pharmacokinetic or exposure levels, considering that in the baboon PET study [^{11}C]BPN uptake at cerebellum peaked within 2-minute post tracer injection and eliminated rapidly [44]. Further, unlike previous rodent and human BOLD fMRI studies [21,43], we used a CBV-based approach in the current work. For the CBV-based approach, changes in MRI signal reflect changes in CBV, rather than the concentration of deoxyhemoglobin as in BOLD imaging [54]. While it could depend on the resting state blood volume at specific brain regions, BOLD and CBV contrasts are known to be spatially [54] and temporally [55] coupled. Overall, our data highlight the importance and utility of awake imaging in NHP.

In anesthetized animals, brain activation patterns induced by buprenorphine challenge differ from the previous PET μ–opioid receptor data. In comparison with the vehicle treatment, buprenorphine challenge did not elicit any significant changes in brain activity (see Fig. 5), possibly due to the effect of anesthesia. Also, ROI analyses indicate that the rank order of regional rCBV changes induced by buprenorphine infusion was different between anesthetized and awake imaging (see Fig, 7). For example, in awake NHP the highest rCBV change was found in frontal cortex and followed by thalamus, caudate, putamen, cingulate cortex, and cerebellum, while the rank order (descending) became frontal cortex, cerebellum, putamen, cingulate cortex, thalamus, and caudate under anesthetized imaging. Anesthetic-drug interactions on brain activity has been investigated by several groups [14,16,18,19], and it was concluded that drug-induced brain activation pattern can vary among the anesthetics used. The extent of anesthesia confounds likely pivots on the particular mechanism of action associated with selected anesthetics and test drugs, which might or might not be an issue, depending on the neurotransmitter system investigated. Considering the observed drug-induced activation can result from drug-receptor downstream biological effects, the use of anesthesia can modulate both direct and indirect neuronal pathways. As such, it is more desirable to perform imaging in preclinical species without anesthesia that enables qualification of imaging biomarkers which represent a closer scenario to that of clinical investigation.

One of the key challenges for awake imaging is to ensure animals remain still during the data acquisition. Significant efforts have been made to establish comprehensive habituation procedures and specialized animal restrainers in order to minimize head and body motion during data acquisition [16,17,24,27,35, 37,56,57]. For example, Keliris et al. have developed a sophisticated MRI-compatible training chair and head-post restrainer to image alert monkeys in a natural upright sitting position, and they

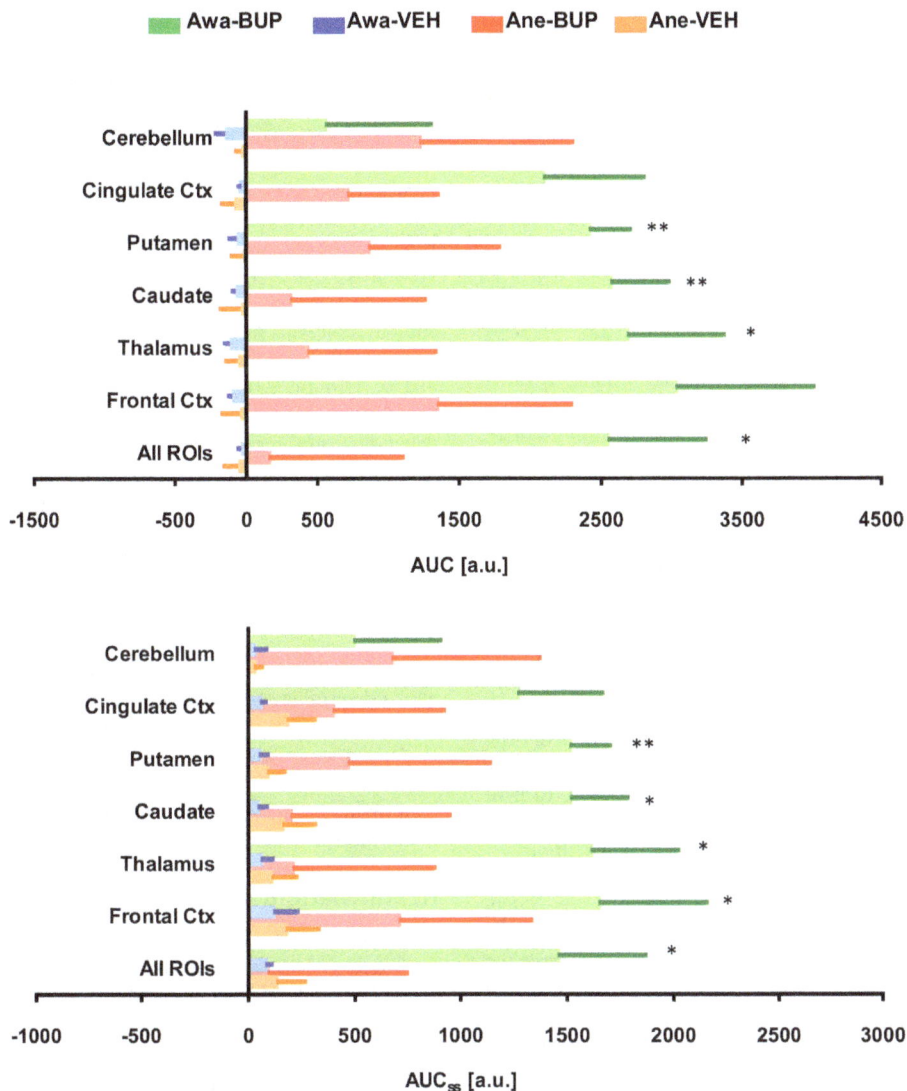

Figure 7. Area-under-curve of regional time-course rCBV change during post-drug infusion derived from the region-of-interest analysis. Results obtained from region-of-interest (ROI) analyses of rCBV time-course data showing the area-under-curve (mean $\pm$ SEM) of the entire post-drug infusion period (AUC) or only the steady-state time period (AUC$_{ss}$). Animals ($n = 4$) were imaged under awake (Awa) or anesthetized (Ane) conditions and treated with either buprenorphine (BUP at 0.03 mg/kg i.v.) or vehicle (VEH). Our data indicated that in awake animals AUC and AUC$_{ss}$ calculated from thalamus, caudate nucleus, and putamen are significantly higher in buprenorphine-treated animals (paired t-test, *$p < 0.05$, **$p < 0.01$ vs vehicle).

found jaw and body movements are the major causes for the fluctuation of fMRI signals [56]. Alternatively, Chen et al. have proposed another approach of integrating an MRI-compatible chair, head-post holder, and volume coil for awake imaging, where in-plane movements can be limited within 80 μm [37]. We have adopted the awake imaging apparatus developed by Andersen et al. [35] and used a custom-made NHP phased-array head coil that can be attached to the head-post for better signal-to-noise ratio (SNR). Without a dedicated NHP MRI scanner [37,56], we have successfully imaged animals in a sphinx position instead. Improved data acquisition and analysis methods have been also developed to enhance the sensitivity to detect targeted drug responses; for example, USPIO imaging contrast agents have been previously exploited to amplify signal changes [36,38] as well as advanced data analysis pipeline for motion correction [39].

To minimize the amount of stress during awake imaging, our study cohort has been trained over several months to acclimatize to the restrainer and scanner environment (see Fig. 1). Some animals showed signs of gradual adaptation to the training, as indicated by the decreased plasma cortisol concentration and behavioral scores (see Fig. 2). This finding is consistent with the results reported by Lee et al. [58], where a weekly decline in cortisol levels was observed in animals receiving chair training for a month. Cortisol levels were also measured in our study, as animals progressed to Phase 1b. We found no significant difference in cortisol concentrations measured at pre- and post- 90-minute training from the trained cohort, whilst in the untrained animals cortisol concentrations elevated significantly (see Fig 3), suggesting that trained animals have been acclimated to the restrainer.

It is noteworthy that in most awake imaging models, a head-post is surgically implanted for the purpose of head fixation. This invasive procedure is however not ideal since the head-post placement requires surgery and can become loose or even detach over time. While this method might be sub-optimal for a longitudinal study, alternative non-invasive approaches have been recently implemented [27,36]. For example, Shrihasam and his colleagues have developed a non-invasive vacuum helmet technique for imaging alert monkeys, and they found that the degrees of translational and rotational head motion during awake imaging are comparable to the same monkey's movements when restrained by a head-post [36]. Likewise, using the expandable foam in combination with a plastic helmet, Murnane et al. have shown the feasibility of imaging conscious monkeys under cocaine challenge without a head-post [27]. There are also disadvantages for this awake imaging approach. For example, awake training is time-consuming and often requires significant effort and resources to habituate the animal. For the current study, it took more than 10 months to complete the awake training protocol and only a sub-group of animals was suitable for the actual imaging study. Although the stress level can be alleviated by extensive training procedures, this factor cannot be completely eliminated.

To develop novel treatments for neurological diseases or psychiatric disorders, PET or single photon emission computed tomography (SPECT) imaging techniques have proved to be useful tools to confirm blood-brain barrier penetration and drug target engagement in the brain, and derived receptor occupancy–drug concentration curves can guide dose selection in clinical development [59,60]. Conversely, biological consequences of drug actions depicted by awake phMRI can offer complimentary pharmacodynamic biomarkers to PET/SPECT imaging. In light of the low success rate associated with the development of novel compounds to treat neurological diseases or psychiatric disorders, phMRI in alert, behaving NHP can serve as a translational imaging platform that affords pharmacodynamic or safety biomarkers, attributed to targeted mechanisms of action. While animal movement and stress during awake imaging increases the noise associated with this approach, the absence of unwanted anesthetic-drug interactions can outweigh efforts needed to overcome these technical hurdles. For the development of CNS compounds, this requirement can be particularly crucial to assess novel experimental therapeutics.

There are limitations for this current study. First, only four animals progressed to the actual imaging experiments and therefore inter-subject variability cannot be properly evaluated.

Second, to fully evaluate the utility of this awake phMRI platform, test-retest study of buprenorphine infusion needs to be explored. Third, in the anesthetized imaging study, buprenorphine did not elicit significant changes in rCBV at brain areas with a high density of μ–opioid receptor (see Figure 5). This observation can be attributed to the level of anesthesia used. Previously, Tinker et al. have reported that the percentage volume of minimum alveolar concentration (MAC) of isoflurane in nonhuman primate is 1.28% and the maintaining dose for most applications is around $1.3 \times$ MAC (i.e. ~1.7%) [61], whereas 2% isoflurane in medical air was selected to anesthetize animals in our study. In combination with paralytics (e.g. vercuronium or mivacurium) or fentanyl, the feasibility of using a lower level of isoflurane (0.3%~1%) in fMRI studies has been demonstrated [62,63]. However, anesthesia protocols could vary among different studies, depending on the experimental design.

In summary, we have shown that, in awake NHP buprenorphine activated brain regions ascribed to high density of μ-opioid receptors, including caudate nucleus, putamen, thalamus, and cingulate cortex. More importantly, in conjunction with previous buprenorphine phMRI studies in conscious rats and humans, our results establish utility of buprenorphine phMRI across species. Further, based on a standard monkey brain atlas, we have established robust phMRI data and ROI analysis pipeline that allows determination of group-level brain activation patterns. Our results indicated that in the same animal, buprenorphine-induced rCBV changes in awake animals are significantly higher than those obtained under the anesthetized condition. Taken together, our data highlight the utility and importance of awake NHP imaging platform as a translational imaging biomarker for drug research.

Acknowledgments

The authors wish to extend our gratitude to Marie A. Holahan and Fuqiang Zhao for insightful discussion. We would also like to thank Htoon Win, Myoe Lynn and Hamzah Isa for their technical support for this work.

Author Contributions

Conceived and designed the experiments: SS DSW TR BH JLE CLC. Performed the experiments: SS ABMAA EM JDB CLC. Analyzed the data: SS ABMAA RB DF CLC. Wrote the paper: SS ABMAA CLC TR EM.

References

1. Wise RG, Tracey I (2006) The role of fMRI in drug discovery. J Magn Reson Imaging 23: 862–876.
2. Borsook D, Becerra L, Hargreaves R (2006) A role for fMRI in optimizing CNS drug development. Nat Rev Drug Discov 5: 411–424.
3. Leslie RA, James MF (2000) Pharmacological magnetic resonance imaging: a new application for functional MRI. Trends Pharmacol Sci 21: 314–318.
4. Jenkins BG (2012) Pharmacologic magnetic resonance imaging (phMRI): imaging drug action in the brain. Neuroimage 62: 1072–1085.
5. Gozzi A, Schwarz A, Reese T, Bertani S, Crestan V, et al. (2006) Region-specific effects of nicotine on brain activity: a pharmacological MRI study in the drug-naive rat. Neuropsychopharmacology 31: 1690–1703.
6. Mueggler T, Baumann D, Rausch M, Rudin M (2001) Bicuculline-induced brain activation in mice detected by functional magnetic resonance imaging. Magn Reson Med 46: 292–298.
7. Chin CL, Tovcimak AE, Hradil VP, Seifert TR, Hollingsworth PR, et al. (2008) Differential effects of cannabinoid receptor agonists on regional brain activity using pharmacological MRI. Br J Pharmacol 153: 367–379.
8. Chen YC, Galpern WR, Brownell AL, Matthews RT, Bogdanov M, et al. (1997) Detection of dopaminergic neurotransmitter activity using pharmacologic MRI: correlation with PET, microdialysis, and behavioral data. Magn Reson Med 38: 389–398.
9. Schwarz AJ, Becerra L, Upadhyay J, Anderson J, Baumgartner R, et al. (2011) A procedural framework for good imaging practice in pharmacological fMRI studies applied to drug development #2: protocol optimization and best practices. Drug Discov Today 16: 671–682.
10. De Simoni S, Schwarz AJ, O'Daly OG, Marquand AF, Brittain C, et al. (2013) Test-retest reliability of the BOLD pharmacological MRI response to ketamine in healthy volunteers. Neuroimage 64: 75–90.
11. Wise RG, Williams P, Tracey I (2004) Using fMRI to quantify the time dependence of remifentanil analgesia in the human brain. Neuropsychopharmacology 29: 626–635.
12. Leppa M, Korvenoja A, Carlson S, Timonen P, Martinkauppi S, et al. (2006) Acute opioid effects on human brain as revealed by functional magnetic resonance imaging. NeuroImage 31: 661–669.
13. Austin VC, Blamire AM, Allers KA, Sharp T, Styles P, et al. (2005) Confounding effects of anesthesia on functional activation in rodent brain: a study of halothane and alpha-chloralose anesthesia. Neuroimage 24: 92–100.
14. Gozzi A, Schwarz A, Crestan V, Bifone A (2008) Drug-anaesthetic interaction in phMRI: the case of the psychotomimetic agent phencyclidine. Magn Reson Imaging 26: 999–1006.
15. Hodkinson DJ, de Groote C, McKie S, Deakin JF, Williams SR (2012) Differential Effects of Anaesthesia on the phMRI Response to Acute Ketamine Challenge. Br J Med Med Res 2: 373–385.
16. Ferris CF, Smerkers B, Kulkarni P, Caffrey M, Afacan O, et al. (2011) Functional magnetic resonance imaging in awake animals. Rev Neurosci 22: 665–674.

17. Liu JV, Hirano Y, Nascimento GC, Stefanovic B, Leopold DA, et al. (2013) fMRI in the awake marmoset: Somatosensory-evoked responses, functional connectivity, and comparison with propofol anesthesia. Neuroimage 78: 186–195.

18. Zhang Z, Andersen AH, Avison MJ, Gerhardt GA, Gash DM (2000) Functional MRI of apomorphine activation of the basal ganglia in awake rhesus monkeys. Brain Res 852: 290–296.

19. Chin CL, Pauly JR, Surber BW, Skoubis PD, McGaraughty S, et al. (2008) Pharmacological MRI in awake rats predicts selective binding of alpha4beta2 nicotinic receptors. Synapse 62: 159–168.

20. Lahti KM, Ferris CF, Li F, Sotak CH, King JA (1999) Comparison of evoked cortical activity in conscious and propofol-anesthetized rats using functional MRI. Magn Reson Med 41: 412–416.

21. Becerra L, Upadhyay J, Chang PC, Bishop J, Anderson J, et al. (2013) Parallel Buprenorphine phMRI Responses in Conscious Rodents and Healthy Human Subjects. J Pharmacol Exp Ther 345: 41–51.

22. Febo M, Segarra AC, Nair G, Schmidt K, Duong TQ, et al. (2005) The neural consequences of repeated cocaine exposure revealed by functional MRI in awake rats. Neuropsychopharmacology 30: 936–943.

23. Baker S, Chin CL, Basso AM, Fox GB, Marek GJ, et al. (2012) Xanomeline modulation of the blood oxygenation level-dependent signal in awake rats: development of pharmacological magnetic resonance imaging as a translatable pharmacodynamic biomarker for central activity and dose selection. J Pharmacol Exp Ther 341: 263–273.

24. Vanduffel W, Fize D, Mandeville JB, Nelissen K, Van Hecke P, et al. (2001) Visual motion processing investigated using contrast agent-enhanced fMRI in awake behaving monkeys. Neuron 32: 565–577.

25. Stefanacci L, Reber P, Costanza J, Wong E, Buxton R, et al. (1998) fMRI of monkey visual cortex. Neuron 20: 1051–1057.

26. Dubowitz DJ, Chen DY, Atkinson DJ, Grieve KL, Gillikin B, et al. (1998) Functional magnetic resonance imaging in macaque cortex. Neuroreport 9: 2213–2218.

27. Murnane KS, Howell LL (2010) Development of an apparatus and methodology for conducting functional magnetic resonance imaging (fMRI) with pharmacological stimuli in conscious rhesus monkeys. J Neurosci Methods 191: 11–20.

28. Mandeville JB, Choi JK, Jarraya B, Rosen BR, Jenkins BG, et al. (2011) FMRI of cocaine self-administration in macaques reveals functional inhibition of basal ganglia. Neuropsychopharmacology 36: 1187–1198.

29. McClure HM (1984) Nonhuman primate models for human disease. Adv Vet Sci Comp Med 28: 267–304.

30. Petrides M, Pandya DN (2002) Comparative cytoarchitectonic analysis of the human and the macaque ventrolateral prefrontal cortex and corticocortical connection patterns in the monkey. Eur J Neurosci 16: 291–310.

31. Nakahara K, Adachi Y, Osada T, Miyashita Y (2007) Exploring the neural basis of cognition: multi-modal links between human fMRI and macaque neurophysiology. Trends Cogn Sci 11: 84–92.

32. Mansour A, Khachaturian H, Lewis ME, Akil H, Watson SJ (1988) Anatomy of CNS opioid receptors. Trends Neurosci 11: 308–314.

33. Smith HR, Beveridge TJ, Porrino LJ (2006) Distribution of norepinephrine transporters in the non-human primate brain. Neuroscience 138: 703–714.

34. Reuning RH, Ashcraft SB, Wiley JN, Morrison BE (1989) Disposition and pharmacokinetics of naltrexone after intravenous and oral administration in rhesus monkeys. Drug Metab Dispos 17: 583–589.

35. Andersen AH, Zhang Z, Barber T, Rayens WS, Zhang J, et al. (2002) Functional MRI studies in awake rhesus monkeys: methodological and analytical strategies. J Neurosci Methods 118: 141–152.

36. Srihasam K, Sullivan K, Savage T, Livingstone MS (2010) Noninvasive functional MRI in alert monkeys. Neuroimage 51: 267–273.

37. Chen G, Wang F, Dillenburger BC, Friedman RM, Chen LM, et al. (2012) Functional magnetic resonance imaging of awake monkeys: some approaches for improving imaging quality. Magn Reson Imaging 30: 36–47.

38. Leite FP, Tsao D, Vanduffel W, Fize D, Sasaki Y, et al. (2002) Repeated fMRI using iron oxide contrast agent in awake, behaving macaques at 3 Tesla. NeuroImage 16: 283–294.

39. Stoewer S, Goense JB, Keliris GA, Bartels A, Logothetis NK, et al. (2011) Realignment strategies for awake-monkey fMRI data. Magn Reson Imaging 29: 1390–1400.

40. Sadee W, Rosenbaum JS, Herz A (1982) Buprenorphine: differential interaction with opiate receptor subtypes in vivo. J Pharmacol Exp Ther 223: 157–162.

41. Heel RC, Brogden RN, Speight TM, Avery GS (1979) Buprenorphine: a review of its pharmacological properties and therapeutic efficacy. Drugs 17: 81–110.

42. Lewis JW (1985) Buprenorphine. Drug Alcohol Depend 14: 363–372.

43. Upadhyay J, Anderson J, Schwarz AJ, Coimbra A, Baumgartner R, et al. (2011) Imaging Drugs with and without Clinical Analgesic Efficacy. Neuropsychopharmacology 36: 2659–2673.

44. Galynker I, Schlyer DJ, Dewey SL, Fowler JS, Logan J, et al. (1996) Opioid Receptor Imaging and Displacement Studies with [6-O-[11C]methyl] Buprenorphine in Baboon Brain. Nuclear Medicine & Biology 23: 325–331.

45. Greenwald MK, Johanson CE, Moody DE, Woods JH, Kilbourn MR, et al. (2003) Effects of buprenorphine maintenance dose on mu-opioid receptor availability, plasma concentrations, and antagonist blockade in heroin-dependent volunteers. Neuropsychopharmacology 28: 2000–2009.

46. Mandeville JB, Marota JJ, Kosofsky BE, Keltner JR, Weissleder R, et al. (1998) Dynamic functional imaging of relative cerebral blood volume during rat forepaw stimulation. Magn Reson Med 39: 615–624.

47. Frey S, Pandya DN, Chakravarty MM, Bailey L, Petrides M, et al. (2011) An MRI based average macaque monkey stereotaxic atlas and space (MNI monkey space). Neuroimage 55: 1435–1442.

48. Nunamaker EA, Halliday LC, Moody DE, Fang WB, Lindeblad M, et al. (2013) Pharmacokinetics of 2 formulations of buprenorphine in macaques (Macaca mulatta and Macaca fascicularis). J Am Assoc Lab Anim Sci 52: 48–56.

49. Wu EX, Tang H, Jensen JH (2004) Applications of ultrasmall superparamagnetic iron oxide contrast agents in the MR study of animal models. NMR Biomed 17: 478–483.

50. Andaluz A, Moll X, Abellan R, Ventura R, Carbo M, et al. (2009) Pharmacokinetics of buprenorphine after intravenous administration of clinical doses to dogs. Vet J 181: 299–304.

51. Jenkinson M, Beckmann CF, Behrens TE, Woolrich MW, Smith SM (2011) Fsl. Neuroimage.

52. Thrall M, Weiser G, Allison R, Campbell T, editors (2012) Veterinary hematology and clinical chemistry 2ed: John Wiely & Sons, Inc.

53. Pfeiffer A, Pasi A, Mehraein P, Herz A (1982) Opiate receptor binding sites in human brain. Brain Res 248: 87–96.

54. Mandeville JB, Marota JJ (1999) Vascular filters of functional MRI: spatial localization using BOLD and CBV contrast. Magn Reson Med 42: 591–598.

55. Shen Q, Ren H, Duong TQ (2008) CBF, BOLD, CBV, and CMRO(2) fMRI signal temporal dynamics at 500-msec resolution. J Magn Reson Imaging 27: 599–606.

56. Keliris GA, Shmuel A, Ku SP, Pfeuffer J, Oeltermann A, et al. (2007) Robust controlled functional MRI in alert monkeys at high magnetic field: effects of jaw and body movements. Neuroimage 36: 550–570.

57. Pinsk MA, Moore T, Richter MC, Gross CG, Kastner S (2005) Methods for functional magnetic resonance imaging in normal and lesioned behaving monkeys. J Neurosci Methods 143: 179–195.

58. Lee JI, Shin JS, Lee JE, Jung WY, Lee G, et al. (2012) Changes of N/L ratio and cortisol levels associated with experimental training in untrained rhesus macaques. J Med Primatol 42: 10–14.

59. Wong DF, Tauscher J, Grunder G (2009) The role of imaging in proof of concept for CNS drug discovery and development. Neuropsychopharmacology 34: 187–203.

60. Hargreaves RJ (2008) The role of molecular imaging in drug discovery and development. Clin Pharmacol Ther 83: 349–353.

61. Fish R, Danneman PJ, Brown M, Karas A (2011) Anesthesia and Analgesia in Laboratory Animals. Elsevier Science: 350.

62. Logothetis NK, Pauls J, Augath M, Trinath T, Oeltermann A (2001) Neurophysiological investigation of the basis of the fMRI signal. Nature 412: 150–157.

63. Wey HY, Li J, Szabo CA, Fox PT, Leland MM, et al. (2010) BOLD fMRI of visual and somatosensory-motor stimulations in baboons. Neuroimage 52: 1420–1427.

16

Combination of TRAIL with Bortezomib Shifted Apoptotic Signaling from DR4 to DR5 Death Receptor by Selective Internalization and Degradation of DR4

Maxim L. Bychkov, Marine E. Gasparian*, Dmitry A. Dolgikh, Mikhail P. Kirpichnikov

Department of Bioengineering, Shemyakin and Ovchinnikov Institute of Bioorganic Chemistry, Moscow, Russia

Abstract

TRAIL (tumor necrosis factor-related apoptosis-inducing ligand) mediates apoptosis in cancer cells through death receptors DR4 and DR5 preferring often one receptor over another in the cells expressing both receptors. Receptor selective mutant variants of TRAIL and agonistic antibodies against DR4 and DR5 are highly promising anticancer agents. Here using DR5 specific mutant variant of TRAIL - DR5-B we have demonstrated for the first time that the sensitivity of cancer cells can be shifted from one TRAIL death receptor to another during co-treatment with anticancer drugs. First we have studied the contribution of DR4 and DR5 in HCT116 p53+/+ and HCT116 p53−/− cells and demonstrated that in HCT116 p53+/+ cells the both death receptors are involved in TRAIL-induced cell death while in HCT116 p53−/− cells prevailed DR4 signaling. The expression of death (DR4 and DR5) as well as decoy (DcR1 and DcR2) receptors was upregulated in the both cell lines either by TRAIL or by bortezomib. However, combined treatment of cells with two drugs induced strong time-dependent and p53-independent internalization and further lysosomal degradation of DR4 receptor. Interestingly DR5-B variant of TRAIL which do not bind with DR4 receptor also induced elimination of DR4 from cell surface in combination with bortezomib indicating the ligand-independent mechanism of the receptor internalization. Eliminatory internalization of DR4 resulted in activation of DR5 receptor thus DR4-dependent HCT116 p53−/− cells became highly sensitive to DR5-B in time-dependent manner. Internalization and degradation of DR4 receptor depended on activation of caspases as well as of lysosomal activity as it was completely inhibited by Z-VAD-FMK, E-64 and Baf-A1. In light of our findings, it is important to explore carefully which of the death receptors is active, when sensitizing drugs are combined with agonistic antibodies to the death receptors or receptor selective variants of TRAIL to enhance cancer treatment efficiency.

Editor: Stacey A. Rizza, Mayo Clinic, United States of America

Funding: This work was supported by the Program of Molecular and Cellular Biology, Russian Academy of Sciences. The funders had no role in study design, data collection and analysis, decision to publish, or preparation of the manuscript.

Competing Interests: The authors have declared that no competing interests exist.

* Email: marine_gasparian@yahoo.com

Introduction

Tumor necrosis factor-related apoptosis-inducing ligand (TRAIL) triggers programmed cell death in various types of cancer cells without causing toxicity to normal cells [1]. Binding of TRAIL with death receptors (DR4 and DR5) induces death signals to the intracellular apoptotic machinery [2]. By contrast, two other receptors, decoy receptor DcR1 and DcR2 are unable to initiate apoptotic cell death and antagonize TRAIL-induced apoptosis [3,4]. Many cancer cell lines express both DR4 and DR5, and each of these receptors can initiate apoptosis independently of the other. The affinity of TRAIL to the both death receptors is equal (K_D 0.5–0.9 nM) [5,6]. However, cancer cell lines expressing DR4 and DR5 receptors at the same level often prefer one receptor to another for TRAIL signaling. The molecular basis for this selective activation via the two receptors is unknown, but the data using the receptor-specific mAbs implicated independent regulation of TRAIL signaling via homotrimeric DR4 and DR5 receptors [7,8]. On the other hand, tumor-derived

mutations in DR5 inhibited TRAIL signaling through the DR4 receptor in BJAB cells by competing for ligand binding [9].

The contribution of one death receptor versus another to apoptotic signaling is different in various tumors. Bortezomib upregulated DR5 but not DR4 receptors cell surface expression in NSCLC cell lines increasing the cell death at the same level with both DR4 and DR5 agonistic antibodies [10]. Sensitive to DR4 and DR5 agonistic antibodies chronic lymphocytic leukemia cells undergo predominantly DR4 mediated apoptosis when were pretreated with histone deacetylase inhibitors [11]. DR5-selective mutant variant of TRAIL DR5-8 exhibited greater potency in colon and breast cancer cell lines [12].

Many cancer cell lines and primary tumors are partially or fully resistant to DR4 and DR5 agonists despite the detectable expression of these receptors in cancer cells and in most tissues [13]. Anticancer drugs such as proteasome inhibitors, doxorubicin, cisplatin, HDAC inhibitors, topotecan, paclitaxel, etoposide upregulated death receptors expression in various tumor cells and sensitized cells to killing by TRAIL [14,15]. However, these drugs usually were unable to overcome acquired resistance to

TRAIL. The proteasome inhibitors can be an important exception since they allow overcoming diverse resistance mechanisms [16,17].

Bortezomib affects TRAIL signaling at multiple levels including enhancement of TRAIL-induced caspase 8 cleavage and activation, inhibition of the cell cycle, changes in cell adherence, inhibition of NF-κB activation and overcomes TRAIL resistance in various tumor cells [18]. Induction of DR5 and/or DR4 and enhancement of TRAIL induced apoptosis by bortezomib have been demonstrated in certain types of cancer cells [19–21]. The maximal synergistic increase of the apoptosis by simultaneous treatment of non-small-cell lung carcinoma [21] and ovarian cancer cells [22] with bortezomib and TRAIL achieved at 16 to 24 h of exposure. Experimental results concerning the role of tumor suppressor protein p53 in stimulation of apoptosis by bortezomib are ambiguous. Bortezomib-induced apoptosis was reported to occur in a p53-independent manner in several works [23–25] while in a recent study [26] the sensitivity to bortezomib has been associated with p53 status.

In the present study we have demonstrated that bortezomib and TRAIL alone upregulated death and decoy receptors expression in HCT116 cells while combination of two drugs caused almost complete internalization of DR4 receptor in ligand-independent and time-dependent manner. As a result, the sensitivity of HCT116 p53$^{-/-}$ cells shifted from DR4 to DR5 receptor. DR4 internalization was caspase dependent and lysosomal pathway of cell death was involved in this process. Our results demonstrated for the first time that the preferential receptor utilization of cancer cells during co-treatment with TRAIL and anti-neoplastic agents could be changed as regulation of receptors expression can differ from that induced by the same agents separately.

Materials and Methods

Cell culture and reagents

Human colorectal carcinoma cell line HCT116 p53$^{+/+}$ and breast adenocarcinoma MDA-MB-231 cell line was from ATCC. HCT116 p53$^{-/-}$ were kindly provided by Prof. B. Vogelstein (Johns Hopkins University School of Medicine) [27].

Cells culture medium DMEM was from PAN Biotech (Aidenbach, Germany) and fetal bovine serum (FBS) was from Hyclone (Cramlington, UK). The proteasome inhibitor bortezomib was obtained from Santa Cruz Biotechnology (Santa-Cruz, USA). General caspase inhibitor Z-VAD-FMK and inhibitor to lysosomal cathepsins E-64 were from MP Biomedicals (Eschwege, Germany), Bafilomycin A1 was from Cayman Chemicals (Ann Arbor, USA). Neutralizing antibodies to TRAIL death and decoy receptors were from Enzo Life Sciences (Farmingdale, USA) and R&D systems (Minneapolis, USA), respectively. FITC-conjugated antibodies to DR4, DR5, DcR1 and DcR2 receptor were obtained from Abnova (Walnut, USA), isotype control antibody was from Immunotech (Marcelle, France). For western blot biotinylated goat antibodies to TRAIL death and decoy receptors were purchased from R&D Systems (Minneapolis, USA), HRP streptavidin and antibodies to actin were from Sigma-Aldrich (St. Lotus, USA).

Recombinant TRAIL preparation

Wild type and mutant variant DR5-B (containing 6 amino acid substitutions Y189N, R191K, Q193R, H264R, I266L and D269H) of TRAIL (114–281) were expressed in E. coli BL21(DE3) strain and purified as we previously described with some modifications [6]. Briefly, the synthetic genes of wild type and DR5-B variant were constructed into bacterial expression vector pET-32a. High-level expression of Trx/TRAIL (thioredoxin/

TRAIL) fusions (approximately 150 mg from 100 ml culture) in E. coli strain BL-21(DE3) was induced by 0.02 mM IPTG at 28°C. Trx/TRAIL and Trx/DR5-B fusions were purified from cytoplasmic protein fraction on Ni-Sepharose high performance (GE Healthcare). After cleavage of fusions with recombinant human enteropeptidase light chain the target proteins were separated from thioredoxin on Ni-NTA agarose. To increase the yield of target proteins and reduce the amount of enteropeptidase for fusions cleavage the amino acids residue of lysine was substituted by arginine in enzyme cleavage site (Asp)$_4$Lys as it was described in our previous work [28].

MTT assay

The cytotoxic effect of wild type TRAIL, DR5 specific mutant variant DR5-B alone or in combination with bortezomib was determined by MTT assay. Briefly, cells were seeded in 96-well plates (SPL Lifesciences) at a density of 1×10^4 per well in 200 µl culture medium (DMEM) and incubated for 16 h at 37°C. Culture medium was aspirated and 200 µl of fresh medium containing indicated concentrations of TRAIL variants and bortezomib were added to cells. Cells were incubated for indicated periods, washed with medium and MTT reagent was added at concentration 0.5 mg/ml. After incubation for 3 h, cells were centrifuged at 2000 rpm for 5 min. The supernatants were aspirated and DMSO was added to each well for formazan solubilization. Absorbance of formazan solution in wells was measured at a wavelength 540 nm using microplate reader (Bio–Rad 680) with background subtraction at 655 nm. Apoptotic cell death was confirmed by assessment of nuclear morphology after cell staining with Hoerst 33344 and propidium iodide.

Flow cytometry

Cells were detached from culture flasks using 0.05% Trypsin-EDTA solution (PanEco), washed in ice cold PBS, and resuspended in FACS buffer (PBS with 0.1% BSA). To confirm that the trypsin does not cleave the receptors additional experiments with 0.6 mM EDTA in PBS (pH = 7.4) or Citric saline buffer (135 mM KCl, 15 mM sodium citrate, pH = 7.4) were performed (Fig. S1). TRAIL receptors cell surface expression was analyzed using FITC-conjugated mouse anti-TRAIL-R1 (DR4), anti-TRAIL-R2 (DR5), anti-TRAIL-R3 (DcR1) and anti-TRAIL-R4 (DcR2) antibodies (Abnova). Mouse IgG (Immunotech) was used as isotype control. Cells (at least 1×10^5 cells for each sample) were incubated with 1 µg of antibodies for 1 h at 4°C, washed in ice-cold PBS twice, resuspended in FACS buffer containing 0.5 µg/ml propidium iodide and analyzed by FACS-can flow cytometer using Cellquest software (Becton Dickinson).

Western blot analysis

Cells (1×10^6) were seeded on 100 mm cell culture dishes, trypsinized and washed by ice cold PBS twice and lysed on ice with RIPA buffer (25 mM Tris-HCl, 150 mM NaCl, 0.1% Triton X-100, 1% NP-40, 0.5% sodium deoxycholate, 0.1% SDS) supplemented with protease inhibitors. Proteins were separated by Tris-glycine SDS-PAGE (12% gel) and transferred to nitrocellulose membranes (GE Healthcare). The membrane was blocked in TBST (50 mM Tris-HCl, 150 mM NaCl with 0.01% of Tween-20) containing 5% of non-fat milk for 2 h and consequently incubated with biotinylated antibodies to TRAIL receptors and with streptavidin-HRP (Sigma) for 1 h. ECL Prime substrate (GE Healthcare) and Versa Doc MP4000 documentation system (Bio Rad) were used for visualization of TRAIL receptors. The intensity of protein bands was calculated using the ImageJ software (http://rsbweb.nih.gov/ij/, NIH, Bethesda, Maryland) by option "gel analyzer" tools.

Analysis of TRAIL receptors internalization by confocal microscopy

To detect the localization of TRAIL receptors 5×10^4 tumor cells were seeded overnight on glass slides in $37°C$ and 5% of CO_2. Next, the culture media were replaced by a fresh one supplemented with 25 mM Baf A1 and after 1 h incubation 1 ng/mL of TRAIL variants and 1 nM of bortezomib were adjusted to the growth medium. Cells were growth for different periods in the presence of indicated reagents, washed with PBS, fixed in 3% paraformaldehyde for 30 min, permeabilized with 0.1% Triton X-100 in PBS for 10 min and blocked in 3% BSA for 30 min. FITC-conjugated antibodies to death and decoy receptors (Abnova) were added at dilution 1:100 and cells were incubated for 1 h in the presence of Hoerst 33342 for visualization of cell nuclei. Then Non-specific bound antibodies were washed with blocking buffer containing 0.1% of Triton X-100. Cells were visualized in 0.6- μm sections using an inverted Nikon Eclipse TE2000-E laser scanning confocal microscope under a ×60 oil immersion objective.

Statistical analysis

Data are presented as mean ± SD from at least three independent experiments. Differences between treated cells and control were assessed with the Student's t test, a p-value less than 0.05 was considered as statistically significant. Statistical analyses were done using Microsoft Office Excel software (Microsoft, Redmond, USA).

Results

Combination of bortezomib and TRAIL shifted sensitivity of HCT116 cells from DR4 to DR5 receptor in time dependent manner

We have chosen human colon carcinoma p53$^{+/+}$ and p53$^{-/-}$ HCT116 cells to investigate the contribution of death and decoy receptors in TRAIL and bortezomib induced cell death signaling. First we have analyzed the expression of the death and decoy receptors at the cells surface (Fig. 1A). TRAIL death receptors were highly expressed in these cells and the ratio of DR4 to DR5 was higher in HCT116 p53$^{-/-}$ cells (1.7 and 2.3 for p53$^{+/+}$ and p53$^{-/-}$ cells, respectively). Both HCT116 p53$^{+/+}$ and HCT116 p53$^{-/-}$ cells expressed decoy receptors DcR1 and DcR2 at the cell surface and the level of these receptors was almost twice higher in HCT116 p53$^{-/-}$ cells.

To investigate the contribution of DR4 and DR5 receptors to TRAIL mediated cell death we used DR5-specific mutant variant of TRAIL – DR5-B, generated in our laboratory. Earlier we have demonstrated that the dissociation constant of DR5-B to DR5 receptor was comparable to wild type TRAIL while it practically did not bind to DR4 or DcR1 receptors and its affinity to DcR2 was much lower (400 fold) in comparison to TRAIL [6]. The contribution of each receptor was analyzed using antagonistic antibodies to the death and decoy receptors (Fig. 1B). This approach revealed that TRAIL mediated cell death through both death receptors in HCT116 p53$^{+/+}$ cells. Blocking of decoy receptors significantly increased DR5 but not DR4 signaling indicating that decoy receptors mainly inhibited the DR5 signaling in these cells. In contrast DR4 signaling was higher in HCT116 p53$^{-/-}$ cells even when both decoy receptors were blocked by antagonistic antibodies. DR5-B variant demonstrated high spec-

ificity to DR5 receptor and was more potent in HCT116 p53$^{+/+}$ but not in p53 null cells in comparison to TRAIL. As it was expected, blocking of decoy receptors did not affect the efficiency of the DR5-B.

Further, we have investigated time dependent combined action of TRAIL and bortezomib. Sensitization of TRAIL mediated cell death by bortezomib depended on ligand concentration and incubation period (Fig. 2A, 2B). In HCT116 p53$^{+/+}$ cells the effect of bortezomib became pronounced at 8 h and reached its maximum at 24 h. In all the time points, DR5-B was more potent cell death inducer in comparison with wild type TRAIL in these cells. In HCT116 p53$^{-/-}$ cells the behavior of DR5-B was extraordinary. Bortezomib during 16 h practically did not altered DR5-B mediated cell death but significantly increased TRAIL induced cell death. However, the efficiency of DR5-B rose strongly with time and became practically equal to TRAIL at 20 h. Moreover at 24 h of treatment DR5-B surpassed TRAIL with the half maximal effective concentration (EC$_{50}$) 0.05±0.005 ng/ml which was almost 10 fold lower in comparison to wild type TRAIL (0.5±0.04 ng/ml) (Fig. 2D). These data indicated that combined treatment of HCT116 p53$^{-/-}$ cells with TRAIL and bortezomib slowly (more than 16 h) shifted contribution of the receptors mediated TRAIL-induced cell death from DR4 to DR5. It should be noted that cytotoxity of bortezomib was higher in HCT116 p53$^{+/+}$ cells in comparison to HCT116 p53$^{-/-}$ (Fig. 2C). However its effect on TRAIL mediated cell death was higher in HCT116 p53$^{-/-}$ cells (Fig. 2D).

Combined treatment of HCT116 cell with bortezomib and TRAIL promotes strong DR4 receptor internalization and degradation

To understand the nature of the shift in receptor specificity we have investigated expression of the death and the decoy cell surface receptors in HCT116 cells during treatment with bortezomib and TRAIL. Surprisingly bortezomib strongly upregulated not only the death receptors but also the decoy receptors (DcR2 more than DcR1) in HCT116 p53$^{+/+}$ cells (Fig. 3A and B). In HCT116 p53$^{-/-}$ cells upregulation of the receptors (with exception of DcR1) by bortezomib was less pronounced. Both TRAIL and DR5-B upregulated the decoy receptors expression in p53 independent manner (Fig. 3B). DR5 receptor was upregulated by TRAIL variants in HCT116 p53$^{+/+}$ but not in HCT116 p53$^{-/-}$ cells at low concentration of ligands (1 ng/ml). However at higher concentrations of ligands (more than 10 ng/ml) upregulation of DR5 receptor was detected also in HCT116 p53$^{-/-}$ cells (data not shown).

Combined treatment with TRAIL and bortezomib induced strong increase of DR4 membrane expression during 16 h of treatment. However, during further incubation with the two drugs DR4 receptor was practically vanished from cell surface of the both HCT116 p53$^{+/+}$ and HCT116 p53$^{-/-}$ cells. Interestingly DR5-B, which has no affinity to DR4 receptor, induced the same effect indicating that DR4 can be internalized without ligand due to activation of DR5 signaling. These observations can explain why HCT116 p53$^{-/-}$ cells which preferred TRAIL signaling through DR4 receptor (Fig. 1B) became DR5 sensitive after prolonged combined treatment with bortezomib and TRAIL (Fig. 2B). Finally, after 24 h of combined treatment with bortezomib, DR5-B became more effective in comparison to TRAIL in both HCT116 p53$^{+/+}$ and HCT116 p53$^{-/-}$ cells (Fig. 2D). This can be explained by significant increase of the relative level of the decoy and death receptors at the cell surface (Fig. 3C). Slight reduction of cell surface DR5 receptor induced by combined action of TRAIL and bortezomib could be the result of

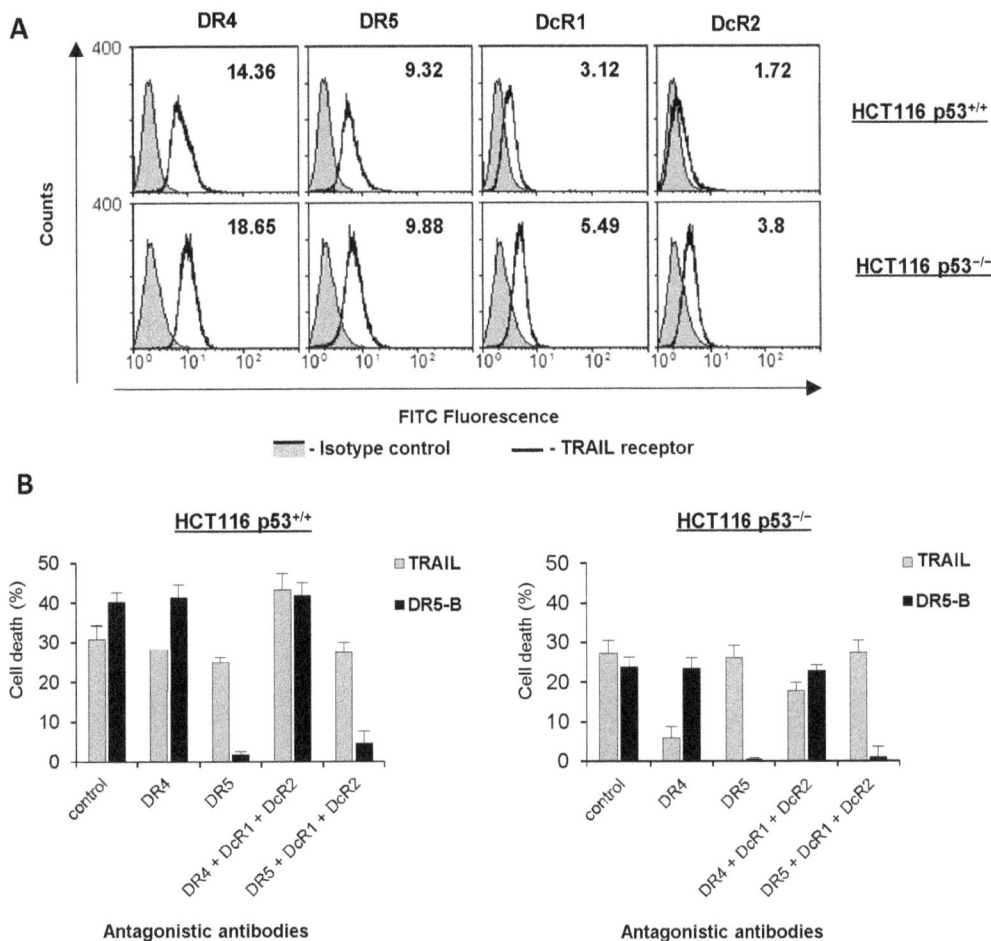

Figure 1. Contribution of death receptors DR4 and DR5 in TRAIL-mediated cell death in HCT116 p53$^{+/+}$ and HCT116 p53$^{-/-}$ cells. (A) Levels of constitutive surface expression of the death and the decoy receptors in HCT116 cells as determined by flow cytometry. (B) Cells were pre-incubated with 20 µg/ml antagonistic antibodies to death and decoy receptors or IgG1 control for 1 h following 4 h treatment with TRAIL or DR5-B (1 µg/ml) and cell death was determined by MTT test. Values are mean ± SD of at least three independent experiments.

some heterotrimeric DR4/DR5 complexes internalization (Fig. 3A).

The similar phenotypic effects of specific DR4 receptor internalization during long period of combined treatment with TRAIL and bortezomib was observed in breast cancer cells MDA-MB-231where almost 5 fold reduction of DR4 receptor on the cell surface was observed after 24 h incubation (Fig. S2). In the same conditions the level of DR5 as well as decoy receptors practically were not affected. As a result, the DR4 dependent MDA-MB-231cells as it was demonstrated using antagonistic receptors to death receptors (Fig. S3A) became more sensitive to DR5-B variant in comparison to TRAIL after 16 h of incubation with bortezomib (Fig. S3B).

Changes of the death and the decoy receptors expression profile in total cellular extract determined by western blot analysis practically coincided with the cell surface expression during treatment with bortezomib and TRAIL (Fig. 4A, 4B). The amount of DR4 receptor after 20 h of incubation was significantly reduced in co-treatment experiments in p53-independent manner, while the levels of DR5 and DcR1 remained almost the same as in non-treated cells. Only the level of DcR2 in total cell extract remained higher after prolonged treatment with the two drugs.

The confocal microscopy experiments with FITC-conjugated antibodies to DR4 receptor conformed the internalization and degradation of DR4 during long treatment of cells in the presence of TRAIL and bortezomib (Fig. 5). In 20 h the major part of DR4 receptor was transported from membrane to the cytoplasm as a part of endosomes. Further incubation of the cells with two drugs (24 h of co-treatment) resulted to dramatic degradation of DR4. Partial internalization but not degradation of DR5, DcR2 and DcR1 receptors was observed during long period of incubation of the cells with bortezomib and TRAIL (Fig. 3 and 5).

General caspase inhibitor z-VAD-FMK inhibited cell death and abrogated bortezomib and TRAIL induced disappearance of DR4 receptor from the cell surface indicating the essential role of caspases activation in DR4 internalization (Fig. 6). The similar effects were observed with DR5-B variant in the both HCT116 p53$^{+/+}$ and HCT116 p53$^{-/-}$ cells (data not shown).

Inhibition of lysosomal activity prevented TRAIL and bortezomib induced DR4 internalization and degradation

Next, we have investigated the molecular mechanisms of bortezomib and TRAIL induced DR4 internalization and degradation by inhibition of lysosomal activity with highly selective inhibitor to lysosomal cathepsins B, H, and L E-64 and specific

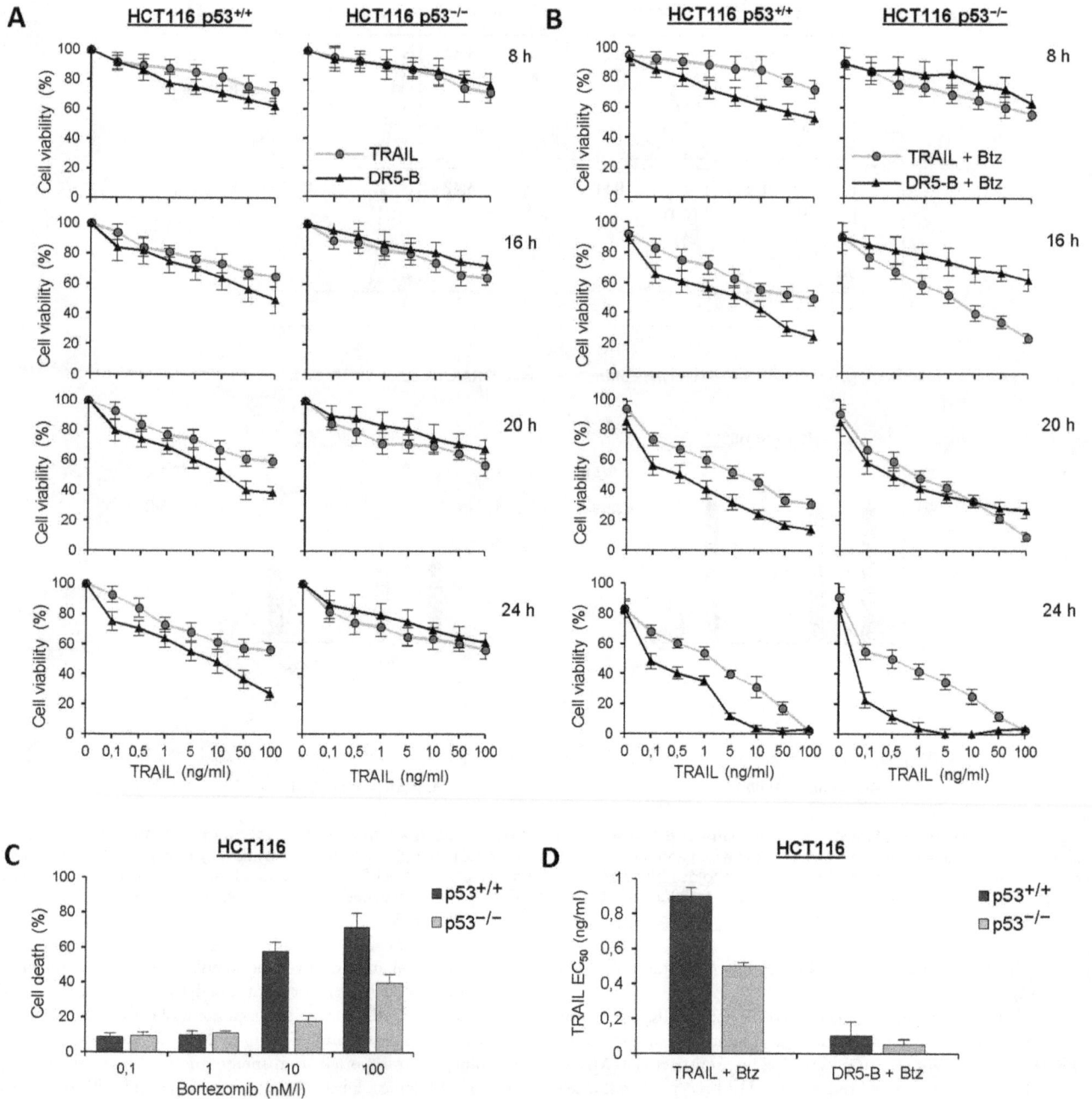

Figure 2. Time-depended influence of bortezomib on TRAIL or DR5-B mediated cell death in HCT116 p53$^{+/+}$ and HCT116 p53$^{-/-}$ cells. (A) Viability of the cells treated with different concentrations of TRAIL or DR5-B during 8, 16, 20 and 24 h of incubation. (B) Viability of the cells treated with 1 nM bortezomib and different concentrations of TRAIL or DR5-B during 8, 16, 20 and 24 h of incubation. (C) Cells were incubated with different concentrations of bortezomib and cell death was measured after 24 h of incubation. (D) Calculation of effective concentrations of TRAIL variants after 24 h treatment of cells with 1 nM bortezomib. Values are mean ± SD of at least three independent experiments.

inhibitor of the vacuolar H(+)-ATPase bafilomycin A1 (Baf-A1) which blocks the endosome acidification. Both inhibitors prevented internalization of DR4 receptor (Fig. 7A, 8A). In the same experiments, E-64 did not affect DR5 receptor cell surface expression while Baf-A1 protected slight reduction of DR5 from cell surface induced by combined action of TRAIL and bortezomib (Fig. 3A, 8A). Probably Baf-A1 prevented not only DR4 but also some heterotrimeric DR4/DR5 complexes internalization.

Prevention of DR4 internalization by Baf-A1 and E-64 strongly inhibited the enhancing effect of bortezomib on DR5-B mediated cell death while the action of wild type TRAIL and bortezomib was only slightly decreased (Fig. 7C, 8B). E-64 itself in combination with bortezomib induced almost 30% cell death but did not significantly affect apoptosis induced by TRAIL or DR5-B (Fig. 8A, 8B). At the same time, E-64 completely inhibited the effect of bortezomib on DR5-B mediated cell death in HCT116 p53$^{-/-}$ cells while TRAIL signaling was only partially inhibited

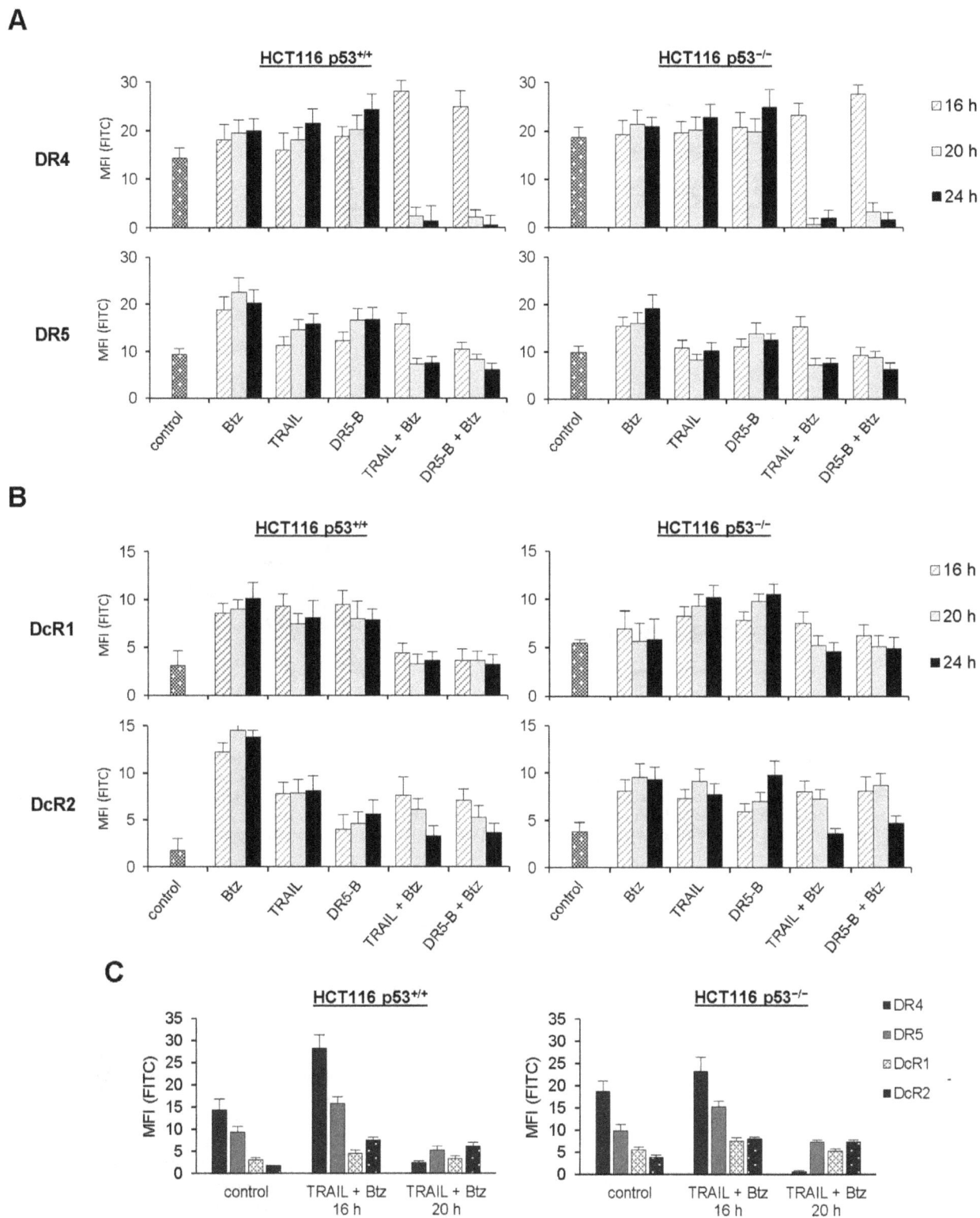

Figure 3. Time-dependent expression of the death and the decoy receptors at the surface of HCT116 p53$^{+/+}$ and p53 null cells treated by bortezomib and TRAIL (or DR5-B). In all experiments, cells were treated with 1 nM bortezomib and 1 ng/ml TRAIL variants alone or in combination. (A) Profiles of the death receptors at the cell surface. (B) Profiles of the decoy receptors at the cell surface. (C) Relative level of death and decoy receptors membrane expression in cells during combined treatment with TRAIL variants and bortezomib. Values in all experiments are mean ± SD of at least three independent experiments.

A

HCT116 p53 +/+

B

HCT116 p53-/-

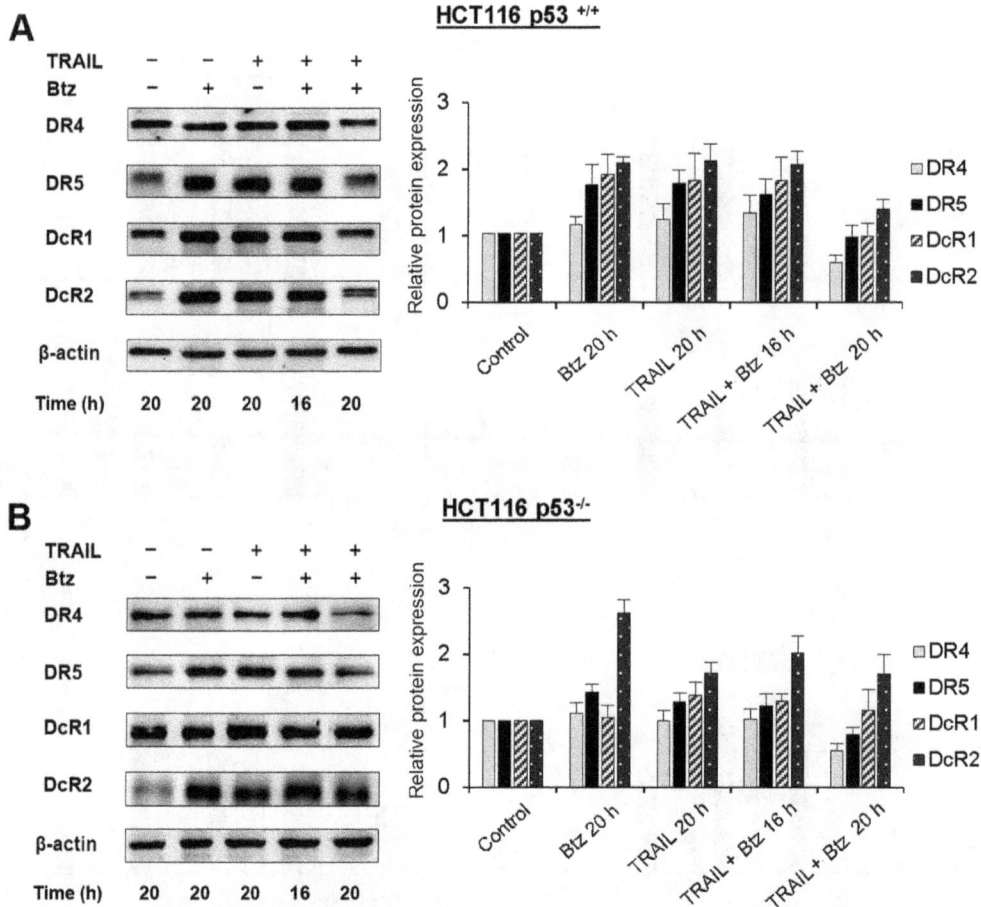

Figure 4. The content of death and decoy receptors in total cell extracts of HCT116 p53$^{+/+}$ and HCT116 p53$^{-/-}$ cells treated by TRAIL, bortezomib or by combination of both drugs. HCT116 p53$^{+/+}$ (A) and HCT116 p53$^{-/-}$ (B) cells were treated with TRAIL (1 ng/ml), bortezomib (1 nM), or by combination of both drugs for various time periods and the content of receptors in total cell extract was determined by Western blot analysis using appropriate biotinylated antibodies to each receptor. Densitometric analysis of three independent experiments was performed using ImageJ software. Values in all experiments are mean ± SD of at least three independent experiments.

(Fig. 7C). These are strong arguments to suggest that DR4 internalization is required for DR5 activation.

Summarizing obtained data it may be suggested that Baf-A1 and E-64 inhibited bortezomib and TRAIL/ or DR5-B mediated cell death indicating that activation of lysosomal cell death pathway is involved in combined action of two agents.

Discussion

Despite numerous studies on modulation of the death and the decoy receptors expression by cytotoxic drugs, the effects of combined treatment with TRAIL and the sensitizers were not investigated in details. In the present study, we have demonstrated for the first time that the sensitivity of cancer cells can be shifted from one TRAIL death receptor to another by chemotherapeutic drug. We have shown that DR4-dependent HCT116 p53$^{-/-}$ and MDA-MB-231 cells became highly sensitive to DR5 specific mutant TRAIL variant DR5-B after prolonged combined treatment with bortezomib by selective internalization of DR4 receptor (Fig. 1, 2, S2A, B). We have found that combined treatment of HCT116 cells with bortezomib and TRAIL changed the death and the decoy receptors profile and these changes differed from that induced by these drugs separately. Bortezomib itself strongly upregulated not only the expression of DR5 but also

DcR2 decoy receptor in HCT116 cells in p53-independent manner. DcR1 decoy receptor was also upregulated by this drug but the effect depended on p53 status (Fig. 3, 4). TRAIL alone upregulated DR5 expression at the cell surface in p53-dependent and the decoy receptors expression in p53-independent manner. Death receptor DR4 was also slightly upregulated by TRAIL or bortezomib in both HCT116 p53$^{+/+}$ and HCT116 p53$^{-/-}$ cells when these drugs were used separately. However, combination of these two drugs resulted in strong increase of DR4 expression at the cell surface during 16 h of treatment with following dramatic decrease in longer incubation period (more than 16 h) independently of p53 status (Fig. 3A). Importantly DR5 specific mutant variant of TRAIL DR5-B, which demonstrated no affinity to DR4 and DcR1 receptors and highly reduced affinity to DcR2 receptor [6], modulated the death and the decoy receptors expression in the same way as wild type TRAIL either alone or in combination with bortezomib. These observations indicated that modulation of the death and the decoy receptors by TRAIL can be induced without binding of the ligand to DR4 receptor. The detailed mechanism of ligand-independent selective internalization of DR4 remained unknown. Recently it was shown that DR4 is a substrate for ubiquitination by membrane-associated RING-CH-8 (MARCH-8) ligase, which had little impact on DR5 in breast carcinoma and melanoma cell lines [29]. To our knowledge selective caspase-

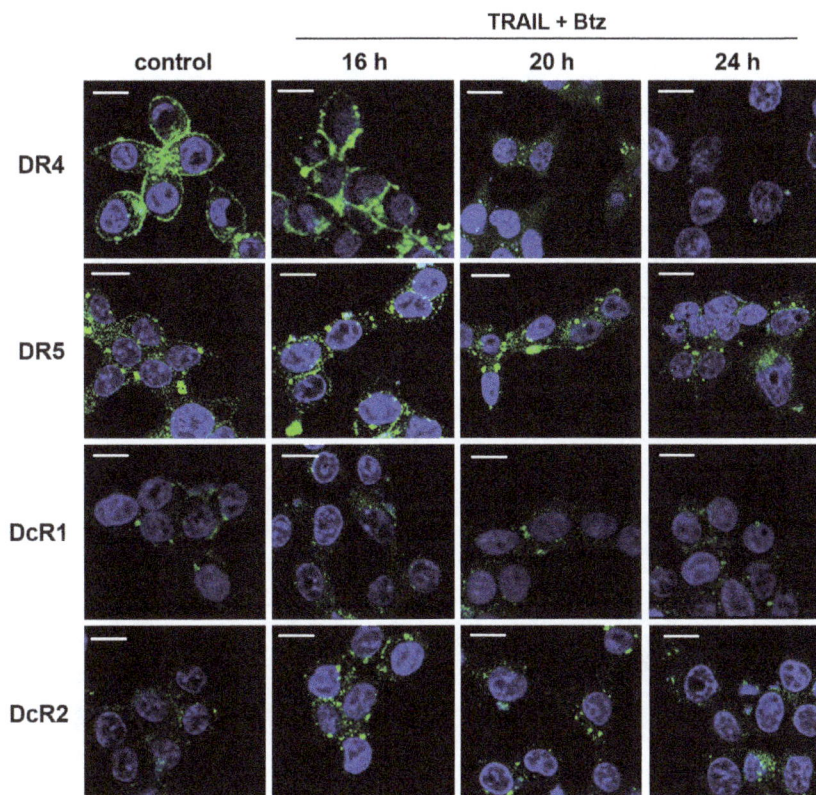

Figure 5. Confocal microscopic analysis of death and decoy receptors localization in HCT116 p53$^{-/-}$ cells treated with TRAIL and bortezomib for indicated periods. Scale bar = 10 μm. Cells were grown for different periods in the presence of indicated reagents, washed with PBS, fixed in 3% paraformaldehyde for 30 min, permeabilized with 0.1% Triton X-100 in PBS for 10 min and blocked in 3% BSA for 30 min. FITC-conjugated antibodies to DR4, DR5, DcR1 and DcR2 receptors (Abnova) were added at dilution 1:100 and cells were incubated for 1 h in the presence of Hoerst 33342 for visualization of cell nuclei. Then non-specific bound antibodies were washed with blocking buffer containing 0.1% of Triton X-100. Cells were visualized in 0.6- μm sections using an inverted Nikon Eclipse TE2000-E laser scanning confocal microscope under a ×60 oil immersion objective.

dependent and ligand-independent depletion was never described before for any kind of receptor. The caspase-8 dependent internalization of CD95 death receptor upon binding of the ligand was observed for the first time in 2002 [30].

General caspase inhibitor Z-VAD-FMK prevented bortezomib and TRAIL induced loss of DR4 from the cell surface and inhibited cell death indicating that activation of caspases was essential for DR4 internalization (Fig. 6A). This observation allows explaining the ligand-independent mechanism of DR4 internalization, which could be caused by DR5-mediated activation of caspases. Irreversible specific inhibitor of lysosomal cathepsins E-64 and specific inhibitor of the vacuolar H(+)-ATPase Baf-A1 also

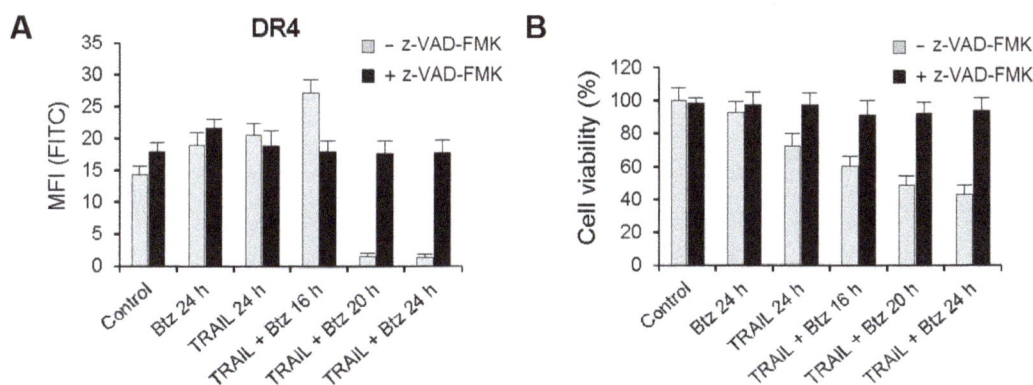

Figure 6. Inhibition of bortezomib and TRAIL induced DR4 internalization by z-VAD-FMK. DR4 receptor cell surface expression and viability of the HCT116 p53$^{+/+}$ cells were analyzed after incubation with 10 μM z-VAD-FMK for 1 h following treatments with TRAIL (1 ng/ml) and bortezomib (1 nM) or in combination of the two drugs.

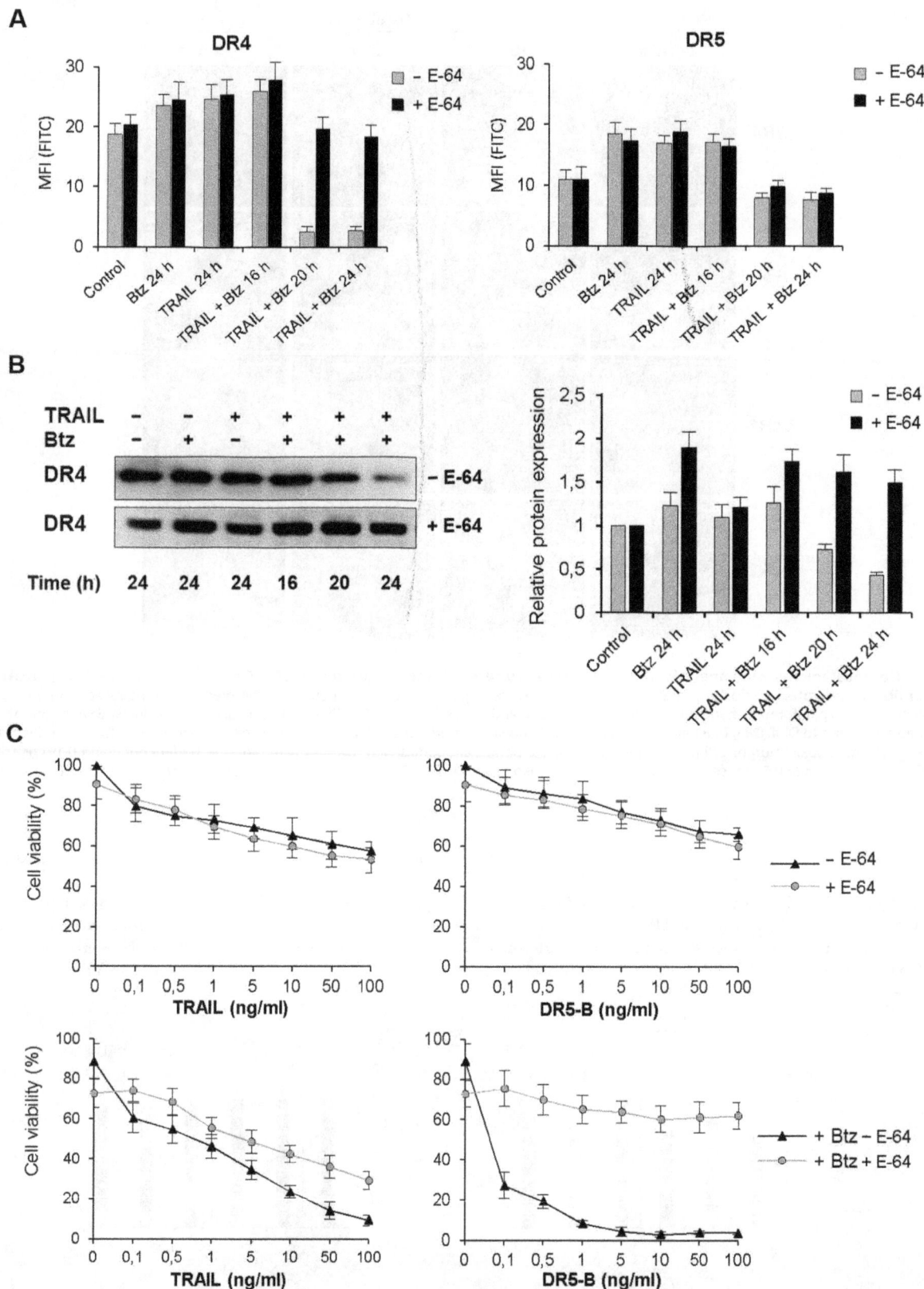

Figure 7. Inhibition of bortezomib and TRAIL induced DR4 internalization by E-64 in HCT116 p53$^{-/-}$ cells. (A) DR4 and DR5 receptors cell surface expression was analyzed after incubation of the cells with E-64 (25 μM) for 1 h following medium change and treatment with TRAIL (1 ng/ml), bortezomib (1 nM) or in combination of the two drugs for 24 h. (B) Cells were treated as in (A) and the expression of DR4 and DR5 receptors in total cell extract was determined by Western blot analysis using appropriate biotinylated antibodies. Densitometric analysis of three independent experiments was performed using ImageJ software. (C) Inhibition of bortezomib and TRAIL induced cell death by E-64 in the cells was determined by MTT test. Values in all experiments are mean ± SD of at least three independent experiments.

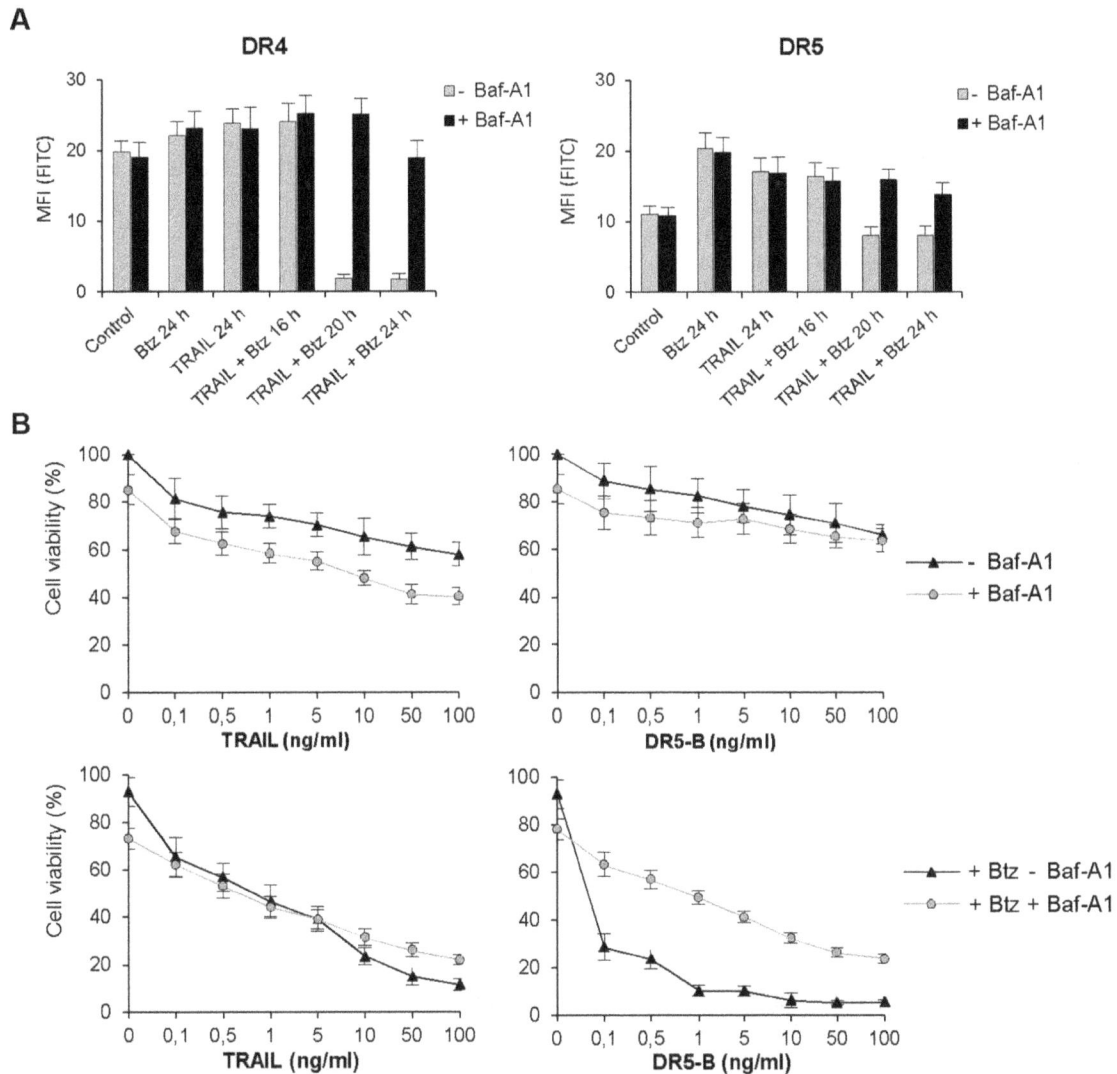

Figure 8. Inhibition of lysosomal activity by Baf-A1 prevented TRAIL and bortezomib induced DR4 internalization. (A) DR4 and DR5 receptors cell surface expression was analyzed in HCT116 $p53^{-/-}$ cells pretreated with Baf-A1 (25 µM) for 1 h following bortezomib (1 nM) and TRAIL (1 ng/ml) treatment alone or in combination for 24 h. (B) Viability of the cells treated as in (A) was determined by MTT test. Values in all experiments are mean ± SD of at least three independent experiments.

suppressed DR4 surface depletion and further degradation (Fig. 7A, 8A) and strongly inhibited DR5-B and bortezomib induced cell death (Fig. 7B, 8B). These observations are indicating that bortezomib in combination with TRAIL activated lysosomes, which contributed to DR4 receptor internalization and degradation. Probably lysosomal proteases stimulated DR4 internalization via activation of caspases and their contribution became insignificant when DR5-dependent caspase activation reached maximum. There is growing evidence that non-caspase proteases, in particular lysosomal cathepsins, can play an important role in the regulation of apoptosis [31]. It was shown that in human pancreatic carcinoma cells bortezomib disrupted lysosomes with release of cathepsin B to the cytosol where it cleaved caspase-2 and induced mitochondrial apoptotic pathway [32]. Redistribution of the cathepsin B from lysosomes to the cytosol in cholangiocarcinoma cells was induced by TRAIL and contributed significantly to apoptosis [33,34]. In our model E-64 and Baf-A1 did not significantly affected cell death induced by TRAIL but strongly

inhibited the sensitizing effect of bortezomib for either TRAIL or DR5-B variant mediated cell death (Fig. 7). Probably activation of cathepsins amplified DR5-dependent apoptotic pathway.

It is paradoxical but our results indicated that the depletion of DR4 receptor was necessary for DR5 activation. This hypothesis is supported by the observed time-dependent increase in efficiency of DR5-B variant induced by bortezomib in HCT116 $p53^{-/-}$ cells (Fig. 2B). During 16 h of co-treatment with TRAIL and bortezomib the level of DR4 at the cell surface remained high and sensitizing effect of bortezomib was negligible for DR5-B in comparison to wild type TRAIL. However, after 16 h when DR4 receptor was practically vanished from the cell surface proapoptotic efficiency of DR5-B became 10 fold higher than of wild type TRAIL. In agreement with our hypothesis it was shown recently that silencing of DR4 in HCT116 $p53^{+/+}$ cells significantly stimulated apoptosis induced by TRAIL in combination with 5-Fluorouracil [35]. The same phenotypic effect was observed in MDA-MB-231 cells (Fig. S2, S3). It is not clear why evolution has created two death receptor with the same function. Although it was demonstrated that combined treatment of cancer cells with monoclonal antibodies to both death receptors only slightly enhanced the efficiency of cell death comparing when they were used separately [36]. Even our data are not strong evidence but we would hypothesize that DR4 receptor can play some regulatory role in DR5 mediated apoptosis.

In conclusion, it should be mentioned that when combination of bortezomib and TRAIL strongly stimulated HCT116 cell death the surviving cells became even more resistant to TRAIL since the ratio of the death and the decoy receptors dramatically decreased independently of p53 status (Fig. 3C). These observations support the therapeutic strategy to choose higher doses of TRAIL to kill as much cells as possible and to escape the residual resistance (Fig. 2B). Our results indicated that before application of the death receptor specific agents (either monoclonal antibodies or receptor specific mutant variants of TRAIL) in combination with chemotherapeutic drugs the receptor selectivity of the cells should be checked carefully. It is clear from our study that modification of the receptors expression induced by combined treatment can strongly differ from that induced by the same agents separately. It is important to investigate the molecular determinants of this phenomenon to choose optimal death receptor targeting agents and sensitizers in combined treatment of cancer.

Supporting Information

Figure S1 Trypsin does not cleave TRAIL receptors at the cell surface. HCT116 p53$^{+/+}$ cells were detached by trypsin-EDTA solution, 0.6 mM EDTA or by citric saline buffer and the level of constitutive surface expression of the death and decoy receptors were determined by flow cytometry. TRAIL receptors cell surface expression was analyzed using FITC-conjugated mouse anti-TRAIL-R1 (DR4), anti-TRAIL-R2 (DR5), anti-TRAIL-R3 (DcR1) and anti-TRAIL-R4 (DcR2) antibodies (Abnova). Mouse IgG (Immunotech) was used as isotype control. Cells (at least 1×10^5 cells for each sample) were incubated with 1 µg of antibodies for 1 h at 4°C, washed in ice-cold PBS twice, resuspended in FACS buffer containing 0.5 µg/ml propidium iodide and analyzed by FACScan flow cytometer using

Cellquest software (Becton Dickinson). Values in all experiments are mean ± SD of at least three independent experiments.

Figure S2 Time-dependent expression of the death and the decoy receptors at the surface of MDA-MB-231 cells treated by bortezomib and TRAIL. In all experiments, cells were treated with 25 nM bortezomib and 1 ng/ml TRAIL alone or in combination at indicated periods and the level of death and decoy receptors cell surface expression was analyzed using FITC-conjugated mouse anti-TRAIL-R1 (DR4), anti-TRAIL-R2 (DR5), anti-TRAIL-R3 (DcR1) and anti-TRAIL-R4 (DcR2) antibodies (Abnova) by FACScan flow cytometer using Cellquest software (Becton Dickinson). Values in all experiments are mean ± SD of at least three independent experiments.

Figure S3 Time-depended influence of bortezomib on TRAIL or DR5-B mediated cell death in MDA-MB-231 cells. (A) Contribution of death receptors DR4 and DR5 in TRAIL-mediated cell death in MDA-MB-231 cells. Cells were pre-incubated with 20 µg/ml antagonistic antibodies to death receptors or IgG1 control for 1 h following 4 h treatment with TRAIL or DR5-B (500 ng/ml) and cell death was determined by MTT test. Values are mean ± SD of at least three independent experiments. (B) Viability of the cells treated with different concentrations of TRAIL or DR5-B with or without bortezomib (25 nM) during 8, 16, 20 and 24 h of incubation. Values are mean ± SD of at least three independent experiments.

Acknowledgments

The authors would like to thank I.S. Litvinov and E.I. Kovalenko from Shemyakin and Ovchinnikov Institute of Bioorganic Chemistry, RAS for technical help in flow cytometry experiments.

Author Contributions

Conceived and designed the experiments: MEG DAD. Performed the experiments: MLB MEG DAD. Analyzed the data: MLB. Contributed reagents/materials/analysis tools: MLB. Wrote the paper: MEG MPK.

References

1. Ashkenazi A, Pai RC, Fong S, Leung S, Lawrence DA, et al. (1999) Safety and antitumor activity of recombinant soluble Apo2 ligand. J Clin Invest 104: 155–162.
2. LeBlanc HN, Ashkenazi A (2003) Apo2L/TRAIL and its death and decoy receptors. Cell Death Differ 10: 66–75.
3. Clancy L, Mruk K, Archer K, Woelfel M, Mongkolsapaya M, et al. (2005) Preligand assembly domain-mediated ligand independent association between TRAIL receptor 4 (TR4) and TR2 regulates TRAIL-induced apoptosis. PNAS 102: 18099–18104.
4. Merino D, Lalaoui N, Morizot A, Schneider P, Solary E, et al. (2006) Differential inhibition of TRAIL-mediated DR5-DISC formation by decoy receptors 1 and 2. Mol Cell Biol 26: 7046–7055.
5. Hymowitz SG, O'Connell MP, Ultsch MH, Hurst A, Totpal K, et al. (2000) A unique zinc-binding site revealed by a high-resolution X-ray structure of homotrimeric Apo2L/TRAIL. Biochemistry 39: 633–640.
6. Gasparian ME, Chernyak BV, Dolgikh DA, Yagolovich AV, Popova EN, et al. (2009) Generation of new TRAIL mutants DR5-A and DR5-B with improved selectivity to death receptor 5. Apoptosis 14: 778–787.
7. Georgakis GV, Li Y, Humphreys R, Andreeff M, O'Brien S, et al. (2005) Activity of selective fully human agonistic antibodies to the TRAIL death receptors TRAIL-R1 and TRAIL-R2 in primary and cultured lymphoma cells: induction of apoptosis and enhancement of doxorubicin- and bortezomib-induced cell death. Br J Haematol 130: 501–510.
8. Griffith TS, Rauch CT, Smolak PJ, Waugh JY, Boiani N, et al. (1999) Functional analysis of TRAIL receptors using monoclonal antibodies. J Immunol 162: 2597–2605.
9. Bin L, Thorburn J, Thomas LR, Clark PE, Humphreys R, et al. (2007) Tumor-derived mutations in the TRAIL receptor DR5 inhibit TRAIL signaling through

the DR4 receptor by competing for ligand binding. J Biol Chem 282: 28189–28194.
10. Luster TA, Carrell JA, McCormick K, Sun D, Humphreys R (2009) Mapatumumab and lexatumumab induce apoptosis in TRAIL-R1 and TRAIL-R2 antibody-resistant NSCLC cell lines when treated in combination with bortezomib. Mol Cancer Ther 8: 292–302.
11. MacFarlane M, Inoue S, Kohlhaas SL, Majid A, Harper N, et al. (2005) Chronic lymphocytic leukemic cells exhibit apoptotic signaling via TRAIL-R1. Cell Death Differ 12: 773–782.
12. Kelley RF, Totpal K, Lindstrom SH, Mathieu M, Billeci K, et al. (2005) Receptor selective mutants of apoptosis-inducing ligand 2/tumor necrosis factor-related apoptosis-inducing ligand reveal a greater contribution of death receptor (DR) 5 than DR4 to apoptosis signaling. J Biol Chem 280: 2205–2212.
13. Yang A, Wilson NS, Ashkenazi A (2010) Proapoptotic DR4 and DR5 signaling in cancer cells: toward clinical translation. Curr. Opin. Cell Biol 22: 837–844.
14. Elrod HA, Sun SY. (2008) Modulation of death receptors by cancer therapeutic agents. Cancer Biol Ther 7: 163–173.
15. Mahalingam D, Szegezdi E, Keane M, de Jong S, Samali A (2009) TRAIL receptor signalling and modulation: Are we on the right TRAIL? Cancer Treat Rev 35: 280–288.
16. Menke C, Bin L, Thorburn J, Behbakht K, Ford HL, et al. (2011) Distinct TRAIL resistance mechanisms can be overcome by proteasome inhibition but not generally by synergizing agents. Cancer Res 71: 1883–1892.
17. de Wilt LH, Kroon J, Jansen G, de Jong S, Peters GJ, et al. (2013) Bortezomib and TRAIL: a perfect match for apoptotic elimination of tumour cells? Crit Rev Oncol Hematol 85: 363–372.
18. Chen KF, Yeh PY, Hsu C, Hsu CH, Lu YS, et al. (2009) Bortezomib overcomes tumor necrosis factor-related apoptosis-inducing ligand resistance in hepatocel-

lular carcinoma cells in part through the inhibition of the phosphatidylinositol 3-kinase/Akt pathway. J Biol Chem 284: 1112–1133.

19. Koschny R, Holland H, Sykora J, Haas TL, Sprick MR, et al. (2007) Bortezomib sensitizes primary human astrocytoma cells of WHO grades I to IV for tumor necrosis factor-related apoptosis-inducing ligand-induced apoptosis. Clin Cancer Res 13: 3403–3412.

20. Seki N, Toh U, Sayers TJ, Fujii T, Miyagi M, et al. (2010) Bortezomib sensitizes human esophageal squamous cell carcinoma cells to TRAIL-mediated apoptosis via activation of both extrinsic and intrinsic apoptosis pathways. Mol Cancer Ther 9: 1842–1851.

21. Voortman J, Resende TP, Abou El, Hassan MA, Giaccone G, et al. (2007) TRAIL therapy in non-small cell lung cancer cells: sensitization to death receptor-mediated apoptosis by proteasome inhibitor bortezomib. Mol Cancer Ther 6: 2103–2112.

22. Saulle E, Petronelli A, Pasquini L, Petrucci E, Mariani G, et al. (2007) Proteasome inhibitors sensitize ovarian cancer cells to TRAIL induced apoptosis. Apoptosis 12: 635–655.

23. An WG, Hwang SG, Trepel JB, Blagosklonny MV (2000) Protease inhibitor induced apoptosis: accumulation of wt p53, p21WAF1/CIP1, and induction of apoptosis are independent markers of proteasome inhibition. Leukemia 14: 1276–1283.

24. Brooks AD, Ramirez T, Toh U, Onksen J, Elliott PJ, et al. (2005) The proteasome inhibitor bortezomib (Velcade) sensitizes some human tumor cells to Apo2L/TRAIL-mediated apoptosis. Ann NY Acad Sci 1059: 160–167.

25. Strauss SJ, Higginbottom K, Jüliger S, Maharaj L, Allen P, et al. (2007) The proteasome inhibitor bortezomib acts independently of p53 and induces cell death via apoptosis and mitotic catastrophe in B-cell lymphoma cell lines. Cancer Res 67: 2783–2790.

26. Ling X, Calinski D, Chanan-Khan AA, Zhou M, Li F (2010) Cancer cell sensitivity to bortezomib is associated with survivin expression and p53 status but not cancer cell types. J Exp Clin Cancer Res 29: 8.

27. Bunz F, Hwang PM, Torrance C, Waldman T, Zhang Y, et al. (1999) Disruption of p53 in human cancer cells alters the responses to therapeutic agents. J Clin Invest 104: 263–269.

28. Gasparian ME, Bychkov ML, Dolgikh DA, Kirpichnikov MP (2011) Strategy for improvement of enteropeptidase efficiency in tag removal processes. Protein Expr Purif 79: 191–196.

29. van de Kooij B, Verbrugge I, de Vries E, Gijsen M, Montserrat V, et al. (2013) Ubiquitination by the membrane-associated RING-CH-8 (MARCH-8) ligase controls steady-state cell surface expression of tumor necrosis factor-related apoptosis inducing ligand (TRAIL) receptor 1. J Biol Chem 288: 6617–6628.

30. Algeciras-Schimnich A, Shen L, Barnhart BC, Murmann AE, Burkhardt JK, et al. (2002) Molecular ordering of the initial signaling events of CD95. Mol Cell Biol 22: 207–220.

31. Conus S, Simon HU (2008) Cathepsins: key modulators of cell death and inflammatory responses. Biochem Pharmacol 76: 1374–1382.

32. Yeung BH, Huang DC, Sinicrope FA (2006) PS-341 (bortezomib) induces lysosomal cathepsin B release and a caspase-2-dependent mitochondrial permeabilization and apoptosis in human pancreatic cancer cells. J Biol Chem 281: 11923–11932.

33. Werneburg NW, Guicciardi ME, Bronk SF, Kaufmann SH, Gores GJ (2007) Tumor necrosis factor-related apoptosis-inducing ligand activates a lysosomal pathway of apoptosis that is regulated by Bcl-2 proteins. J Biol Chem 282: 28960–28970.

34. Nagaraj NS, Vigneswaran N, Zacharias W (2006) Cathepsin B mediates TRAIL-induced apoptosis in oral cancer cells. J Cancer Res Clin Oncol 132: 171–183.

35. Yu R, Deedigan L, Albarenque SM, Mohr A, Zwacka RM (2013) Delivery of sTRAIL variants by MSCs in combination with cytotoxic drug treatment leads to p53-independent enhanced antitumor effects. Cell Death Dis 4: e503.

36. Marini P, Denzinger S, Schiller D, Kauder S, Welz S, et al. (2006) Combined treatment of colorectal tumours with agonistic TRAIL receptor antibodies HGS-ETR1 and HGS-ETR2 and radiotherapy: enhanced effects in vitro and dose-dependent growth delay in vivo. Oncogene 25: 5145–5154.

17

Acid Suppression Therapy Does Not Predispose to *Clostridium difficile* Infection: The Case of the Potential Bias

Lena Novack[1]*, **Slava Kogan**[2], **Larisa Gimpelevich**[1], **Michael Howell**[3], **Abraham Borer**[4], **Ciarán P. Kelly**[5], **Daniel A. Leffler**[6], **Victor Novack**[2]

1 Department of Epidemiology, Faculty of Health Sciences, Ben-Gurion University of the Negev, Beer-Sheva, Israel, 2 Clinical Research Center, Soroka University Medical Center, Ben-Gurion University of the Negev, Beer-Sheva, Israel, 3 The University of Chicago Medicine, Chicago, Illinois, United States of America, 4 Infectious Diseases Unit, Soroka University Medical Center, Beer-Sheva, Israel, 5 Division of Gastroenterology, Beth Israel Deaconess Medical Center, Harvard Medical School, Boston, Massachusetts, United States of America, 6 The Celiac Center at BIDMC, Division of Gastroenterology, Beth Israel Deaconess Medical Center, Boston, Massachusetts, United States of America

Abstract

Objective: An adverse effect of acid-suppression medications on the occurrence of *Clostridium difficile* infection (CDI) has been a common finding of many, but not all studies. We hypothesized that association between acid-suppression medications and CDI is due to the residual confounding in comparison between patients with infection to those without, predominantly from non-tested and less sick subjects. We aimed to evaluate the effect of acid suppression therapy on incidence of *CDI* by comparing patients with CDI to two control groups: not tested patients and patients suspected of having CDI, but with a negative test.

Methods: We conducted a case-control study of adult patients hospitalized in internal medicine department of tertiary teaching hospital between 2005–2010 for at least three days. Controls from each of two groups (negative for CDI and non-tested) were individually matched (1:1) to cases by primary diagnosis, Charlson comorbidity index, year of hospitalization and gender. Primary outcomes were diagnoses of International Classification of Diseases (ICD-9)–coded CDI occurring 72 hours or more after admission.

Results: Patients with CDI were similar to controls with a negative test, while controls without CDI testing had lower clinical severity. In multivariable analysis, treatment by acid suppression medications was associated with CDI compared to those who were not tested (OR = 1.88, p-value = 0.032). Conversely, use of acid suppression medications in those who tested negative for the infection was not associated with CDI risk as compared to the cases (OR = 0.66; p = 0.059).

Conclusions: These findings suggest that the reported epidemiologic associations between use of acid suppression medications and CDI risk may be spurious. The control group choice has an important impact on the results. Clinical differences between the patients with CDI and those not tested and not suspected of having the infection may explain the different conclusions regarding the acid suppression effect on CDI risk.

Editor: Markus M. Heimesaat, Charité, Campus Benjamin Franklin, Germany

Funding: The authors have no support or funding to report.

Competing Interests: The authors have declared that no competing interests exist.

* Email: novack@bgu.ac.il

Background

The morbidity and mortality rates caused by *Clostridium difficile* have increased lately, reflecting increased antibiotic use, the aging population and the emergence of high-level resistant strains [1,2] Outbreaks of CDI have been registered in hospitals worldwide [1,3], with reports of increased severity of disease, more frequent community acquired disease and rising CDI-associated healthcare costs [4,5]. The Centers for Disease Control (CDC)

have reported that the annual burden of CDI in the US is > 350,000 new cases with 14,000 CDI-related deaths. [6]

Antibiotic treatment has been shown to be the main risk factor for development of CDI. [6,7] Additional, well-established, risk factors include advancing age (e.g. older than 65), hospital admission, severe underlying disease, [8] prolonged hospitalization [9] and invasive gastrointestinal procedures. [10]

During the last decade studies have reported marked overuse of proton pump inhibitors (PPIs). As many as 60% of prescriptions may not follow the criteria of the National Institute for Clinical

Excellence, but are administered for non-indicated, prophylactic reasons [11–13]. Gastric acid suppression treatment has been shown repetitively to be associated with an increased risk of hospital and community-acquired CDI. [14–18]. This association has been explained by the loss of the defensive effect of gastric acid. [12,19] While this mechanism appears reasonable for vegetative enteric pathogens it is less plausible for CDI where the inoculum is believed to be predominantly in the form of acid-resistant spores. Also, the association between acid suppression therapy and CDI has not been universal and was not found in some studies. [12,20]

One of the major limitations of these pharmaco-epidemiological studies is a potential bias inherently associated with this type of analysis: despite the multivariate adjustment the two comparison groups (with and without acid suppression) might differ significantly. Patients who develop CDI are known to be more ill than most other hospital patients. Thus they may be more likely to carry risk factors and exposures that lead to the use of acid suppression therapy. Put differently, the epidemiologic association may result from severe underlying disease being associated with CDI and, in parallel, leading to increased PPI use.

We hypothesize that the comparison groups used to examine the association between acid suppression therapy and CDI are intrinsically unsuited due to their very different clinical characteristics leading to bias. Therefore, to address this concern, we conducted a nested case-control study of CDI patients with two separate matched control groups: one with suspected CDI but negative stool testing and a second without suspected CDI.

Methods

Study Population and Study Groups Definition

The study population comprised adult patients hospitalized in internal medicine wards of Soroka University Medical Center (SUMC) during the period 2005–2010. SUMC is a 1100-bed tertiary teaching hospital and the only provider of in-hospital care for the population of 700,000 in southern Israel. Patients included in the study had to spend at least 3 days in the hospital and cases had to be hospitalized 3 days before infection was detected (to qualify as a hospital-acquired infection). We chose not to include patients hospitalized after 2010 in light of growing awareness in our hospital of the reported risk of CCDI associated with use of acid-suppressor medications, supported by the FDA safety announcement issued in Feb 2, 2012 [21].

Cases were defined as a first incidence of a positive stool *C. difficile* toxin (by enzyme-linked immunosorbent assay) in a patient with diarrhea. For each case we matched one control with a negative C. difficile toxin test and one who was not suspected to have CDI and was not tested. Both types of controls were matched by gender, age (with a caliper of 5 years) and hospitalization within 12 months before or after the date of the case hospitalization. Controls with a negative test for CDI were also matched by the primary diagnosis.

Definitions

Treatment by acid-suppressors was defined as use of a H_2 receptor antagonist (H_2RA) or PPI three months prior to admission and during the index hospitalization. The H_2RA medications included famotidine and ranitidine; PPI medications included omeprazole, lansoprazole and pantoprazole. We further defined exposure to acid suppression by three levels of intensity: (a) patients not receiving acid-suppressor medications, (b) patients receiving only H_2RA medications, and (c) patients receiving one daily dose of PPI treatment.

Antibiotic treatment was defined by the extent of exposure to antibiotics and was analyzed in 3 groups by the expected risk of CDI: i.e. no antibiotics administered, low-risk and high-intermediate risk antimicrobials. The group of high-intermediate risk antibiotics included fluoroquinolones, cephalosporins, beta-lactams, macrolides, carbapenems, sulfonomides and clindamycin. All other types of antibiotics were included in the low-risk category. This breakdown of antibiotics medications follow the definitions set in our previous investigation [22], as well as by UpToDate web site [23].

Primary diagnosis and co-morbidities were defined by the International Classification of Diseases, 9th Revision (ICD-9). We used the Charlson index to compute the burden of co-morbid conditions. The overall comorbidity score reflects the cumulative increased likelihood of one-year mortality; the higher the score, the more severe the burden of comorbidities. [24]

No informed consent was required, as the current research was based only on patients' medical records collected from the hospital admission-discharge-transfer (ATD) database. Patients' records were anonymized and de-identified prior to analysis. This approach, as well as the protocol of the study, has been approved by the Soroka University Medical Center IRB committee.

Statistical Analysis

Continuous variables were presented as means±standard deviation (sd), median, minimum and maximum; they were compared between study groups using Wilcoxon and t-test, depending on the variable distribution. Categorical variables were presented as percent out of available cases and compared between study groups using univariate conditional logistic regression technique. Cases were compared separately to each type of control. Multivariate analysis for identifying independent factors affecting CDI was performed using conditional logistic regression. We restricted the study population in the multivariable analysis to those cases with matched controls to keep the comparisons balanced. We performed sensitivity analysis on a sub-set of the study population, where each case was matched to both types of controls.

Results

Overview

During the study period (2005–2010) the SUMC laboratory tested 2,343 stool samples for CDI, 337 were positive (Figure 1) and 212 out of 337 were found eligible for the study (main reasons for non-eligibility were: hospital stay shorter than 72 hours, age below 18, not primary case of CDI). There were 185 patients with a negative stool test and 159 patients without a test who could be matched to the cases. Both types of controls were matched only to 132 cases.

The study population

Approximately half of the patients were women (51.4%) and on average 69 years old (Table 1). As matching by age was performed with a caliper of 5 years, there was a small discrepancy in age between the study groups; controls with a negative test result were one year older and controls without a test were 2 years older compared to their cases. Even though being clinically marginally important, the two-years difference in age between cases and the controls without a test was statistically significant (p-value<0.001). Of note, 19.3% of the CDI patients lived in nursing homes, compared to 10.8% in the 2 groups of controls (p-value = 0.042). Treatment by antibiotics was more intense within the CDI group than in patients without CDI (Table 2).

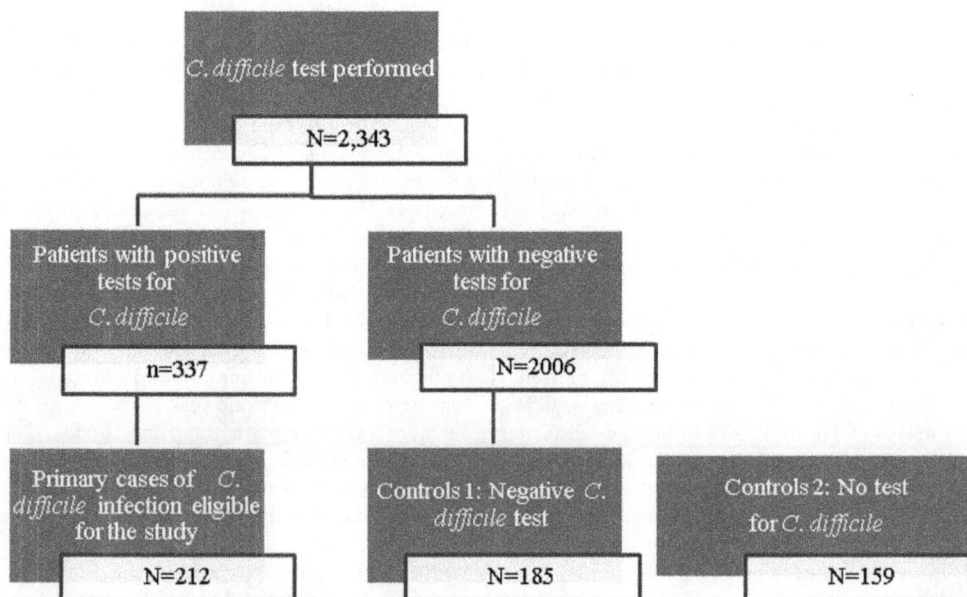

Figure 1. Flowchart of enrolled patients.

Distribution of primary diagnoses is shown in table 3, and was not different between the study groups. The majority of patients were hospitalized due to an infectious disease (62.8%), followed by 17.3% with a diagnosis of a cardiovascular disorder and 9.4% patients hospitalized due to a neoplasm. The group of CDI cases was similar to the group of controls with a negative *C. difficile* test by their co-morbidities and Charlson score (Table 3). Controls without a test had significantly lower rates of pneumonia and anemia (p-value = 0.030 and p-value<0.001, respectively). The proportion of patients fed by nasogastric tube was similar in CDI cases (25.5%) and in controls with a negative test (31.9%) but was lower in control patients without a test (12.6%). To summarize, patients with CDI were similar to controls with a negative test, while controls without a suspicion for CDI had lower clinical severity in several respects. These clinical differences were reflected in a longer hospitalization and higher mortality rate within the patients with a test compared to the patients without (median length of stay was 15 days and 1-year mortality rate reached 49.6% in the group with the test (controls and cases), compared to 5 days of stay (p-value<0.001) and mortality rate 37.7% (p-value = 0.11) in the group without the test.

Acid suppression therapy

Treatment by acid-suppression medication prior to hospitalization was recorded in 38% patients, without differences between the study groups (table 4). However, as we noticed previously with clinical characteristics, the frequency of treatment by acid suppression medications was similar between cases and controls with a negative test but different from the controls without a test. Administering of H_2RA was more common within patients with a *C. difficile* test, 21.7% and 20.0% for those with a positive or negative result, respectively, compared to 13.8% for those with no test. In other words, CDI cases were not different from the controls suspected for having CDI (and thus tested) in terms of their exposure to H_2RA (p-value = 0.511), but their exposure to H_2RA was higher compared to the controls without a test (at borderline significance level of 0.074). Of note, exposure to PPI therapy was

more frequent within those who tested negative for CDI than in the group of CDI cases (48.6% vs. 36.8%, p-value = 0.004).

Results of a multivariable analysis of factors associated with the *C.Difficile* infection are presented in table 5. After adjusting for well-established risk factors, i.e. Charlson index, residence in a nursing home and treatment by antibiotics, treatment by acid suppression medications showed a protective trend on risk for CDI (OR = 0.66; p-value = 0.059) within the group of patients suspected for infection (i.e. tested for CDI). However, as reported by other studies, treatment with these medications was associated with an increased likelihood of the infection when CDI cases were compared to the controls that were not tested (OR = 1.88, p-value = 0.032). Similar trends were obtained for the effect of H_2RA and PPI medications, when tested separately. Treatment by H_2RA showed no risk increase whereas the administration of a PPI significantly reduced the likelihood of CDI within the patients who were tested (OR = 0.54; p-value = 0.019). Each medication was associated with an increased likelihood of CDI when CDI cases were compared to untested controls, however with p-values approaching significance (OR_{H2RA} = 1.99, p-value = 0.075 and OR_{PPI} = 1.82, p-value = 0.077).

Sensitivity and Missing Data Analysis

Not all 212 CDI cases were matched to both types of controls. Sensitivity analysis on a fully matched set of 132 cases with both controls available showed no difference in study conclusions.

Furthermore, 27 CDI cases had no tested negative controls and 53 CDI had no controls from the group without a test. Closer inspection of distribution of exposure within "not-paired" CDI cases reveal that 27 cases without negative tested controls to the rest of the sample used in the analysis. However, 53 cases without a match in non-suspected group had lower exposure to acid-suppression therapy (47% in non-paired cases vs. 62% in the paired cases used in the main analysis). We have simulated a univariable conditional logistic regression analysis on 1000 samples assuming inclusion of the group of unpaired cases, which would have resulted in overall 58.2% of exposure in all cases. The analysis showed that the risk estimate would have decreased from

Table 1. Demographic Characteristics of the Study Population.

Demographic characteristics	Cases: Patients testing positive for *C. difficile* (N = 212)	Patients without *C. difficile* infection	
		Patients negative on *C. difficile* test - Controls type 1 (N = 185)	Patients without a *C. difficile* test - Controls type 2 (N = 159)
Age, years			
Mean±SD	68.2±16.9	69.0±16.9	71.2±17.5
Median	72.0	74.0	77.0
Min; Max	18.0–92.0	18.0–92.0	22.0–97.0
(pv vs. cases)		(pv = 0.084)	(pv<0.001)
Female Gender, % (n/N)	53.3% (112)	55.7% (103)	51.6% (82)
(pv vs. cases)		(pv = 1.000)	(pv = 1.000)
Family status, %(n/N)			
Married	62.5%(130/208)	58.3%(98/168)	58.5%(93)
Divorced	3.4%(7/208)	5.4%(9/168)	3.8%(6)
Widow	9.1%(19/208)	7.7%(13/168)	12.6%(20)
Not Married	7.2%(15/208)	7.1%(12/168)	7.5%(12)
(pv vs. cases)		(pv = 1.000)	(pv = 0.330)
Country of birth, %(n/N)			
Israel	21.2%(45)	19.5%(36)	20.8%(33)
Former USSR	25.0%(53)	25.4%(47)	30.2%(48)
Asia	33.5%(71)	28.6%(53)	23.9%(38)
Europe	7.5%(16)	9.2%(17)	19.5%(31)
North America	4.7%(10)	4.3%(8)	1.9%(3)
Africa	4.7%(10)	2.7%(5)	3.1%(5)
(pv vs. cases)		(pv = 0.143)	(pv = 0.596)
Residence %(n/N)			
Home	78.3%(166)	86.5%(160)	86.8%(138)
Nursing Home	19.3%(41)	10.3%(19)	11.3%(18)
Other	2.4%(5)	3.2%(7)	1.9%(3)
(pv vs. cases)		(pv = 0.087)	(pv = 0.143)
Type of Residency, %(n/N)			
City	79.4%(167)	75.8%(138)	85.8%(133)
Non-urban settlement	7.1%(15)	7.0%(13)	7.0%(11)
Kibbutz	3.8%(8)	1.6%(3)	3.9%(6)
Bedouin-Arab village	8.1%(17)	6.6%(12)	4.5%(7)
(pv vs. cases)		(pv = 0.132)	(pv = 0.067)

1.88 (table 4) to 1.60, and would have maintained the statistical significance.

Discussion

In this study we hypothesized that the comparison of CDI cases to all hospital patients without CDI, as adopted in a majority of studies, brings bias to the results based on the overall severity of illness in the CDI patients. Severely ill patients may be more likely to receive acid suppression medications leading to an apparent association of these medications with CDI. We assessed our hypothesis in a case-control setting, in which patients with a positive test for *C. difficile* (CDI cases) were compared separately to patients suspected of CDI but with a negative test (a group that may be clinically more similar to CDI patients) and controls in whom CDI was not suspected or tested for.

The data obtained in our study brought us to a different understanding of the association between acid-suppression medications and CDI. From the comparison of demographical, clinical and procedural characteristics of the study groups – it became apparent that the group of cases is similar to the group of controls with suspected CDI but having a negative test. Furthermore, both are very different from the patients without a test. The CDI cases and the controls with a negative test are united by a clinical suspicion for having CDI (and therefore being tested for it). This clinical suspicion identifies a group of subjects with high underlying disease burdens and high subsequent death rates. The similarity between CDI cases and controls with a negative test for CDI and their difference from patients not suspected of CDI is statistically evident for the diagnoses of pneumonia and/or anemia, more prevalent co-morbidities, as well as more frequent procedures compared to patients in whom the test was not

Table 2. Clinical Characteristics of the study population during hospitalization, by study groups.

Clinical Characteristics	Cases: Patients testing positive for *C. difficile* (N = 212)	Patients without *C. difficile* infection	
		Patients negative on *C. difficile* test - Controls type 1 (N = 185)	Patients without a *C. difficile* test - Controls type 2 (N = 159)
Procedure during Hospitalization, % (n) *(pv vs. cases)*			
Colonoscopy	6.1% (13)	7.1%(13) (pv = 1.000)	2.5%(4) (pv = 0.092)
Surgery	22.9% (47/205)	28.2%(51/181) (pv = 0.590)	3.8%(6) (pv<0.001)
Feeding, %(n)			
Oral	71.2% (151)	67.6%(125)	85.6%(136)
Nasogastric tube	25.5% (54)	31.9%(59)	12.6%(20)
PEG	3.3% (7)	0.5%(1)	1.9%(3)
(pv vs. cases)		(pv = 0.925)	(pv = 0.003)
Antibiotics 3 months prior to or during hospitalization, % (n) *(pv vs. cases)*	96.7% (205)	91.9% (170) (pv = 0.064)	66.0% (105) (pv<0.001)
Before Hospitalization	45.8% (97)	20.0% (37) (pv<0.001)	19.5% (31) (pv<0.001)
During Hospitalization	93.4% (198)	88.1% (163) (pv = 0.151)	64.2% (102)(pv<0.001)
WBC			
Mean±SD	15.7±18.6	11.9±7.9	11.6±7.7
Positive result obtained for test in, % (n) *(pv vs. cases)*			
Bacteriology	54.7%(116)	48.1%(89) (pv = 0.271)	25.3%(40) (pv<0.001)
Blood	19.3% (41)	23.8% (44) (pv = 0.499)	9.4% (15) (pv = 0.002)
Sputum	9.1% (19)	11.4%(21) (pv = 0.398)	0.6% (1) (pv<0.001)
Urine	40.6%(86)	27.5%(51) (pv = 0.014)	14.5%(23) (pv<0.001)
Length of stay, days			
Median	16.0	13.0	5.0
Min-Max	0.0–440.0	1.0–127.0 (pv = 0.078)	1.0–69.0 (pv<0.001)
Mortality, %(n) *(pv vs. cases)*			
In-hospital	21.2% (45)	18.4%(34) (pv = 0.409)	13.2%(21) (pv = 0.010)
At 1 year follow-up	53.3%(113)	45.4%(84) (pv = 0.110)	37.7%(60) (pv<0.001)

performed. The patients suspected for CDI also more frequently required nasogastric feeding and more frequently had a positive bacterial culture in blood, sputum or urine, compared to controls without a CDI test. These markers of increased underlying disease severity were also associated with adverse clinical outcomes including longer hospitalizations and higher mortality rates.

Prior exposures to acid-suppressing medications in the community was not different between the study groups, but changed following hospitalization, when patients not suspected of having CDI were less likely to receive acid-suppressing medication compared to those with suspected or proven CDI. This discrepancy resulted in an estimated independent adverse effect for exposure to H₂RA and PPI medications, with OR = 1.88 (p-value = 0.032) for those with CDI compared to the controls that were not tested. Quite remarkably, the patients with a negative *C. difficile* test were more likely to be exposed to intensive acid suppression treatment (48.6% exposed to PPI) compared to those with CDI (36.7% exposed to PPI). In keeping with this finding, the multivariable analysis did not show a detrimental effect of acid suppression medications (OR = 0. 66, p-value = 0.059) in comparison between patients with CDI and those with suspected CDI. Based on the contradictory findings we cannot conclude that there

is an adverse effect of exposure to acid-suppressing medication and CDI risk.

Acid anti-secretory medications and particularly PPIs may lead to diarrhea. [25] Thus, patients taking PPIs may be more likely to be tested for CDI but be negative, as most of the patients would have PPI-induced diarrhea, in comparison to general population of patients with more prevalent CDI-induced diarrhea. To illustrate this let us consider the following hypothetical example, where we have 100 patients with diarrhea and no PPI treatment with CDI prevalence of 5% (5 cases); and let us assume that PPI treatment is associated with 2 folds increase in diarrhea risk, leading to a situation where in the same hospital population, but now treated with PPI we will have twice as many patients with diarrhea – 200. Assuming that PPI treatment does not increase CDI risk, among these 200 subjects we will still have the same 5 cases of CDI (2.5%). We might conclude that statistically speaking PPI treatment is associated with a protective effect against CDI – a decrease from 5% to 2.5% incidence. This may, in part, account for the protective, but spurious PPI effect observed in our study.

Our findings disagree directly with the widely held opinion that acid suppression medications are a risk factor for CDI. This discrepancy inevitably leads to questions regarding the validity of

Table 3. Clinical Characteristics of the study population at admission, by study groups.

Clinical Characteristics	Cases: Patients testing positive for *C. difficile* (N=212)	Patients without *C. difficile* infection	
		Patients negative on *C. difficile* test - Controls type 1 (N=185)	Patients without a *C. difficile* test - Controls type 2 (N=159)
Primary Diagnosis, % (n)			
Cardiovascular	16.5% (34)	17.8% (33)	18.2% (29)
Infectious	67.0% (142)	58.9% (109)	61.6% (98)
Neoplasm	8.0% (17)	11.4% (21)	8.8% (14)
Orthopedics	3.3% (7)	2.7% (5)	0.6% (1)
Renal	2.8 (6)	2.7% (5)	6.9 (11)
Others	2.8 (6)	6.5% (12)	3.8 (6)
(pv vs. cases)		(pv=0.370)	(pv=0.199)
Co-morbidities, % (n) *(pv vs. cases)*			
History MI	19.8%(42)	27.6%(51) (pv=0.182)	25.2%(40) (pv=0.532)
Heart failure	43.3%(94)	40.5%(75) (pv=0.177)	40.3%(64) (pv=0.306)
Chronic Pulmonary Disease	8.0%(17)	8.6%(16) (pv=0.839)	11.3%(18) (pv=0.850)
Pneumonia	30.2% (17)	30.3% (56) (pv=1.000)	20.8% (33) (pv=0.030)
Diabetes	34.4%(73)	37.3%(69) (pv=1.000)	34.6%(55) (pv=0.810)
Hypertension	46.2%(98)	48.1%(89) (pv=0.644)	52.2%(83) (pv=0.550)
Chronic Renal Failure	13.7%(29)	14.1%(26) (pv=0.880)	13.2%(21) (pv=0.424)
Peptic Ulcer Disease	4.7%(10)	4.9%(9) (pv=1.000)	2.5%(4) (pv=0.344)
Cancer	19.3%(41)	26.5%(49) (pv=0.057)	19.5%(31) (pv=1.000)
Anemia	40.1%(85)	37.8%(70) (pv=1.000)	28.3%(43) (pv=0.001)
Charlson Index			
Mean±SD	5.0±3.3	5.6±3.9	5.0±3.3
Median	5.0	6.0	5.0
Min-Max *(pv vs. cases)*	0.0–19.0	0.0–18.0 (pv=0.114)	0.0–15.0 (pv=0.520)

our methodology. For example, possible inaccuracies of the *C. difficile* tests might have concealed the effect. However, the assessed effect is in fact significantly opposite, which cannot be fully explained by laboratory error. Our results showing an adverse effect of acid-suppression medications in comparison with controls not tested for CDI, is in fact, consistent with the published research by Pohl [18], Howell et al [22], Bavishi and Dupont [26] or by Pakyz et al [27], where the control group consisted of all

Table 4. Exposure to Acid-suppression medications, by study groups.

Acid suppression medication	Cases: Patients testing positive for *C. difficile* (N=212)	Patients without *C. difficile* infection	
		Patients negative on *C. difficile* test - Controls type 1 (N=185)	Patients without a *C. difficile* test - Controls type 2 (N=159)
Acid suppression % (n/N)			
Within 3 months prior to hospitalization			
H₂RA	8.5% (18)	11.4% (21) (pv=0.275)	6.9% (11) (pv=0.283)
PPI	26.4% (56)	31.3% (58) (pv=0.223)	29.6% (47)(pv=0.892)
Acid suppression % (n/N)			
During hospitalization	58.5% (124)	68.7% (127) (pv=0.041)	47.2% (75) (pv=0.008)
By type of medication (pv vs. cases)			
H₂RA	21.7% (46)	20.0%(37) (pv=0.511)	13.8%(22) (pv=0.074)
PPI	36.8% (78)	48.6%(90) (pv=0.004)	33.3%(53) (pv=0.222)

Table 5. Factors affecting *C. difficile* infection, results of a multivariate analysis by conditional logistic regression.

Patients' Characteristics[1]	Patients negative on *C. difficile* test - Controls type 1 (N = 185)		Patients without a *C. difficile* test - Controls type 2 (N = 159)	
	Odds Ratio (CI 95%)	p-value	Odds Ratio (CI 95%)	p-value
Acid suppression during hospitalization	0.66 (0.44–1.02)	0.059	1.88 (1.06–3.36)	0.032
Antibiotic Therapy (before and during hospitalization)	3.03 (1.07–8.62)	0.037	12.97 (4.59–36.61)	<0.001
Residing in a nursing home	1.98 (1.07–3. 669)	0.029	2.59 (1.09–6.18)	0.031

[1]The model included adjustment to Charlson Index.

patients not-positive for CDI. In those studies the group of patients with a negative CDI test was diluted by the majority who were not tested. Therefore, the published data parallels the results in our study whereby untested controls show reduced use of acid suppression medications compared to those with CDI. Of note, few studies comparing cases to patients with negative CDI results, e.g. by Shah et al in 2000 [28] or McFarland et al in 2007 [29], found no association between exposure to acid-suppression and the infection.

Previous research [30] and our data support the hypothesis that the administration of acid-suppressors and testing for CDI (whether positive or negative) are both markers of an unmeasured severity of illness. Comparing cases and controls within a group of patients with the test, who are similar in their degrees of disease severity, could produce the level of adjustment needed to unmeasured confounders. A cohort strategy might lack this necessary level of adjustment and result in biased estimates.

Our analyses confirmed several well-established risk factors for the development of CDI including antibiotic therapy and residence in a nursing home. Conversely, in our study acid suppression therapy was not associated with an increased risk for CDI when patients with similar levels of disease severity were compared. Acid suppression therapy and CDI both track patients with more severe disease leading to an apparent association that does not appear to be primary or causative. Furthermore, these results draw into question the recent Drug Safety Labeling Changes made by the US FDA warning about an association between PPI use and risk for CDI as well as similar warnings in current CDI treatment guidelines. [31]

The study findings, however, have to be treated with caution in view of its limitations. Not all CDI cases were matched to both types of controls; however sensitivity analysis on a fully matched set (132 cases + 2 controls) did not changed conclusions from the main analysis. Likewise, sensitivity analysis of cases without negatively tested controls (27 cases) and cases without non-suspected controls (53 cases) resulted in the same statistical inference. These findings support the internal validity of the study.

We assume that some of the questionable findings in the study may have roots in a possible bias, e.g. the spurious protective effect of PPIs, as discussed previously. The positive effect of PPIs use could have been inflicted by a synergistic interaction that becomes prominent when antibiotics and PPIs are used together [32]. However, the interaction should not affect our findings since the rates of the antibiotics exposure were similar in tested controls (88.1%) and cases (93.4%).

The results might be not fully generalizable, as the study was conducted in a single hospital. On the other hand, the point estimates obtained throughout the analysis is within the range of the effect reported in other studies, which supports the external validity of the results.

To conclude, the potential study bias described in the current analysis needs to be addressed in future research by a careful selection of the relevant control groups for CDI patients.

Author Contributions

Conceived and designed the experiments: LN LG MH VN. Performed the experiments: SK LG. Analyzed the data: LN LG. Wrote the paper: LN LG MH AB CK DL VN.

References

1. Kelly CP, LaMont JT (2008) Clostridium difficile–more difficult than ever. New England Journal of Medicine 359 (18): 1932–40.
2. O'Connor JR, Johnson S, Gerding DN (2009) Clostridium difficile infection caused by the epidemic BI/NAP1/027 strain. Gastroenterology 136 (6): 1913–24.
3. Warmy M, Pepin J, Fang A, Killgore G, Thompson A, et al. (2005) Toxin production by an emerging strain of Clostridium difficile associated with outbreaks of severe disease in North America and Europe. Lancet 366: 9491.
4. Miller MA, Hyland M, Ofner-Agostini M, Gourdeau M, Ishak M, et al Canadian Hospital Epidemiology Committee. Canadian Nosocomial Infection Surveillance. (2002) Morbidity, mortality, and healthcare burden of nosocomial Clostridium difficile-associated diarrhea iMorbidity, mortality, and healthcare burden of nosocomial Clostridium difficile-associated diarrhea in Canadian hospitals. Infect Control Hosp Epidemiol 23 (3): 137–40.
5. McFarland LV (2008) Update on the changing epidemiology of Clostridium difficile-associated disease. Nat Clin Pract Gastroenterol Hepatol 5 (1): 40–8.
6. Owens RC Jr, Donskey CJ, Gaynes RP, Loo VG, Muto CA (2008) Antimicrobial-associated risk factors for Clostridium difficile infection. Clin Infect Dis 46 (Suppl 1): S19–31.
7. Gujja D, Friedenberg FK (2009) Predictors of serious complications due to Clostridium difficile infection. Aliment Pharmacol Ther 29 (6): 635–42.

8. Kyne L, Sougioultzis S, McFarland LV, Kelly CP (2002) Underlying disease severity as a major risk factor for nosocomial Clostridium difficile diarrhea. Infect Control Hosp Epidemio 23(11): 653–9.
9. Bignardi GE (1998) Risk factors for Clostridium difficile infection. J Hosp Infect 40: 1–15.
10. Pierce PF Jr, Wilson R, Silva J Jr, Garagusi VF, Rifkin GD, et al. (1982) Antibiotic-associated pseudomembranous colitis: an epidemiologic investigation of a cluster of cases. J Infect Dis 145: 269–74.
11. Choudhry MN, Soran H, Ziglam HM (2008) Overuse and inappropriate prescribing of proton pump inhibitors in patients with Clostridium difficile-associated disease. QJM. 101 (6): 445–8.
12. Cunningham R, Dial S (2008) Is over-use of proton pump inhibitors fuelling the current epidemic of Clostridium difficile-associated diarrhoea? J Hosp Infect 70 (1): 1–6.
13. Rashid S, Rajan D, Iqbal J, Lipka S, Jacob R, et al. (2012) Inappropriate Use of Gastric Acid Suppression Therapy in Hospitalized Patients with Clostridium difficile-Associated Diarrhea: A Ten-Year Retrospective Analysis. ISRN Gastroenterol: 902320.
14. Aseeri M, Schroeder T, Kramer J, Zackula R (2008) Gastric acid suppression by proton pump inhibitors as a risk factor for clostridium difficile-associated diarrhea in hospitalized patients. Am J Gastroenterol 103 (9): 2308–13.

15. Dial S, Delaney JA, Barkun AN, Suissa S (2005) Use of gastric acid-suppressive agents and the risk of community-acquired Clostridium difficile-associated disease. JAMA 294 (23): 2989–95.

16. Cadle RM, Mansouri MD, Logan N, Kudva DR, Musher DM (2007) Association of proton-pump inhibitors with outcomes in Clostridium difficile colitis. Am J Health Syst Pharm 64 (22): 2359–63.

17. Dalton BR, Lye-Maccannell T, Henderson EA, Maccannell DR, Louie TJ (2009) Proton pump inhibitors increase significantly the risk of Clostridium difficile infection in a low-endemicity, non-outbreak hospital setting. Aliment Pharmacol Ther 29 (6): 626.

18. Pohl JF (2012) Clostridium difficile infection and proton pump inhibitors. Curr Opin Pediat 24 (5): 627–31.

19. Jump RL, Pultz MJ, Donskey CJ (2007) Vegetative Clostridium difficile survives in room air on moist surfaces and in gastric contents with reduced acidity: a potential mechanism to explain the association between proton pump inhibitors and C. difficile-associated diarrhea? Antimicrob Agents Chemother 51 (8): 2883–7.

20. Pépin J, Saheb N, Coulombe MA, Alary ME, Corriveau MP, et al. (2005) Emergence of fluoroquinolones as the predominant risk factor for Clostridium difficile-associated diarrhea: a cohort study during an epidemic in Quebec. Clin Infect Dis 41 (9): 1254–60.

21. Administration, U.S. Food and Drug (2012) FDA Drug Safety Communication: Clostridium difficile-associated diarrhea can be associated with stomach acid drugs known as proton pump inhibitors (PPIs). U.S. Food and Drug Administration. Availebl: http://www.fda.gov/Drugs/DrugSafety/ucm290510.htm#sa. Accessed: September 8, 2014.

22. Howell MD, Novack V, Grgurich P, Soulliard D, Novack L, et al. (2010) Iatrogenic gastric acid suppression and the risk of nosocomial Clostridium difficile infection. Arch Intern Med 170 (9): 784–90.

23. Antibiotics C diff PPI. UpToDate. Available: www.uptodate.com/store. Accessed September 8, 2014.

24. Charlson ME, Pompei P, Ales KL, MacKenzie CR (1987) A new method of classifying prognostic comorbidity in longitudinal studies: development and validation. J Chronic Dis 40 (5): 373–83.

25. Yearsley KA, Gilby LJ, Ramadas AV, Kubiak EM, Fone DL, et al. (2006) Proton pump inhibitor therapy is a risk factor for Clostridium difficile-associated diarrhoea. Aliment Pharmacol Ther 24 (4): 613–9.

26. Bavishi C, Dupont HL (2011) Systematic review: the use of proton pump inhibitors and increased susceptibility to enteric infection. Aliment Pharmacol Ther 34 (11–12): 1269–81.

27. Pakyz AL, Jawahar R, Wang Q, Harpe SE (2014) Medication risk factors associated with healthcare-associated Clostridium difficile infection: a multilevel model case-control study among 64 US academic medical centres. J Antimicrob Chemother 69(4):1127–31.

28. Shah S, Lewis A, Leopold D, Dunstan F, Woodhouse K (2000) Gastric acid suppression does not promote clostridial diarrhoea in the elderly. QJM 93 (3): 175–81.

29. McFarland LV, Clarridge JE, Beneda HW, Raugi GJ (2007) Fluoroquinolone use and risk factors for Clostridium difficile-associated disease within a Veterans Administration health care system. Clin Infect Dis 45 (9): 1141–51.

30. Oake N, Taljaard M, van Walraven C, Wilson K, Roth V, et al. (2010) The effect of hospital-acquired Clostridium difficile infection on in-hospital mortality. Arch Intern Med 170 (20): 1804–10.

31. Surawicz CM, Brandt LJ, Binion DG, Ananthakrishnan AN, Curry SR, et al. (2013) Guidelines for diagnosis, treatment, and prevention of Clostridium difficile infections.

32. Kwok CS, Arthur AK, Anibueze CI, Singh S, Cavallazzi R, et al. (2012) Risk of Clostridium difficile infection with acid suppressing drugs and antibiotics: meta-analysis. Am J Gastroenterol 107(7):1011–9.

18

Down Regulation of Wnt Signaling Mitigates Hypoxia-Induced Chemoresistance in Human Osteosarcoma Cells

Donald J. Scholten II[1,2], Christine M. Timmer[1], Jacqueline D. Peacock[2], Dominic W. Pelle[1,2,3], Bart O. Williams[2], Matthew R. Steensma[1,2,3]*

1 Michigan State University College of Human Medicine, Grand Rapids, Michigan, United States of America, 2 Van Andel Research Institute, Grand Rapids, Michigan, United States of America, 3 Helen DeVos Childen's Hospital, Spectrum Health System, Grand Rapids, Michigan, United States of America

Abstract

Osteosarcoma (OS) is the most common type of solid bone cancer and remains the second leading cause of cancer-related death for children and young adults. Hypoxia is an element intrinsic to most solid-tumor microenvironments, including that of OS, and is associated with resistance to therapy, poor survival, and a malignant phenotype. Cells respond to hypoxia through alterations in gene expression, mediated most notably through the hypoxia-inducible factor (HIF) class of transcription factors. Here we investigate hypoxia-induced changes in the Wnt/β-catenin signaling pathway, a key signaling cascade involved in OS pathogenesis. We show that hypoxia results in increased expression and signaling activation of HIF proteins in human osteosarcoma cells. Wnt/β-catenin signaling is down-regulated by hypoxia in human OS cells, as demonstrated by decreased active β-catenin protein levels and axin2 mRNA expression ($p<0.05$). This down-regulation appears to rely on both HIF-independent and HIF-dependent mechanisms, with HIF-1α standing out as an important regulator. Finally, we show that hypoxia results in resistance of human OS cells to doxorubicin-mediated toxicity (6–13 fold increase, $p<0.01$). These hypoxic OS cells can be sensitized to doxorubicin treatment by further inhibition of the Wnt/β-catenin signaling pathway ($p<0.05$). These data support the conclusion that Wnt/β-catenin signaling is down-regulated in human OS cells under hypoxia and that this signaling alteration may represent a viable target to combat chemoresistant OS subpopulations in a hypoxic niche.

Editor: Chunming Liu, University of Kentucky, United States of America

Funding: The authors thank the Van Andel Research Institute and Spectrum Health for financial support of this work. The funders had no role in study design, data collection and analysis, decision to publish, or preparation of the manuscript.

Competing Interests: B.O. Williams has commercial research support from Genentech. The other authors have no conflicts of interest to disclose.

* Email: matt.steensma@vai.org

Introduction

Osteosarcoma (OS) is the most common type of solid bone cancer, mainly arising in children and young adults, and it remains the second leading cause of cancer-related death in this age group [1]. Osteosarcomas are aggressive, high-grade tumors, with about 20% of patients presenting with metastases [1]. OS is a genomically unstable and heterogeneous tumor, and therapeutic options have not improved over the past four decades [2,3].

Hypoxia is intrinsic to most solid-tumor microenvironments and is associated with resistance to therapy, poor survival, and a malignant phenotype [4]. Cells respond to hypoxia through alterations in gene expression, mediated most notably through the hypoxia-inducible factor (HIF) class of transcription factors [5]. HIF itself is a heterodimeric transcription factor comprising an oxygen-sensitive α-subunit and a constitutively expressed β-subunit [6]. Under normoxia, prolyl hydroxylases hydroxylate the HIFα subunit using O_2 as a substrate, and the hydroxylated HIFα can interact with the von Hippel-Lindau protein to ubiquitinate it and target it for degradation [7,8]. Under hypoxic conditions, the lack of O_2 prevents this hydroxylation, and heterodimerized HIF enters the nucleus to bind to hypoxia

response elements and function as a transcription factor by interacting with other coactivators such as CBP/p300 [7]. Hypoxic regions have been identified in human osteosarcomas, and increased levels of HIF-1α are correlated with decreased disease-free survival and overall survival, as well as increased microvessel density and surgical stage [9,10]. In OS cell lines, hypoxia increases cell migration and promotes chemoresistance independent of HIF-1α [11,12]. Although signaling responses governed by HIFs have been studied extensively in different cancers, little is known about the contributing mechanisms of hypoxia-associated therapy resistance in OS and whether or not they are related to HIFs.

The Wnt/β-catenin signaling pathway contributes to the pathogenesis of numerous diseases including OS [13,14,15,16,17]. In the absence of Wnts, β-catenin undergoes phosphorylation at key serine and threonine residues via the "destruction complex", which includes adenomatous polyposis coli (APC), axin2, casein kinase 1 (CK1), and glycogen synthase kinase 3 (GSK3). This targets β-catenin for subsequent ubiquitinylation and proteasomal degradation. Binding of Wnts to the Frizzled family of receptors and the LDL-receptor-related proteins

(LRP) 5 and 6 co-receptors serves to inhibit the destruction complex, allowing β-catenin to enhance TCF/LEF-mediated transcription [14]. Wnt/β-catenin signaling activation contributes to chemoresistance in OS cells, and increased β-catenin expression has been correlated with shorter cumulative survival in OS patients [18,19].

Although studies in colorectal cancer cells have demonstrated hypoxic interactions between HIFs and β-catenin, results are conflicting in terms of defining Wnt/β-catenin signaling alterations in response to hypoxia in osteoblasts [20,21,22]. Furthermore, no studies have examined whether Wnt/β-catenin signaling is involved in the cellular adaptation to hypoxia in OS. Here we show that that hypoxia results in increased expression and signaling activation of HIF proteins in human osteosarcoma cells. We also show that Wnt/β-catenin signaling is down-regulated under hypoxic conditions, and this down-regulation appears to receive contributions that are both HIF-independent and HIF-dependent. Finally, we show that hypoxia results in robust resistance of OS cells to doxorubicin treatment, which is part of the mainstay chemotherapy regimen for OS patients. This hypoxia-induced chemotherapy resistance can be reduced by further inhibition of the Wnt/β-catenin signaling pathway, suggesting a role for Wnt signaling antagonism in targeting hypoxic OS cell subpopulations.

Materials and Methods

General cell culture and hypoxia chamber

Human osteosarcoma cells (143B, MNNG/HOS, MG-63) were obtained from the ATCC (Manassas, VA). The human OS cell line 206-2 was derived from a consenting OS patient according to protocols approved by the local ethics committee (IRB full name: Spectrum Health Institutional Review Board; part of the Spectrum Health Research Protection Program). Written informed consent was obtained from human research subjects under an IRB-approved (IRB full name: Spectrum Health Institutional Review Board), musculoskeletal tumor and tissue acquisition protocol at Spectrum Health (2011-002). The 143B cells were cultured in Dulbecco's Modified Eagle Medium (DMEM; Gibco) supplemented with 1% L-glutamine, 1% penicillin/streptomycin, and 10% fetal calf serum (FCS); MNNG/HOS cells in Minimum Essential Medium with Earle's Salts (EMEM) supplemented with 1% L-glutamine, 1% penicillin/streptomycin, and 10% FCS; MG-63 cells in EMEM supplemented with 1% L-glutamine, 1% penicillin/streptomycin, 1% nonessential amino acids, 1% sodium pyruvate, and 10% FCS; and 206-2 cells in Minimum Essential Medium (MEM-α) supplemented with 1% L-glutamine, 1% penicillin/streptomycin, and 10% FCS. These cells were cultured under standard incubation conditions (37°C, 5% CO_2) and were subcultured every 3–4 days. Incubation under hypoxic conditions was in a 856-HYPO model hypoxia chamber (PLAS Labs, Lansing, MI) set to 0.5% O_2, 5% CO_2, and 37°C.

Silencing of HIF-1α and HIF-2α

Bacterial glycerol stocks containing the shRNA plasmid of interest were purchased from Sigma Aldrich. shRNA sequences used were as follows: HIF-1α; TRCN0000003810, TRCN0000003811; HIF-2α; TRCN0000003804, TRCN0000003806. Lentiviral particles were produced in the 293FT packaging cell line using the ViraPower Lentiviral Packaging Mix (Invitrogen) according to the manufacturer's guidelines. Lentiviral infection of MNNG/HOS cells was done in the presence of 8 µg/mL polybrene (Millipore) according to the manufacturer's guidelines

before puromycin selection (2 µg/mL). A non-targeting shRNA was used as a control (Sigma Aldrich; SHC002V).

Quantitative reverse transcription PCR (qrt-PCR)

Total RNA was extracted from OS cells using TRIzol reagent (Invitrogen). Complementary DNA synthesis was performed using 500 ng RNA according to the instructions with the High Capacity cDNA Reverse Transcription Kit (Invitrogen). 18S primers (F:CCGCAGCTAGGAATAATGGA; R:CGGTCCAAGAATTTCACCTC), axin2 primers (F:AAGCAAGCGATGAGTTTG-CCTGTG; R:ACAGCCAAGACAGTTCACAAGAGC), and c-myc primers (published previously) were obtained from Integrated DNA Technologies (Coralville, IA) [23]. Quantitative polymerase chain reactions were performed using SYBR Select Mastermix (Applied Biosystems, Carlsbad, CA) in 10 µL reactions. Polymerase chain reaction was performed according to the manufacturer's instructions using a StepOnePlus cycler (Applied Biosystems). Data were analyzed using the $2^{-\Delta\Delta C_T}$ method [24]. Data were presented as mean and standard deviation using Microsoft Excel, with statistical significance being determined using a two-tailed, one-sample t-test with $\mu = 1$ using R and significance set at $\alpha = 0.05$ [25].

Western blot analysis

Whole-cell lysates were washed with PBS and scraped on ice in lysis buffer (RIPA lysis buffer) supplemented with complete Protease Inhibitor Cocktail (Roche). Protein concentration was measured using the BCA assay (Pierce), and 20 µg of whole-cell lysate was run on a 10% SDS/polyacrylamide gel. The proteins were transferred onto a nitrocellulose membrane, and membranes were probed overnight at 4°C with the appropriate primary antibody; antibodies used were as follows: active β-catenin, β-catenin, Oct4 (Cell Signaling Technologies); HIF-1α (R&D Systems), HIF-2α (Abcam), β-tubulin (Santa Cruz), and actin (Millipore). Membranes were then probed with a horseradish-peroxidase-conjugated secondary antibody for 1.5 hours at room temperature before detection using an enhanced chemiluminescence (ECL) detection system (Pierce). Images shown are representative of 2 independent experiments. Western blot densitometry was performed using ImageJ software (Rasband, W.S., ImageJ, U. S. National Institutes of Health, Bethesda, Maryland, USA, http://imagej.nih.gov/ij/, 1997–2014).

Chemoresistance assay

Cells were plated into 96-well white-walled plates (Greiner Bio-One) at 1×10^3 cells/well and allowed to adhere for 24 hours before drug treatments. The cells were then exposed to serial dilutions of doxorubicin (0–10 µM, LC Labs) and were placed in either normoxic or hypoxic conditions (as described above). After an additional 72 hours, cell viability was determined using the CellTiter-Glo Luminescent Cell Viability assay (Promega). Data were normalized to an untreated control well and graphed, and half maximal inhibitory concentration (IC_{50}) values were calculated from the dose-response curve as the concentration of doxorubicin that produced a 50% decrease in the mean luminescence relative to untreated control wells. Statistical tests (two-tailed paired t-test and two-tailed two-sample t-test) were performed using R with significance set at $\alpha = 0.05$. The tankyrase inhibitor XAV939 (Santa Cruz) and porcupine inhibitor IWP-2 (Sigma Aldrich) were used at a 10 µM concentration, with dimethyl sulfoxide (DMSO; Fischer) alone used as a control.

Results

HIFs are present and can be induced via hypoxia in human OS cells

The goal of this study was to identify targetable signaling changes taking place under hypoxic conditions related (or unrelated) to the HIF transcription factors in human OS cells. We first needed to validate the presence of HIFs and examine their activity and induction under normoxic and hypoxic conditions. We cultured human OS cell lines (143B, MG-63, MNNG/HOS) under hypoxic (0.5% O_2) or normoxic conditions for 72 hours and examined the protein levels of HIF-1α, HIF-2α, and a downstream target of HIF-2α, Oct4, by western blot. The expression of HIF-2α and Oct4 in the MG-63 and 143B cell lines increased under the hypoxic conditions relative to normoxic conditions (Figure 1A). When we examined HIF protein expression at shorter time points in the MNNG/HOS cell line, we found that both HIF-1α and HIF-2α were induced by culturing cells under hypoxic conditions for increasing time periods (Figure 1B). Results of two independent replicates were quantified, showcasing the increase in HIF protein levels (Figure S1). These results show that hypoxia stimulates both the expression and signaling activity of HIF proteins in human OS cells.

Wnt/β-catenin signaling is down-regulated in response to hypoxia

Previous reports have described interactions between β-catenin and HIF-1α, thereby linking the Wnt signaling pathway to the hypoxic response [22]. Furthermore, there have been conflicting reports on the role of changes in Wnt/β-catenin signaling in response to hypoxia in osteoblasts [20,21]. We set out to characterize alterations to Wnt/β-catenin signaling in response to hypoxia in human OS cells. In MG-63 cells, we examined protein expression for different durations of hypoxia via western blots and again noticed increased HIF-1α and HIF-2α expression (Figure 2A). We also noticed decreased protein levels of active β-catenin throughout the hypoxic time course, suggesting that Wnt/β-catenin signaling was down-regulated (Figure 2A). This finding was supported through western blot quantification of active β-catenin protein levels (Figure S2). This active (hypophosphorylated) β-catenin antibody recognizes the stabilized form of β-catenin that has not been phosphorylated by GSK-3β, which thereby is active in cell-cell adhesion and canonical Wnt signaling. Levels of active β-catenin strongly correlate with its transcriptional activity [26]. As an alternative measure of Wnt/β-catenin signaling activity, we assessed axin2 mRNA expression using

qrt-PCR. Axin2 is a well-established target of β-catenin-dependent transcription, and its mRNA expression is routinely used as a marker of Wnt/β-catenin signaling [27]. After 72 hours of hypoxia, axin2 mRNA was reduced to 49% in the MG-63 cell line and 44% in the 143B cell line relative to their respective normoxic controls (Figure 2B, p<0.05). These results using active β-catenin protein levels and axin2 mRNA expression indicate that Wnt/β-catenin signaling activity is decreased under hypoxic conditions in human OS cells.

Hypoxic Wnt/β-catenin signaling alterations show evidence of both HIF-dependent and HIF-independent mechanisms

The observed down-regulation in Wnt/β-catenin signaling raises mechanistic questions, especially regarding the potential involvement of HIF proteins. To determine whether the expression of either HIF protein is needed for the decrease in Wnt/β-catenin signaling, we stably transduced MNNG/HOS cells with shRNA targeting either HIF-1α or HIF-2α. We confirmed knockdown at the mRNA (80–90% knockdown) and protein level specific to each HIF protein relative to a non-targeting shRNA control for two independent shRNA's targeting each HIFα subunit (data not shown). Next we examined Wnt/β-catenin signaling activity under hypoxic conditions between the shHIF and non-targeting shRNA MNNG/HOS cells. Active β-catenin protein levels were decreased under hypoxic conditions in both the non-targeting shRNA and the shHIFα cell lines (Figure 3A), as was seen before in the MG-63 cell line (see Fig. 2A). There was also a decrease in total β-catenin at the 72 hour time point (Figure 3A). We assessed axin2 mRNA expression across the shHIF-modified cell lines, comparing normoxic to hypoxic conditions to determine whether β-catenin transcriptional activity was truly altered, or whether the decrease in active β-catenin protein only reflected a decrease in total β-catenin. There was a statistically significant decrease in axin2 mRNA expression under hypoxic conditions in the non-targeting shRNA MNNG/HOS cell line (Figure 3B, p< 0.01), just as noted earlier for the MG-63 and 143B lines (see Figure 2B). That decrease was also consistent in the shHIF-1α- and shHIF-2α-treated MNNG/HOS cell lines, indicating that HIF-independent mechanisms contribute to Wnt/β-catenin signaling down-regulation under hypoxia (Figure 3B, p<0.05). However, when the data were normalized to the hypoxia shnon control, axin2 mRNA expression in both hypoxia shHIF-1α cell lines was increased, implying that HIF-1α contributes to Wnt/β-catenin signaling down-regulation (Figure 3C, p<0.05). Thus, this

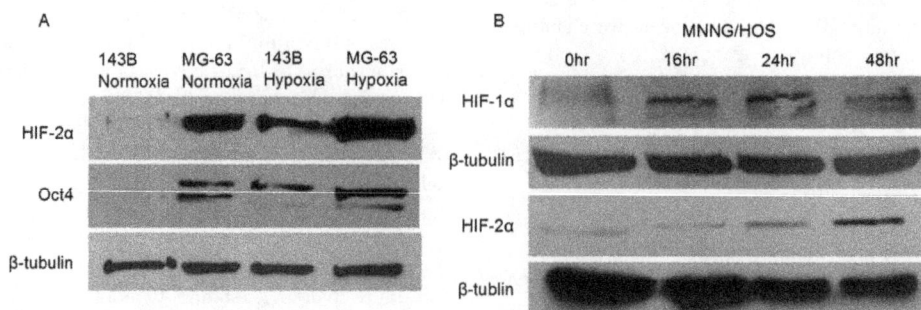

Figure 1. HIFs are present and active in human OS cells. A, 143B and MG-63 human OS cells showed increases in HIF-2α protein expression by western blot when cultured for 72 hour under hypoxic conditions (0.5% O_2). The HIF-2α downstream target, Oct4, was also increased, indicating HIF signaling activity. β-tubulin was the loading control. B, MNNG/HOS human OS cells were cultured under hypoxia for up to 48 hour and compared to a normoxia (0 hour) control. Both HIF-1α and HIF-2α levels were increased as seen by western blot. β-tubulin was used as a loading control.

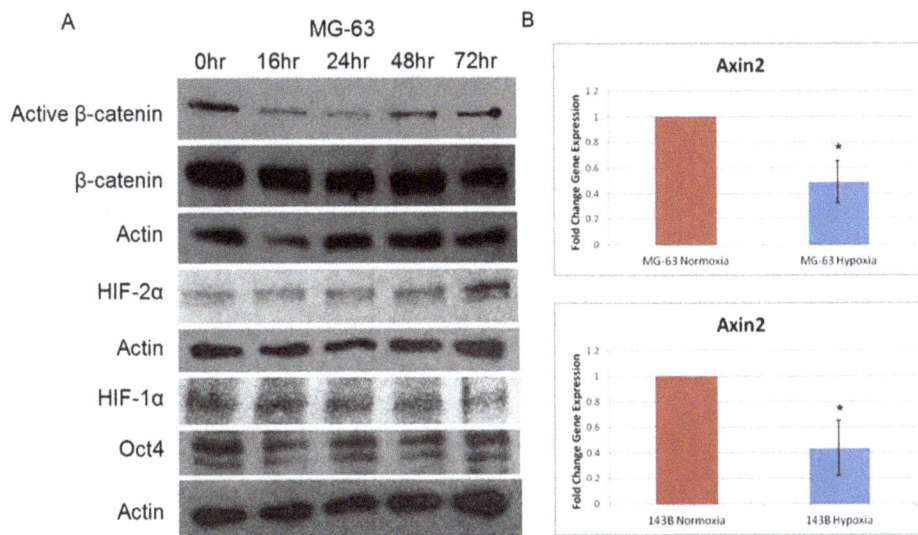

Figure 2. Hypoxia down-regulates Wnt/β-catenin signaling in human OS cells. A, MG-63 human OS cells were cultured under hypoxia over 72 hour, and increased HIF protein expression was observed by western blot. Protein levels of active β-catenin were decreased under hypoxic conditions relative to normoxic conditions (0 hour). Actin was the loading control. B, Axin2 mRNA levels were determined as a measure of Wnt/β-catenin signaling under hypoxic conditions (72 hour, 0.5% O_2) via quantitative reverse-transcription PCR (qrt-PCR) normalized to normoxia. Asterisks indicate statistical significance (*p<0.05).

data suggests that both HIF-dependent and HIF-independent mechanisms contribute to the hypoxia-mediated down-regulation of Wnt/β-catenin signaling in human OS cells.

Hypoxia results in chemoresistance of human OS cells to doxorubicin

Hypoxia has been shown to promote resistance to cytotoxic drugs in other human OS cell lines [12]. Thus we asked whether a more broad panel of OS cell lines, and particularly a patient-derived cell line isolate, show resistance under hypoxia to doxorubicin treatment, which is part of the mainstay chemotherapy regimen for OS patients [28]. We cultured both MNNG/HOS cells and 143B cells under normoxic and hypoxic conditions for 72 hours in the presence of increasing concentrations of doxorubicin. In both cell lines we saw a dramatic right shift in the dose–response curve under hypoxic conditions, indicating that these cells were more resistant to doxorubicin-mediated growth inhibition (Figure 4A). We calculated the average half maximal

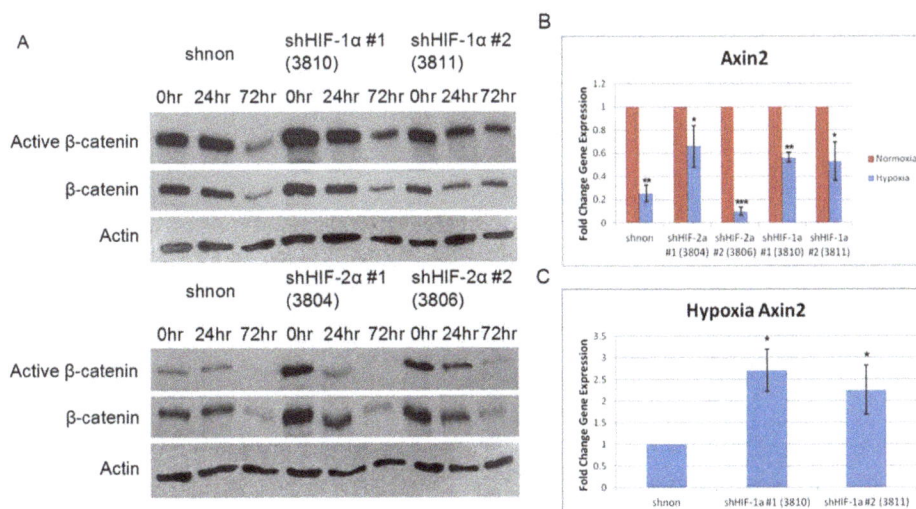

Figure 3. Wnt/β-catenin signaling down-regulation is both dependent and independent of HIF expression. A, Levels of active β-catenin were determined by western blot at different hypoxia time points for each of the shRNA in MNNG/HOS cells. Overall levels of active β-catenin decreased regardless of HIF expression, although the magnitude of decrease was not equal across all lines. Active and total β-catenin protein levels were decreased at the 72 hour time point. Actin was the loading control. B, Decreased Wnt/β-catenin signaling activity under hypoxia was confirmed by measuring axin2 mRNA levels via qrt-PCR in MNNG/HOS cells. Hypoxia (72 hour, 0.5% O_2) resulted in decreased axin2 mRNA expression relative to normoxia. C, When analyzed relative to the shnon hypoxia mRNA, axin2 mRNA was increased in the shHIF-1α MNNG/HOS cell lines. Asterisks indicate statistical significance (*p<0.05, **p<0.01, ***p<0.001). shNON: non-targeting shRNA; HIF shRNAs used are indicated in parentheses.

inhibitory concentration (IC$_{50}$) between normoxic and hypoxic conditions for each cell line and found that hypoxia resulted in a statistically significant increase in the doxorubicin IC$_{50}$ (MNNG/HOS, 5.9-fold increase; 143B, 13.6-fold increase, Figure 4B, p< 0.01). We tested a patient-derived OS cell line (206-2) and found that it too was significantly more resistant to doxorubicin treatment under hypoxic conditions (7.5-fold increase, Figure 4B, p<0.01). We also examined the response to doxorubicin treatment under hypoxia and normoxia in MNNG/HOS cells in the context of either HIF-1 or HIF-2 knockdown. We were not able to determine any statistically significant difference between the non-targeting shRNA and the HIFα shRNA cell lines (Figure S3).

Wnt/β-catenin signaling inhibitors sensitize hypoxic human OS cells to doxorubicin

Coupled with the findings of hypoxic Wnt/β-catenin down-regulation and the hypoxia-induced chemoresistance, we asked whether survival in the face of chemotherapy for a hypoxic OS cell depended on a threshold of Wnt/β-catenin signaling activity, and whether further inhibition of this pathway would sensitize the cell to chemotherapy. We chose to attenuate Wnt/β-catenin signaling under hypoxic conditions using the tankyrase inhibitor XAV939 [29]. XAV939 works by stabilizing axin2 and preventing its tankyrase-mediated degradation, thereby promoting the degradation of β-catenin and decreasing Wnt/β-catenin-dependent gene expression [29,30]. We first validated

that treatment with XAV939 results in decreased protein levels of active β-catenin and decreased mRNA expression of Wnt target genes axin2 and c-myc in MG-63 cells (Figure S4). We then treated MG-63 human OS cells under hypoxic conditions with 10 μM XAV939 (or DMSO alone as a control); treatment with XAV393 resulted in a 23% reduction in the 72-hour doxorubicin IC$_{50}$ (Figure 5, p<0.05).

As another approach, we antagonized Wnt secretion using the porcupine inhibitor IWP-2 [31]. Porcupine is a member of the membrane-bound O-acyltransferase family of enzymes that is needed to add a palmitoyl group to Wnts. Such addition is required for Wnt secretion, and the inhibition of porcupine results in decreased Wnt secretion [31]. Treatment of MG-63 cells with IWP-2 resulted in decreased protein levels of active β-catenin and decreased mRNA expression of Wnt target genes axin2 and c-myc (Figure S4). Subsequently, treatment of MG-63 cells under hypoxic conditions with 10 μM IWP-2 resulted in a reduction in the 72-hour doxorubicin IC$_{50}$ similar to that with XAV393 (24%; Figure 5, p<0.05). These data suggest that inhibition of Wnt/β-catenin signaling may serve as a target in effectively sensitizing hypoxic OS cell subpopulations to chemotherapy.

Discussion

Tumor hypoxia and HIF expression are found in a wide range of solid tumors and are often associated with a poor prognosis [8]. Hypoxia can drive many processes that contribute to cancer

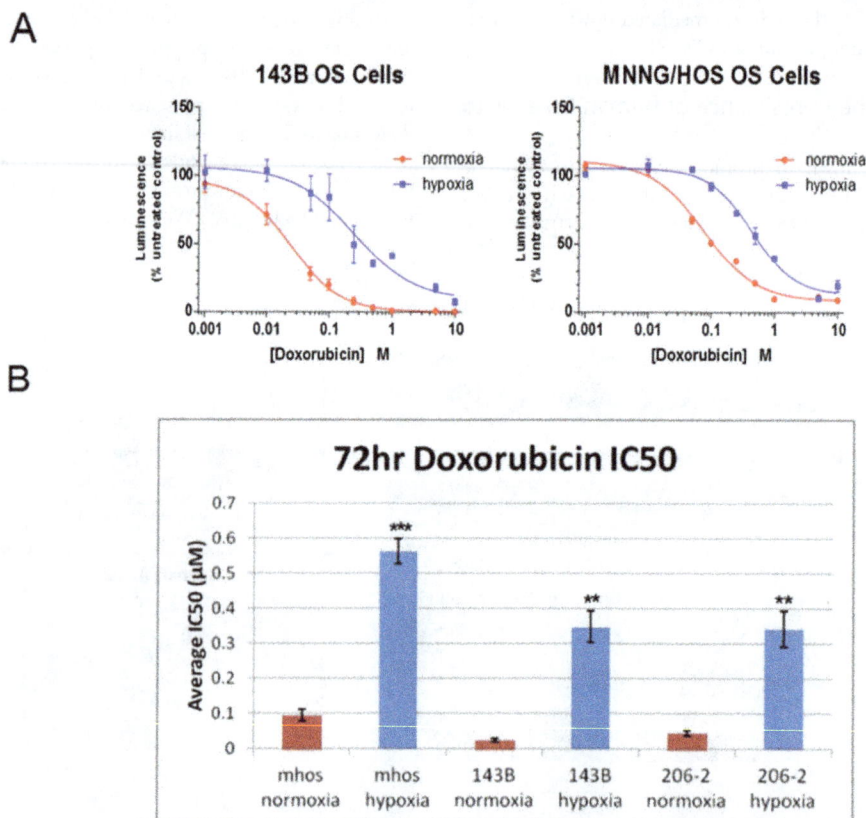

Figure 4. Hypoxia results in chemoresistance of human OS cells to doxorubicin. A, Dose-response curves for the 143B and MNNG/HOS (mHOS) cell lines treated with increasing concentrations of doxorubicin under normoxic and hypoxic conditions (72 hour, 0.5% O$_2$). Luminescence (viability) was determined as a percent of untreated control (0 μM doxorubicin). B, Average half maximal inhibitory concentration (IC$_{50}$) values were obtained from the dose-response curves and compared between normoxic and hypoxic conditions for the cell lines MNNG/HOS (mHOS), 143B, and a patient-derived OS cell line, 206-2. Asterisks indicate statistical significance (**p<0.01, ***p<0.001).

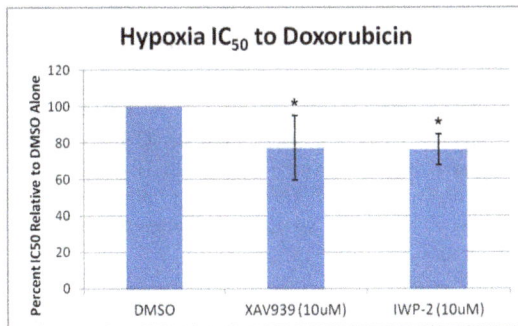

Figure 5. Further Wnt/β-catenin signaling inhibition sensitizes hypoxic OS cells to doxorubicin. MG-63 OS cells were treated with increasing concentrations of doxorubicin under hypoxic conditions in the presence of the tankyrase inhibitor XAV939, the porcupine inhibitor IWP-2, or DMSO alone. Half maximal inhibitory concentrations (IC_{50}) were calculated, and the percent IC_{50} relative to DMSO alone was determined. Asterisks indicate statistical significance (*$p < 0.05$).

progression, including altered metabolism, angiogenesis, pH regulation, and cell proliferation [32]. Many of these responses are mediated through the HIF class of transcription factors, because both HIF-1α and HIF-2α can influence the expression of key target genes for tumor growth and progression. It is no surprise that clinical data highlights the importance of increases in HIF on parameters of poor outcome in OS patients [9,10]. So far, inhibition strategies targeting the HIF proteins directly have suffered from a lack of specificity [33]. It may be a more viable option to target the key downstream mediators of the hypoxic response. *VEGFA*, a well-characterized HIF target gene, is associated with poor prognosis in OS patients [34]. A single clinical trial is ongoing targeting VEGFA with bevacizumab in osteosarcoma (NCT00667342), however it is unclear whether this therapy is effective [35]. Downstream hypoxia/HIF targets have shown promise in other cancers, including VEGFA in various cancers and GLUT1 in renal cell carcinoma [36,37,38].

Although signaling mediated by HIFs constitutes a potent hypoxia response mechanism, there are many instances of hypoxia responses that are considered HIF-independent. Crucial signaling pathways other than HIFs, such as RAS and PI3K/mTOR, can function in hypoxia-induced angiogenesis [39]. These pathways can be activated under hypoxia through inhibition of the suppressive activity of PTEN and MAPK phosphatases via reactive oxygen species (ROS) [40,41,42]. Alternative signaling pathways and ROS mediators can in turn regulate HIF expression and activity, adding further complexity to the response to hypoxia [43,44]. An understanding of crucial, downstream, HIF-independent signaling pathways that are regulated by hypoxia could lead to new therapeutic targets.

In this study, we tested the hypothesis that Wnt/β-catenin signaling is altered under hypoxic conditions in human OS cells, and we sought contributions of HIFs to such alteration. Other studies in osteoblasts, using exogenous HIF-1α and siRNAs targeting HIF-1α under normoxic conditions, have noted that HIF-1α inhibits Wnt signaling, but we used physiologic hypoxia-induced HIF-1α or HIF-2α in the context of their knockdown to examine Wnt signaling differences [45]. Through our work we were able to conclude Wnt/β-catenin signaling is down-regulated under hypoxia in OS cells, and that both HIF-independent and HIF-dependent mechanisms contribute to this finding, with HIF-1α standing out as an important mediator. Although the baseline β-catenin levels and the magnitude of its subsequent alteration

under hypoxia differ among the cell lines used (MG-63 in Figure 2A, MNNG/HOS in Figure 3A), the general trend of β-catenin and canonical Wnt signaling decrease remained consistent. It may be that this baseline results from differences intrinsic to the origin and behavior of the cell lines themselves [46]. HIF-independent mechanisms explaining our findings could involve the Siah-1-p53 axis; Siah-1 increases under hypoxia in other cancer cell lines and results in the degradation of β-catenin dependent on p53 [47]. Studies in osteoblasts have specifically focused on HIF-1α driving a decrease in Wnt/β-catenin signaling through activation of sclerostin [20]. Future work will be needed to identify whether these or additional mechanisms are responsible for hypoxic Wnt/β-catenin signaling down-regulation in OS cells. It is also possible that since 100% knockdown of HIF expression was not achieved using RNA interference, a low level of HIF activity could be sufficient to govern canonical Wnt signaling changes, or that redundancy between HIF-1 and HIF-2 could result in compensation. This is an area of current ongoing investigation.

We also examined the chemoresistance of OS cells under hypoxic conditions, and assessed the efficacy of Wnt signaling inhibitors on sensitizing hypoxic OS cells to chemotherapy. Our results show that across multiple OS cell lines, including a patient-derived clinical sample, hypoxia promotes robust resistance to doxorubicin, and hypoxic OS cells can be sensitized to doxorubicin by simultaneously antagonizing the Wnt signaling pathway. This is not to say that hypoxia-mediated chemoresistance in OS cells is driven by down-regulated Wnt signaling per se, but instead that homeostasis of hypoxic OS cells may be susceptible to a second hit of Wnt signaling antagonism. Similar strategies for targeting a signaling pathway from multiple directions have proven effective in other cancers, as one study highlights that mTORC and HDAC inhibition mechanistically converged on the PI3K/AKT/mTOR pathway to reduce breast cancer cell viability [48]. Future directions would include determining if any synergism exists between doxorubicin and Wnt signaling antagonism. Others have shown that hypoxia promotes cell cycle arrest, which could be a contributing mechanism for hypoxia-induced chemoresistance [49]. We chose to normalize our chemoresistance assays to an untreated control under either normoxia or hypoxia to focus more closely on signaling pathway inhibition rather than proliferation differences. Future work examining hypoxia-induced proliferation differences and the signaling pathways responsible in OS will be important.

XAV939 and IWP-2 differ in their mechanisms of Wnt signaling inhibition, with XAV939 targeting Wnt signaling at the β-catenin level and IWP-2 targeting Wnt signaling at the Wnt secretion and subsequent membrane receptor level. A likely explanation for their similar effects on sensitizing hypoxic OS cells to chemotherapy is that this finding may depend on the presence of Wnts for β-catenin signaling. It will be important to identify which Wnt ligands are important for the hypoxic response, and their downstream effects on canonical and non-canonical Wnt signaling. Additionally, more potent and specific inhibitors of the Wnt signaling pathway than the ones used in this study are being used currently in clinical trials (NCT01351103). Our work serves as an *in-vitro* model demonstration of how cells under oxygen tensions similar to those in the tumor microenvironment may be susceptible to Wnt signaling antagonism. More work will need to be done to examine the biological efficacy of more potent and specific Wnt signaling inhibitors on hypoxic OS cells.

The clinical importance of our findings is clear, as a range of oxygen tensions (0–5% O_2) can be observed within a solid tumor [50,51,52]. By targeting mechanisms that allow osteosarcoma cells to adapt to hypoxia within the solid tumor microenvironment, it is conceivable that the emerging pipeline of Wnt-targeted therapies can be leveraged to increase the effectiveness of current osteosarcoma drug regimens. Osteosarcoma is a very heterogeneous cancer, and data regarding the role of Wnt signaling in osteosarcoma is conflicting [2]. A recent genomic analysis of 46 early stage osteosarcoma specimens confirmed deletion of key genes in the canonical Wnt signaling pathway [53]. In this study and others, β-catenin activation has not been readily demonstrable by immunohistochemistry in human specimens [54]. Other studies confirm that osteosarcoma is responsive to Wnt signaling inputs, both within the canonical and non-canonical pathways [17,55]. Using a systems biology approach, Wnt signaling pathways were identified as common mechanisms in human metastatic osteosarcoma models, suggesting a role for Wnt signaling antagonism in advanced stage OS [56]. Our experimental approach utilized metastatic cell lines and a chemoresistant patient-derived cell isolate to model advanced stage disease, and thus may be an important setting to investigate the use of Wnt-targeted therapies. Despite the complexity of signaling pathway alterations under hypoxia, whether related or unrelated to HIFs, the Wnt signaling pathway may serve as a viable target for hypoxia-induced chemoresistant OS cell subpopulations.

Supporting Information

Figure S1   Quantification of HIF protein levels under hypoxia. Western blots from two independent experiments culturing MNNG/HOS cells under hypoxia for different time periods were quantified using ImageJ software. Band intensity is shown relative to β-tubulin.

Figure S2   Quantification of active β-catenin protein levels under hypoxia. Western blots from two independent experiments culturing MG-63 cells under hypoxia for different time periods were quantified using ImageJ software. Band intensity is shown relative to actin.

Figure S3   Effects of HIF knockdown on OS cell resistance to doxorubicin. 72 hour doxorubicin IC_{50} values are shown for two independent shRNA's targeting either HIF-1α or HIF-2α in MNNG/HOS cells. No significant difference was noted under hypoxic conditions (n = 3).

Figure S4   Validation of Wnt/β-catenin Signaling Inhibition by XAV939 and IWP-2. MG-63 cells were treated with either 10 μM XAV939 or IWP-2, with DMSO serving as a control. Active β-catenin protein levels were decreased by both XAV939 and IWP-2 compared to DMSO, and XAV939 treatment resulted in decreased in total β-catenin levels as determined by western blot. Treatment with XAV939 and IWP-2 also resulted in decreased mRNA expression of Wnt target genes axin2 and c-myc.

Acknowledgments

The authors thank the members of the Laboratory of Musculoskeletal Oncology, David Nadziejka for writing assistance, and Dr. Ben Alman of Duke University for intellectual feedback.

Author Contributions

Conceived and designed the experiments: DJS MRS. Performed the experiments: DJS CMT. Analyzed the data: DJS CMT JDP. Contributed reagents/materials/analysis tools: DJS JDP. Wrote the paper: DJS JDP DWP BOW MRS.

References

1. Siclari VA, Qin L (2010) Targeting the osteosarcoma cancer stem cell. J Orthop Surg Res 5: 78.
2. Kuijjer ML, Hogendoorn PC, Cleton-Jansen AM (2013) Genome-wide analyses on high-grade osteosarcoma: making sense of a genomically most unstable tumor. Int J Cancer 133: 2512–2521.
3. Anninga JK, Gelderblom H, Fiocco M, Kroep JR, Taminiau AH, et al. (2011) Chemotherapeutic adjuvant treatment for osteosarcoma: where do we stand? Eur J Cancer 47: 2431–2445.
4. Vaupel P, Mayer A (2007) Hypoxia in cancer: significance and impact on clinical outcome. Cancer Metastasis Rev 26: 225–239.
5. Mazumdar J, Dondeti V, Simon MC (2009) Hypoxia-inducible factors in stem cells and cancer. J Cell Mol Med 13: 4319–4328.
6. Michaylira CZ, Nakagawa H (2006) Hypoxic microenvironment as a cradle for melanoma development and progression. Cancer Biol Ther 5: 476–479.
7. Lu X, Kang Y (2010) Hypoxia and hypoxia-inducible factors: master regulators of metastasis. Clin Cancer Res 16: 5928–5935.
8. Keith B, Johnson RS, Simon MC (2012) HIF1alpha and HIF2alpha: sibling rivalry in hypoxic tumour growth and progression. Nat Rev Cancer 12: 9–22.
9. Yang QC, Zeng BF, Dong Y, Shi ZM, Jiang ZM, et al. (2007) Overexpression of hypoxia-inducible factor-1alpha in human osteosarcoma: correlation with clinicopathological parameters and survival outcome. Jpn J Clin Oncol 37: 127–134.
10. El Naggar A, Clarkson P, Zhang F, Mathers J, Tognon C, et al. (2012) Expression and stability of hypoxia inducible factor 1alpha in osteosarcoma. Pediatr Blood Cancer 59: 1215–1222.
11. Knowles HJ, Schaefer KL, Dirksen U, Athanasou NA (2010) Hypoxia and hypoglycaemia in Ewing's sarcoma and osteosarcoma: regulation and phenotypic effects of Hypoxia-Inducible Factor. BMC Cancer 10: 372.
12. Adamski J, Price A, Dive C, Makin G (2013) Hypoxia-induced cytotoxic drug resistance in osteosarcoma is independent of HIF-1Alpha. PLoS One 8: e65304.
13. Cai Y, Cai T, Chen Y (2014) Wnt pathway in osteosarcoma, from oncogenic to therapeutic. J Cell Biochem 115: 625–631.
14. Moon RT, Kohn AD, De Ferrari GV, Kaykas A (2004) WNT and beta-catenin signalling: diseases and therapies. Nat Rev Genet 5: 691–701.
15. Lin CH, Guo Y, Ghaffar S, McQueen P, Pourmorady J, et al. (2013) Dkk-3, a secreted wnt antagonist, suppresses tumorigenic potential and pulmonary metastasis in osteosarcoma. Sarcoma 2013: 147541.
16. Rubin EM, Guo Y, Tu K, Xie J, Zi X, et al. (2010) Wnt inhibitory factor 1 decreases tumorigenesis and metastasis in osteosarcoma. Mol Cancer Ther 9: 731–741.
17. Guo Y, Rubin EM, Xie J, Zi X, Hoang BH (2008) Dominant negative LRP5 decreases tumorigenicity and metastasis of osteosarcoma in an animal model. Clin Orthop Relat Res 466: 2039–2045.
18. Ma Y, Ren Y, Han EQ, Li H, Chen D, et al. (2013) Inhibition of the Wnt-beta-catenin and Notch signaling pathways sensitizes osteosarcoma cells to chemotherapy. Biochem Biophys Res Commun 431: 274–279.
19. Deng Z, Niu G, Cai L, Wei R, Zhao X (2013) The prognostic significance of CD44V6, CDH11, and beta-catenin expression in patients with osteosarcoma. Biomed Res Int 2013: 496193.
20. Chen D, Li Y, Zhou Z, Wu C, Xing Y, et al. (2013) HIF-1alpha inhibits Wnt signaling pathway by activating Sost expression in osteoblasts. PLoS One 8: e65940.
21. Genetos DC, Toupadakis CA, Raheja LF, Wong A, Papanicolaou SE, et al. (2010) Hypoxia decreases sclerostin expression and increases Wnt signaling in osteoblasts. J Cell Biochem 110: 457–467.
22. Kaidi A, Williams AC, Paraskeva C (2007) Interaction between beta-catenin and HIF-1 promotes cellular adaptation to hypoxia. Nat Cell Biol 9: 210–217.
23. Kumar N, Basundra R, Maiti S (2009) Elevated polyamines induce c-MYC overexpression by perturbing quadruplex-WC duplex equilibrium. Nucleic Acids Res 37: 3321–3331.
24. Livak KJ, Schmittgen TD (2001) Analysis of relative gene expression data using real-time quantitative PCR and the 2(-Delta Delta C(T)) Method. Methods 25: 402–408.
25. Team RC (2013) R: A Language and Environment for Statistical Computing. Vienna, Austria: R Foundation for Statistical Computing.
26. Staal FJ, Noort Mv M, Strous GJ, Clevers HC (2002) Wnt signals are transmitted through N-terminally dephosphorylated beta-catenin. EMBO Rep 3: 63–68.

27. Jho EH, Zhang T, Domon C, Joo CK, Freund JN, et al. (2002) Wnt/beta-catenin/Tcf signaling induces the transcription of Axin2, a negative regulator of the signaling pathway. Mol Cell Biol 22: 1172–1183.

28. Bielack S, Carrle D, Casali PG (2009) Osteosarcoma: ESMO clinical recommendations for diagnosis, treatment and follow-up. Ann Oncol 20 Suppl 4: 137–139.

29. Huang SM, Mishina YM, Liu S, Cheung A, Stegmeier F, et al. (2009) Tankyrase inhibition stabilizes axin and antagonizes Wnt signalling. Nature 461: 614–620.

30. Riffell JL, Lord CJ, Ashworth A (2012) Tankyrase-targeted therapeutics: expanding opportunities in the PARP family. Nat Rev Drug Discov 11: 923–936.

31. Chen B, Dodge ME, Tang W, Lu J, Ma Z, et al. (2009) Small molecule-mediated disruption of Wnt-dependent signaling in tissue regeneration and cancer. Nat Chem Biol 5: 100–107.

32. Bertout JA, Patel SA, Simon MC (2008) The impact of O_2 availability on human cancer. Nat Rev Cancer 8: 967–975.

33. Onnis B, Rapisarda A, Melillo G (2009) Development of HIF-1 inhibitors for cancer therapy. J Cell Mol Med 13: 2780–2786.

34. Chen D, Zhang YJ, Zhu KW, Wang WC (2013) A systematic review of vascular endothelial growth factor expression as a biomarker of prognosis in patients with osteosarcoma. Tumour Biol 34: 1895–1899.

35. Turner DC, Navid F, Daw NC, Mao S, Wu J, et al. (2014) Population pharmacokinetics of bevacizumab in children with osteosarcoma: implications for dosing. Clin Cancer Res 20: 2783–2792.

36. Vacchelli E, Aranda F, Eggermont A, Galon J, Sautes-Fridman C, et al. (2014) Trial Watch: Tumor-targeting monoclonal antibodies in cancer therapy. Oncoimmunology 3: e27048.

37. Liao D, Johnson RS (2007) Hypoxia: a key regulator of angiogenesis in cancer. Cancer Metastasis Rev 26: 281–290.

38. Chan DA, Sutphin PD, Nguyen P, Turcotte S, Lai EW, et al. (2011) Targeting GLUT1 and the Warburg effect in renal cell carcinoma by chemical synthetic lethality. Sci Transl Med 3: 94ra70.

39. Mizukami Y, Kohgo Y, Chung DC (2007) Hypoxia inducible factor-1 independent pathways in tumor angiogenesis. Clin Cancer Res 13: 5670–5674.

40. Hamanaka RB, Chandel NS (2010) Mitochondrial reactive oxygen species regulate cellular signaling and dictate biological outcomes. Trends Biochem Sci 35: 505–513.

41. Kwon J, Lee SR, Yang KS, Ahn Y, Kim YJ, et al. (2004) Reversible oxidation and inactivation of the tumor suppressor PTEN in cells stimulated with peptide growth factors. Proc Natl Acad Sci U S A 101: 16419–16424.

42. Kamata H, Honda S, Maeda S, Chang L, Hirata H, et al. (2005) Reactive oxygen species promote TNFalpha-induced death and sustained JNK activation by inhibiting MAP kinase phosphatases. Cell 120: 649–661.

43. Agani F, Jiang BH (2013) Oxygen-independent regulation of HIF-1: novel involvement of PI3K/AKT/mTOR pathway in cancer. Curr Cancer Drug Targets 13: 245–251.

44. Tormos KV, Chandel NS (2010) Inter-connection between mitochondria and HIFs. J Cell Mol Med 14: 795–804.

45. Chen D, Li Y, Zhou Z, Xing Y, Zhong Y, et al. (2012) Synergistic inhibition of Wnt pathway by HIF-1alpha and osteoblast-specific transcription factor osterix (Osx) in osteoblasts. PLoS One 7: e52948.

46. Mohseny AB, Machado I, Cai Y, Schaefer KL, Serra M, et al. (2011) Functional characterization of osteosarcoma cell lines provides representative models to study the human disease. Lab Invest 91: 1195–1205.

47. Wang D, Wang Y, Kong T, Fan F, Jiang Y (2011) Hypoxia-induced beta-catenin downregulation involves p53-dependent activation of Siah-1. Cancer Sci 102: 1322–1328.

48. Wilson-Edell KA, Yevtushenko MA, Rothschild DE, Rogers AN, Benz CC (2014) mTORC1/C2 and pan-HDAC inhibitors synergistically impair breast cancer growth by convergent AKT and polysome inhibiting mechanisms. Breast Cancer Res Treat 144: 287–298.

49. Goda N, Ryan HE, Khadivi B, McNulty W, Rickert RC, et al. (2003) Hypoxia-inducible factor 1alpha is essential for cell cycle arrest during hypoxia. Mol Cell Biol 23: 359–369.

50. Brown JM, Wilson WR (2004) Exploiting tumour hypoxia in cancer treatment. Nat Rev Cancer 4: 437–447.

51. Hockel M, Vaupel P (2001) Tumor hypoxia: definitions and current clinical, biologic, and molecular aspects. J Natl Cancer Inst 93: 266–276.

52. Martin SK, Diamond P, Gronthos S, Peet DJ, Zannettino AC (2011) The emerging role of hypoxia, HIF-1 and HIF-2 in multiple myeloma. Leukemia 25: 1533–1542.

53. Du X, Yang J, Yang D, Tian W, Zhu Z (2014) The genetic basis for inactivation of Wnt pathway in human osteosarcoma. BMC Cancer 14: 450.

54. Cai Y, Mohseny AB, Karperien M, Hogendoorn PC, Zhou G, et al. (2010) Inactive Wnt/beta-catenin pathway in conventional high-grade osteosarcoma. J Pathol 220: 24–33.

55. Enomoto M, Hayakawa S, Itsukushima S, Ren DY, Matsuo M, et al. (2009) Autonomous regulation of osteosarcoma cell invasiveness by Wnt5a/Ror2 signaling. Oncogene 28: 3197–3208.

56. Flores RJ, Li Y, Yu A, Shen J, Rao PH, et al. (2012) A systems biology approach reveals common metastatic pathways in osteosarcoma. BMC Syst Biol 6: 50.

19

Mucosal Healing Did Not Predict Sustained Clinical Remission in Patients with IBD after Discontinuation of One-Year Infliximab Therapy

Cong Dai, Wei-Xin Liu, Min Jiang, Ming-Jun Sun*

Department of Gastroenterology, First Affiliated Hospital, China Medical University, Shenyang City, Liaoning Province, China

Abstract

Aim: To assess the endoscopic activity and Clinical activity after a one-year period of infliximab therapy and to evaluate the association between mucosal healing and need for retreatment after stopping infliximab in patients with Inflammatory bowel disease (IBD).

Methods: The data from 109 patients with Crohn's disease (CD) and 107 patients with Ulcerative colitis (UC) received one-year infliximab were assessed. The primary endpoint of the study was the proportion of clinical remission, mucosal healing and full remission in IBD after the one-year period of maintenance infliximab therapy. The secondary endpoint was the frequency of relapses in the next year.

Results: A total of 84.4% (92/109) CD patients and 81.3% (87/107) UC patients achieved clinical remission, 71.56% (78/109) of CD patients and 69.16% (74/107) UC patients achieved mucosal healing, 56.88% (62/109) of CD patients and 54.21% (58/107) of UC patients achieved full remission at the end of the year of infliximab therapy. Infliximab therapy was restarted in the 10.19% (22/216) patients (13 CD, 9 UC) who achieved mucosal healing, and 13.89% (30/216) patients (18 CD, 12 UC) who achieved clinical remission and 6.48% (14/216) patients (8 CD, 6 UC) who achieved full remission had to be retreated within the next year. Neither clinical remission nor mucosal healing was associated with the time to restarting Infliximab therapy in IBD.

Conclusion: Mucosal healing did not predict sustained clinical remission in patients with IBD in whom the infliximab therapies had been stopped. And stopping or continuing infliximab therapy may be determined by assessing the IBD patient's general condition and the clinical activity.

Editor: Mathias Chamaillard, INSERM, France

Funding: The authors have no support or funding to report.

Competing Interests: The authors have declared that no competing interests exist.

* Email: 273159833@qq.com

Introduction

Inflammatory bowel disease (IBD) is a chronic recurrent disease, which mainly consists of ulcerative colitis (UC) and Crohn's disease (CD) [1]. And it is a growing worldwide health burden especially in many developing countries. Although not completely defined, the aetiopathology of IBD is thought to be a consequence of immune dysregulation, impaired mucosal integrity, enteric bacterial dysbiosis and genetic susceptibility factors [2,3,4]. The aims of treatment in IBD are to induce and maintain remission, to improve quality of life and to prevent the development of complications and the need for surgery. Now the pharmaceutical therapies have included corticosteroids, 5-aminosalicylic acids (5-ASAs), immunomodulators such as azathioprine, 6-mercaptopurine (6-MP), methotrexate, and biological therapy such as infliximab, adalimumab [5,6].

Colonoscopies play an important role in the diagnosis, management and monitoring of IBD. Now the most important goals in the treatment of IBD is mucosal healing, because some studies have demonstrated that mucosal healing can alter the course of IBD due to its association with sustained clinical remission and reduced rates of hospitalization and surgery [7]. And mucosal healing at the time of treatment withdrawal may predict better outcomes in IBD [8].

The endoscopy provides a direct evaluation of the mucosal lesions in IBD and intestinal activity may be quantified by indices of endoscopic activity, but a clear definition of mucosal healing is still lacking. Most of the clinical trials define mucosal healing as the total disappearance of mucosal ulcerations. The Simplified Endoscopic Activity Score for Crohn's Disease (SES-CD) is a relatively easy tool to evaluate the endoscopic activity in CD [9], and the Mayo endoscopic score is common indices to evaluate the endoscopic activity in UC [10,11]. The weaknesses of these endoscopic activity indices include the absence of a clear definition and the lack of validation of mucosal healing [12]. At the same time, routine endoscopic follow-up is recommended for all IBD patients who have achieved clinical remission with medical therapy; for those with persistent complaints, in order to rule out post-inflammatory irritable bowel syndrome; for those still within their first year after surgery; and for those who are stopping biological therapies but continuing immunosuppressants [13,14].

The introduction of monoclonal anti-TNF-α drugs revolutionised the management of IBD. Although the precise mechanism of action is unknown, it is thought that anti-TNF-α drugs cause apoptosis of inflammatory cells carrying membrane-bound TNF-α, an important cytokine in the pathogenesis of IBD. And anti-TNF-α drugs have proven their efficacy in inducing and maintaining clinical and endoscopic remission in both CD and UC. For example, Good data exist demonstrating the efficacy of anti-TNF-α drugs for inducing and sustaining remission for patients with moderate to severely CD, with approximately 60% of patients showing overall clinical improvement [15,16]. Long-term data have shown infliximab to be beneficial, in initial responders, over a median follow-up period of 4.6 years [17]. The efficacy of anti-TNF-α drugs in the treatment of UC is less impressive than their effect in CD. The ACT UC Trials were large, multicentre RCTs that compared infliximab with placebo in the treatment of moderate to severe active UC [13]. There was a modest, but significant benefit in clinical improvement over placebo.

According to the Consensus Statement on Diagnoses and Treatment of IBD in China, biological therapies (infliximab approved for the treatment of CD and UC) have to be discontinued after a one-year maintaining clinical remission treatment period. The endoscopic healing of the mucosa is commonly evaluated at the end of the one-year treatment period with biological therapies. In the present study, we want to assess the endoscopic activity and the rate of mucosal healing after a one-year period of infliximab therapy and to evaluate how the endoscopic findings of the mucosa predict the frequency of relapses and the need for restarting infliximab therapy.

Materials and Methods

Study design

This was a prospective observational study conducted in the Department of Gastroenterology, First Affiliated Hospital, China Medical University between January 2010 and December 2013. The study was approved by China Medical University Regional and Institutional Committee of Science and Research Ethics and by the Regional and Institutional Human Medical Biological Research Ethics Committee of China Medical University. All participants have provided their written informed consent to participate in our study. The ethics committees have approved this consent procedure. We have also obtained informed consent from the next of kin, caretakers, or guardians on behalf of the minors/children enrolled in our study.

The analysis focused on patients who underwent an ileocolonoscopy before and after the one-year maintenance infliximab therapy and in whom infliximab therapy were discontinued at the end of the year. Endoscopies were performed by two experienced gastroenterologists after stopping the one-year infliximab therapy.

One hundred and nine CD patients (59 females, 41 males, mean disease duration at the beginning of biological therapy: 6.2 years) and 107 UC patients (59 females, 48 males, mean disease duration at the beginning of biological therapy: 11.4 years) were prospectively followed up in this study. Twelve CD patients (8 females, 4 males, mean disease duration at the beginning of biological therapy: 5.8 years) and 8 UC patients (5 females, 3 males, mean disease duration at the beginning of biological

therapy: 9.9 years) were lost in the follow-up. There was no significant difference about the basic clinical characteristics of patients between included and not included in the study. All patients received maintenance infliximab therapy for one year in accordance with the Consensus Statement on Diagnoses and Treatment of IBD in China. CD disease phenotypes were determined according to the Montreal Classification [18]. These patients received the last dose of infliximab therapy at least 3 month before the repeated one-year therapy. Seventy-three patients were naive to biological therapy (did not receive biological therapy before the one-year treatment period analyzed in the study) in the CD group, and 68 patients in the UC group. The concomitant immunosuppression during the induction therapy was corticosteroids in 100 (CD: 66, UC: 34) and azathioprine in 66 (CD: 45, UC: 21) patients. The clinical characteristics of the patients are presented in Table 1. Patients' data regarding smoking status, previous appendectomy, perianal involvement, presence of extraintestinal manifestation, outcome of induction therapy, previous surgical procedures, and previous biological therapy were collected.

Assessment of clinical and endoscopic remission

Clinical activities, as determined by the Crohn's Disease Activity Index (CDAI) [19] in CD and by the Mayo score [10] in UC, were calculated at the end of infliximab therapy when the endoscopic assessment was performed, while partial Mayo scores were calculated when infliximab therapy needed to be restarted. Clinical remission was defined as a CDAI of <150 points and a Mayo score of <2 points. Sustained clinical remission was defined as a stable, steroid-free clinical remission during the 1-year follow-up period. The definition of relapse and indication for restarting biologicals were an increase of >100 points in CDAI and a CDAI of >150 points and a partial Mayo score of >3 points.

The endoscopic severity of CD was quantified with SES-CD in CD [8] and with Mayo endoscopic subscore in UC [10]. The endoscopic scores were prospectively assessed by two investigators (Min Jiang and Ming-Jun Sun). Mucosal healing was defined using the endoscopic indices as SES-CD between 0 and 3 and Mayo endoscopic subscore as 0.

Endpoints

Data collection and analysis were performed at the Department of Gastroenterology, First Affiliated Hospital, China Medical University. The primary endpoint of the study was the proportion of mucosal healing in IBD after the one-year period of maintenance infliximab therapy. The secondary endpoint was the frequency of relapses in the next year.

Statistical analysis

Variables were tested for normality using Shapiro-Wilk's W test. The χ^2-test and logistic regression analysis were used to assess the association between categorical clinical variables and clinical/endoscopic outcomes. The variables analyzed were gender, disease duration, active smoking, appendectomy, location/extent, behavior, associated perineal disease, extraintestinal manifestations, previous surgery, previous biological therapy, clinical activities, CRP levels, and outcomes of induction therapy. The difference between patients with mucosal healing and those who failed to achieve endoscopic remission was assessed by chi-square or Fisher's exact tests. Kaplan-Meier survival curves were plotted for analysis with the Log-Rank and Breslow tests. For the statistical analysis, SPSS 11.5 was used. And $P<0.05$ was considered significant.

Table 1. Demographic and clinical characteristics of patients.

	CD patients (*n* = 109)	UC patients (*n* = 107)
Female/male	68/41	59/48
Mean age at diagnosis (yr)	26 (14–63)	31 (12–57)
Mean age at the beginning of infliximab therapy (yr)	32 (19–64)	42 (15–65)
Age at diagnosis		
<20 years (A1)	15	17
20–40 years (A2)	73	68
>40 years (A3)	21	22
Location		
Ileal (L1)	20	-
Colonic (L2)	31	-
Ileocolonic (L3)	56	-
Upper GI (L4)	2	-
Proctitis	-	0
Left-sided colitis	-	64
Extensive colitis	-	43
Behaviour		
Inflammatory (B1)	53	-
Stricturing (B2)	17	-
Penetrating (B3)	35	-
Perianal manifestation	41	-
Extraintestinal manifestation	39	12
Surgery before infliximab therapy	23	5
Previous biological therapy	17	3
Median CDAI/pMayo at the start of infliximab therapy	328	9.8
Median CRP level at the start of infliximab therapy (mg/l)	13.8	11.2
Current smokers	74	21
Appendectomy	13	1

Results

Clinical activity of IBD after the one-year period of infliximab therapy

The median CDAI was 72 (interquartile range: 36.8–97.5) ($P < 0.01$) and the partial Mayo score was 1.4 (interquartile range: 0–5.2) ($P < 0.01$) at the end of the treatment period. A total of 92/109 patients with CD (84.4%) and 87/107 with UC (81.3%) achieved clinical remission at the end of the year of infliximab therapy.

Endoscopic activity of IBD before and after the one year period of infliximab therapy

Colonoscopies reached the terminal ileum in each patient. The median values of the SES-CD and the Mayo endoscopic subscores significantly improved after infliximab therapy [18 (interquartile range: 11–25) vs 6 (interquartile range: 2–11), $P < 0.01$, and 3 (interquartile range: 2–4) vs 1 (interquartile range: 0–3), $P < 0.01$]. Mucosal healing was achieved in 71.56% (78/109) of CD patients and 69.16% (74/107) of UC patients. Full remission – both mucosal healing and clinical remission - was achieved in 56.88% (62/109) of CD patients and 54.21% (58/107) of UC patients.

The frequency of relapses in the next year

During the next year follow up period, 13.89% (30/216) of patients (18 CD, 12 UC) in the clinical remission group and 6.48% (14/216) patients (8 CD, 6 UC) in the full remission group had to be retreated. In CD, infliximab therapy was restarted due to clinical relapse in 21.1% (23/109) of patients after a median 4.8 month (interquartile range: 3.2–6.3 month). The median CDAI was 327 (interquartile range: 115–369) at the time of relapse. In UC, infliximab therapy needed to be restarted in 14.02% (15/107) patients after a median 6.7 month (interquartile range: 2.8–9.7 month). The median partial Mayo score was 5.9 (interquartile range: 4.5–7.2) at the time of retreatment. Of note, infliximab therapy was restarted in the 10.19% (22/216) patients (13 CD, 9 UC) who achieved mucosal healing, and 13.89% (30/216) patients (18 CD, 12 UC) who achieved clinical remission and 6.48% (14/216) patients (8 CD, 6 UC) who achieved full remission had to be retreated within the next year. Endoscopic activity was not assessed in each patient when the infliximab therapy was restarted. The response rates for retreatment were 78.26% (18/23) in CD and 66.67% (10/15) in UC within an average of three months after the reintroduction of infliximab therapy.

In a univariate or Kaplan-Meier analysis using the Log-Rank and Breslow tests, neither clinical remission nor mucosal healing was associated with the time to restarting infliximab therapy in either CD (Figure 1) or UC (Figure 2). In univariate analysis or logistic regression analysis, none of the investigated parameters (e.g., gender, disease duration, smoking status, history of appendectomy, location/extent, behavior, extraintestinal manifestations, previous surgery, previous biological therapy, CRP level, or the effect of induction therapy) was associated with the need to restart infliximab therapy in either CD or UC (Table 2).

Discussion

In this prospective observational study conducted in patients with CD and UC receiving infliximab therapy for one year, mucosal healing was observed in 71.56% and 69.16% of the patients, respectively. Full remission, including both clinical and endoscopic remission, was detected in 56.88% and 54.21% of patients with CD and UC. Retreatment with infliximab therapy was necessary in 16.67% (13/78) of CD patients and in 12.16% (9/74) of UC patients, despite their achieving mucosal healing at the end of the year of infliximab therapy. Our results showed that mucosal healing after one year of infliximab treatment was not associated with sustained clinical remission.

Regarding the therapeutic approach of IBD, anti-TNF-α drugs proved to be the most effective in inducing mucosal healing. For example, The ACT trials confirmed the efficacy of infliximab in inducing and maintaining mucosal healing in active UC [20]. And The ACCENT I study confirmed that scheduled infliximab therapy is more effective in achieving mucosal healing than episodic treatment [21] for CD. In our study, infliximab therapy proved to be more effective in achieving mucosal healing in CD than in UC. This result may be due to the difference in the sizes of the inflamed area and the proportion of patients with previous biological therapy in the CD and UC groups. Now mucosal healing is very important for patients with IBD, because it seems to

be associated with better outcomes (reduced rate of complications, surgery and hospitalization) in CD [21,22]. In a Norwegian study, mucosal healing was associated with lower colectomy rate in UC and decreased need for steroid treatment in CD [23]. The STORI trial suggested that one of the most important predictors of relapse was the absence of mucosal healing at the time of drug withdrawal [14]. The study of Baert *et al* [24] confirmed that complete mucosal healing in patients with early stage CD predicted sustained steroid-free remission 3 and more years. At the same time, Ananthakrishnan have found that mucosal healing as an endpoint is cost effective in CD patients [25].

Now an important question is when mucosal healing should be established. International guidelines recommend assessing endoscopic mucosal healing before stopping the therapy with anti-TNF agents. But our results do not support the guidelines because more than 13.82% of the patients with mucosal healing relapsed and needed retreatment after one-year infliximab therapy. At the same time, there is no established guideline on when anti-TNF agents can be discontinued. Different studies have concluded different views. For example, In the STORI study, infliximab therapy was terminated in 115 CD patients in clinical remission after treatment with scheduled infliximab for at least one year [14]. But Forty-five percent of patients relapsed following withdrawal from infliximab. In a Danish single-center study, 24% of CD patients and 30% of UC patients discontinued infliximab while in clinical steroid-free remission [26]. The proportion of patients in remission declined steadily, with 61% of CD patients and 75% of UC patients remaining in remission after 1 year. Half of these patients maintained their remission after a median of 2 years. In total, 96% of CD patients and 71% of UC patients experienced complete clinical remission when retreated with infliximab after their relapses. In our study, the relapsed rate of the full remission patients was 11.67%, and the response rates for retreatment were

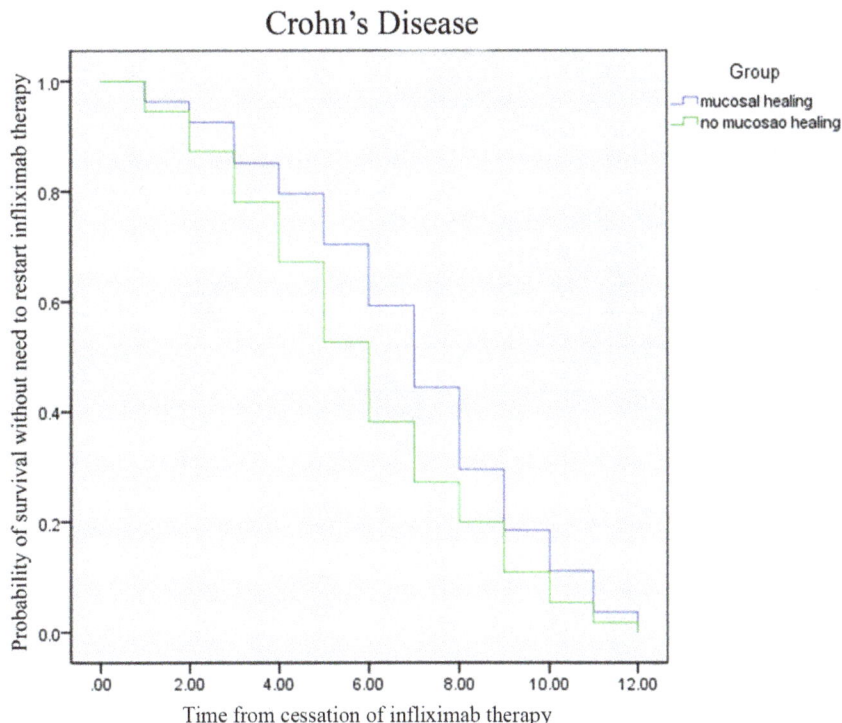

Figure 1. Kaplan-Meier analysis using Log-Rank and Breslow tests (clinical remission or mucosal healing was not associated with the time to restarting infliximab therapy in Crohn's disease).

Ulcerative Colitis

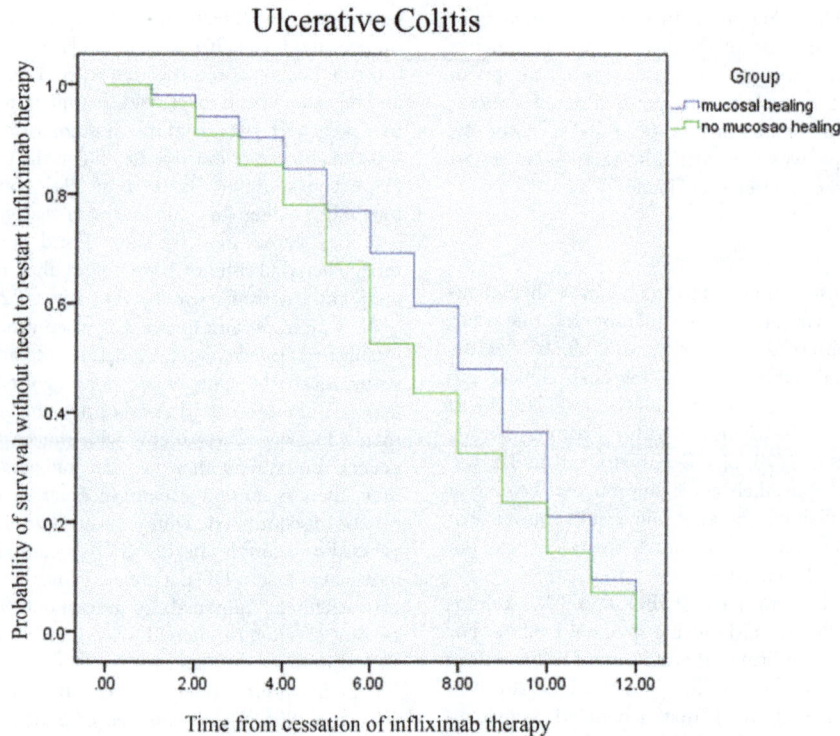

Figure 2. Kaplan-Meier analysis using Log-Rank and Breslow tests (clinical remission or mucosal healing was not associated with the time to restarting infliximab therapy in Ulcerative colitis).

78.26% in CD and 66.67% in UC at the end of the year of infliximab therapy.

There are some limitations in our study. Firstly, biopsy samples were not taken routinely to assess microscopic activity of patients with IBD. Theoretically, the microscopic evaluation of the mucosa reflects the therapeutic response more accurately than an endoscopy, but it should be noted that the histological assessment of biopsy samples demonstrates only mucosal abnormalities. For example, the transmural pattern of CD is difficult to evaluate [27] by biopsy. And Laharie *et al* [28] did not find any correlation between histologically confirmed microscopic inflammation and endoscopic activity indices in patients with IBD. Therefore, the necessity for microscopic evaluation in the assessment of mucosal healing in IBD may be worthy of further consideration. Secondly, there is no widespread agreement regarding an acceptable definition of mucosal healing. The disappearance of mucosal ulcers and erosions may be used for mucosal healing more frequently in clinical practice. In our study, mucosal healing was evaluated on the basis of endoscopic activity indices. Finally, the sample size of our study is not particularly large, but we think that the tendency of our results is worth considering.

Table 2. Univariate regression analysis of need for retreatment with infliximab therapy.

Factor	CD-P value	UC-P value
Gender	0.87	0.63
Disease duration	0.12	0.15
Smoking status	0.96	0.53
Appendectomy	0.98	-
Location/extent	0.92	0.87
Behaviour	0.98	-
Extraintestinal manifestations	0.37	-
Steroid therapy at inclusion	0.19	0.13
Previous surgery	0.98	-
Previous biological therapy	0.42	-
Elevated CRP level	0.51	0.86
Outcome of induction therapy	0.29	0.23

Now the primary goals of treatment in IBD are not only the induction and maintenance of clinical remission but also the induction of mucosal healing in an attempt to alter the course of IBD. And mucosal healing represents a more reliable and objective marker in the assessment of therapeutic response than clinical activity indices. Macroscopic findings of the mucosa represent its real alterations of patients with IBD, so endoscopy is the gold standard method of assessing mucosa lesions of patients with IBD.

But none of the studies support that mucosal healing correlates with clinical activity of IBD. Our results have revealed a high proportion of patients who relapsed even after mucosal healing. The higher relapse rates in patients with IBD who achieved mucosal healing may be explained by the shorter duration of their infliximab therapy. Therefore, the necessity of the routine endoscopic examinations at the end of the one-year period of infliximab therapy is worth considering. In conclusion, we think that stopping or continuing infliximab therapy may be determined by assessing the IBD patient's general condition and the clinical activity. At the same time, we have concluded that the long-term advantages of mucosal healing can be achieved only if we continue previous effective therapies, even after mucosal healing by the endoscopic examination. In future, large controlled clinical trials are required to confirm these results.

Author Contributions

Conceived and designed the experiments: CD MS. Performed the experiments: CD WL. Analyzed the data: MJ. Contributed reagents/materials/analysis tools: CD MJ. Contributed to the writing of the manuscript: CD MS.

References

1. Baumgart DC, Sandborn WJ (2007) Inflammatory bowel disease: clinical aspects and established and evolving therapies. Lancet 369: 1641–1657.
2. Wardle RA, Mayberry JF (2014) Patient knowledge in inflammatory bowel disease: the Crohn's and Colitis Knowledge Score. Eur J Gastroenterol Hepatol 26: 1–5.
3. Ye L, Cao Q, Cheng J (2013) Review of Inflammatory Bowel Disease in China. ScientificWorldJournal 2013: 296470.
4. Mulder DJ, Noble AJ, Justinich CJ, Duffin JM (2013) A tale of two diseases: The history of inflammatory bowel disease. J Crohns Colitis.
5. Speight RA, Mansfield JC (2013) Drug advances in inflammatory bowel disease. Clin Med 13: 378–382.
6. Danese S (2012) New therapies for inflammatory bowel disease: from the bench to the bedside. Gut 61: 918–932.
7. Pineton de Chambrun G, Peyrin-Biroulet L, Lemann M, Colombel JF (2010) Clinical implications of mucosal healing for the management of IBD. Nat Rev Gastroenterol Hepatol 7: 15–29.
8. Armuzzi A, Van Assche G, Reinisch W, Pineton de Chambrun G, Griffiths A, et al. (2012) Results of the 2nd scientific workshop of the ECCO (IV): therapeutic strategies to enhance intestinal healing in inflammatory bowel disease. J Crohns Colitis 6: 492–502.
9. Daperno M, D'Haens G, Van Assche G, Baert F, Bulois P, et al. (2004) Development and validation of a new, simplified endoscopic activity score for Crohn's disease: the SES-CD. Gastrointest Endosc 60: 505–512.
10. Dave M, Loftus EV Jr (2012) Mucosal healing in inflammatory bowel disease-a true paradigm of success? Gastroenterol Hepatol (N Y) 8: 29–38.
11. Schroeder KW, Tremaine WJ, Ilstrup DM (1987) Coated oral 5-aminosalicylic acid therapy for mildly to moderately active ulcerative colitis. A randomized study. N Engl J Med 317: 1625–1629.
12. Rutgeerts P, Vermeire S, Van Assche G (2007) Mucosal healing in inflammatory bowel disease: impossible ideal or therapeutic target? Gut 56: 453–455.
13. Rutgeerts P, Sandborn WJ, Feagan BG, Reinisch W, Olson A, et al. (2005) Infliximab for induction and maintenance therapy for ulcerative colitis. N Engl J Med 353: 2462–2476.
14. Louis E, Mary JY, Vernier-Massouille G, Grimaud JC, Bouhnik Y, et al. (2012) Maintenance of remission among patients with Crohn's disease on antimetabolite therapy after infliximab therapy is stopped. Gastroenterology 142: 63–70 e65; quiz e31.
15. Hanauer SB, Feagan BG, Lichtenstein GR, Mayer LF, Schreiber S, et al. (2002) Maintenance infliximab for Crohn's disease: the ACCENT I randomised trial. Lancet 359: 1541–1549.
16. Hanauer SB, Sandborn WJ, Rutgeerts P, Fedorak RN, Lukas M, et al. (2006) Human anti-tumor necrosis factor monoclonal antibody (adalimumab) in Crohn's disease: the CLASSIC-I trial. Gastroenterology 130: 323–333; quiz 591.
17. Schnitzler F, Fidder H, Ferrante M, Noman M, Arijs I, et al. (2009) Long-term outcome of treatment with infliximab in 614 patients with Crohn's disease: results from a single-centre cohort. Gut 58: 492–500.
18. Silverberg MS, Satsangi J, Ahmad T, Arnott ID, Bernstein CN, et al. (2005) Toward an integrated clinical, molecular and serological classification of inflammatory bowel disease: report of a Working Party of the 2005 Montreal World Congress of Gastroenterology. Can J Gastroenterol 19 Suppl A: 5A–36A.
19. Best WR, Becktel JM, Singleton JW, Kern F Jr (1976) Development of a Crohn's disease activity index. National Cooperative Crohn's Disease Study. Gastroenterology 70: 439–444.
20. Rutgeerts P, Feagan BG, Lichtenstein GR, Mayer LF, Schreiber S, et al. (2004) Comparison of scheduled and episodic treatment strategies of infliximab in Crohn's disease. Gastroenterology 126: 402–413.
21. Rutgeerts P, Diamond RH, Bala M, Olson A, Lichtenstein GR, et al. (2006) Scheduled maintenance treatment with infliximab is superior to episodic treatment for the healing of mucosal ulceration associated with Crohn's disease. Gastrointest Endosc 63: 433–442; quiz 464.
22. Schnitzler F, Fidder H, Ferrante M, Noman M, Arijs I, et al. (2009) Mucosal healing predicts long-term outcome of maintenance therapy with infliximab in Crohn's disease. Inflamm Bowel Dis 15: 1295–1301.
23. Froslie KF, Jahnsen J, Moum BA, Vatn MH (2007) Mucosal healing in inflammatory bowel disease: results from a Norwegian population-based cohort. Gastroenterology 133: 412–422.
24. Baert F, Moortgat L, Van Assche G, Caenepeel P, Vergauwe P, et al. (2010) Mucosal healing predicts sustained clinical remission in patients with early-stage Crohn's disease. Gastroenterology 138: 463–468; quiz e410–461.
25. Ananthakrishnan AN, Korzenik JR, Hur C (2013) Can Mucosal Healing Be a Cost-effective Endpoint for Biologic Therapy in Crohn's Disease? A Decision Analysis. Inflamm Bowel Dis 19: 37–44.
26. Steenholdt C, Molazahi A, Ainsworth MA, Brynskov J, Ostergaard Thomsen O, et al. (2012) Outcome after discontinuation of infliximab in patients with inflammatory bowel disease in clinical remission: an observational Danish single center study. Scand J Gastroenterol 47: 518–527.
27. Freeman HJ (2010) Limitations in assessment of mucosal healing in inflammatory bowel disease. World J Gastroenterol 16: 15–20.
28. Laharie D, Filippi J, Roblin X, Nancey S, Chevaux JB, et al. (2013) Impact of mucosal healing on long-term outcomes in ulcerative colitis treated with infliximab: a multicenter experience. Aliment Pharmacol Ther 37: 998–1004.

20

Molecular Integrative Clustering of Asian Gastric Cell Lines Revealed Two Distinct Chemosensitivity Clusters

Meng Ling Choong[1], Shan Ho Tan[1], Tuan Zea Tan[2], Sravanthy Manesh[1], Anna Ngo[1], Jacklyn W. Y. Yong[1], Henry He Yang[2], May Ann Lee[1]*

1 Experimental Therapeutics Centre, Agency for Science Technology and Research, Singapore, Singapore, **2** Bioinformatics Core, Cancer Science Institute of Singapore, National University of Singapore, Singapore

Abstract

Cell lines recapitulate cancer heterogeneity without the presence of interfering tissue found in primary tumor. Their heterogeneous characteristics are reflected in their multiple genetic abnormalities and variable responsiveness to drug treatments. In order to understand the heterogeneity observed in Asian gastric cancers, we have performed array comparative genomic hybridization (aCGH) on 18 Asian gastric cell lines. Hierarchical clustering and single-sample Gene Set Enrichment Analysis were performed on the aCGH data together with public gene expression data of the same cell lines obtained from the Cancer Cell Line Encyclopedia. We found a large amount of genetic aberrations, with some cell lines having 13 fold more aberrations than others. Frequently mutated genes and cellular pathways are identified in these Asian gastric cell lines. The combined analyses of aCGH and expression data demonstrate correlation of gene copy number variations and expression profiles in human gastric cancer cells. The gastric cell lines can be grouped into 2 integrative clusters (ICs). Gastric cells in IC1 are enriched with gene associated with mitochondrial activities and oxidative phosphorylation while cells in IC2 are enriched with genes associated with cell signaling and transcription regulations. The two clusters of cell lines were shown to have distinct responsiveness towards several chemotherapeutics agents such as PI3 K and proteosome inhibitors. Our molecular integrative clustering provides insight into critical genes and pathways that may be responsible for the differences in survival in response to chemotherapy.

Editor: Surinder K. Batra, University of Nebraska Medical Center, United States of America

Funding: The authors have no support or funding to report.

Competing Interests: The authors have declared that no competing interests exist.

* Email: malee@etc.a-star.edu.sg

Introduction

Gastric cancer is the second leading cause of cancer death worldwide, and is particularly common in East Asia [1]. It does not get as much attention as other cancers because of its lower incidence in the West. There is a decreasing trend in the incidence of this cancer. However, rates in Asia are among the highest in the world. It is the third most common cancer in males in Singapore and the fifth most common cancer in females in Singapore [2]. It claimed approximately 330 lives every year in Singapore. Diagnosis of gastric cancer usually occurs at late stage of the disease when treatment options are limited and often unsuccessful. Therefore it is critical to improve on early detection and treatment of the cancer.

Traditionally, classification of gastric cancers is based on histopathological findings. The widely used Lauren's classification divides gastric cancers into two major histological types, namely intestinal type or diffuse type [3]. Intestinal type cancers have recognizable gland formation which ranges from well to poorly differentiated. The tumors grow in expanding, rather than infiltrative, patterns. They are believed to arise from chronic atrophic gastritis. In contrast, diffuse type cancers have non-cohesive tumor cells diffusely infiltrating the stroma of the stomach and often exhibit deep infiltration of the stomach wall with little or no gland formation. They may arise out of single-cell mutations within normal gastric glands, and are associated with worse prognosis [4]. Advances in molecular biology have made available molecular classifications based either on genomic aberrations or gene expression profiles, or an integration of both [5–10].

Cell lines formed the foundation of cancer biology and the quest for drug treatments. Common alterations in cell lines, which include gains and losses of entire arms of chromosomes, are often the same ones found in primary tissue [11]. Cell lines also do not contain non-cancerous cells found in primary tumor tissues, making the cultivated lines ideal for finding mutations in the cancer genome [12]. Thus, comparing signatures between cell lines would more likely reflect intrinsic differences between tumor cells with minimal potentially confounding effects from neighboring non-cancer cells [5].

Many Asian gastric cell lines are available commercially and they have contributed to the progress in gastric cancer biology and treatment. Despite being relatively homogenous and devoid of tissue complexity, these Asian gastric cell lines are found to have heterogeneous response or susceptibility to drug treatment (personal unpublished data, and public data in CCLE and Sanger COSMIC). We reasoned that subtle genomic variations may contribute to the underlying differences observed among these gastric cell lines. Unlike tumor tissue, these differences would be intrinsic and a signature to the biology of the particular gastric cell line since there is no interference from other cell types.

We analyzed the gene copy number and LOH in 18 Asian gastric cell lines. Coupling our results to gene expression profiles of these cell lines available from CCLE, we identified two distinct genomic signatures based on genetic aberrations among these Asian gastric cancer cell lines. The clustering was further validated by in vitro chemotherapy sensitivity study done in our lab and with data publicly available from CCLE and Sanger COSMIC databases. A molecular classification on gastric cancer patients would have great clinical impact as it leads to more accurate prediction of prognosis, allowing targeted therapy based on the underlying biology of each subgroup.

Materials and Methods

Cell lines

Asian gastric cell lines SNU-1, SNU-5, SNU-16 and Kato-III, were purchased from the American Type Culture Collection. MKN1, MKN7, MKN45, MMKN74, Fu97, AZ-521, SCH, OCUM-1, NUGC-3, NUGC-4, IM95 and IM95 m were purchased from Japan Health Sciences Foundation. SNU-216 was purchased from Korea Cell Line Bank. YCC-3 [5] was a gift from Patrick Tan, Genome Institute of Singapore.

Array comparative genomic hybridization (aCGH) and copy number determination

CGH array was performed by Origen Labs (Singapore) using the Affymetrix CytoScan HD array platform. Cell pellets containing 1×10^6 cells were used for the aCGH hybridization. The genomic DNA quality, hybridization signal strengths and internal controls satisfied Affymetrix required standard at each step before proceeding to the next. Data from the 18 gastric cell lines on Affymetrix Cytoscan HD array were pre-processed using Affymetrix Chromosome Suite 1.2.2.271 using the single sample analysis workflow and default settings. Hidden Markov model segmentation was applied to call DNA copy number gain, loss or loss of heterozygosity (LOH) status. For matching purposes, the Entrez Gene ID was assigned to each gene name in this data set using the NCBI's Entrez Gene Database [13]. DNA copy number gain, loss or LOH was compiled by counting the number of mutation for each cell line and mutation type. The kinome gene list and human pathways were downloaded from public databases [14,15].

Public microarray data pre-processing

Affymetrix U133 Plus2 DNA microarray gene expressions of 27 gastric cancer cell lines (Kato-III, IM95, SNU-620, SNU-16, OCUM-1, NUGC-4, 2313287, HUG1N, MKN45, NCIN87, KE39, AGS, SNU-5, SNU-216, NUGC-3, NUGC-2, MKN74, MKN7, RERFGC1B, GCIY, KE97, Fu97, SH10TC, MKN1, SNU-1, Hs746 T, HGC27) were downloaded from Cancer Cell Line Encyclopedia (CCLE) [16] in March 2013. Robust Multi-array Average (RMA) normalization was performed. Principal component analysis plot show no obvious batch effect. The normalized data is then collapsed by taking the probe sets with highest gene expression.

Hierarchical clustering and single-sample Gene Set Enrichment Analysis (ssGSEA)

Unsupervised hierarchical clustering (1-Spearman distance, average linkage) was performed on the cell lines using the aCGH data. Putative driver genes of which copy number aberrations correlated to mRNA gene expression were identified to determine subtypes or clusters that are driven by different mechanisms. This was done using Mann Whitney U-test with $p < 0.05$, and Spearman Correlation Coefficient test with Rho > 0.6. We then performed consensus clustering [17] on the gene expression data of the 27 gastric cancer cell lines from CCLE using these putative driver genes. We selected $k = 2$ as it gives sufficiently stable similarity matrix. In order to assign new samples to this integrative cluster, significance analysis of microarray (SAM) [18] with threshold $q < 2.0$ was used to generate subtype signature based on the mRNA expression data of the 1762 genes from the 27 gastric cancer cell lines in CCLE.

ssGSEA was used to estimate pathway activities of the gastric cancer cell line in the Molecular Signature Database v3.1 (Msigdb v3.1) [19,20]. The pathway activities are represented in enrichment scores which were rank normalized to [0.0, 1.0]. SAM analysis was performed with threshold $q < 0.2$, and fold change > 2.0 (for up-regulated pathways), or < 0.5 (for down-regulated pathways) to obtain subtype-specific pathways from the 27 gastric cell lines in CCLE.

Drug treatment

A panel of 39 compounds against various cellular targets was obtained from Selleck Chemicals (Table S1 in File S1). Cells were seeded in 50 µl medium in 96-well plates at 8000 cells/well and incubated overnight. Serial dilutions of compounds were performed starting from 200 µM with 1: 4 dilutions for subsequent dilutions. Serially diluted compounds (50 µl) were added to cells and incubated for 48 hours. To measure cell viability, CellTiter-Glo (Promega) was added to the wells at 1:1 ratio. After 10 minutes of incubation at room temperature, luminescence was measured with Safire II plate reader (Tecan). The experiments were carried out in triplicates for each dose dilution point and independently replicated on a separate occasion. Data was analyzed with Graphpad Prism software to determine the half maximal inhibitory concentration (IC_{50}). P-values were computed from Mann Whitney U-test.

Results and Discussions

Genetic aberrations in the Asian gastric cell lines

In this study, we analyzed the copy number aberrations and LOH in Asian gastric cell lines by aCGH. Genes that are frequently gain, loss or have LOH are identified. Though continuous cell lines tend to harbor more mutations than the primary tumor where it was originally derived [6], cell lines are able to recapitulate major patterns of tumor heterogeneity [21,22]. We detected total genetic aberrations (gain, loss and LOH) in the Asian gastric cell lines ranging from 1724 in AZ-521 to 22631 in NUGC-3 (Table 1). Reflecting this trend, we found that AZ-521 has the least number of genetic aberrations in the human kinome (37 out of a total of 531 kinases) [14] while NUGC-3 has the most number of gene aberrations (510) in its kinome (Table 1).

We found that 72% of the Asian gastric cell lines have gene copy number gain in *CDK13, EGFR, PAK1* and *STK17A* kinases (Table 2). Amplification of *CDK13* was found to associate with gastric and liver cancers [23]. High *EGFR* and *PAK1* expression levels are closely correlated to the incidence and development of gastric cancer in East Asians [24,25] while an unanticipated role

Table 1. Total and kinome genetics aberrations (consisting of gain, loss and LOH) in the 18 Asian gastric cell lines.

Name	Total Genetic Aberrations				Kinome Genetic Aberrations			
	Gain	Loss	LOH	Total	Gain	Loss	LOH	Total
AZ-521	1	1582	141	1724	0	35	2	37
SNU-1	611	1718	76	2405	13	41	1	55
IM95	1819	2137	1155	5111	73	0	35	108
IM95 m	1828	2236	1161	5225	45	48	24	117
Kato-III	3135	0	2131	5266	45	51	24	120
SNU-5	3646	0	1983	5629	89	0	50	139
SNU-16	3195	2621	1130	6946	101	0	47	148
Fu97	4826	0	2319	7145	78	60	25	163
MKN45	2015	0	5339	7354	40	0	129	169
YCC-3	5767	0	2036	7803	134	0	37	171
NUGC-4	7151	0	664	7815	83	0	94	177
MKN7	3859	0	4047	7906	165	0	22	187
OCUM-1	6045	4416	57	10518	143	116	3	262
SCH	3048	8130	1803	12981	71	195	49	315
MKN1	4687	7885	2808	15380	115	174	64	353
MKN74	5733	9792	1935	17460	139	238	47	424
SNU-216	3574	12481	1834	17889	82	307	40	429
NUGC-3	7202	15355	74	22631	154	354	2	510

Table 2. Frequently mutated kinase genes in the 18 Asian gastric cell lines.

Gain		Loss		LOH	
Kinase	Number of cell lines	Kinase	Number of cell lines	Kinase	Number of cell lines
CDK13	13 (72%)	MAP3K15	8 (44%)	GUCY2F	11 (61%)
EGFR	13	RPS6KA6	8	PAK3	11
STK17A	13	PRKX	8	CDKL5	11
PHKG1	12	GUCY2F	8	MYLK3	10
CAMK2B	12	RPS6KA3	8	RPS6KA3	10
STK31	12	MST4	8	RPS6KA6	10
HCK	11	NRK	8	MAP3K15	10
SRC	11	BMX	7	WNK3	10
AURKA	11	TAF1	7	PIM2	9
ADCK5	10	PDK3	7	BTK	9
STK3	10	JAK2	7	CASK	9
SGK2	10	CASK	7	CDK16	9
PAK1	10	CDK16	6	PDK3	9
SRMS	10	ALPK2	6	ARAF	9
EIF2AK1	10	PAK3	6	PRKX	9

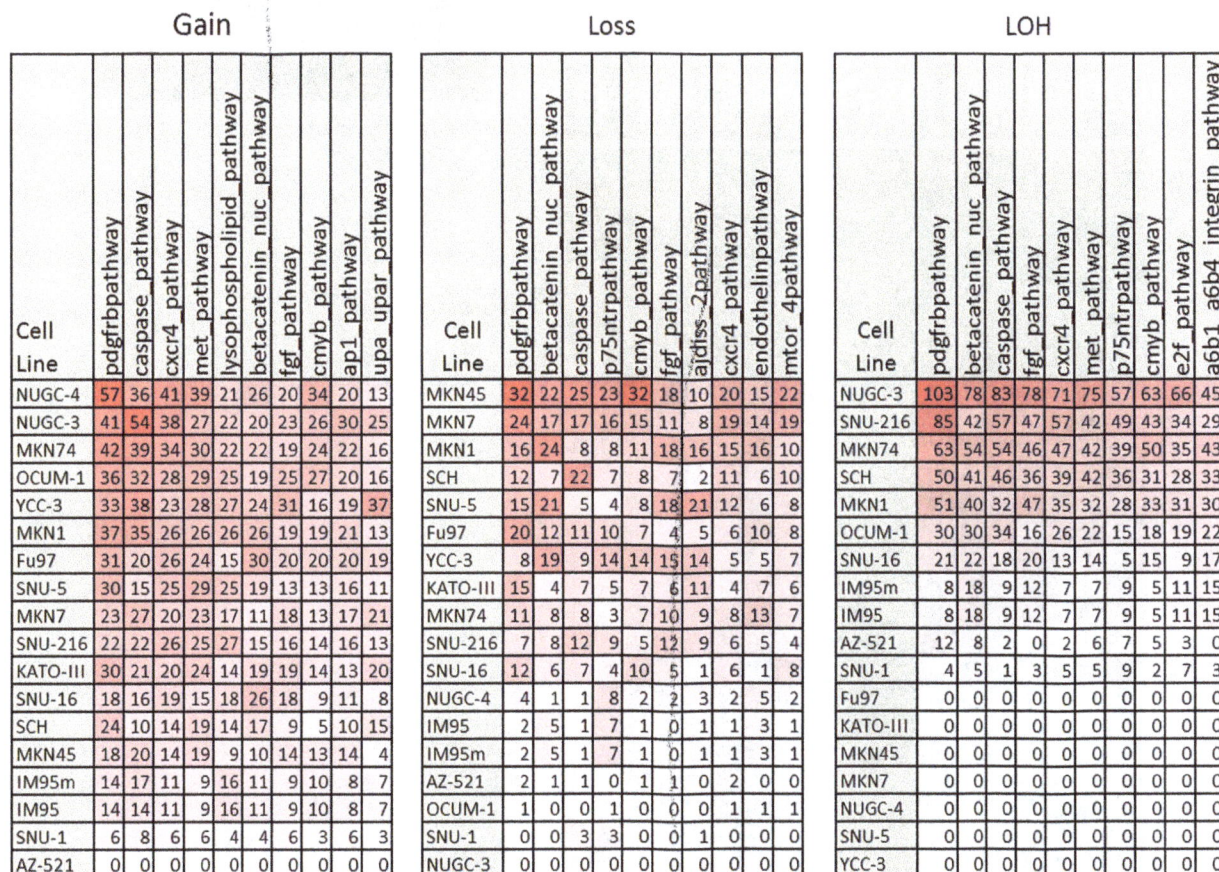

Gain

Cell Line	pdgfrbpathway	caspase_pathway	cxcr4_pathway	met_pathway	lysophospholipid_pathway	betacatenin_nuc_pathway	fgf_pathway	cmyb_pathway	ap1_pathway	upa_upar_pathway
NUGC-4	57	36	41	39	21	26	20	34	20	13
NUGC-3	41	54	38	27	22	20	23	26	30	25
MKN74	42	39	34	30	22	22	19	24	22	16
OCUM-1	36	32	28	29	25	19	25	27	20	16
YCC-3	33	38	23	28	27	24	31	16	19	37
MKN1	37	35	26	26	26	26	19	19	21	13
Fu97	31	20	26	24	15	30	20	20	20	19
SNU-5	30	15	25	29	25	19	13	13	16	11
MKN7	23	27	20	23	17	11	18	13	17	21
SNU-216	22	22	26	25	27	15	16	14	16	13
KATO-III	30	21	20	24	14	19	19	14	13	20
SNU-16	18	16	19	15	18	26	18	9	11	8
SCH	24	10	14	19	14	17	9	5	10	15
MKN45	18	20	14	19	9	10	14	13	14	4
IM95m	14	17	11	9	16	11	9	10	8	7
IM95	14	14	11	9	16	11	9	10	8	7
SNU-1	6	8	6	6	4	4	6	3	6	3
AZ-521	0	0	0	0	0	0	0	0	0	0

Loss

Cell Line	pdgfrbpathway	betacatenin_nuc_pathway	caspase_pathway	p75ntrpathway	cmyb_pathway	fgf_pathway	a|diss-2pathway	cxcr4_pathway	endothelinpathway	mtor_4pathway
MKN45	32	22	25	23	32	18	10	20	15	22
MKN7	24	17	17	16	15	11	8	19	14	19
MKN1	16	24	8	8	11	18	16	15	16	10
SCH	12	7	22	7	8	7	2	11	6	10
SNU-5	15	21	5	4	8	18	21	12	6	8
Fu97	20	12	11	10	7	4	5	6	10	8
YCC-3	8	19	9	14	14	15	14	5	5	7
KATO-III	15	4	7	5	7	6	11	4	7	6
MKN74	11	8	8	3	7	10	9	8	13	7
SNU-216	7	8	12	9	5	12	9	6	5	4
SNU-16	12	6	7	4	10	5	1	6	1	8
NUGC-4	4	1	1	8	2	2	3	2	5	2
IM95	2	5	1	7	1	0	1	1	3	1
IM95m	2	5	1	7	1	0	1	1	3	1
AZ-521	2	1	1	0	1	1	0	2	0	0
OCUM-1	1	0	0	1	0	0	0	1	1	1
SNU-1	0	0	3	3	0	0	1	0	0	0
NUGC-3	0	0	0	0	0	0	0	0	0	0

LOH

Cell Line	pdgfrbpathway	betacatenin_nuc_pathway	caspase_pathway	fgf_pathway	cxcr4_pathway	met_pathway	p75ntrpathway	cmyb_pathway	e2f_pathway	a6b1_a6b4_integrin_pathway
NUGC-3	103	78	83	78	71	75	57	63	66	45
SNU-216	85	42	57	47	57	42	49	43	34	29
MKN74	63	54	54	46	47	42	39	50	35	43
SCH	50	41	46	36	39	42	36	31	28	33
MKN1	51	40	32	47	35	32	28	33	31	30
OCUM-1	30	30	34	16	26	22	15	18	19	22
SNU-16	21	22	18	20	13	14	5	15	9	17
IM95m	8	18	9	12	7	7	9	5	11	15
IM95	8	18	9	12	7	7	9	5	11	15
AZ-521	12	8	2	0	2	6	7	5	3	0
SNU-1	4	5	1	3	5	5	9	2	7	3
Fu97	0	0	0	0	0	0	0	0	0	0
KATO-III	0	0	0	0	0	0	0	0	0	0
MKN45	0	0	0	0	0	0	0	0	0	0
MKN7	0	0	0	0	0	0	0	0	0	0
NUGC-4	0	0	0	0	0	0	0	0	0	0
SNU-5	0	0	0	0	0	0	0	0	0	0
YCC-3	0	0	0	0	0	0	0	0	0	0

Figure 1. Top 10 cellular pathways having the most genetic aberrations in the Asian gastric cell lines. The numerics in red boxes are the number of aberrations. Increased intensity of red corresponds to increased number of aberrations.

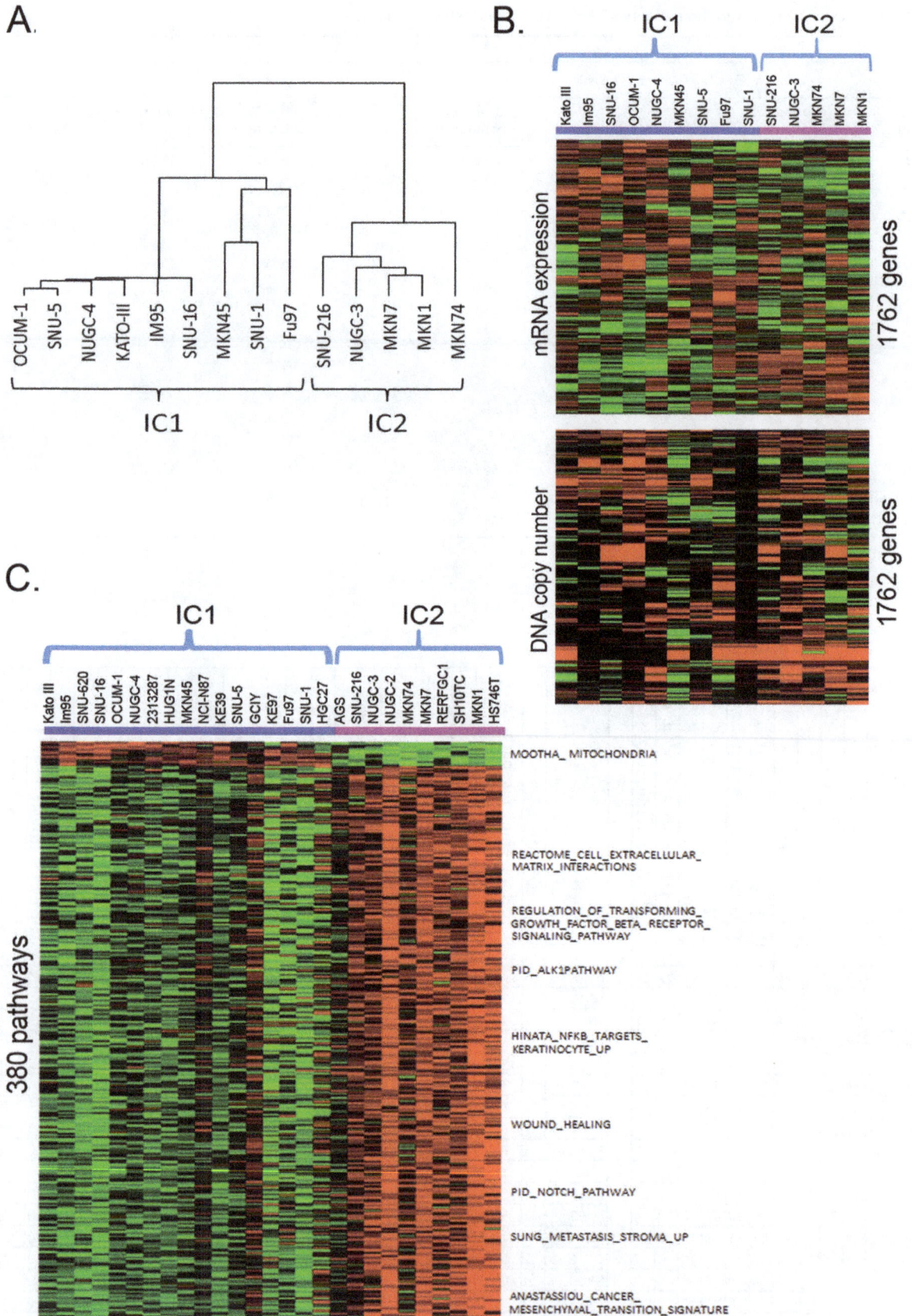

Figure 2. Molecular clustering of the Asian gastric cancer cell lines. (A) Hierarchical clustering using cell lines with both DNA copy number and mRNA expression data. (B) mRNA expression (mean-centered, normalized) heatmap (upper panel) and copy number (lower panel) of 1,762

putative driver genes from 14 gastric cell lines. (C) ssGSEA pathway enrichment score (mean-centered) heatmap for 380 subtype-specific pathways using 27 gastric cell lines from CCLE. Only selected pathway/genesets are labeled. Color code for mRNA expression: red = high expression, green = low expression. Color code for copy number: green = copy number loss, red = copy number gain, black = normal copy number. Color code for pathway enrichment: red = high enrichment, green = low enrichment.

for STK17A as a candidate promoter of cell proliferation and survival was recently identified [26]. On the other hand, 44% of these cell lines have gene copy number loss in *MAP3K15*, an apoptosis-facilitating factor [27], and *RPS6KA6*, a potent tumor suppressor in multiple cancers [28]. LOH is associated with inactivation or loss of a normal allele. We detected LOH of *GUCY2F* in 61% of the Asian gastric cancer cell lines. *GUCY2F* is needed to repress transcription of several growth factor genes and inhibits growth of gastric carcinoma [29]. LOH of *MYLK3* is found in 56% of the Asian gastric cell lines. *MYLK3* is implicated in gastric acid secretion (KEGG entry 91807) and reduced secretion of gastric acid due to atrophic mucosa is observed in gastric cancer.

The NCI-Nature Pathway Interaction Database [15] has 137 human pathways representing 9248 interactions. The top 10 pathways with the most number of gain, loss and LOH for each cell line from our array CGH analysis are summarized in Fig. 1. We found that genes in the PDGFR-beta and the caspase pathways contained the most number of genetic aberrations (gain,

loss and LOH). Deregulation of the PDGFR-beta pathway affects angiogenesis in gastric cancer and depth of cancer cell invasion into the gastric subserosal layer [30]. Down-regulation of caspase activities has been detected in various human gastric cancer-derived cell lines [31]. On the other hand, genes in the nuclear beta-catenin pathway have the most number of loss and LOH with no gain of genetic materials in these Asian cell lines. Deregulation of the Wnt/beta-catenin pathway due to loss of membranous E-cadherin has been reported in gastric cancers [32].

Integrative cluster identification and signature generation

Additionally, we investigated the correlation between copy number aberrations and gene expression data of these cell lines in the public domain. The integrated analysis of DNA copy number variations and corresponding gene expression data would allow identification of significant genes and cellular pathways critical to the gastric cancer pathophysiology. Of the 18 gastric cell lines that we have performed aCGH, only 14 cell lines have corresponding

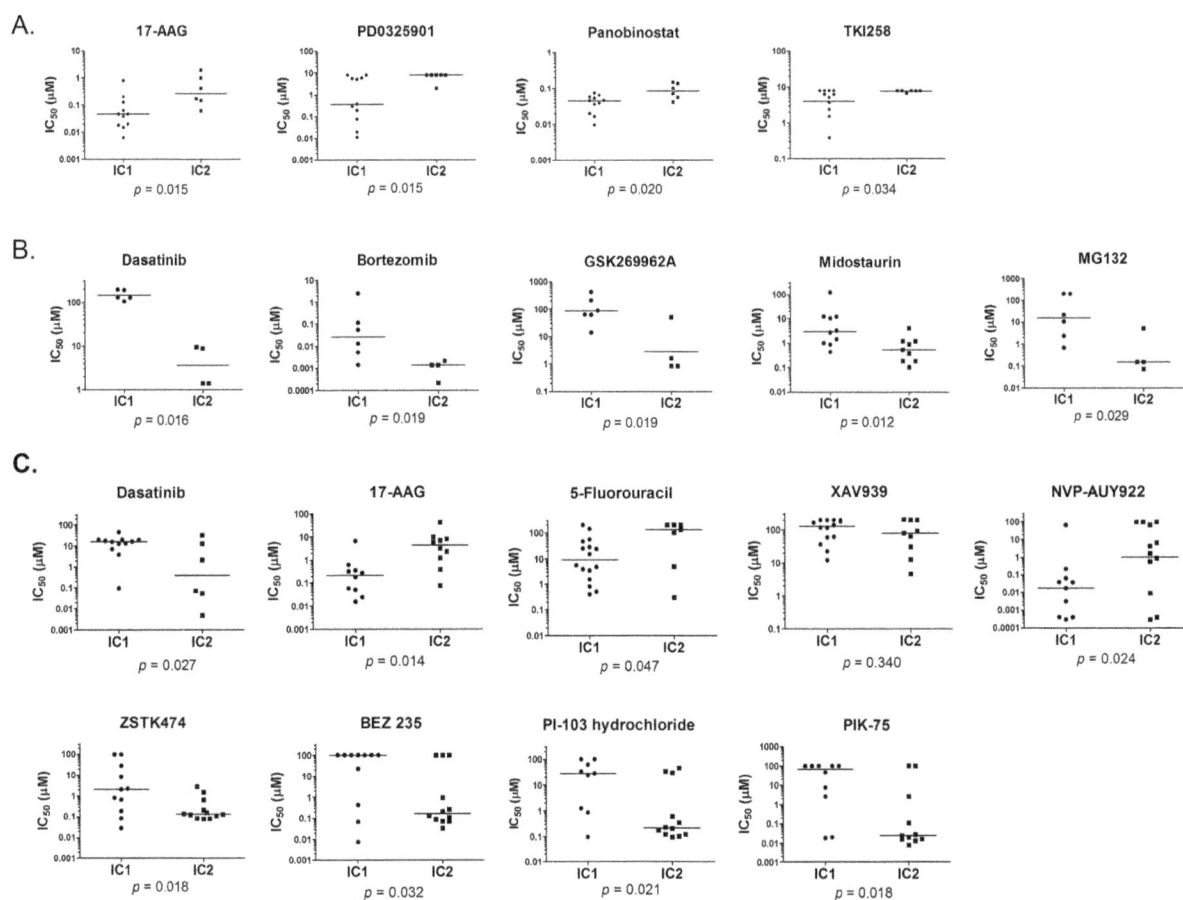

Figure 3. Dot plots of IC$_{50}$ values for targeted inhibitors that have significant differences in toxicity to the Asian gastric cancer cells between the two integrated clusters. (A) Targeted inhibitors from the CCLE database. (B) Targeted inhibitors from the Sanger COSMIC database. (C) Selected targeted inhibitors in our lab showing significant differences in sensitivity (except XAV939) towards the two clusters of cell lines. Y-axis is the IC$_{50}$ values in log10 scale. P-value is computed by Mann Whitney U-test. Horizontal bars are medians for sample distributions.

mRNA expression data in CCLE. CCLE has a total of 27 Asian gastric cell lines at the time of analysis (March 2013). We used Mann Whitney U-test and Spearman Correlation Coefficient test to identify 1762 putative driver genes of which copy number aberrations correlate to mRNA gene expression (Table S2 in File S1). Consensus clustering using these putative driver genes revealed 2 clusters of gastric cell lines. We named them integrated clusters (IC) 1 and 2 (Fig. 2A).

An overall strong correlation between DNA copy number and mRNA expression was observed (Fig. 2B). A similar study with human gastric tumor samples [6] also noted the correlation. These findings suggest that DNA copy number variation is a key contributor to the expression variation of these genes. Cells in IC1 have higher expression of genes involved in oxidoreductase and mitochondria activities. Cells in IC2 have higher expression of genes involved in diverse cellular signaling functions. The roles of these genes in the two clusters of gastric cancer would need to be explored further. SAM was then performed to generate 114 subtype signature genes based on the mRNA expression data of the 1762 genes from the 27 gastric cancer cell lines in CCLE (Table S3 in File S1).

The cell lines in our two integrative clusters correlated strongly with a molecular clustering system reported by Tan et al. [5]. Cell lines in our IC1 and IC2 groups are almost identical to cell lines in their G-INT and G-DIF groups, respectively. The only differences are cell lines Fu-97 and SNU-1 in our IC1 are grouped into G-DIF instead of G-INT. Tan et al. performed the classification based on gene expression data only while we incorporated both in-house aCGH data with public gene expression data. The additional genomic information from aCGH may result in re-arrangement of the hierarchical tree. Tan et al. also found that their data associated significantly with Lauren's classification but remained distinct with overall concordance of 64% with Lauren's histopathological classification. The discrepancies between molecular and histological classification could be due to the ability of genetic classification to capture salient features of the tumor that are less likely to be discerned by light microscopy [5].

Pathway analysis for the Integrative Clusters

ssGSEA was used to estimate pathway activities of the gastric cancer cell line in the Msigdb v3.1. SAM analysis revealed 380 subtype-specific pathways (Table S4 in File S1). The pathway enrichment score heatmap of the 380 subtype-specific pathways from the 27 gastric cell lines in CCLE is shown in Fig. 2C. Cell lines in the IC1 cluster have enrichment of genes associated with oxidative phosphorylation and mitochondria functions. On the other hand, cell lines in the IC2 cluster have enrichment of genes associated with higher inflammatory response, epithelial-mesenchymal transition, TGF-beta, Notch, RAS, and NFκB signaling. Clustering of gastric cancers to IC1 emphasizes on metabolism and energy generation while IC2 emphasizes on cell signaling and regulation of transcriptions suggesting that there are two mechanistically very distinct groups of gastric cancers.

Drug sensitivity of Asian gastric cell lines based on the integrative clustering

Drug sensitivity data (50% growth inhibitory concentration, IC_{50}) were obtained from CCLE (Fig. 3A) and Sanger COSMIC (Fig. 3B). In both CCLE and COSMIC [33], cells were treated with compounds for approximately 72 hours. In-house drug sensitivity assay was performed for 48 hours (Table S5 in File S1). Growth inhibition between the two clusters of Asian gastric cancer cell lines was compared. Only compounds showing significant differential sensitivity between the two molecular clusters in

CCLE, COSMIC and our in-house data are shown. We verified that the effect of 17-AAG and dasatinib in our collection of cell lines are similar to the results obtained from CCLE and COSMIC even though the length of incubation time with the compounds were different between our data and the public data (Fig. 3C).

5-Fluorouracil, a thymidylate synthase inhibitor which is the current treatment for gastric cancer, was found to be slightly more effective in cell lines in IC1 compared to IC2 (p = 0.047) (Fig. 3C). Similar results were also observed by Tan et al. [5] where cells in G-INT are more sensitive towards 5-fluorouracil than G-DIF. A significant benefit from adjuvant 5′-fluorouracil therapy in G-INT subtype compared to G-DIF subtype in retrospective patient cohorts has also been reported by Tan et al. Furthermore, a 10-year follow-up study found that 5-fluorouracil therapy with radiation could benefit all but the diffuse subtype based on Lauren's classification [34].

Since we observed gene loss and LOH in the nuclear beta-catenin pathway, we postulate that targeting this pathway may have a therapeutic effect in gastric cancer [35]. However, we found that gastric cell lines in both IC1 and IC2 clusters are generally not responsive (IC_{50} ~100 μM) towards XAV939, a tankyrase inhibitor [36] which selectively inhibit beta-catenin mediated transcription (Fig. 3C). This suggests that genetic aberrations in the beta-catenin pathway may be superfluous to the survival of the gastric cancer cells.

Cells in IC1 have enrichment of genes associated with oxidative phosphorylation and mitochondria functions. We found that cells in IC1 are more resistant to proteosome inhibitors bortezomib and MG132 (Fig. 3B). Proteosome inhibitors induce reactive oxygen species generation [37] which contribute to oxidative damage and cell death. Enrichment of genes associated with mitochondria function in cells in IC1 may enhance the ability of these cells to withstand oxidative damage. In contrast, the Hsp90 inhibitors, NVP-AUY922 and 17-AAG, are found to be more effective in inhibiting growth of cell lines in IC1 (p = 0.024 and 0.014, respectively). Mitochondrial Hsp90 is involved in complex signaling pathway that prevents initiation of induced apoptosis. The increased sensitivity of cells in the IC1 towards Hsp90 inhibitors further suggests that mitochondria activity is important in the survival of this cluster of cell lines [38].

Interestingly, we found that a subset of gastric cells within the IC1 are more sensitive towards the MEK/ERK inhibitor PD0325901 (p = 0.015; Fig. 3A). The MEK-ERK pathway is required for the S727 phosphorylation of mitochondrial STAT3 which is critical for electron transport chain activity and ATP abundance [39]. The pan histone deacetylase inhibitor panobinostat is also more toxic to gastric cells in IC1 (p = 0.020). On top of its mitochondrial modulatory effect and induction of apoptosis, panobinostat could also undermine the chaperon function of Hsp90 through hyperacetylation of Hsp90 [40]. Gastric cells in IC1 are also more sensitive towards TKI258 compared to cells in IC2 (p = 0.034). TKI258 is a multi-targeted receptor tyrosine kinase inhibitor with activity against FGFR, VEGFR, PDGFR, FLT3, and KIT. These will indirectly decrease Y243 phosphorylation of mitochondrial pyruvate dehydrogenase kinase 1, leading to inactivation of pyruvate dehydrogenase complex and decreased cell proliferation [41].

In support of our findings that the gastric cells in IC2 are enriched for genes involved in cell signalling, we found that cells in IC2 are generally more sensitive to kinase inhibitors than cells in IC1. Cell lines in IC2 are more sensitive to treatment with PI3 K inhibitors BEZ235, ZSTK424, PI-103 and PIK-75 (p = 0.032, 0.018, 0.021 and 0.018 respectively) (Figure 3C). This reflects a central role for the PI3 K pathway in cancer cell proliferation

[42]. Targeting the PI3 K/AKT pathway may represent an important therapeutic target for gastric cancer [43]. We also found significantly lower IC_{50} values with gastric cells in IC2 compared to cells in IC1 when treated with kinase inhibitors dasatinib (Bcr-abl and Src inhibitor) (p = 0.027), GSK269962A (Rho kinase inhibitor) (p = 0.019), and midostaurin (Flt3 and multiple kinase inhibitor) (p = 0.012).

The absolute magnitude of the differential drug sensitivities ranges from 2–10 fold in the gastric cell lines based on our clustering. The modest differences may still be clinically meaningful given the small therapeutic windows associated with cytotoxicity even in targeted chemotherapy. A large patient cohort study will be needed to confirm the value of the molecular clustering strategies by us or others in predicting chemosensitivity and prognosis.

In conclusion, combination of aCGH and gene expression analysis to identify potential candidate oncogenes or tumor suppressor genes is a powerful and proven approach that has been reported in other cancer studies. This study provides insight into DNA copy number variations and their correlation to gene expression profiles in Asian gastric cell lines. A schematic diagram of the overall workflow is shown in Fig. S1 located in File S1. We report here the discovery of signature genes and cellular pathways associated with two genomic clusters of these cell lines. The two clusters of cell lines responded differentially to targeted therapeutic agents. Our results provide new insights into the molecular

pathogenesis of this malignancy and could potentially augment the conventional histological classification of gastric cancers.

Supporting Information

File S1 Table S1: A panel of target-specific compounds for chemosensitivity study in the Asian gastric cell lines. Table S2: Putative driver genes selected using correlated genes between copy number aberration and mRNA gene expression (Mann Whitney test, p<0.05, Spearman correlation coefficient, Rho >0.6). Table S3: Integrative cluster signature (Copy number and mRNA correlated genes). Table S4: Integrative cluster-specific pathway. Table S5: Compounds showing significant differences in sensitivity between the two integrative clusters of Asian gastric cell lines. Figure S1: A schematic diagram of the analysis workflow.

Acknowledgments

We acknowledge the excellent cell culture technical support by Sifang Wang and Yu Wang, Experimental Therapeutics Centre.

Author Contributions

Conceived and designed the experiments: MLC MAL. Performed the experiments: MLC SM AN JY. Analyzed the data: MLC SHT TZT. Contributed reagents/materials/analysis tools: MLC SHT TZT HY. Contributed to the writing of the manuscript: MLC SHT TZT.

References

1. Leung WK, Wu MS, Kakugawa Y, Kim JJ, Yeoh KG, et al. (2008) Screening for gastric cancer in Asia: current evidence and practice. Lancet Oncol 9: 279–287.
2. Singapore Cancer Registry (2011) Cancer Survival in Singapore 1968–2007. Singapore: National Registry of Diseases Office: Health Promotion Board.
3. Lauren P (1965) The Two Histological Main Types of Gastric Carcinoma: Diffuse and So-Called Intestinal-Type Carcinoma. An Attempt at a Histo-Clinical Classification. Acta Pathol Microbiol Scand 64: 31–49.
4. Dicken BJ, Bigam DL, Cass C, Mackey JR, Joy AA, et al. (2005) Gastric adenocarcinoma: review and considerations for future directions. Ann Surg 241: 27–39.
5. Tan IB, Ivanova T, Lim KH, Ong CW, Deng N, et al. (2011) Intrinsic subtypes of gastric cancer, based on gene expression pattern, predict survival and respond differently to chemotherapy. Gastroenterology 141: 476–485, 485 e471–411.
6. Fan B, Dachrut S, Coral H, Yuen ST, Chu KM, et al. (2012) Integration of DNA copy number alterations and transcriptional expression analysis in human gastric cancer. PLoS One 7: e29824.
7. Tay ST, Leong SH, Yu K, Aggarwal A, Tan SY, et al. (2003) A combined comparative genomic hybridization and expression microarray analysis of gastric cancer reveals novel molecular subtypes. Cancer Res 63: 3309–3316.
8. Kim B, Bang S, Lee S, Kim S, Jung Y, et al. (2003) Expression profiling and subtype-specific expression of stomach cancer. Cancer Res 63: 8248–8255.
9. Chen X, Leung SY, Yuen ST, Chu KM, Ji J, et al. (2003) Variation in gene expression patterns in human gastric cancers. Mol Biol Cell 14: 3208–3215.
10. Boussioutas A, Li H, Liu J, Waring P, Lade S, et al. (2003) Distinctive patterns of gene expression in premalignant gastric mucosa and gastric cancer. Cancer Res 63: 2569–2577.
11. Beroukhim R, Mermel CH, Porter D, Wei G, Raychaudhuri S, et al. (2010) The landscape of somatic copy-number alteration across human cancers. Nature 463: 899–905.
12. Bignell GR, Greenman CD, Davies H, Butler AP, Edkins S, et al. (2010) Signatures of mutation and selection in the cancer genome. Nature 463: 893–898.
13. Coordinators NR (2014) Database resources of the National Center for Biotechnology Information. Nucleic Acids Res 42: D7–17.
14. Manning G, Whyte DB, Martinez R, Hunter T, Sudarsanam S (2002) The protein kinase complement of the human genome. Science 298: 1912–1934.
15. Schaefer CF, Anthony K, Krupa S, Buchoff J, Day M, et al. (2009) PID: the Pathway Interaction Database. Nucleic Acids Res 37: D674–679.
16. Barretina J, Caponigro G, Stransky N, Venkatesan K, Margolin AA, et al. (2012) The Cancer Cell Line Encyclopedia enables predictive modelling of anticancer drug sensitivity. Nature 483: 603–607.
17. Wilkerson MD, Hayes DN (2010) ConsensusClusterPlus: a class discovery tool with confidence assessments and item tracking. Bioinformatics 26: 1572–1573.
18. Tusher VG, Tibshirani R, Chu G (2001) Significance analysis of microarrays applied to the ionizing radiation response. Proc Natl Acad Sci U S A 98: 5116–5121.

19. Subramanian A, Tamayo P, Mootha VK, Mukherjee S, Ebert BL, et al. (2005) Gene set enrichment analysis: a knowledge-based approach for interpreting genome-wide expression profiles. Proc Natl Acad Sci U S A 102: 15545–15550.
20. Verhaak RG, Tamayo P, Yang JY, Hubbard D, Zhang H, et al. (2013) Prognostically relevant gene signatures of high-grade serous ovarian carcinoma. J Clin Invest 123: 517–525.
21. Neve RM, Chin K, Fridlyand J, Yeh J, Baehner FL, et al. (2006) A collection of breast cancer cell lines for the study of functionally distinct cancer subtypes. Cancer Cell 10: 515–527.
22. Hoshida Y, Toffanin S, Lachenmayer A, Villanueva A, Minguez B, et al. (2010) Molecular classification and novel targets in hepatocellular carcinoma: recent advancements. Semin Liver Dis 30: 35–51.
23. Kim HE, Kim DG, Lee KJ, Son JG, Song MY, et al. (2012) Frequent amplification of CENPF, GMNN and CDK13 genes in hepatocellular carcinomas. PLoS One 7: e43223.
24. Gao M, Liang XJ, Zhang ZS, Ma W, Chang ZW, et al. (2013) Relationship between expression of EGFR in gastric cancer tissue and clinicopathological features. Asian Pac J Trop Med 6: 260–264.
25. Li LH, Luo Q, Zheng MH, Pan C, Wu GY, et al. (2012) P21-activated protein kinase 1 is overexpressed in gastric cancer and induces cancer metastasis. Oncol Rep 27: 1435–1442.
26. Mao P, Hever-Jardine MP, Rahme GJ, Yang E, Tam J, et al. (2013) Serine/threonine kinase 17A is a novel candidate for therapeutic targeting in glioblastoma. PLoS One 8: e81803.
27. Kaji T, Yoshida S, Kawai K, Fuchigami Y, Watanabe W, et al. (2010) ASK3, a novel member of the apoptosis signal-regulating kinase family, is essential for stress-induced cell death in HeLa cells. Biochem Biophys Res Commun 395: 213–218.
28. Li Q, Jiang Y, Wei W, Ji Y, Gao H, et al. (2014) Frequent epigenetic inactivation of RSK4 by promoter methylation in cancerous and non-cancerous tissues of breast cancer. Med Oncol 31: 793.
29. Kitadai Y, Yamazaki H, Yasui W, Kyo E, Yokozaki H, et al. (1993) GC factor represses transcription of several growth factor/receptor genes and causes growth inhibition of human gastric carcinoma cell lines. Cell Growth Differ 4: 291–296.
30. Suzuki S, Dobashi Y, Hatakeyama Y, Tajiri R, Fujimura T, et al. (2010) Clinicopathological significance of platelet-derived growth factor (PDGF)-B and vascular endothelial growth factor-A expression, PDGF receptor-beta phosphorylation, and microvessel density in gastric cancer. BMC Cancer 10: 659.
31. Philchenkov A, Zavelevich M, Kroczak TJ, Los M (2004) Caspases and cancer: mechanisms of inactivation and new treatment modalities. Exp Oncol 26: 82–97.
32. Cheng XX, Wang ZC, Chen XY, Sun Y, Kong QY, et al. (2005) Frequent loss of membranous E-cadherin in gastric cancers: A cross-talk with Wnt in determining the fate of beta-catenin. Clin Exp Metastasis 22: 85–93.

33. Garnett MJ, Edelman EJ, Heidorn SJ, Greenman CD, Dastur A, et al. (2012) Systematic identification of genomic markers of drug sensitivity in cancer cells. Nature 483: 570–575.

34. Macdonald JS, Benedetti J, Smalley S, Haller D, Hundahl S, et al. (2009) Chemoradiation of resected gastric cancer: A 10-year follow-up of the phase III trial INT0116 (SWOG 9008). Journal of Clinical Oncology 27: abstr 4515.

35. Wu WK, Cho CH, Lee CW, Fan D, Wu K, et al. (2010) Dysregulation of cellular signaling in gastric cancer. Cancer Lett 295: 144–153.

36. Huang SM, Mishina YM, Liu S, Cheung A, Stegmeier F, et al. (2009) Tankyrase inhibition stabilizes axin and antagonizes Wnt signalling. Nature 461: 614–620.

37. Ling YH, Liebes L, Zou Y, Perez-Soler R (2003) Reactive oxygen species generation and mitochondrial dysfunction in the apoptotic response to Bortezomib, a novel proteasome inhibitor, in human H460 non-small cell lung cancer cells. J Biol Chem 278: 33714–33723.

38. Siegelin MD (2013) Inhibition of the mitochondrial Hsp90 chaperone network: a novel, efficient treatment strategy for cancer? Cancer Lett 333: 133–146.

39. Gough DJ, Koetz L, Levy DE (2013) The MEK-ERK pathway is necessary for serine phosphorylation of mitochondrial STAT3 and Ras-mediated transformation. PLoS One 8: e83395.

40. Rao R, Nalluri S, Fiskus W, Savoie A, Buckley KM, et al. (2010) Role of CAAT/enhancer binding protein homologous protein in panobinostat-mediated potentiation of bortezomib-induced lethal endoplasmic reticulum stress in mantle cell lymphoma cells. Clin Cancer Res 16: 4742–4754.

41. Hitosugi T, Fan J, Chung TW, Lythgoe K, Wang X, et al. (2011) Tyrosine phosphorylation of mitochondrial pyruvate dehydrogenase kinase 1 is important for cancer metabolism. Mol Cell 44: 864–877.

42. Porta C, Paglino C, Mosca A (2014) Targeting PI3 K/Akt/mTOR Signaling in Cancer. Front Oncol 4: 64.

43. Ye B, Jiang LL, Xu HT, Zhou DW, Li ZS (2012) Expression of PI3 K/AKT pathway in gastric cancer and its blockade suppresses tumor growth and metastasis. Int J Immunopathol Pharmacol 25: 627–636.

21

Dual Effects of Ketoconazole *cis*-Enantiomers on CYP3A4 in Human Hepatocytes and HepG2 Cells

Aneta Novotná[1][9], Kristýna Krasulová[2][9], Iveta Bartoňková[1], Martina Korhoňová[1], Petr Bachleda[3], Pavel Anzenbacher[2], Zdeněk Dvořák[1]*

1 Regional Centre of Advanced Technologies and Materials, Faculty of Science, Palacky University, Olomouc, Czech Republic, **2** Institute of Pharmacology, Faculty of Medicine and Dentistry, Palacky University, Olomouc, Czech Republic, **3** 2nd Department of Surgery, University Hospital Olomouc, Olomouc, Czech Republic

Abstract

Antifungal drug ketoconazole causes severe drug-drug interactions by influencing gene expression and catalytic activity of major drug-metabolizing enzyme cytochrome P450 CYP3A4. Ketoconazole is administered in the form of racemic mixture of two *cis*-enantiomers, i.e. (+)-ketoconazole and (−)-ketoconazole. Many enantiopure drugs were introduced to human pharmacotherapy in last two decades. In the current paper, we have examined the effects of ketoconazole *cis*-enantiomers on the expression of CYP3A4 in human hepatocytes and HepG2 cells and on catalytic activity of CYP3A4 in human liver microsomes. We show that both ketoconazole enantiomers induce CYP3A4 mRNA and protein in human hepatocytes and HepG2 cells. Gene reporter assays revealed partial agonist activity of ketoconazole enantiomers towards pregnane X receptor PXR. Catalytic activity of CYP3A4/5 towards two prototypic substrates of CYP3A enzymes, testosterone and midazolam, was determined in presence of both (+)-ketoconazole and (−)-ketoconazole in human liver microsomes. Overall, both ketoconazole *cis*-enantiomers induced CYP3A4 in human cells and inhibited CYP3A4 in human liver microsomes. While interaction of ketoconazole with PXR and induction of CYP3A4 did not display enantiospecific pattern, inhibition of CYP3A4 catalytic activity by ketoconazole differed for ketoconazole *cis*-enantiomers ((+)-ketoconazole IC_{50} 1.69 μM, K_i 0.92 μM for testosterone, IC_{50} 1.46 μM, K_i 2.52 μM for midazolam; (−)-ketoconazole IC_{50} 0.90 μM, K_i 0.17 μM for testosterone, IC_{50} 1.04 μM, K_i 1.51 μM for midazolam).

Editor: Bandana Chatterjee, University of Texas Health Science Center, United States of America

Funding: This research was supported by the Czech Science Agency [Grant GACR 13-01809S] and by the student project from Palacky University [PrF-2014-004]. The funders had no role in study design, data collection and analysis, decision to publish, or preparation of the manuscript.

Competing Interests: The authors have declared that no competing interests exist.

* Email: moulin@email.cz

9 These authors contributed equally to this work.

Introduction

Ketoconazole is an imidazole antifungal drug that is used both systemically and topically, in the treatment of various fungal infections. While oral ketoconazole was discontinued in many countries, there is increasing evidence that it might be a drug of choice in the therapy of systemic infections, if the first line treatment with other antifungals fails. Various topical formulations of ketoconazole, such as creams or shampoos are massively used. Ketoconazole is also used as prophylactic agens in immune-suppressed patients (oncologic, transplant etc.). Molecular mechanism of ketoconazole action is an inhibition of fungal cytochrome P450 CYP51A, which is lanosterol-14α-demethylase that catalyzes conversion of lanosterol to ergosterol in fungi [1].

There is a myriad of potential drugs that ketoconazole can interact with, including statins, tricyclic antidepressants, antivirotics, anticonvulsives and many others. The clinical relevance of ketoconazole-drug interactions varies substantially. While certain interactions are benign and result in little or no clinical outcomes, others can produce significant toxicity or compromise efficacy if not properly managed through monitoring and dosage adjustment. Some interactions produce significant toxicity or compro-

mise efficacy to such an extent that they cannot be managed and the particular combination of ketoconazole and interacting medicine should be avoided [2]. The mechanisms of ketoconazole-drug interactions are multiple and the most frequently, they are caused by inhibition of catalytic activity of main biotransformation enzyme CYP3A4, and also CYP2C9 [3]. Ketoconazole can disturb pharmacokinetics of drugs by interactions with transcriptional regulators of drug-metabolizing enzymes [4]. Numerous data were published regarding the effects of ketoconazole on pregnane X receptor PXR, which is a master regulator of CYP3A4 expression. We described that ketoconazole up-regulates CYP3A4 mRNA and down-regulates PXR mRNA in LS174T cells. Ketoconazole also activated CYP3A4 promoter, but it inhibited rifampicin-inducible activity of reporter gene. Binding of the ligand to PXR, and interaction of PXR with SRC1 was diminished by ketoconazole [5,6]. Ketoconazole also blocks interactions between PXR and its transcriptional co-activator HNF4α [7]. The transcriptional activation of genes regulating biotransformation and transport by the liganded PXR was inhibited by ketoconazole. Mutations at the AF-2 surface of the human PXR ligand-binding domain indicated that ketoconazole may interact with specific residues outside the ligand-binding pocket [8]. From receptor theory point of view, this behavior indicates partial agonism of ketoconazole against PXR [9]. Structure-function as well as computational docking analysis suggested a putative binding region containing critical charge clamp residues Gln-272, and Phe-264 on the AF-2 surface of PXR. Recent study confirmed that a residue Ser-208, which is on the opposite side of the protein from the AF-2 region critical for receptor regulation, is involved in interactions between ketoconazole and PXR. The identification of new locations for antagonist binding on the surface or buried in PXR indicates novel allosteric aspects to the mechanism of receptor antagonism [10]. It was demonstrated that ketoconazole is an antagonist not only for PXR, but also for many other nuclear and steroid receptors, including glucocorticoid receptor GR [11,12], liver X receptor LXR, constitutive androstane receptor CAR, farnesoid X receptor FXR and peroxisome proliferator-activated receptor gamma PPARγ [6]. Recently, ketoconazole was identified as an activator

and ligand of aryl hydrocarbon receptor and inducer of CYP1A enzymes [12,13].

Ketoconazole contains two chiral centers in its molecule, therefore, it forms four enantiomers. The therapeutically used ketoconazole (KET) is a racemic mixture consisting of two *cis*-enantiomers; (2R,4S)-(+)-KET and (2S,4R)-(−)-KET. Individual enantiomers of the drug may display quantitatively and/or qualitatively different pharmaco−/toxico-kinetics and pharmaco−/toxico-dynamics. The examples are numerous [14]. Logically, a concept of enantiopure drugs emerged and many enantiopure drugs were introduced to human pharmacotherapy during last two decades. Enantiospecific effects of KET on catalytic activities of CYP3A4/5 [15,16] were reported. However, it was demonstrated that inhibition parameters of separate enantiomers for CYP3A4 are substrate-dependent and the data should be interpreted with care [17]. A phase II clinical study was conducted with compound DIO-902 (which is ketoconazole enantiomer (−)-KET), as a candidate drug for the treatment of

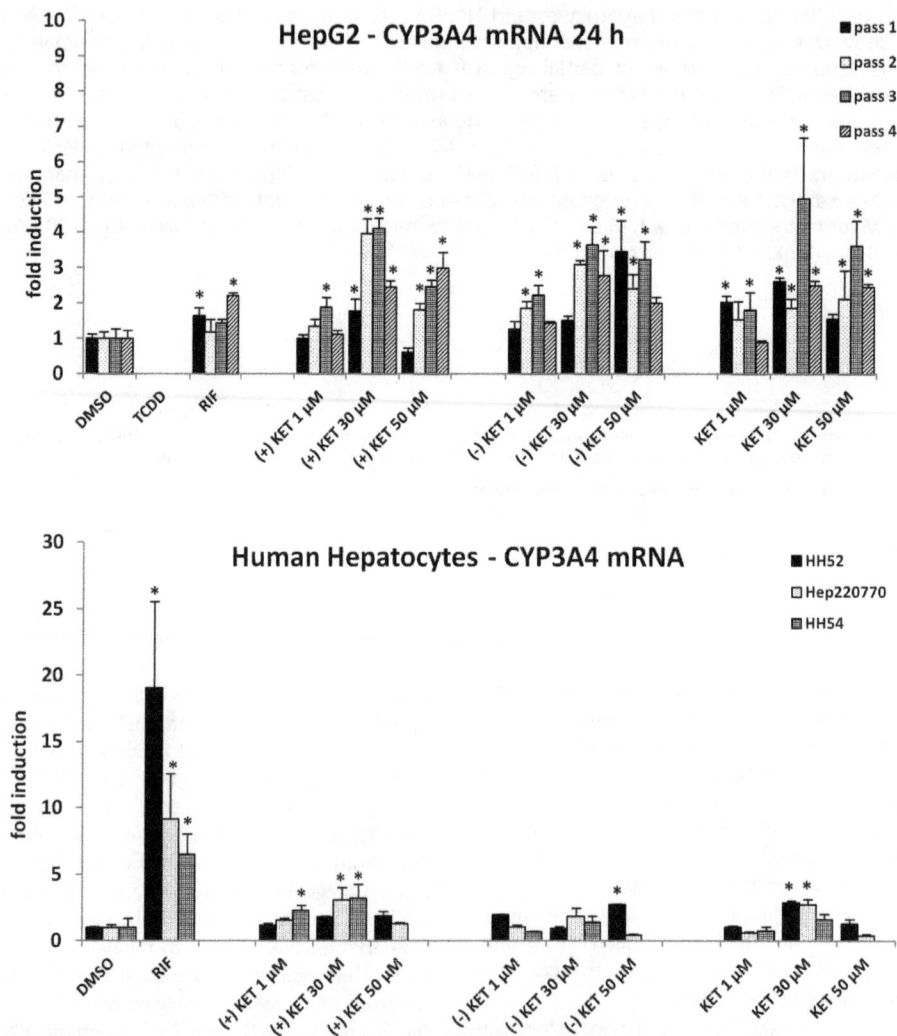

Figure 1. Effects of ketoconazole *cis*-enantiomers on CYP3A4 mRNA expression in HepG2 cells and human hepatocytes. (i) HepG2 cells were seeded in 6-well plates and stabilized for 16 h. Experiments were performed in four consecutive cell passages. (ii) Primary human hepatocytes from three different donors (HH52, HH54 and Hep220770) were used. Cells were incubated for 24 h with RIF (10 µM), vehicle (DMSO; 0.1% v/v) and ketoconazole ((+), (−), (rac); 1 µM, 30 µM, 50 µM). RT-PCR analyses of CYP3A4 mRNA are shown. The data are the mean ± SD from triplicate measurements and are expressed as a fold induction over vehicle-treated cells. The data were normalized to GAPDH mRNA levels. An asterisk (*) indicates that the value is significantly different from the activity of vehicle-treated cells.

Diabetes mellitus Type II [18]. However, due to the side effects, a study was interrupted and DIO-902 was suspended [19].

Taking in account massive use of ketoconazole, its chiral structure and numerous drug interactions, it is of value to study enantiospecific interactions between ketoconazole and drug-metabolizing pathways. We have recently described enantiospecific effects of ketoconazole *cis*-enantiomers on transcriptional activity of AhR and induction of CYP1A genes in human hepatocytes and cancer cell lines [12]. In the current paper, we have examined the effects of ketoconazole *cis*-enantiomers on the expression of CYP3A4 in human hepatocytes and HepG2 cells and on catalytic activity of CYP3A4 in human liver microsomes.

Materials and Methods

Compounds and reagents

Dimethylsulfoxide (DMSO), rifampicin (RIF) and hygromycin B were purchased from Sigma-Aldrich (Prague, Czech Republic). *Cis*-enantiomers of ketoconazole (2R, 4S)-(+)-KET and (2S, 4R)-(−)-KET were isolated from commercial ketoconazole by preparative HPLC at Department of Analytical Chemistry,

Faculty of Science, Palacky University Olomouc. Luciferase lysis buffer was from Promega (Hercules, CA).

Cell culture

Human Caucasian colon adenocarcinoma cells LS174T (ECACC No. 87060401) and human Caucasian hepatocellular carcinoma cells HepG2 (ECACC No. 85011430) were purchased from ECACC and were cultured in as recommended by manufacturer. Primary human hepatocytes used in this study were obtained from two sources: (i) from multiorgan donors HH52 (female; 60 years) and LH54 (male; 71 years); the use of liver cells of donors HH52 and HH54 was approved by "Ethical committee at the Faculty Hospital Olomouc", and it was in accordance with Transplantation law #285/2002 Sb; "Ethical committee at the Faculty Hospital Olomouc" waived the authors from obtaining consent from the next of kin, regarding human hepatocytes obtained from liver donors HH52 and HH54. (ii) long-term human hepatocytes in monolayer Batch HEP220770 (female; 35 years) were purchased from Biopredic International (Biopredic International, Rennes, France). Cells were cultured in serum-free medium. Cultures were maintained at 37°C and 5% CO2 in a humidified incubator.

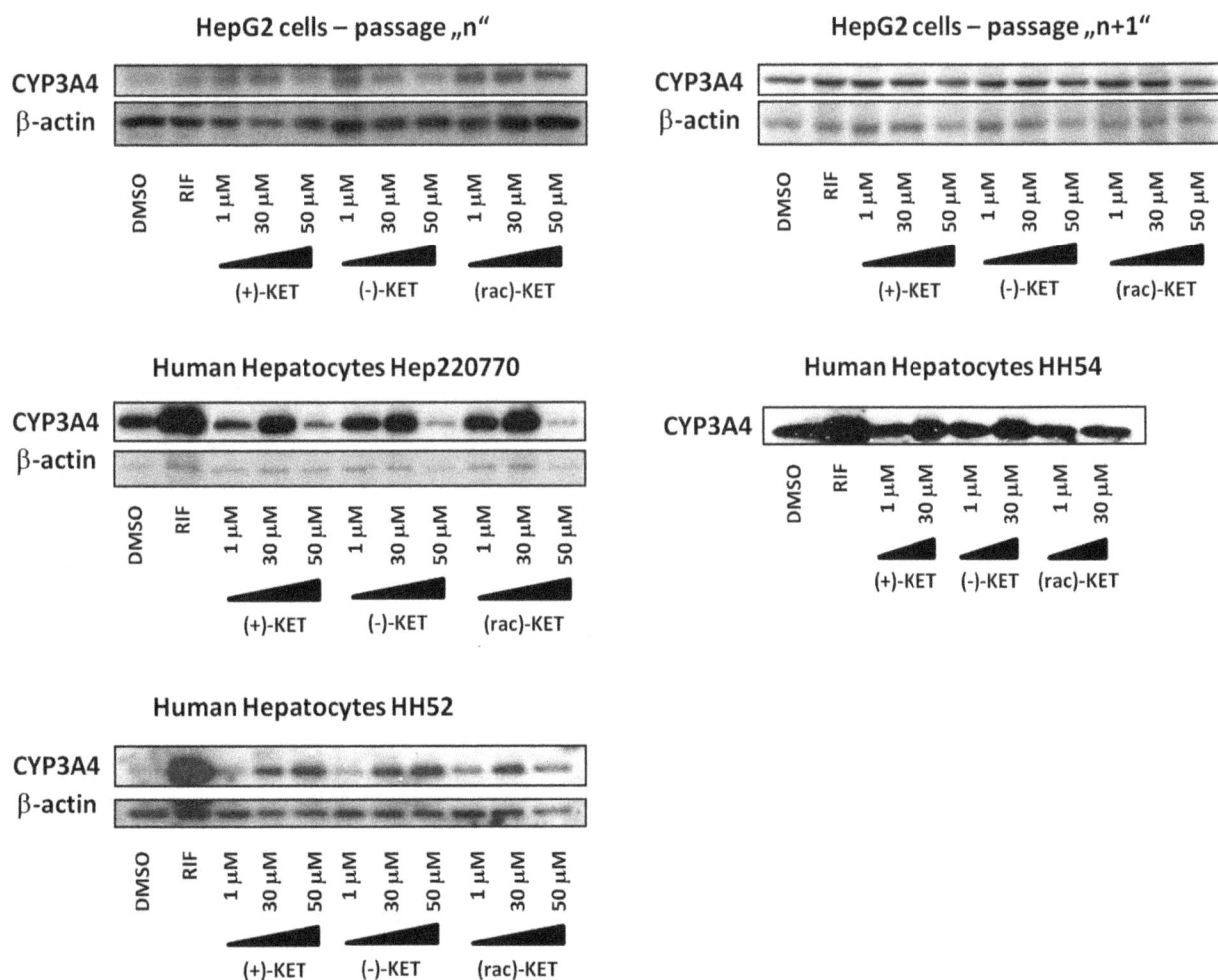

Figure 2. Effects of ketoconazole *cis*-enantiomers on CYP3A4 protein expression in HepG2 cells and human hepatocytes. Western blots of CYP3A4 and β-actin from three different human hepatocytes cultures (HH52, HH54 and Hep220770) and from two consecutive passages of HepG2 cells are shown. Cells were incubated for 48 h with RIF (10 μM), vehicle (DMSO; 0.1% v/v) and ketoconazole ((+), (−), (rac); 1 μM, 30 μM, 50 μM). Density of bands was quantified by densitometry.

MTT test

PXR agonist

PXR antagonist

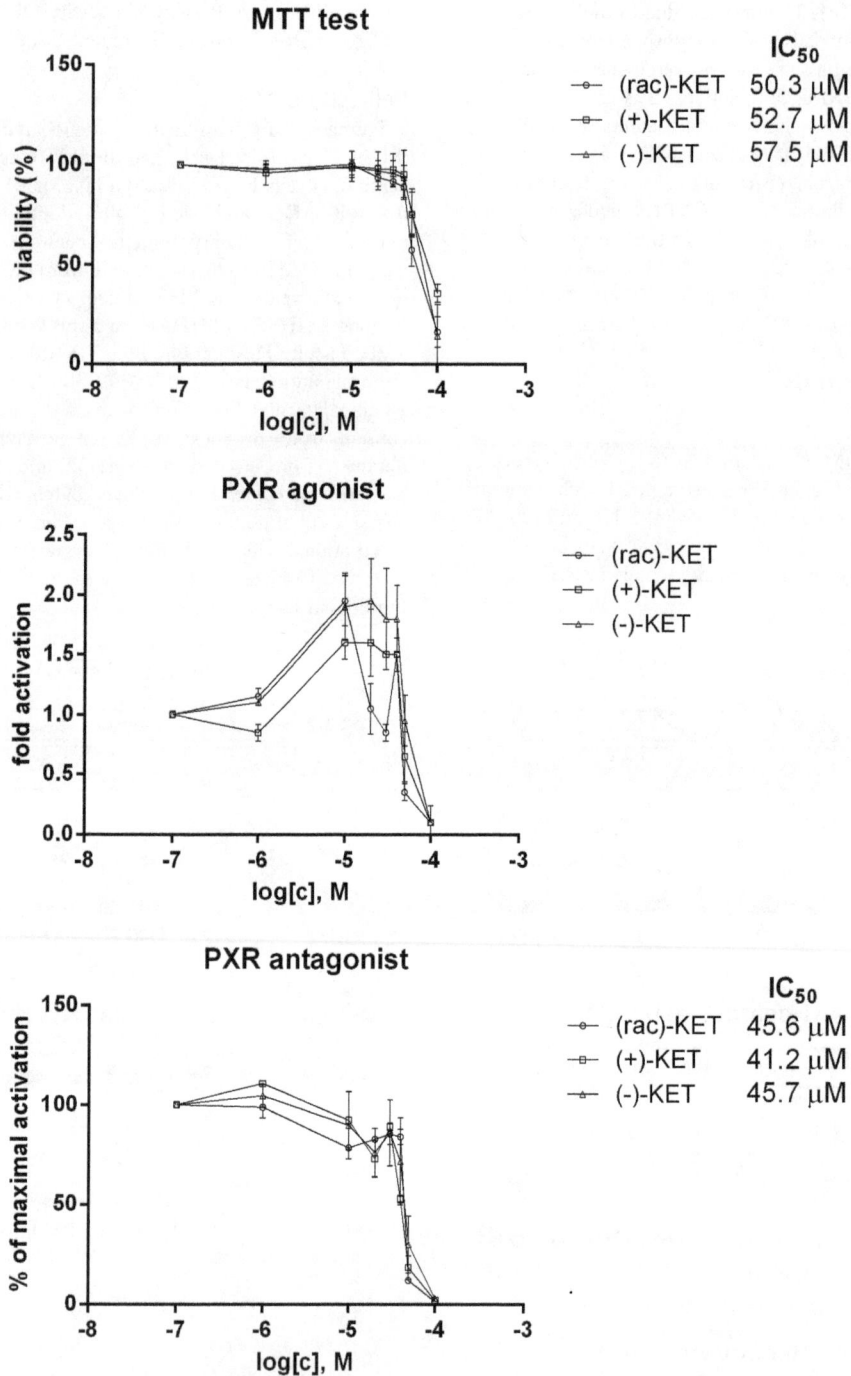

Figure 3. Effect of ketoconazole *cis*-enantiomers on transcriptional activity of pregnane X receptor PXR in transiently transfected LS174T cells. LS174T cells, transiently transfected with *p3A4-luc* reporter, were seeded in 24-well plates, stabilized for 16 h and then incubated for 24 h with (+)-KET, (−)-KET and rac-KET at concentrations ranging from 0.1 μM to 100 μM. The vehicle was DMSO (0.1% v/v). Model activator of PXR was rifampicin (RIF; 10 μM). Treatments were performed in triplicates. ***Upper panel:*** MTT test; The data are the mean from experiments from three consecutive passages of cells and are expressed as a percentage of viability of control cells. The values of IC_{50} were calculated and are indicated in a figure. ***Middle panel:*** *Agonist mode* - Transfected LS174T cells were incubated with KET in the absence of RIF (10 μM). The data are the mean from experiments from two consecutive passages of cells and are expressed as a fold induction of luciferase activity over control cells. ***Lower panel:*** *Antagonist mode* - Transfected LS174T cells were incubated with KET in the presence of RIF (10 μM). The data are the mean from experiments from two consecutive passages of cells and are expressed as a percentage of maximal induction attained by RIF. The values of IC_{50} were calculated and the average values are indicated in figures.

Table 1. Enzyme kinetics parameters for *in vitro* biotransformation two prototypic CYP3A4/5 substrates, testosterone and midazolam, with ketoconazole and two cis enantiomers, (+)-KET and (−)-KET, as inhibitors.

Ketoconazole (μM)	IC_{50} (μM)		K_i (μM)	
	TST	MDZ	TST	MDZ
(rac)-KET	0.84 ± 0.05	1.06 ± 0.18	0.27 ± 0.13	2.28 ± 1.70
(+)-KET	1.69 ± 0.27	1.46 ± 0.28	0.92 ± 0.47	2.52 ± 1.80
(−)-KET	0.90 ± 0.16	1.04 ± 0.11	0.17 ± 0.05	1.51 ± 0.99

TST, testosterone; MDZ, midazolam.

mRNA determination and quantitative reverse transcriptase polymerase chain reaction

Total RNA was isolated using TRI Reagent (Molecular Research Center, Cincinnati, OH, USA). cDNA was synthesized using M-MLV Reverse Transcriptase (Finnzymes, Espoo, Finland) in the presence of random hexamers (Takara, Shiga, Japan). qRT-PCR was carried out using LightCycler FastStart DNA Master-

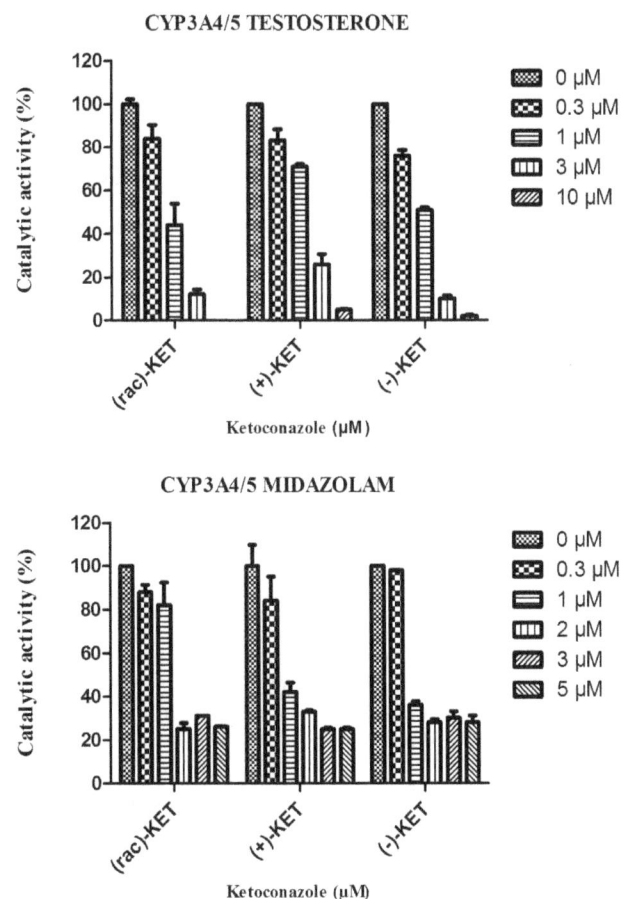

Figure 4. Effect of ketoconazole *cis*-enantiomers on catalytic activity of CYP3A4/5 in human liver microsomes. Inhibition of the CYP3A4/5 catalytic activity in assay with specific substrate testosterone (upper panel) and midazolam (lower panel) in human liver microsomes. Racemate, (+)-KET and (−)-KET were used in concentrations 0.3 μM, 1 μM, 2 μM, 3 μM, 5 μM and 10 μM. Inhibition of activity is determined as the mean ± SD and expressed in per cent as activity remaining relative to control (100%, without ketoconazole).

PLUS SYBR Green I (Roche Diagnostic Corporation, Prague, Czech Republic) on a Light Cycler 480 II apparatus (Roche Diagnostic Corporation). CYP3A4 and GAPDH mRNAs were determined as described previously [20]. Measurements were performed in triplicates. Gene expression was normalized to GAPDH as a housekeeping gene.

Protein detection and Western blotting

Total protein extracts were prepared as described elsewhere [21]. SDS-PAGE gels (10%) were run according to the general procedure followed by the protein transfer onto PVDF membrane. The membrane was saturated with 5% non-fat dried milk. Blots were probed with primary antibodies against CYP3A4 (mouse monoclonal; sc-53850, HL3) and actin (goat polyclonal; sc-1616, 1–19), both purchased from Santa Cruz Biotechnology (Santa Cruz, CA, USA). Chemiluminescent detection was performed using horseradish peroxidase-conjugated secondary antibodies (Santa Cruz Biotechnology) and Western blotting Luminol kit (Santa Cruz Biotechnology). The density of bands was measured by densitometry.

Gene reporter assay and cytotoxicity assay

A transiently transfected LS174T human colon adenocarcinoma cells were used for assessment of PXR transcriptional activity. A chimera *p3A4-luc* reporter construct containing the basal promoter (−362/+53) with proximal PXR response element and the distal xenobiotic responsive enhancer module (−7836/−7208) of the *CYP3A4* gene 5'-flanking region inserted to pGL3-Basic reporter vector was used. The reporter plasmid was transiently transfected to LS174T cells by lipofection (FuGENE 6). Cells were incubated for 24 h with tested compounds and/or vehicle (DMSO; 0.1% v/v), in the presence or absence of RIF (10 μM; LS174T cells). After the treatments, cells were lysed and luciferase activity was measured. In parallel, cell viability was determined by conventional MTT test [MTT = 3-(4,5-dimethylthiazol-2-yl)-2,5-diphenyltetrazolium bromide]; briefly: After the treatment, culture medium was replaced with fresh one and 100 μL of MTT reagent (5 mg/mL PBS) was added. Three hours later, the medium was removed, and cells were washed with PBS and lysed for 5 min with 1 mL of DMSO containing 1% ammonia. The lysate was diluted 20 times with DMSO (+1% ammonia) and absorbance at 540 nm was measured against blank (DMSO+1% ammonia) (TECAN, Schoeller Instruments LLC). Results were normalized to the control value (i.e. $100 \times A_{sample}/A_{control}$) and expressed as percentage of control.

Catalytic activity of CYP3A4 in human liver microsomes

Chemical reagents used for microsomal incubations and HPLC analysis were purchased from commercial sources. Testosterone

and 1′-hydroxymidazolam were obtained from Sigma-Aldrich CZ (Prague, Czech Republic) and 6β-hydroxytestosterone was purchased from Ultrafine (Manchester, UK). Midazolam was purchased from Abcam (Cambridge, UK).

Human liver microsomes were delivered from Xenotech (Lenexa, KS). Details of the CYP3A4/5 enzymatic activity of the mixture can be accessed from the Xenotech Web site (www.xenotechllc.com). The CYP3A4/5 activity was determined according to established protocols by using two specific substrates. Assays were based on testosterone 6β-hydroxylation and midazolam 1′-hydroxylation. Monitoring of formed metabolites from specific substrates was performed by HPLC using the Prominence system (Shimadzu, Kyoto, Japan) using reverse phase C-18 columns (LiChroCART or Chromolith-HighResolution from Merck, Darmstadt, Germany) and UV detection, according to [22]. The substrate concentrations were corresponding to the K_m values of measured enzymes. In the case of inhibition, K_i values were determined by additional measurements using extra substrate concentration (adequate to $1/2\ K_m$, K_m, $2\ K_m$ and $4\ K_m$). Assays were performed with eight concentrations (0.3; 1, 2, 3, 5 and 10 µM) of racemic ketoconazole and its (−)-KET and (+)-KET isomers plus ketoconazole-free controls. Incubations were performed in two independent experiments at 37°C. All reaction mixtures were buffered by 100 mM K/PO_4 (pH 7.4) and contained an NADPH generating system consisting of isocitrate dehydrogenase, $NADP^+$, isocitric acid and $MgSO_4$.

Inhibition of CYP3A4/5 catalytic activities by individual ketoconazole forms was evaluated by plotting the remaining activity against the inhibitor concentration using GraphPad Prism (La Jolla, CA). The values of IC_{50} were obtained using Sigma Plot 12 scientific graphing software (SPSS, Chicago, IL). Determination of K_i was performed in two steps: First, the type of inhibition was assessed from Dixon plot, then, a GraphPad Prism 6 software for mixed inhibition fitted to the data points by nonlinear regression based on Henri-Michaelis-Menten equation.

Statistics

Experiments in cell cultures were performed at least in three different cell passages. In each passage, treatments of cells were performed in triplicates. For measurement of luminescence (luciferase activity) and absorbance (MTT), triplicates from each sample were run. One-way analysis of variance followed by Dunnett's multiple comparison post hoc test or Student's t test were used for statistical analyses of data.

Results

Effects of ketoconazole *cis*-enantiomers on CYP3A4 mRNA and protein expression in HepG2 cells and human hepatocytes

We examined the effects of ketoconazole *cis*-enantiomers on the expression of CYP3A4 in two experimental *in vitro* systems, i.e. in human hepatoma cells HepG2 and in primary human hepatocytes. Cells were incubated for 24 h (mRNA expression) and 48 h (protein expression) with RIF (10 µM), vehicle (DMSO; 0.1% v/v) and ketoconazole ((+), (−), (rac); 1 µM, 30 µM, 50 µM). Rifampicin, a model activator of PXR and an inducer of CYP3A4 induced CYP3A4 mRNA in two of four passages of HepG2 cells by factor approx. 2-fold. All forms of ketoconazole ((+), (−), (rac)) induced CYP3A4 mRNA in HepG2 cells. The induction profiles slightly varied between four consecutive passages of HepG2 cells, and we observed either dose-dependent induction or a drop in CYP3A4 mRNA induction at 50 µM concentrations of KET, probably due to cytotoxicity issues. The effects of ketoconazole

were not enantiospecific. The fold inductions of CYP3A4 mRNA by ketoconazole were comparable with those by RIF, or higher (Figure 1; upper panel). Induction of CYP3A4 mRNA by rifampicin in human hepatocytes cultures HH52, HH54 and Hep220770 was 19-fold, 7-fold and 9-fold, respectively. Induction of CYP3A4 mRNA by ketoconazole in human hepatocytes was significant (p<0.05) for following samples: culture HH52 ((−)-KET 50 µM; (rac)-KET 30 µM); culture HH54 ((+)-KET 1 µM and 30 µM); culture Hep220770 ((+)-KET 30 µM; (rac)-KET 30 µM). The induction profiles of CYP3A4 mRNA in human hepatocytes by ketoconazole were not enantiospecific and the observed differences between cultures and enantiomers are rather due to the inter-individual variability (Figure 1; lower panel). We did not find convincing induction of CYP3A4 protein in HepG2 cells incubated for 48 h with ketoconazole. All forms of ketoconazole strongly and dose-dependently (with drop of CYP3A4 protein at 50 µM of KET in some samples) induced CYP3A4 protein in three human hepatocytes cultures, but the effects were not enantiospecific (Figure 2). Overall, ketoconazole induced CYP3A4 in HepG2 cells and human hepatocytes, but the effects were not enantiospecific.

Effects of ketoconazole *cis*-enantiomers on transcriptional activity of pregnane X receptor PXR in human LS174T gene reporter cell line

In next series of experiments, the effects of ketoconazole *cis*-enantiomers on transcriptional activity of PXR were assessed in human colon adenocarcinoma cells LS174T transiently transfected with *p3A4-luc* reporter construct. First, a cytotoxicity of tested compounds after 24 h of incubation was assessed by MTT test. We observed dose-dependent cytotoxicity of all ketoconazole forms tested, with IC_{50} values of 50.3 µM ((rac)-KET), 52.7 µM ((+)-KET) and 57.5 µM ((−)-KET). Cytotoxic effects of *cis*-enantiomers of ketoconazole were not enantiospecific (Figure 3; upper panel). In gene reporter assays, an induction of PXR-dependent luciferase activity by rifampicin varied from 20-fold to 27-fold, as compared to vehicle-treated cells. All forms of ketoconazole dose-dependently activated PXR, with maximal inductions approx. 2-fold, for 10 µM –20 µM concentrations of ketoconazole. The half-maximal effective concentrations (EC_{50}) were not calculated, because of decline in luciferase activity for concentration of ketoconazole 30 µM and higher, probably due to the intrinsic cytotoxicity (Figure 3; middle panel). In antagonist mode, all forms of ketoconazole dose-dependently inhibited the activation of PXR by rifampicin. The decrease of luciferase activity was in large part caused by cytotoxic effects of ketoconazole. However, antagonistic effects of ketoconazole towards PXR were demonstrated as well, because half-maximal inhibitory concentrations IC_{50} were significantly lower as compared to those from MTT test, i.e. 45.6 µM ((rac)-KET), 41.2 µM ((+)-KET) and 45.7 µM ((−)-KET) (Figure 3; lower panel).

Collectively, ketoconazole increased basal and inhibited ligand-activated PXR transcriptional activity, and its effects were not enantiospecific.

Effects of ketoconazole *cis*-enantiomers on catalytic activity of CYP3A in human liver microsomes

The catalytic activity of CYP3A enzymes (CYP3A4 and CYP3A5, with overlapping substrate specificity and prototypic substrates testosterone and midazolam [3] in human liver microsomes was determined to get a complete picture of the influence of ketoconazole on the properties of the CYP3A4/5 enzyme system. Both activities were reduced to values below 50%;

the highest inhibition was observed with substrate testosterone (inhibition down to 3% of the initial activity at the KET concentration of 10 μM, Figure 4). To determine the K_i values, experiments were repeated with 4 different concentrations of substrates (corresponding to $1/2$ K_m, 1 K_m, 2 K_m and 4 K_m). The K_i was obtained from a nonlinear regression based on mixed type of inhibition. The IC_{50} and K_i data for the inhibition of CYP3A4 by racemate, (+)-KET and (−)-KET using testosterone and midazolam as substrates are shown in the Table 1. According to the IC_{50} and K_i values and regardless of substrate, data indicate that effect of ketoconazole is enantiospecific. The (−)-KET exhibits in all cases higher inhibitory potential than the (+)-KET. According to the result of experiment with testosterone as substrate of CYP3A, the difference between particular enantiomers is approximately 5-fold. In the case of midazolam as a specific substrate of CYP3A, the (−)-KTZ was about 1.5-fold more potent inhibitor. According to IC_{50} and K_i, racemate usually acts similarly as (−)-KET. In this respect, the results presented here are similar to those obtained in the previous study showing the IC_{50} for inhibition of CYP3A/5-mediated testosterone and methadone metabolism by ketoconazole cis-enantiomers [15].

Discussion

Chiral pharmacology has advanced significantly during last two decades. FDA initial guidance on chiral drugs was released in 1992, as the differential actions and toxicities of enantiomers became more evident. Racemates have virtually disappeared from development of new molecular entities. Single enantiomer or achiral drugs now dominate newly approved drugs worldwide [14]. In addition, racemic drugs previously granted patents are expiring, so they become candidates for a "chiral switch", i.e. development of single enantiomer or paired enantiomers in case of diastereomers [23]. This permits additional years of market exclusivity, and pharmaceutical companies are sometimes suspected from "evergreening" the drugs. Ideally, therapeutic activity would reside in one enantiomer (eutomer) and adverse effects in the other (dystomer). However, there is a range of possibilities, and the combined actions of the individual enantiomers may actually make the racemate or enantiomer combinations even desirable [14].

In the current paper, we have studied the effects of ketoconazole cis-enantiomers on the expression and catalytic activity of CYP3A4 in human in vitro systems. Ketoconazole exists in the form of four enantiomers. The therapeutically used ketoconazole is a racemic mixture consisting of two cis-enantiomers; (2R,4S)-(+)-KET and (2S,4R)-(−)-KET. Since numerous ketoconazole-drug interactions were reported, it is certainly of value to investigate, whether one of the ketoconazole enantiomers exerts less interaction potential against CYP3A4 as compared to other enantiomer. We have recently examined antifungal activities of ketoconazole cis-enantiomers against 7 strains of Candida spp. and we demonstrated that (+)-KET is two times more potent than (−)-KET for strains C. albicans and C. tropicalis, while (−)-KET is seven times more potent than (+)-KET for other five tested strains [12], which was in line with observations of other authors [24]. These data imply enantiospecific pattern of clinical (desirable) activities of ketoconazole. We have also observed enantiospecific effect of ketoconazole on AhR-CYP1A signaling pathway, the

activation of which may be considered as undesired effect of ketoconazole [12]. On the other hand, antagonistic effects of ketoconazole against glucocorticoid receptor GR were not enantiospecific [12]. In the present paper we show that ketoconazole partial agonist activity against pregnane X receptor PXR (Figure 3), as well as ketoconazole-mediated induction of CYP3A4 (Figure 1, Figure 2) are not enantiospecific, i.e. both cis-enantiomers ((+), (−)) were equipotent.

As the aim of this paper was to examine the possible enantiospecific differences in the interactions of the KET cis-enantiomers with the CYP3A enzyme system, we studied also the possible changes in the inhibition of CYP3A enzyme in human liver microsomes by these compounds. Ketoconazole is generally considered as CYP3A4/5 -specific inhibitor [25]. According to our results, as well as by data from the literature [15,16], both the (+)-KET and (−)-KET exhibit distinct, moderate differences in the values of the IC_{50} parameters characterizing the testosterone, alprazolam, quinidine and midazolam metabolism with the (−)-KET being more potent. Here, for prediction of the drug-drug interaction mediated by (−)- KET and (+)-KET by CYP3A in more detail, the K_i values of cis-enantiomers were estimated for the first time. On the other hand, there are several studies discussing inhibition of CYP3A by racemic ketoconazole; the extent of inhibition is usually expressed both as the IC_{50} and K_i. It is however known that the inhibitory potency of ketoconazole is highly variable (K_i values may range, for different CYP3A substrates, from 0.001 to 25 μM) [3]. In this study, we have found the K_i for racemic KET 0.27 μM for testosterone 6β-hydroxylation and 2.28 μM for midazolam 1'-hydroxylation, which fits into this range. In general, the differences may be caused by various factors. The most important factor is apparently an incorrect assignment of inhibition mechanism. According to our data analysis, the mixed model of inhibition mechanism was used which was found also by another study [25]. For the (−)-KET, 5-fold stronger inhibitory potency in testosterone metabolism and 1.5-fold in case of midazolam was found. Racemate acted similarly as the (−)-KET, being, in other words, more potent inhibitor of CYP3A4/5 than the (+)-KET. Hence, for the ability to inhibit the CYP3A enzymes, the (−)-KET enantiomer is more responsible. Interestingly, as it has been shown in our previous paper (discussed above), antifungal activity of cis-enantiomers on several strains was determined with a result describing enantiospecificity of the biological effect of this drug [12]. The (−)-KET seems to be more potent inhibitor of CYP51 in most fungi. In conclusion, the enzyme activity data presented in this paper, support enantiospecific clinical pattern of ketoconazole effect.

In conclusion, we show that ketoconazole inhibits enantiospecifically CYP3A4/5 catalytic activity, while its effects of CYP3A4 expression and PXR activity are not enantiospecific. Regarding PXR-CYP3A4 signaling and metabolic cascade, the potential enantiopure preparations of ketoconazole in human pharmacotherapy are not of interest.

Author Contributions

Conceived and designed the experiments: AN ZD PA KK. Performed the experiments: AN KK IB MK. Analyzed the data: AN KK PA ZD PB. Contributed reagents/materials/analysis tools: PA ZD PB. Contributed to the writing of the manuscript: ZD PA.

References

1. Heeres J, Meerpoel L, Lewi P (2010) Conazoles. Molecules 15: 4129–4188.
2. Gubbins PO, Heldenbrand S (2010) Clinically relevant drug interactions of current antifungal agents. Mycoses 53: 95–113.
3. Greenblatt DJ, Venkatakrishnan K, Harmatz JS, Parent SJ, von Moltke LL (2010) Sources of variability in ketoconazole inhibition of human cytochrome P450 3A in vitro. Xenobiotica 40: 713–720.

4. Dvorak Z (2011) Drug-drug interactions by azole antifungals: Beyond a dogma of CYP3A4 enzyme activity inhibition. Toxicol Lett 202: 129–132.

5. Svecova L, Vrzal R, Burysek L, Anzenbacherova E, Cerveny L, et al. (2008) Azole antimycotics differentially affect rifampicin-induced pregnane X receptor-mediated CYP3A4 gene expression. Drug Metab Dispos 36: 339–348.

6. Huang H, Wang H, Sinz M, Zoeckler M, Staudinger J, et al. (2007) Inhibition of drug metabolism by blocking the activation of nuclear receptors by ketoconazole. Oncogene 26: 258–268.

7. Lim YP, Kuo SC, Lai ML, Huang JD (2009) Inhibition of CYP3A4 expression by ketoconazole is mediated by the disruption of pregnane X receptor, steroid receptor coactivator-1, and hepatocyte nuclear factor 4alpha interaction. Pharmacogenet Genomics 19: 11–24.

8. Wang H, Huang H, Li H, Teotico DG, Sinz M, et al. (2007) Activated pregnenolone X-receptor is a target for ketoconazole and its analogs. Clin Cancer Res 13: 2488–2495.

9. Venkatesh M, Wang H, Cayer J, Leroux M, Salvail D, et al. (2011) In vivo and in vitro characterization of a first-in-class novel azole analog that targets pregnane X receptor activation. Mol Pharmacol 80: 124–135.

10. Li H, Redinbo MR, Venkatesh M, Ekins S, Chaudhry A, et al. (2013) Novel yeast-based strategy unveils antagonist binding regions on the nuclear xenobiotic receptor PXR. J Biol Chem 288: 13655–13668.

11. Duret C, Daujat-Chavanieu M, Pascussi JM, Pichard-Garcia L, Balaguer P, et al. (2006) Ketoconazole and miconazole are antagonists of the human glucocorticoid receptor: consequences on the expression and function of the constitutive androstane receptor and the pregnane X receptor. Mol Pharmacol 70: 329–339.

12. Novotna A, Korhonova M, Bartonkova I, Soshilov AA, Denison MS, et al. (2014) Enantiospecific Effects of Ketoconazole on Aryl Hydrocarbon Receptor. PLoS One 9: e101832.

13. Korashy HM, Shayeganpour A, Brocks DR, El-Kadi AO (2007) Induction of cytochrome P450 1A1 by ketoconazole and itraconazole but not fluconazole in murine and human hepatoma cell lines. Toxicol Sci 97: 32–43.

14. Smith SW (2009) Chiral toxicology: it's the same thing…only different. Toxicol Sci 110: 4–30.

15. Dilmaghanian S, Gerber JG, Filler SG, Sanchez A, Gal J (2004) Enantioselectivity of inhibition of cytochrome P450 3A4 (CYP3A4) by ketoconazole: Testosterone and methadone as substrates. Chirality 16: 79–85.

16. Allqvist A, Miura J, Bertilsson L, Mirghani RA (2007) Inhibition of CYP3A4 and CYP3A5 catalyzed metabolism of alprazolam and quinine by ketoconazole as racemate and four different enantiomers. Eur J Clin Pharmacol 63: 173–179.

17. Stresser DM, Blanchard AP, Turner SD, Erve JC, Dandeneau AA, et al. (2000) Substrate-dependent modulation of CYP3A4 catalytic activity: analysis of 27 test compounds with four fluorometric substrates. Drug Metab Dispos 28: 1440–1448.

18. Schwartz SL, Rendell M, Ahmann AJ, Thomas A, Arauz-Pacheco CJ, et al. (2008) Safety profile and metabolic effects of 14 days of treatment with DIO-902: results of a phase IIa multicenter, randomized, double-blind, placebo-controlled, parallel-group trial in patients with type 2 diabetes mellitus. Clin Ther 30: 1081–1088.

19. Arakaki R, Welles B (2010) Ketoconazole enantiomer for the treatment of diabetes mellitus. Expert Opin Investig Drugs 19: 185–194.

20. Vrzal R, Knoppova B, Bachleda P, Dvorak Z (2013) Effects of oral anorexiant sibutramine on the expression of cytochromes P450s in human hepatocytes and cancer cell lines. J Biochem Mol Toxicol 27: 515–521.

21. Novotna A, Srovnalova A, Svecarova M, Korhonova M, Bartonkova I, et al. (2014) Differential effects of omeprazole and lansoprazole enantiomers on aryl hydrocarbon receptor in human hepatocytes and cell lines. PLoS One 9: e98711.

22. Phillips IR Shephard EA, editors (2006) Cytochrome P450 Protocols. 2nd ed. Totowa: Humana Press.

23. Caner H, Groner E, Levy L, Agranat I (2004) Trends in the development of chiral drugs. Drug Discov Today 9: 105–110.

24. Rotstein DM, Kertesz DJ, Walker KA, Swinney DC (1992) Stereoisomers of ketoconazole: preparation and biological activity. J Med Chem 35: 2818–2825.

25. Greenblatt DJ, Zhao Y, Venkatakrishnan K, Duan SX, Harmatz JS, et al. (2011) Mechanism of cytochrome P450-3A inhibition by ketoconazole. J Pharm Pharmacol 63: 214–221.

22

Methadone Induction in Primary Care for Opioid Dependence: A Pragmatic Randomized Trial (ANRS Methaville)

Patrizia Maria Carrieri[1,2,3]*, **Laurent Michel**[4,5,6], **Caroline Lions**[1,2,3], **Julien Cohen**[1,2,3], **Muriel Vray**[7,8], **Marion Mora**[1,2,3], **Fabienne Marcellin**[1,2,3], **Bruno Spire**[1,2,3], **Alain Morel**[9], **Perrine Roux**[1,2,3] **and the Methaville Study Group**¶

1 INSERM UMR912 (SESSTIM), Marseille, France, **2** Aix Marseille Université, UMR_S912, Marseille, France, **3** ORS PACA, Observatoire Régional de la Santé Provence Alpes Côte d'Azur, Marseille, France, **4** INSERM, Research Unit 669, Paris, France, **5** Univ Paris-Sud and Univ Paris Descartes, UMR-S0669, Paris, France, **6** Centre Pierre Nicole, Paris, France, **7** Unité de Recherche et d'Expertise en Epidémiologie des Maladies Emergentes, Institut Pasteur, Paris, France, **8** Institut National de la Santé et de la Recherche Médicale (INSERM), Paris, France, **9** Oppelia, Paris, France

Abstract

Objective: Methadone coverage is poor in many countries due in part to methadone induction being possible only in specialized care (SC). This multicenter pragmatic trial compared the effectiveness of methadone treatment between two induction models: primary care (PC) and SC.

Methods: In this study, registered at ClinicalTrials.Gov (NCT00657397), opioid-dependent individuals not on methadone treatment for at least one month or receiving buprenorphine but needing to switch were randomly assigned to start methadone in PC (N = 155) or in SC (N = 66) in 10 sites in France. Visits were scheduled at months M0, M3, M6 and M12. The primary outcome was self-reported abstinence from street-opioids at 12 months (M12) (with an underlying 15% non-inferiority hypothesis for PC). Secondary outcomes were abstinence during follow-up, engagement in treatment (i.e. completing the induction period), retention and satisfaction with the explanations provided by the physician. Primary analysis used intention to treat (ITT). Mixed models and the log-rank test were used to assess the arm effect (PC vs. SC) on the course of abstinence and retention, respectively.

Results: In the ITT analysis (n = 155 in PC, 66 in SC), which compared the proportions of street-opioid abstinent participants, 85/155 (55%) and 22/66 (33%) of the participants were classified as street-opioid abstinent at M12 in PC and SC, respectively. This ITT analysis showed the non-inferiority of PC (21.5 [7.7; 35.3]). Engagement in treatment and satisfaction with the explanations provided by the physician were significantly higher in PC than SC. Retention in methadone and abstinence during follow-up were comparable in both arms (p = 0.47, p = 0.39, respectively).

Conclusions: Under appropriate conditions, methadone induction in primary care is feasible and acceptable to both physicians and patients. It is as effective as induction in specialized care in reducing street-opioid use and ensuring engagement and retention in treatment for opioid dependence.

Trial registration: Number Eudract 2008-001338-28; ClinicalTrials.gov: NCT00657397; International Standard Randomized Controlled Trial Number Register ISRCTN31125511

Editor: John E. Mendelson, California Pacific Medical Center Research Institute, United States of America

Funding: The study received external funding by the French National Agency for Research on Aids and Viral Hepatitis (ANRS) and the French Ministry of Health. The funders had no role in study design, data collection and analysis, decision to publish, or preparation of the manuscript.

Competing Interests: The authors have declared that no competing interests exist.

* Email: pmcarrieri@aol.com

¶ Membership of the Methaville Study Group is provided in the Acknowledgments.

Introduction

Methadone is included in the WHO list of essential medicines thanks to its effectiveness in treating opioid dependence, preventing HIV [1] and improving adherence to antiretroviral treatment in HIV-infected individuals [2]. Despite this, access to methadone remains limited because of the risk of overdose during induction, especially in countries where the need for methadone is even greater.

While access to buprenorphine in primary care has been possible since 1996 thanks to its safety profile [3,4], methadone induction in France, as in most countries, is currently possible only in specialized centers caring for substance dependence (located in *ad hoc* sites or in hospitals) (hereafter specialized care or SC). In France these centers can refer patients to PC only after the end of methadone induction, i.e. when methadone doses are stabilized (after at least 14 days).

The specific model of care for regulating methadone induction can greatly influence its safety as the risk of overdose during the induction phase remains a major concern. Internationally, the regulations governing the extent to which methadone induction (i.e. until dosage stabilization) is authorized in primary care (PC) differ considerably. For example, methadone induction in PC is legal in the UK, in Switzerland and in Canada under different models of care. In contrast, France, the United States but also other countries have no such system currently in place.

This means that in the many geographic areas underserved by SC, opioid-dependent individuals seeking treatment have no access to methadone. To tackle this situation, one of the objectives of the French public health authorities' national strategic plan for prevention and care of Hepatitis was to consider using primary care as an entry point for methadone treatment, based on the results of a pragmatic trial. The trial, entitled Methaville, was designed both to evaluate the feasibility of methadone induction in PC and to compare outcomes in participants randomized into PC induction with those randomized into SC induction. Being a pragmatic trial, the objectives were to verify the feasibility and acceptability of the PC induction model to physicians and patients, and also to show that the main patient outcome (street-opioid abstinence after one year of treatment) and secondary outcomes (abstinence during follow-up, engagement in treatment, retention in treatment and satisfaction with the explanations provided by the physician) were all comparable between both induction arms.

Methods

The protocol for this trial and supporting CONSORT checklist are available as Checklist S1 and English protocol S1.

Ethics

The Methaville ANRS trial is registered with the French Agency of Pharmaceutical Products (AFSSAPS) under the number 2008-A0277-48, the European Union Drug Regulating Authorities Clinical Trials: Number Eudract 2008-001338-28, the ClinicalTrials.gov Identifier: NCT00657397 and the International Standard Randomized Controlled Trial Number Register ISRCTN31125511. The study protocol was approved by the Ethics Committee of Persons Protection in Paris, France. All individuals provided written, informed consent before participating in the study.

Physicians and Participants

In this multicenter, pragmatic, randomized trial, for each study site we selected an SC physician and nearby PC physicians who already had field experience in care for opioid dependence and/or training in care for drug dependence, and who were willing to participate. Only PC physicians with patients potentially eligible for enrollment in the study were selected because if methadone induction in PC is officially adopted in France in the future, only PC physicians meeting the above criteria will be targeted by authorities as methadone prescribers. Ten sites in four geographic areas (North, North-Eastern, South-Western and South-Eastern France) were included, with each site having at least one SC and

one PC physician. These four geographical areas were chosen to better target the different types of populations who would benefit from access to methadone in primary care, as each geographical area is characterized by different drug markets and drug user practices/needs. Physicians (in PC and SC) enrolled opioid-dependent individuals who were randomized to start methadone either in PC or in SC.

Inclusion criteria were chosen to target a population representative of drug users needing/seeking methadone treatment in France as follows: aged over 18 years old, seeking care for opioid dependence and not prescribed methadone for at least one month or receiving buprenorphine but needing to switch to methadone for medical reasons (side effects, treatment misuse, etc.). Non-inclusion criteria were similar to those in other studies involving methadone prescription in PC [5,6] as follows: could not be reached by phone for an interview and screening positive for opioids/benzodiazepines/alcohol triple co-dependence, as assessed by the MINI [7] (as this condition exposed participants to a high risk of overdose [8,9]) and finally, for women, being pregnant.

Study design

The first visit took place when a patient seeking care for opioid dependence or needing to switch treatment from buprenorphine to methadone went to see a PC or SC physician participating in the trial. After providing consent to participate the patient was randomized into the PC or SC arm by this physician. To make patient randomization feasible, each site had one SC with at least one PC physician in the nearby vicinity. All PC and SC physicians involved underwent a one-day training course both to standardize methadone induction practices according to trial guidelines and to acquaint them with trial procedures [10]. Trial guidelines stipulated that the starting dose should be on average 30 mg and not exceed 40 mg, with 10 mg increases every 2–4 days thereafter until dose stabilization. This is comparable to methadone induction protocols used in other trials [5,11].

The "intervention" provided by trained physicians consisted in at least fourteen-day supervised methadone induction either in PC or in SC according to trial guidelines (Table 1). Thereafter, supervision was required only for patients who were deemed to be at risk of overdose. One main difference between both arms in the model of care was that delays in initiating treatment were more common in SC (see Table 1).

Participants were also followed up over one year through medical visits and phone interviews at months 0 (M0, enrolment), at 3, 6 and 12 months (M3, M6 and M12, respectively).

To emulate current care practices in France, patients could choose to change arm after the induction phase, i.e. SC physicians could refer their patient to a PC colleague who would prescribe methadone and vice versa. Accordingly, arm changes (PC to SC or SC to PC) were not considered as deviations from the protocol. Further details and the pre-trial phase of the protocol are described elsewhere [10].

Data sources and outcomes

The following 5 sources provided study data: a pre-enrollment medical questionnaire, a medical questionnaire at each scheduled visit (enrolment (M0), months 3, 6 and 12, respectively M3, M6 and M12), a short self-administered questionnaire (completed during scheduled visits), a Computer Assisted Telephone Interview (CATI) (conducted just after each scheduled visit) lasting no more than 30 minutes, and when available, urine rapid tests [10].

Abstinence from street-opioids at M12 was chosen as the primary outcome. Abstinence during the course of treatment, engagement in treatment, retention in methadone maintenance

Table 1. Features of the PC and SC model of care for methadone treatment (ANRS Methaville trial).

Methaville model for Primary Care (PC)	Current Methadone model for specialized care (SC)
• During induction, methadone intake is delivered and supervised daily at the pharmacy (with take home doses only for the weekend). Supervision is compulsory during induction.	• During induction, methadone is delivered daily at the center by the physician, the pharmacist or the nurse or is delivered at the pharmacy (with take home doses only for the weekend). Supervision is compulsory during induction.
• Psychosocial and health status assessment is not a necessary condition to start methadone – referral to specialized center if needed.	• It is recommended that Methadone induction is started after initial visits/interviews carried out by different members of health staff:
	a) A social counselor and/or a psychologist to obtain a psychosocial assessment of the patient;
	b) A physician or a nurse to obtain an assessment of the general health of the patient;
	c) An assessment of his/her social rights (health insurance, accommodation, resources, and previous access to care for drug dependence).
• Referral to psychosocial counseling in SC during methadone treatment if needed.	• Psychosocial counseling provided during methadone treatment.
• Methadone prescription possible the same day as the first medical visit.	• Time before methadone prescription may be delayed by some days after the first medical visit, depending on patient's conditions (withdrawal syndromes, pregnancy, etc.).
• Doses are prescribed according to Methaville guidelines.	• Doses are prescribed according to Methaville guidelines.
• Doses are reassessed at every medical visit (i.e. every 2–3 days) during induction.	• Doses are reassessed at every medical visit (i.e. every 2–3 days) during induction.
• Urine analyses at first dose prescription and monitoring once/twice a week during induction.	• Urine analyses at first dose prescription and monitoring once/twice a week during induction.

treatment and patient satisfaction with the explanations provided by the physician were secondary outcomes. The primary outcome, abstinence from street opioids during the previous month, was measured using a validated question [12], administered during phone interviews by trained non-judgmental staff. This question was also answered in the medical interviews at enrolment, M3, M6 and M12.

Methadone dose was defined as the number of mg/day of methadone prescribed by the physician for each patient at each medical visit.

Engagement in treatment was computed in those randomized to each specific arm as the proportion of patients who actually started methadone and remained in the trial until the stabilization of dosages (i.e. until the end of induction). Follow-up participation rates, i.e. participants who continued participating in study interviews until M12, were computed for each arm.

Retention in methadone maintenance treatment was defined, only for patients who actually started methadone treatment, as the time between the first day of methadone induction and the last known date that the patient was still receiving treatment. For individuals still on methadone at M12, retention was set at 12 months.

A 5-point Likert scale measured patient satisfaction with the explanations provided by his/her prescribing physician during CATI at M6 only. This outcome was then dichotomized (very satisfied vs. other).

There were three main reasons to justify the choice to use patient self-reported street-opioid use as the primary outcome. The first reason was to avoid introducing measures which would not reflect routine practices in the field of care for drug dependence in France (for example neither urine tests nor hair analysis are routinely performed). These alternative measures would have been negatively affected by several missing values. Furthermore, any cases with complete values would most likely have been biased, as urine testing is currently performed at the discretion of the physician if he/she is doubtful about patients' drug use. The second one was to place the patient at the center of

the study and consider his/her self-reported experience with treatment (satisfaction with the explanations provided by the physician) as a major outcome. This choice reflects the work in other trials involving drug users and in other fields of medicine where patient's reported outcomes are considered as main outcome measures [13,14]. Third, patient self-reports are valid as PC physicians rely on them in clinical practice [15].

We chose the endpoint at M12 for the trial phase on the basis that any comparison between arms would not be significant enough immediately after the induction phase or indeed at M3, and that any possible benefit could be confirmed after one year of treatment.

The outcomes used in this pragmatic trial were those typically used in trials assessing the efficacy of a treatment for opioid dependence [5,6]. The only difference here is that they were used to assess methadone effectiveness (and not efficacy) by induction arm.

Safety issues

To ensure safety during induction, we implemented a wide range of strategies minimizing overdose risk in the trial's model of care, including a one-day training session for PC physicians, strict supervision of participants when they took their doses at the pharmacy during treatment initiation, and fostering strong collaboration between all the health professionals involved in the study, including pharmacists (shared-care model) [16]. The non-inclusion of patients with triple co-dependence (alcohol-opioid-benzodiazepine) [8,9] does not constitute a restrictive criterion and reflects standard practice for safety concerns. Methadone initiation in these patients is possible only after benzodiazepine detoxification.

Pharmacists and physicians involved in the trial had to signal overdoses, signs of intoxication and lost-to-follow-up patients to the center of methodology and management (CMM) (ORS PACA- INSERM-IRD UMR912). The latter was required to notify any severe adverse event, such as an overdose, to the French

National Agency for Research on Aids and Viral Hepatitis (ANRS) which in turn notified the French Agency of Pharmaceutical Products (ANSM).

A list of 50 health-related symptoms included in the questionnaire helped document self-reported symptoms during follow-up.

Statistical considerations

Sample size. Although retention in treatment is the most important outcome in patients receiving treatment for opioid dependence [17] and even more important in the context of decision-making by public health authorities, this trial was funded for HCV prevention purposes with opioid abstinence being considered the most pertinent primary outcome. It was therefore designed with an underlying hypothesis of non-inferiority in terms of the proportion of PC-inducted patients who were abstinent from street-opioids at 12 months (M12) of methadone treatment with respect to their SC counterparts.

The study hypothesis was that after one year of treatment, the proportion of patients abstinent from street-opioids would be 70% [18,19] for SC. Selecting an inferiority margin of 15 for patients starting methadone in PC entailed recruiting a minimum of 150 patients in order to show the non-inferiority, if any, of the PC arm for the primary outcome.

The choice of this margin reflected our willingness to accept decreased effectiveness in PC in return for increased attractiveness and engagement in PC treatment.

Randomization and masking. Randomization of patients was performed centrally by the study's methodology and data management center (ORS PACA- INSERM-IRD UMR912), via a secured intranet site, by simple random sampling with no block control on randomization rate. Information about patient randomization was confidentially stored and hidden from the study research team - except statisticians and the data manager - until the end of the last M12 interview, in December 2011. A randomization ratio 2:1 (PC: SC) was chosen to deliberately over-represent patients followed-up in PC to increase the probability of detecting possible intoxications in PC during induction.

Statistical analysis. Medians and interquartile ranges (IQR) and proportions were used to describe the distributions of continuous and categorical variables, respectively. Distributions of variables among the two groups were compared using Mann-Whitney U test for continuous variables, Chi-Squared or Fisher exact test for categorical variables.

The primary analysis used intention-to-treat (ITT) (n = 221) and the primary outcome was measured using a validated question [12] about opioid use during the previous month collected by CATI or medical interview (when CATI data was incomplete). The difference between both arms in the proportion of patients reporting abstinence from street-opioids during the previous month at M12 and the related 95% confidence interval (95% CI) were computed. In this ITT analysis all patients who discontinued follow-up before M12 for any reason (i.e. refused to start methadone after randomization or discontinued follow-up for any reason including treatment interruption, lost to follow-up, incarceration etc.) were classified as "failure" i.e. street-opioid users (see Fig. 1).

A "*per protocol*" analysis was also conducted only on individuals still followed-up at month 12 (n = 162).

Participants still followed up at M12 but with missing values for OTI (Opiate Treatment Index) at M12 were also classified as street-opioid users in both the ITT and *per protocol* analysis. The ITT classification for those who discontinued follow-up for any reason and for those with missing data is particularly pertinent in

this population of opioid-dependent individuals because discontinuation is generally associated with relapse into street-opioid use.

Logistic mixed models assessed the effects of time on methadone and of each arm on the course of abstinence from street-opioids, and took into account whether patients were switching from buprenorphine to methadone at enrolment. Mixed models are currently considered the most appropriate methods to use in clinical trials with missing outcomes, as they meet intention-to-treat criteria [20]. A log-rank test was used to compare Kaplan-Meier curves for retention in treatment among patients who were engaged in treatment, i.e. completed the induction phase (n = 188). SAS (v.9.2) and STATA (v.12) statistical software packages were used for the statistical analyses.

Results

Sites and physicians included in the study

Of 12 sites contacted in France, two refused to participate for organizational reasons. The 10 participating sites each included a SC and between 1 to 3 PC physicians in the nearby vicinity. Among the 57 physicians (SC & PC) who agreed to participate, 32 (56%) enrolled at least one patient who met the inclusion criteria. These 32 physicians were significantly different from the other 25 in that they were significantly older (p = 0.02) and had more years of medical experience (p = 0.002).

Baseline data

The patients included were mainly men (84%), median [IQR] age was 32 [27–38] years and 51% were switching from buprenorphine. Table 2 reports the main patient characteristics for each induction arm.

Patient disposition

From January 2009 to December 2010, the 32 physicians in the 10 trial sites enrolled 221 eligible individuals who were to be followed up for 12 months. The flow of participants through each stage is reported in Figure 1. All participants approached agreed to participate in the trial before randomization. One pregnant woman was excluded.

Among the 221 eligible patients, 66 and 155 were randomly assigned to start methadone in SC and in PC, respectively. However, 18 (27%) and 8 (5%) subsequently refused to be inducted in SC and in PC (p<0.001), respectively. These 26 patients were classified as "failure" in the ITT analysis.

Of the 185 who started treatment, 5 SC and 2 PC patients dropped out (discontinued study visits) during induction (p = 0.026) (Figure 2) and were also classified as "failure" in the ITT analysis. Ten SC and 16 PC patients discontinued follow-up after induction (p = 0.13). They too were classified as "failure" in the ITT analysis.

Overall, 15 (31%) of the 48 SC-inducted patients and 18 (12%) of the 147 PC-inducted patients (p = 0.0023) discontinued follow-up. Reasons for discontinuation are reported in Figure 1.

Finally, 33 SC-inducted and 129 PC-inducted patients were present at M12 for the *per protocol* analysis. Data on the primary outcome was missing for four of these individuals (2 in SC and 2 in PC) who were therefore considered opioid users (i.e. "failure") in the ITT and *per protocol* analyses.

Participants who were switching from buprenorphine were older, more likely male, and, most importantly, had a higher abstinence rate from street-opioids (38% vs. 12.5%) and cocaine (78.5% vs. 68%) at baseline, than those who were out of opioid maintenance treatment. However, as these differences were similar

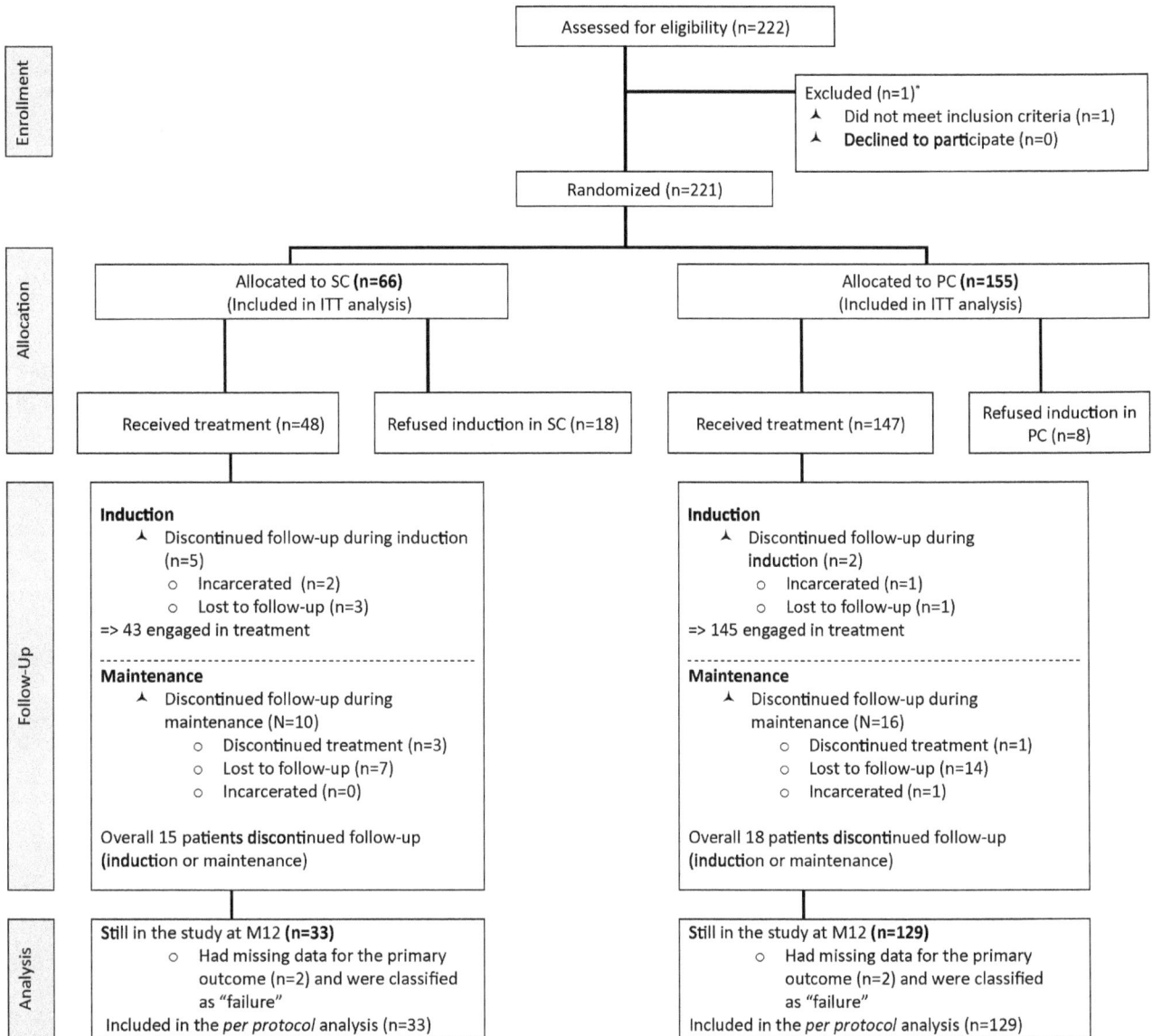

Figure 1. Flow chart of ANRS Methaville trial.

in both induction arms their compatibility in terms of the primary outcome remains unaffected.

Among the 48 SC patients, 18 (14 before M3 and 4 others before M6) changed to PC after induction, while one PC patient changed to SC. Nine patients were re-inducted during the study period after methadone interruption, two of these being re-inducted twice.

Sixty percent of the participants were prescribed methadone doses of between 60 and 80 mg between 11 and 17 days after initiation.

HIV and HCV self-reported prevalence rates were 2% and 19%, respectively.

The end of the study was set for the 1st January 2012 to allow one full year of follow-up for patients enrolled in December 2010.

Outcomes

Primary outcome was street opioid abstinence at 12 months and secondary outcomes: abstinence during follow-up, engagement in

treatment, retention in treatment and satisfaction with the explanations provided by the physician.

The rates of participants included in the study and still in treatment at M12 were $129/155 = 83\%$ for PC, $33/66 = 50\%$ for SC and $162/221 = 73\%$ for total sample.

The ITT and *per protocol* analyses reporting the difference in the proportions of street-opioid abstinent participants are described in Table 3. In the former (n = 155 in PC, 66 in SC), 85/155 (55%) and 22/66 (33%) were classified as street-opioid abstinent at M12 in PC and SC, respectively. The ITT analysis demonstrated the non-inferiority of the PC arm: the difference between the percentages of patients abstinent from street-opioids between both arms at M12 and the 95% CI was 21.5 [7.7; 35.3] in favor of PC. Although a *per protocol* analysis is not generally considered suitable in a pragmatic trial [15], it was computed for the sake of performing a comprehensive analysis. As expected, it provided inconclusive results, as the difference between the

Table 2. Patient characteristics by induction arm (SC and PC) at baseline (ANRS Methaville trial).

	SC (n = 48) % or median [IQR]	PC (n = 147) (%) or median [IQR]	Total % or median [IQR]
Gender	21	14	16
Male	79	86	84
Female	21	14	16
Age - *years*	30 [27–39]	32 [27–38]	32 [27–38]
Employment	44	53	51
High school certificate	43	32	35
Living in a couple	33	31	32
Children	33	39	38
Home owner or renter	56	64	62
Living area			
Urban	59	52	54
Suburban	13	26	23
Rural	28	22	23
Switching from buprenorphine	52	51	51
Age at first drug use - *years* (n = 176)	18 [17–21]	18 [17–22]	18 [17–21]
Age at first regular drug use - *years* (n = 160)	20 [18–24]	20 [18–25]	20 [18–24]
History of drug injection (n = 175)	55	47	49
Age at first drug injection (n = 86) – years	22 [20–25]	21 [19–26]	22 [19–26]
Drug injection (n = 162)*	21	14	15
Drug snorting (n = 162)*	74	61	64
Use of street opioids (n = 187)*	79	69	72
Cocaine use (n = 162)*	26	27	27
Use of psychotropic drugs (n = 162)*	13	23	20
Daily cannabis use (n = 176)*	20	17	18
Hazardous alcohol consumption (n = 172)**	33	32	33
Depressive symptoms (n = 170)***	32	41	39
History of suicide attempts (n = 157)	10	18	17
History of drug overdose (n = 188)	12	12	12
HIV+ (n = 152)****	3	2	2
HCV+ (n = 140) ****	18	19	19

*during the previous 4 weeks.
**AUDIT score ≥7 for males and ≥6 for females.
***CES-D score>17 for males and>23 for females.
****among those who had already done a test.

proportions and the non-inferiority margins was −0.8 [−18.8; 17.3], including the inferiority margin of −15.

Mixed models found no significant arm effect (p = 0.39) on abstinence during follow-up, even when adjusting for the switch from buprenorphine treatment. Abstinence from street-opioids significantly increased between enrolment and M3 and remained stable thereafter (Table 4). These results remained valid even after adjusting for a possible heterogeneity effect among sites (i.e. study sites with more than one PC physician versus sites with only one) which was tested as a random effect factor in the mixed models but which was not found to be statistically significant.

Engagement in treatment among those who were randomized only concerned patients who completed the methadone induction phase, i.e. 65% (43/66*100) for SC and 94% (145/155*100) for PC, p<0.001 (Fig. 1)).

When we computed "retention in treatment" we only focused on patients who had in fact started methadone treatment (i.e. 48 in SC and 147 in PC). At M12, thirty-three (33/48*100 = 69%) patients inducted in SC and 129 (129/147*100 = 88%) inducted in PC were still in treatment.

The Kaplan-Meier curves in Fig. 2 show that retention in methadone maintenance treatment was comparable between both induction arms.

Interestingly, PC-inducted patients reported high satisfaction with the explanations provided by their physician more often than their SC-inducted counterparts (p = 0.01).

Prescribed methadone dose during the study

Regarding the median dose of prescribed methadone, there were no significant differences between both arms. The median [IQR] dose of methadone at M12 was 60 [45–90] mg in primary care and 67.5 [50–82.5] mg in specialized care.

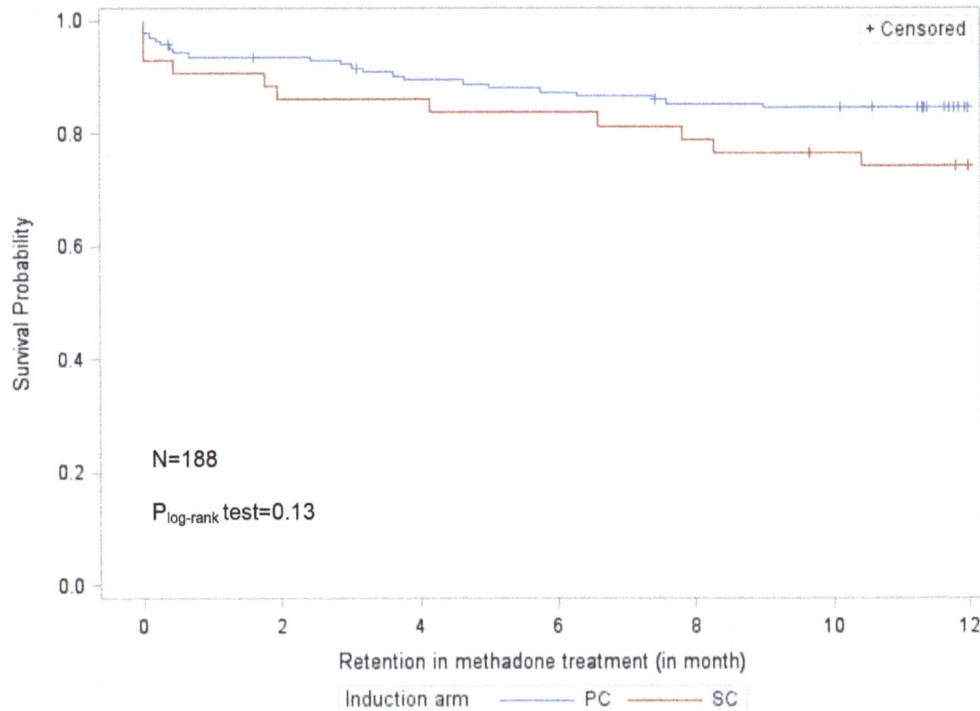

Figure 2. Retention in methadone maintenance treatment in patients (who completed the induction phase) in primary care (PC) versus those who started in specialized care (SC).

Adverse events and self-reported symptoms

No overdose was observed during the induction phase but one patient with a history of suicide attempts did intentionally overdose during methadone maintenance. Apart from this case, no other severe adverse events were reported during the trial.

The following symptoms were reported by more than 20% of patients at month 3: fatigue/energy loss (49%), difficulty sleeping (48%), constipation (40%), shortness of breath (33%), muscle pain (32%), tingling (32%), poor appetite (31%), wheezing (31%), loss of sexual desire (31%), stomach pain (28%), headaches (28%), joint pain (23%), weight loss (20%) and blackouts (20%).

Discussion

This study is the first to randomize methadone initiation in primary care. It was deliberately designed as a pragmatic trial [21,22], i.e. having a real-life context to ensure external validity and to provide information about methadone effectiveness, irrespective of the induction site. It was also designed to provide recommendations about the possible authorization of methadone induction in primary care in France.

The main result of the trial is that induction in primary care is feasible, as patients in primary care are not less likely to be abstinent from street opioids compared with those inducted in specialized care. Another interesting result is that PC appears to be more attractive for opioid-dependent individuals, first because patients randomized into primary care were more likely to accept

Table 3. ITT and *per protocol* analysis for the difference in the percentage of street-opioid abstinent patients by induction arm and its 95% confidence interval.

	Specialized care	Primary care	% [95% CI] of the difference
ITT analysis			
Number of street-opioid abstinent patients at M12	22	85	
Number of patients included	66	155	
Street-opioid abstinent patients	33%	54%	21.5 [7.7; 35.3]
Per protocol analysis			
Number of street-opioid abstinent patients at M12	22	85	
Number of patients at M12	33	129	
Street-opioid abstinent patients at M12	67%	66%	−0.8 [−18.8; 17.3]

Table 4. Odds ratio from the adjusted mixed model for abstinence from opioids use during the treatment (n = 615 visits and 188 patients).

	OR (IC95%)
Time since methadone treatment initiation	
M3 vs. M0	19.62 (8.69–44.33)
M6 vs. M0	16.73 (7.73–36.19)
M12 vs. M0	19.42 (8.98–41.98)
Arm induction	
PC vs. SC	1.58 (0.57–4.37)
switching from buprenorphine	
Yes vs. No	1.99 (0.85–4.67)

treatment than those randomized in specialized centers. Secondly patients who were inducted (after randomization) in primary care were more likely to engage in treatment and report greater satisfaction with medical information provided by their physician. Furthermore, this study highlighted that once methadone treatment was started, retention in treatment was similar in both arms. These last two results reflect the two main criteria generally used for assessing the effectiveness of treatments for opioid dependence - namely retention and non-medical opioid use – and confirm the comparable effectiveness of PC and SC over one year.

Similar results were found in a previous pragmatic trial comparing maintenance in primary care and specialized care. That trial also showed comparable outcomes and better satisfaction with treatment in the primary care maintenance arm [5,19,23].

Engagement in treatment was significantly lower in specialized care than in primary care, with early discontinuation rates significantly higher in the former group. This may be directly attributable to the specific French context, where access to buprenorphine already exists in primary care [4]. Indeed, previous pragmatic trials for other treatments involving primary care [15] have highlighted that strong patient engagement is related to the high motivation of physicians enrolled in the trial. This was also the case for physicians who accepted to participate in the present trial. Indeed this is the population of physicians which will be targeted if methadone induction becomes authorized in France.

In addition, it is important to note that the results of this trial by and large are consistent with those found in previous literature [24]. This shows that patients receiving methadone in primary care have comparable treatment responses in terms of retention and opioid use.

Using primary care as an entry point for opioid dependence care (and also for associated comorbidities) has greatly contributed to the scaling-up of treatment for opioid dependence in countries such as the UK. Even more importantly it helps "normalize" care for drug users. The availability of buprenorphine in primary care has partially contributed to "normalize" care for drug users in France as it means they can initiate a treatment option for opioid dependence "free-of-charge" like any other patient, and do so in structures which also provide care for other medical conditions to the general population.

As the French public health authorities were particularly concerned by the overdose risk during induction, the design of the trial proposed a specific model of care for methadone induction in PC in order to maximize safety. Individuals inducted in PC were over-represented in order to better detect possible

overdoses during induction in the PC arm. As it happened, no overdoses were observed during induction, confirming previous results about the importance of a shared-care model to minimize such a risk [16].

The strengths of this study lie in the following three key points: first the identification of physicians who will likely be authorized to induct methadone by public health authorities; second the choice of a population of patients which was highly representative of individuals seeking care for opioid dependence in France (non-inclusion criteria were based exclusively on clinical practice criteria to control the risk of overdose); third, the adoption of a flexible treatment protocol where patients could choose to change arm after induction reflecting current clinical practice in France.

One reason why equity of access to methadone and buprenorphine is important in France is because primary care physicians regularly have to manage persistent buprenorphine-injection practices and associated complications [25], which are often a consequence of inadequate dosage prescription [26] or patient dissatisfaction with treatment. For this reason it is important for France to also consider patients who need to switch from buprenorphine to methadone for medical reasons. Despite the wide availability of generic buprenorphine in France, switching from buprenorphine to methadone in primary care could result in reduced costs for care of opioid dependence. However, methadone is likely to present more drug-drug interactions than buprenorphine for those on HIV or HCV medication. Consequently, before starting methadone in patients already receiving such medication, physicians should know how to modify methadone doses accordingly. This is why primary care physicians involved in the present trial received training and appropriate guidelines for all possible drug-drug interactions with methadone treatment, together with guidance about the differences between starting methadone in buprenorphine patients compared with methadone induction in street-opioid users.

A substantial portion of the participants starting methadone in SC switched from buprenorphine to methadone. This is the usual treatment chain for opioid-dependent patients in France. This is not so frequent in other countries. However, switching in France is impossible in areas underserved by specialized centers for substance dependence (i.e. non-urban areas) where general methadone initiation is not available.

Although methadone induction is already possible in primary care in some countries including the UK and Switzerland, no previous trial has compared methadone outcomes over one year as a function of the site of induction. The randomization of a specific model of care for drug users has already been performed in other trials [5,27,28] which had similar public health objectives.

The population targeted in this trial is representative of those seeking care for opioid dependence in France [29] and in other countries where similar models of specialized care are available [30–33]. However it is difficult to say to what extent these results remain valid in countries where access to opioid maintenance treatment is not free for drug users. Nevertheless, the study was performed according to standard international guidelines [34,35] in order to make our results as relevant as possible for other contexts.

Among the limitations of the trial, the need for physical proximity between the primary care physician and specialized centers obliged us to target areas where patients' need for methadone was already being substantially met by the specialized centers rather than underserved areas. This resulted in slowed enrolment rates and the enforced extension of the duration of enrolment period. Certainly a larger sample size and longer follow-up would have provided long term comparisons and increased the study's power, but this was not feasible both because of the practical reasons outlined above and cost reasons. The possible effect of heterogeneity between sites (i.e. sites with more than one PC physician versus sites having only one) was tested as a random effect factor in mixed models but was not found to be significant. It is possible that a larger sample size could have altered these results. However, it was important to represent different site sizes (i.e. those with different numbers of participating PC physicians) in the trial for external validity reasons.

Today, many governments of countries with HCV and HIV epidemics driven by drug use are still reluctant to introduce or scale up methadone treatment using alternative models of care, even though such an approach would be cost-effective, especially for controlling HIV and HCV [36].

The model used for primary care in this study may be of interest in other settings where access to methadone is needed for HIV and HCV prevention purposes. However, it is important to remember that our results strongly depend on the specific context of France where primary care already plays an important role in engaging patients in treatment for opioid dependence.

In conclusion, methadone induction in primary care is feasible and acceptable for both physicians and patients. It is as effective as induction in specialized care in reducing street-opioid use and ensuring engagement and retention in treatment for opioid dependence.

Supporting Information

Checklist S1 CONSORT 2010 checklist for the ANRS-Methaville trial.

English protocol S1 Published protocol of ANRS-Methaville trial.

Acknowledgments

We thank all the members of the ANRS-Methaville Study Group. We especially thank all the physicians involved in the trial and all the patients who took part in this study. Finally, we thank Jude Sweeney for the English revision and editing of our manuscript.

The ANRS Methaville Study Group:
Scientific Committee: P.M. Carrieri (project director)[1,2,3], A. Morel (principal investigator)[4], L. Michel[5,6,7], M. Mora[1,2,3], P. Roux[1,2,3], JF. Aubertin[8], S. Robinet[8], JC. Desenclos[9], J. Cohen[1,2,3], A. Herszkowicz[10], C. Paul[11], I. Porteret[11], T. Sainte Marie[12].

Physicians who contributed to the study: Dr Achard (Private practice, Besançon); Dr Aubertin (Private practice, Thionville); Dr Balteau Bijeau (CSST Wads, Metz); Dr Bartolo (Protox, Marseille); Dr Bibette (Private practice; Biarritz); Dr Biderman (Private practice, Meudon); Dr. Bry (Private practice); Dr Cadart (Private practice, Avignon); Dr Dewost (CSST Le trait d'union; Boulogne); Dr. Daulouede (CSST Bizia, Bayonne); Dr Gassmann (Private practice, Strasbourg); Dr Guena (CSST La Boussole, Rouen); Dr Guillet (CSST Le trait d'union; Boulogne); Dr Gutekunst (Private practice, Buchviller); Dr Herouin (CSST La Boussole, Rouen); Dr Herran (CSST Bizia, Bayonne); Dr Jacob (CSST Centre Hospitalier du Jury, Metz); Dr Kerloc'h (CSST Bizia, Bayonne); Dr Khouri; Dr Lasalarié (Private practice, Marseille); Dr Lavignasse (CSST Bizia, Bayonne); Dr Magnin (Private practice, Besançon); Dr Marre (Private practice, Le Havre); Dr. Mauraycaplanne; Dr Michel (Private practice, Lillebonne); Dr. Alain Morel (CSST Le trait d'union; Boulogne); Dr Nemayechi (Private practice, Bordeaux); Dr Paillou (CSST CEID, Bordeaux); Dr Partouche (Private practice, Thionville); Dr Petit (CSST AVAPT, Avignon); Dr Pouclet (CSST Centre Hospitalier du Jury, Metz); Dr Raulin (Private practice, Maromme); Dr Regard (Private practice, Avignon); Dr Roch (Private practice, Besançon); Dr Rouille; Dr Truffy (Private practice, Metz); Dr Vergez (Private practice, Marseille); Dr Vincent (Private practice, Bayonne); Dr Wajsbrot (Private practice, Avignon).

[1] INSERM U912 (SESSTIM), Marseille, France
[2] Université Aix Marseille, IRD, UMR-S912, Marseille, France
[3] ORS PACA, Observatoire Régional de la Santé Provence Alpes Côte d'Azur, Marseille, France
[4] Oppelia, Paris, France
[5] INSERM, Research Unit 669, Paris, France.
[6] Univ Paris-Sud and Univ Paris Descartes, UMR-S0669, Paris, France.
[7] Centre Pierre Nicole, Paris, France.
[8] Private practice
[9] Institut de Veille Sanitaire, Saint Maurice, France.
[10] Ministry of Health, France.
[11] French National Agency of Research on AIDS and hepatitis (ANRS), France.
[12] Hôpital Bicêtre, AP-HP, Le Kremlin-Bicêtre, France.

Safety committee: J. Bachellier, P.Beauverie, M. Vray, B. Stambul, F. Questel.
International committee of experts: R. Baker, H. Catania, M. Gossop, R. Haemmig, M. Torrens, A. Wodak.
Center of Methodology and Management, INSERM U912:
Protocol, guidelines, training: P.M. Carrieri L. Michel, M. Mora, P. Roux.
Phone interviews, training, logistics: G. Maradan, J. Biemar, S. Huguet, C. Bravard
Data collection, management and statistical analyses: P. Kurkdji, C. Taieb, J. Cohen, C. Lions.
Administration: C. Giovannini, MP. Kissikian.
The French National Agency for Research on AIDS and Viral Hepatitis (ANRS): JC. Desenclos, N. Job-Spira, V. Dore, C. Paul, I. Porteret.
French agency for the safety of health products (AFSSPAS): N. Richard.
French Ministry of Health: A.Herszkowicz, N. Prisse.
ASUD association: F. Olivet; AIDES association
Center of evaluation and information on drug dependence (CEIP): J. Arditti

Author Contributions

Conceived and designed the experiments: PMC AM PR LM MV BS. Performed the experiments: AM PMC PR LM MM. Analyzed the data: JC CL FM PMC. Contributed reagents/materials/analysis tools: MM AM LM PR PMC. Wrote the manuscript: PMC. Contributed to the writing of the manuscript: PR.

References

1. Macarthur GJ, Minozzi S, Martin N, Vickerman P, Deren S, et al. (2012) Opiate substitution treatment and HIV transmission in people who inject drugs: systematic review and meta-analysis. Bmj 345: e5945.
2. Roux P, Carrieri MP, Villes V, Dellamonica P, Poizot-Martin I, et al. (2008) The impact of methadone or buprenorphine treatment and ongoing injection on highly active antiretroviral therapy (HAART) adherence: evidence from the MANIF2000 cohort study. Addiction 103: 1828–1836.
3. Carrieri MP, Amass L, Lucas GM, Vlahov D, Wodak A, et al. (2006) Buprenorphine use: the international experience. Clin Infect Dis 43 Suppl 4: S197–215.
4. Auriacombe M, Fatseas M, Dubernet J, Daulouede JP, Tignol J (2004) French field experience with buprenorphine. Am J Addict 13 Suppl 1: S17–28.
5. Fiellin DA, O'Connor PG, Chawarski M, Pakes JP, Pantalon MV, et al. (2001) Methadone maintenance in primary care: a randomized controlled trial. Jama 286: 1724–1731.
6. Strain EC, Bigelow GE, Liebson IA, Stitzer ML (1999) Moderate- vs high-dose methadone in the treatment of opioid dependence: a randomized trial. Jama 281: 1000–1005.
7. Sheehan DV, Lecrubier Y, Sheehan KH, Amorim P, Janavs J, et al. (1998) The Mini-International Neuropsychiatric Interview (M.I.N.I.): the development and validation of a structured diagnostic psychiatric interview for DSM-IV and ICD-10. J Clin Psychiatry 59 Suppl 20: 22–33; quiz 34–57.
8. Brands B, Blake J, Marsh DC, Sproule B, Jeyapalan R, et al. (2008) The impact of benzodiazepine use on methadone maintenance treatment outcomes. J Addict Dis 27: 37–48.
9. Kerr T, Fairbairn N, Tyndall M, Marsh D, Li K, et al. (2007) Predictors of non-fatal overdose among a cohort of polysubstance-using injection drug users. Drug Alcohol Depend 87: 39–45.
10. Roux PD, Michel LD, Cohen J, Mora M, Morel A, et al. (2012) Initiation of Methadone in primary care (ANRS-Methaville): a phase III randomized intervention trial. BMC Public Health 12: 488.
11. Schwartz RP, Jaffe JH, Highfield DA, Callaman JM, O'Grady KE (2007) A randomized controlled trial of interim methadone maintenance: 10-Month follow-up. Drug Alcohol Depend 86: 30–36.
12. Darke S, Hall W, Wodak A, Heather N, Ward J (1992) Development and validation of a multi-dimensional instrument for assessing outcome of treatment among opiate users: the Opiate Treatment Index. Br J Addict 87: 733–742.
13. Coons SJ, Kothari S, Monz BU, Burke LB (2011) The patient-reported outcome (PRO) consortium: filling measurement gaps for PRO end points to support labeling claims. Clin Pharmacol Ther 90: 743–748.
14. Snyder CF, Blackford AL, Aaronson NK, Detmar SB, Carducci MA, et al. (2011) Can patient-reported outcome measures identify cancer patients' most bothersome issues? J Clin Oncol 29: 1216–1220.
15. Fransen GA, van Marrewijk CJ, Mujakovic S, Muris JW, Laheij RJ, et al. (2007) Pragmatic trials in primary care. Methodological challenges and solutions demonstrated by the DIAMOND-study. BMC Med Res Methodol 7: 16.
16. Weinrich M, Stuart M (2000) Provision of methadone treatment in primary care medical practices: review of the Scottish experience and implications for US policy. Jama 283: 1343–1348.
17. Farre M, Mas A, Torrens M, Moreno V, Cami J (2002) Retention rate and illicit opioid use during methadone maintenance interventions: a meta-analysis. Drug Alcohol Depend 65: 283–290.
18. Teesson M, Ross J, Darke S, Lynskey M, Ali R, et al. (2006) One year outcomes for heroin dependence: findings from the Australian Treatment Outcome Study (ATOS). Drug Alcohol Depend 83: 174–180.
19. Wittchen HU, Apelt SM, Soyka M, Gastpar M, Backmund M, et al. (2008) Feasibility and outcome of substitution treatment of heroin-dependent patients in specialized substitution centers and primary care facilities in Germany: a naturalistic study in 2694 patients. Drug Alcohol Depend 95: 245–257.
20. Hamer RM, Simpson PM (2009) Last observation carried forward versus mixed models in the analysis of psychiatric clinical trials. Am J Psychiatry 166: 639–641.
21. Bouvenot G, Vray M (2006) Essais cliniques: théorie, pratique et critique; Medecine-Sciences, editor: Flammarion.
22. Vray M, Schwartz D (1996) Comments on a pragmatic trial. J Clin Epidemiol 49: 949–950.
23. Keen J, Oliver P, Rowse G, Mathers N (2003) Does methadone maintenance treatment based on the new national guidelines work in a primary care setting? Br J Gen Pract 53: 461–467.
24. MacGowan RJ, Swanson NM, Brackbill RM, Rugg DL, Barker T, et al. (1996) Retention in methadone maintenance treatment programs, Connecticut and Massachusetts, 1990–1993. J Psychoactive Drugs 28: 259–265.
25. Del Giudice P (2004) Cutaneous complications of intravenous drug abuse. Br J Dermatol 150: 1–10.
26. Roux P, Villes V, Blanche J, Bry D, Spire B, et al. (2008) Buprenorphine in primary care: Risk factors for treatment injection and implications for clinical management. Drug Alcohol Depend 97: 105–113.
27. O'Connor PG, Oliveto AH, Shi JM, Triffleman EG, Carroll KM, et al. (1998) A randomized trial of buprenorphine maintenance for heroin dependence in a primary care clinic for substance users versus a methadone clinic. Am J Med 105: 100–105.
28. Gibson AE, Doran CM, Bell JR, Ryan A, Lintzeris N (2003) A comparison of buprenorphine treatment in clinic and primary care settings: a randomised trial. Med J Aust 179: 38–42.
29. Cadet-Taïrou A, Cholley D (2004) Rapport 2004 - Approche régionale de la substitution aux opiacés, 1999–2002. OFDT. 28–36 p.
30. McCowan C, Kidd B, Fahey T (2009) Factors associated with mortality in Scottish patients receiving methadone in primary care: retrospective cohort study. Bmj 338: b2225.
31. Nosyk B, Sun H, Evans E, Marsh DC, Anglin MD, et al. (2012) Defining dosing pattern characteristics of successful tapers following methadone maintenance treatment: results from a population-based retrospective cohort study. Addiction 107: 1621–1629.
32. Hser YI, Saxon AJ, Huang D, Hasson A, Thomas C, et al. (2014) Treatment retention among patients randomized to buprenorphine/naloxone compared to methadone in a multi-site trial. Addiction 109: 79–87.
33. Schwartz RP, Kelly SM, O'Grady KE, Gandhi D, Jaffe JH (2012) Randomized trial of standard methadone treatment compared to initiating methadone without counseling: 12-month findings. Addiction 107: 943–952.
34. Fareed A, Casarella J, Amar R, Vayalapalli S, Drexler K (2010) Methadone maintenance dosing guideline for opioid dependence, a literature review. J Addict Dis 29: 1–14.
35. Soyka M, Kranzler HR, van den Brink W, Krystal J, Moller HJ, et al. (2011) The World Federation of Societies of Biological Psychiatry (WFSBP) guidelines for the biological treatment of substance use and related disorders. Part 2: Opioid dependence. World J Biol Psychiatry 12: 160–187.
36. Wolfe D, Carrieri MP, Shepard D (2010) Treatment and care for injecting drug users with HIV infection: a review of barriers and ways forward. Lancet 376: 355–366.

23

Risk Factors for Severe Neutropenia following Intra-Arterial Chemotherapy for Intra-Ocular Retinoblastoma

Ira J. Dunkel[1,2]*, **Weiji Shi**[3], **Kim Salvaggio**[4], **Brian P. Marr**[5,6], **Scott E. Brodie**[7], **Y. Pierre Gobin**[4], **David H. Abramson**[5,6]

1 Department of Pediatrics, Memorial Sloan-Kettering Cancer Center, New York, NY, United States of America, 2 Department of Pediatrics, New York Presbyterian Hospital Weill Cornell Medical College, New York, NY, United States of America, 3 Department of Epidemiology and Biostatistics, Memorial Sloan-Kettering Cancer Center, New York, NY, United States of America, 4 Department of Neurosurgery, New York Presbyterian Hospital Weill Cornell Medical College, New York, NY, United States of America, 5 Department of Surgery, Memorial Sloan-Kettering Cancer Center, New York, NY, United States of America, 6 Department of Ophthalmology, New York Presbyterian Hospital Weill Cornell Medical College, New York, NY, United States of America, 7 Department of Ophthalmology, Mount Sinai Medical Center, New York, NY, United States of America

Abstract

Purpose: Intra-arterial chemotherapy is a promising strategy for intra-ocular retinoblastoma. Neutropenia is the most commonly encountered systemic toxicity and in this study we aimed to determine the risk factors associated with the development of severe ($\geq$ grade 3) neutropenia.

Methods: Retrospective review of 187 evaluable cycles of melphalan-containing intra-arterial chemotherapy from the first three cycles administered to 106 patients with intra-ocular retinoblastoma from May 2006 to June 2011. Cycles were considered to be evaluable if (1) blood count results were available in the 7 to 14 days post-treatment interval and (2) concurrent intravenous chemotherapy was not administered. Toxicity was assessed via the Common Terminology Criteria for Adverse Events version 4.0.

Results: 54 cycles (29%) were associated with grade 3 (n = 43) or grade 4 (n = 11) neutropenia. Multivariate stepwise logistic regression revealed that a higher melphalan dose (>0.40 mg/kg) was significantly associated with severe neutropenia during all 3 cycles (odds ratio during cycle one 4.11, 95% confidence interval 1.33–12.73, p = 0.01), but the addition of topotecan and/or carboplatin were not. Prior treatment with systemic chemotherapy was not associated with severe neutropenia risk in any analysis.

Conclusions: Intra-arterial melphalan-based chemotherapy can cause severe neutropenia, especially when a dose of greater than 0.40 mg/kg is administered. Further study with a larger sample may be warranted.

Editor: John W. Glod, National Cancer Institute, United States of America

Funding: This work was supported by Perry's Promise Fund. The funders had no role in study design, data collection and analysis, decision to publish, or preparation of the manuscript.

Competing Interests: The authors have declared that no competing interests exist.

* Email: dunkeli@mskcc.org

Introduction

Retinoblastoma is the most common primary ocular tumor of childhood. In the United States and other socio-economically advantaged parts of the world, the vast majority of patients have intra-ocular disease at diagnosis. During the past 15 to 20 years advanced intra-ocular disease has most often been treated with enucleation, but super selective intra-arterial chemotherapy appears to be a promising option [1–2]. It is generally well tolerated, but grade 3 and 4 neutropenia may occur. We performed this analysis to try to determine risk factors associated with the development of severe neutropenia and hypothesized that factors associated with development of grade 3 or 4 neutropenia would be (1) the melphalan dose, (2) administration of topotecan and/or carboplatin in addition to melphalan, and (3) prior treatment with systemic chemotherapy.

Methods

Ethics statement

The Memorial Sloan-Kettering Cancer Center's Institutional Review Board/Privacy Board approved this retrospective review of existing data, granting a waiver for this to be done without obtaining consent from the subjects or their parents/legal guardians. All protected health information was handled in accordance with institutional policies that did not require the information to be anonymized and de-identified prior to analysis.

Patients

We retrospectively reviewed the first 106 consecutive patients with intra-ocular retinoblastoma treated with intra-arterial chemotherapy at our centers from May 2006 to June 2011.

Patients most frequently were treated with intra-arterial single-agent melphalan, but some cycles also included treatment with intra-arterial topotecan and/or carboplatin (Table 1). The number of agents to be used and the doses of chemotherapy administered were determined on a case by case basis. In general, patients received more than one agent if they had more severe disease or had been extensively pre-treated with intravenous chemotherapy and/or external beam radiation therapy, especially if we were treating the only remaining eye. In cycle 1, the dose was primarily determined by the patient's age. Patients 3 to 6 months of age generally received 2.5 mg of melphalan, 6 to 12 months of age, 3 mg of melphalan, 1 to 3 years of age, 4 mg of melphalan, and ≥3 years of age, 5 mg of melphalan [1]. In subsequent cycles we would consider increasing the dose(s) if the ophthalmic artery had large extra-ocular branches or if an inadequate response had been encountered without significant toxicity. We would consider decreasing the dose(s) if wedge flow was encountered or significant toxicity was encountered, such as an interval decrease in the eye's electroretinogram or an ocular inflammatory reaction. The median topotecan dose administered was 0.4 mg (range 0.2 to 2 mg) and the median carboplatin dose administered was 30 mg (range 25 to 80 mg).

We asked the parents to have a complete blood count performed 7 to 10 days after each dose of intra-arterial chemotherapy. However, many families did not reside in the New York area and returned home after the treatment, and so compliance was variable. Intra-arterial chemotherapy cycles were considered to be evaluable if (1) blood count results were available in the 7 to 14 days post-treatment interval, and (2) concurrent intravenous chemotherapy was not administered. However, if a blood count was not available within the 7 to 14 day post-treatment window, but grade 3 or 4 neutropenia was documented earlier or later in the cycle, the cycle was considered evaluable. Toxicity was assessed via the Common Terminology Criteria for Adverse Events (CTCAE) version 4.0.

Statistics

A binary melphalan dose is of interest in potential prediction. An optimal cut-off point of the dose was selected using Miller and Siegmund's minimum p-value approach and Altman, Lausen, Sauerbrei, and Schumacher's formula to adjust the minimum p-value selected from the systematic dependent multiple testing [3–4]. The highest and lowest 10% of the melphalan dose data were eliminated from the selection procedure. A univariate analysis of relationship between treatment factors and severe neutropenia (defined as grade 3 or 4 neutropenia) was performed using Chi-square, or Fisher's exact test. A multivariate analysis of the joint relationship was performed using a stepwise logistical regression method. Variables with p-value ≤0.20 on univariate analysis were candidates for the initial multivariate model. The statistical analysis was performed with the software SAS version 9.2 (SAS Institute Cary, NC) and r package ROCR (version 2.9.2). A p-value<0.05 was considered significant.

All analyses were based on evaluable cycles only. Grade 3 and 4 neutropenia were combined into the entity of severe neutropenia due to the small number of grade 4 neutropenia events (n = 5, 3, and 3 during cycles 1, 2 and 3, respectively).

Results

Melphalan dose and analysis of optimal cut-off point

A preliminary analysis showed that a higher melphalan dose (continuous variable) was significantly associated with severe neutropenia during cycles 2 and cycle 3 (p<0.0001, p<0.0001

Table 1. The number of patients treated per cycle with the various chemotherapy agents and the number of patients evaluable for analysis of neutropenia.

Cycle	Patient	M only	M + T	M+T+C	M+C	Inevaluable	Evaluable
1	106	74	21	10	1	33	73
2	100	67	25	7	1	36	64
3	86	53	24	8	1	36	50

M: melphalan; T: topotecan; C: carboplatin.

by t-test, respectively). The minimum p-value approach showed that 0.50 mg/kg was the best cut-off point during cycle 2 (>0.50 versus ≤50 mg/kg, $\chi^2 = 18.55$, adjusted p = 0.0007) and 0.40 mg/kg during cycle 3 (>0.40 versus ≤0.40 mg/kg, $\chi^2 = 26.26$, adjusted p<0.0001). Melphalan dose>0.40 mg/kg was also associated with severe neutropenia during cycle 2 ($\chi^2 = 12.34$, adjusted p = 0.01).

Analyses of treatment factors and severe neutropenia

Cycle 1. A univariate analysis regarding cycle 1 showed that a higher dose of melphalan (>0.40 versus ≤0.40 mg/kg) was significantly associated with severe neutropenia (p = 0.01, Table 2). The univariate analysis also showed that the severe neutropenia rate was significantly different among patients treated with different chemotherapy regimens (melphalan alone versus melphalan and either topotecan or carboplatin versus melphalan, topotecan and carboplatin, p = 0.04). Further pairwise comparison showed that patients treated with three chemotherapy agents more frequently experienced severe neutropenia compared to those treated with two agents (50% versus 9%, p = 0.02). However, a stepwise logistic regression revealed that while higher melphalan dose remained associated with severe neutropenia (odds ratio (OR) 4.11, 95% CI 1.33–12.73, p = 0.01), the number of chemotherapy agents administered did not.

Cycle 2. A univariate analysis revealed that a higher cycle 2 melphalan dose (>0.50 versus ≤0.50 mg/kg) was significantly associated with severe neutropenia (p<0.0001 by Chi-square test, adjusted p = 0.0007, Table 3). A stepwise logistic regression showed melphalan dose remained associated with severe neutropenia during cycle 2 (p = 0.0005, OR 10.86, 95% CI 2.84–41.57).

Cycle 3. A univariate analysis demonstrated that a higher cycle 3 melphalan dose (>0.40 versus ≤0.40 mg/kg) was once again significantly associated with severe neutropenia (p<0.0001, adjusted p<0.0001, Table 4). The univariate analysis and further pairwise comparison also showed that patients who had severe neutropenia during cycle 1 or 2 more frequently experienced severe neutropenia during cycle 3 compared to those who did not (yes versus unknown versus no, p = 0.02; yes versus no, p = 0.01). A stepwise multivariate logistic regression analysis revealed that while the higher melphalan dose remained associated with severe

neutropenia (p = 0.0001, OR 72.0, 95% CI 7.93–653.4), severe neutropenia during cycle 1 or 2 did not.

Impact of inevaluable cycles

A greater proportion of later cycles were inevaluable (31%, 36%, and 42% in cycles 1, 2, and 3, respectively) and that could introduce bias on generalization. However, there was no significant difference in melphalan dose (continuous or binary> 0.40 versus ≤0.40 mg/kg), chemotherapy regimen, prior treatment, and severe neutropenia during cycle 1, 2 or 3 between the patients who had or had no record (at cycle 1, 2, or 3, p = 0.11 to 0.95), except that patients with record received a higher mean melphalan dose during cycle 1 (0.40±0.14 versus 0.34±0.14, p = 0.04). In addition, patients with record received a higher binary melphalan dose (>0.50 versus ≤0.50 mg/kg) during cycle 2 (27% versus vs 8%, p = 0.03).

Clinical consequences of severe neutropenia

Most patients who developed severe neutropenia were asymptomatic. Two patients were admitted to the hospital during three periods of severe neutropenia due to fever and/or mucositis. Both patients made complete recoveries.

Other severe hematological toxicities

Severe (grade 3 or 4) anemia or thrombocytopenia were encountered infrequently. Five patients suffered 1 episode each (5 episodes total) of grade 3 anemia and 2 patients suffered 1 episode each (2 episodes total) of grade 4 thrombocytopenia.

Discussion

Intra-arterial chemotherapy was first introduced into the treatment regimen for patients with intra-ocular retinoblastoma by Reese and colleagues in 1955 when they administered triethylenemelamine via the internal carotid artery [2]. It then fell out of favor due to toxicity concerns (that included death) and lack of clear benefit over other treatments until 1987 when Kaneko and colleagues began to administer selective ophthalmic arterial injection of melphalan using a balloon catheter. Their group recently reported a retrospective series of 343 patients (408

Table 2. Cycle 1: Univariate analysis of severe neutropenia.

Variable	Severe neutropenia (25%)		p-value
	No (n = 55)	Yes (n = 18)	
M dose, mg/kg (mean ± SD)	0.39±0.14	0.43±0.12	
Median (range)	0.35 (0.15–0.89)	0.46 (0.27–0.68)	
≤0.40	37 (67%)	6 (33%)	0.01
>0.40	18 (33%)	12 (67%)	
Chemotherapy agents			0.04
M only	30 (55%)	11 (61%)	
M+ T/C	20 (36%)	2 (11%)	
M+ T + C	5 (9%)	5 (28%)	
Prior treatment[a]			0.77
No	24 (45%)	7 (41%)	
Yes	29 (55%)	10 (59%)	

M: melphalan; T: topotecan; C: carboplatin.
[a]Data not available for 3 patients (2 had and 1 did not have severe neutropenia).

Table 3. Cycle 2: Univariate analysis of severe neutropenia[a].

Variable	Severe neutropenia (30%)		p-value
	No (n = 45)	Yes (n = 19)	
M dose, mg/kg (mean ± SD)	0.36±0.12	0.51±0.13	
Median (range)	0.34 (0.04–0.57)	0.52 (0.26–0.71)	
≤0.50	40 (89)	7 (37)	<0.001[c]
>0.50	5 (11)	12 (63)	
≤0.40	31 (69%)	4 (21%)	0.01[c]
>0.40	14 (31%)	15 (79%)	
Chemotherapy agents			0.26
M only	22 (49%)	9 (47%)	
M+ T/C	20 (44%)	6 (32%)	
M+ T + C	3 (7%)	4 (21%)	
Prior treatment[b]			0.13
No	22 (51%)	5 (29%)	
Yes	21 (49%)	12 (71%)	
Cycle 1 grade 3 or 4 neutropenia			0.66
No	27 (60%)	9 (47%)	
No record	10 (22%)	5 (26%)	
Yes	8 (18%)	5 (26%)	

M: melphalan; T: topotecan; C: carboplatin.
[a]Only one variable was associated with severe neutropenia at p≤0.05 on univariate analysis; multivariate analysis was not performed.
[b]Data not available for 4 patients (2 had and 2 did not have severe neutropenia).
[c]Cut-off point selection adjusted p-value.

Table 4. Cycle 3: Univariate analysis of severe neutropenia.

Variable	Severe neutropenia (34%)		p-value
	No (n = 33)	Yes (n = 17)	
M dose, mg/kg (mean ± SD)	0.34±0.11	0.50±0.08	
Median (range)	0.33 (0.13–0.70)	0.50 (0.33–0.69)	
≤0.40	27 (82%)	1 (6%)	<0.001[b]
>0.40	6 (18%)	16 (94%)	
Chemotherapy agents			0.15
M only	13 (39%)	4 (24%)	
M+ T/C	17 (52%)	8 (47%)	
M+ T + C	3 (9%)	5 (29%)	
Prior treatment[a]			0.83
No	16 (50%)	7 (47%)	
Yes	16 (50%)	8 (53%)	
Cycle 1 or 2, grade 3 or 4 neutropenia			0.02
No	14 (42%)	3 (18%)	
No record	11 (33%)	3 (18%)	
Yes	8 (24%)	11 (65%)	

M: melphalan; T: topotecan; C: carboplatin.
[a]Data not available for 3 patients (1 had and 2 did not have severe neutropenia).
[b]Cut-off point selection adjusted p-value.

eyes) treated with 1452 procedures from 1988 to 2007 [5]. They generally used single-agent melphalan at a dose of 5 to 7.5 mg/m^2 and did not encounter any > grade 1 decrease of white blood cells. Using a 30:1 conversion factor, these doses are approximately 0.17 to 0.25 mg/kg of melphalan.

In the patients reported in this series, we used a higher dose of melphalan (median dose of evaluable cycles 0.36 mg/kg, range 0.04 to 0.89 mg/kg) and have encountered severe neutropenia in 29% of the cycles. Fortunately, most of the episodes of severe neutropenia were grade 3 (n = 43) rather than grade 4 (n = 11) and were generally clinically insignificant. We counseled the parents about the risk of fever and neutropenia, but did not routinely prescribe filgrastim. We did not encounter any severe neutropenia during cycles in which the melphalan dose was ≤0.25 mg/kg (the approximate dose used in Japan). A limitation is that we may have overestimated the risk of neutropenia due to our decision to consider cycles with blood counts performed outside of the 7 to 14 day window without neutropenia to be inevaluable, but to consider cycles evaluable if grade 3 or 4 neutropenia was documented earlier or later in the cycle. We felt that potentially overestimating rather than underestimating the risk of neutropenia associated with the intra-arterial chemotherapy was the more conservative approach.

We hypothesized that (1) adding topotecan and/or carboplatin to the melphalan regimen and (2) a history of prior patient exposure to intravenous chemotherapy might be associated with increased risk for severe neutropenia, but that turned out not to be the case. The only factor that remained significant in analyses was melphalan dose, particularly when a dose of greater than 0.40 mg/kg was administered. Due to the relatively small number of events and sample size, we may not have enough power to detect some difference. We were also unable to select an optimal cut-off point of melphalan dose in a multivariate setting. Further study with a larger sample size may be warranted. This increased risk of neutropenia associated with a melphalan dose of greater than 0.40 mg/kg is comparable to the results in a small series reported by Argentine investigators. They noted that children receiving more than 0.48 mg/kg for bilateral tandem infusions had a significantly higher systemic area under the curve and a 50% probability of grade 3 or 4 neutropenia [6].

These data may help assist in the selection of safe intra-arterial chemotherapy doses for patients with intra-ocular retinoblastoma, but it is important to note that most patients who developed severe neutropenia were asymptomatic and did not require hospital admission for fever and neutropenia or an infection. To minimize the risk of severe neutropenia patients should be treated with a melphalan dose of 0.40 mg/kg or less, but should higher doses be required to adequately treat the retinoblastoma and cure the eye, the risk of severe neutropenia may be acceptable.

Acknowledgments

A preliminary version of this work was presented at the 2009 International Congress of Ocular Oncology meeting in Cambridge, UK.

Author Contributions

Conceived and designed the experiments: IJD BPM SEB YPG DHA. Analyzed the data: IJD WS. Contributed reagents/materials/analysis tools: IJD KS BPM SEB YPG DHA. Wrote the paper: IJD WS KS BPM SEB YPG DHA.

References

1. Gobin YP, Dunkel IJ, Marr BP, Brodie SE, Abramson DH. (2011) Intra-arterial chemotherapy in the management of retinoblastoma: Four-year experience. Arch Ophthalmol 129: 732–737.
2. Reese AB, Hyman GA, Merriam GR Jr, Forrest AW, Kligerman MM. (1954) Treatment of retinoblastoma by radiation and triethylenemelamine. AMA Arch Ophthalmol 53: 505–513.
3. Miller R, Siegmund D. (1982) Maximally selected chi square statistics. Biometrics 38: 1011–1016.
4. Altman DG, Lausen B, Sauerbrei W, Schumacher M. (1994) Dangers of using "optimal" cutpoints in the evaluation of prognostic factors. J Natl Cancer Inst 86: 829–835.
5. Suzuki S, Yamane T, Mohri M, Kaneko A. (2011) Selective ophthalmic arterial injection therapy for intraocular retinoblastoma: The long term prognosis. Ophthalmology 118: 2081–2087.
6. Schaiquevich P, Buitrago E, Taich P, Torbidoni A, Ceciliano A, et al. (2012) Pharmacokinetic analysis of melphalan after superselective ophthalmic artery infusion in preclinical models and retinoblastoma patients. Invest Ophthalmol Vis Sci 53: 4205–4212.

24

A South African Public-Private Partnership HIV Treatment Model: Viability and Success Factors

Jude Igumbor[1]*, Sophie Pascoe[1], Shuabe Rajap[2], Wendy Townsend[3], John Sargent[3], Ernest Darkoh[3]

1 Research and Development Department, BroadReach Healthcare, Cape Town, South Africa, 2 Operations Department, BroadReach Healthcare, Cape Town, South Africa, 3 BroadReach Healthcare, Cape Town, South Africa

Abstract

Introduction: The increasing number of people requiring HIV treatment in South Africa calls for efficient use of its human resources for health in order to ensure optimum treatment coverage and outcomes. This paper describes an innovative public-private partnership model which uses private sector doctors to treat public sector patients and ascertains the model's ability to maintain treatment outcomes over time.

Methods: The study used a retrospective design based on the electronic records of patients who were down-referred from government hospitals to selected private general medical practitioners (GPs) between November 2005 and October 2012. In total, 2535 unique patient records from 40 GPs were reviewed. The survival functions for mortality and attrition were calculated. Cumulative incidence of mortality for different time cohorts (defined by year of treatment initiation) was also established.

Results: The median number of patients per GP was 143 (IQR: 66–246). At the time of down-referral to private GPs, 13.8% of the patients had CD4 count <200 cell/mm^3, this proportion reduced to 6.6% at 12 months and 4.1% at 48 months. Similarly, 88.4% of the patients had suppressed viral load (defined as HIV-1 RNA <400 copies/ml) at 48 months. The patients' probability of survival at 12 and 48 months was 99.0% (95% CI: 98.4%–99.3%) and 89.0% (95% CI: 87.1%–90.0%) respectively. Patient retention at 48 months remained high at 94.3% (95% CI: 93.0%–95.7%).

Conclusions: The study findings demonstrate the ability of the GPs to effectively maintain patient treatment outcomes and potentially contribute to HIV treatment scale-up with the relevant support mechanism. The model demonstrates how an assisted private sector based programme can be effectively and efficiently used to either target specific health concerns, key populations or serve as a stop-gap measure to meet urgent health needs.

Editor: Sten H. Vermund, Vanderbilt University, United States of America

Funding: This paper was developed using part of routinely collected data of a HIV treatment programme that is funded by the U.S. Agency for International Development (USAID) under the Cooperative Agreement No. 674-A-00-08-00008-00. The funding agency had no role in study design, data collection and analysis, decision to publish or preparation of the manuscript, and the paper is not a requirement for the treatment programme funding. Beyond using the data of a funded programme, there was no external funding for this study.

Competing Interests: All of the authors work for BroadReach Healthcare. The authors have tried to remain unbiased by highlighting the strengths and weaknesses of the model and the paper.

* Email: jigumbor@brhc.com

Introduction

With advances in antiretroviral treatment and improved survival of people living with HIV, the South African health system has to contend with an unprecedented demand for HIV/AIDS-related health care resources. Preliminary reports of the South African household HIV prevalence survey already suggest an almost 2% increase in prevalence between 2010 and 2012 [1]. This scenario excludes the continued HIV transmission and increase in the number of people who will require treatment following the new WHO treatment initiation recommendations [2,3]. These factors exacerbate the need for more efficient use of South Africa's total human resources for health to meet the growing demand for treatment.

In spite of the above, there has been an astronomical increase in the number of people living with HIV who are on treatment in South Africa [4]. Estimates show that the number of people on antiretroviral therapy in South Africa increased from less than 600,000 in 2008 to over 2,100,000 in 2013 [4,5]. However, a significant proportion of people requiring treatment still do not have access to it, with the treatment gap estimated to be as high as 45% in certain populations [3–5]. In addition, the current ART coverage success is fraught with challenges of poor patient retention, suboptimal adherence and treatment failure, partly due to insufficient human resources and high patient load for the limited capacities in health facilities [6–9]. Halting and reversing this challenge will require continued innovations to further enhance access to treatment and reduce patient load per service provider. In this regard, it became necessary to explore other options, one of which is to harness skills in the private sector to help address this national challenge with far reaching consequences.

Against this background, this paper describes the outcomes of an innovative public-private-partnership (PPP) model in an attempt to ascertain its ability to maintain patient treatment outcomes and the model's success factors that can be harnessed for future programmes. The model – referred to as the private general medical practitioner (GP) model – assumes the treatment of stable patients who were originally initiated on treatment at public health facilities.

Methodology

The GP model was developed at the request of the North West Provincial Department of Health. The GP model is one of the three models used by BroadReach Healthcare (BRHC) – a private healthcare solutions company – to provide HIV treatment through selected private GPs. The GP model was designed to be sustainable with minimal external financial support. The costs supported by BroadReach Healthcare included the start-up costs of setting up a staffed office within selected public sector wellness clinics, patient data management, adherence support and a negotiated consultation fee for the private GPs. The Department of Health provided ART medication from their district pharmacy, and laboratory services were rendered by National Health Laboratory Services which is a government parastatal. Eligible patients were down-referred to a select group of GPs in the communities where the patients live. The GPs were selected based on their prior training and experience in HIV/AIDS treatment. Patients were considered eligible for down referral if they had been stable on ART for at least 3–6 months with a suppressed viral load, did not have private medical insurance, did not have concurrent illnesses (excluding TB) and voluntarily consented to participate in the programme. The patients were then cared for by the private GPs as an alternative to public sector health service outlets. The patients were initially referred back to the public sector for the management of acute co-morbidities and complications. This was changed after 2012 to allow the GPs to manage co-morbidities. The adherence and treatment support services provided by BroadReach Healthcare were in the form of patient education sessions and adherence/wellness training, which patients attended upon their down-referral and on an annual basis. Other adherence support services provided by BroadReach Healthcare included the use of clinic-based adherence supporters; home visits by adherence supporters and telephonic follow up.

A key component of the model was its patient information management system, referred to as the Disease Management System (DMS). BroadReach Healthcare's DMS is managed by Aid for AIDS (AfA) which is a private data company that is funded through donor funds. The DMS promotes efficient management of complex patient information; it is available both online and offline (for remote use); and provides real-time patient information such as treatment regimen and pick-up history, laboratory information, doctors' consultation notes and adherence support data. The DMS is also automated to send important phone text messages, to remind patients, doctors, pharmacists and laboratory personnel of treatment activities. The reminders included scheduled treatment pick-up and laboratory test dates, details of defaulting patients, undesirable laboratory results and uncollected treatments. Some of these innovations were not part of the routine public sector treatment programme. Figure 1 illustrates the model's implementation processes and scope of services offered. Further information about the model is available from the authors.

This study was based on a retrospective design and used the electronic records of patients enrolled in the GP model. Patients included in this analysis are cared for by 40 GPs. The database used for the study was developed for patient management but contained the minimum scope of variables needed for this study's objectives. The data elements taken from the database for this study were age, sex, treatment initiation dates, treatment regimen, results of routine clinical tests and respective test dates of the patients. Patients younger than 18 years were rarely recruited into the GP model and were thus excluded from the analysis. Outcome variables considered were viral load, CD4 cell counts and patient retention. The treatment outcomes were categorized, for example, viral load status was defined as either suppressed or unsuppressed using 400 copies/ml as the status threshold for suppression. Methods of CD4 count and viral load testing have been described [10]. Loss-to-follow-up in the study was defined as patients on treatment who stopped picking up their treatment and have had no contact with the treatment programme for three months or more after their last scheduled visit date was missed. The deceased and lost-to-follow-ups were further anonymously verified to be actually lost-to-follow-up and not deceased using the national death records. Time in the study for the deceased and those lost-to-follow-up was defined as the time of initiation into the GP model to the last contact date. Data was statistically analysed using STATA 11. The median CD4 count and proportion of patients with suppressed viral load (defined as HIV-1 RNA less than 400 copies/ml) were calculated at baseline and at 6, 12, 24 and 48 months. Cumulative incidence of mortality for different time cohorts (defined by year of treatment initiation) was also established. Prior data of modest quality could not be obtained hence the baseline data referred to in this paper is the data at the point of down referral into the GP model. The median time to death and attrition was established, followed by the calculation of the survival functions for mortality and attrition respectively.

The study is based on data that is collected and stored on DMS (which is managed by a different private company on behalf of BroadReach Healthcare). The database used for this study had no individual patient identifier and the analysis was completely anonymous. Patients in the GP model also signed a consent for their information to be entered into the central database and used for routine decisions on patient and programme management and were made aware that any further analyses will exclude patient identifiers.

Results

The database used for this analysis included 2535 longitudinal patient records from their respective time of down-referral to November 2012. The first group of patients were down-referred into the partnership model in November 2005. The patients' duration in the care of the GPs ranged from 2–84 months with a 28 months median. The median number of patients each GP ever managed in the model was 143 (IQR: 66–246). The median age of the patients was 40 years old (IQR 34–46). About two-thirds (68.4%) of the patients were female. The median CD4 cell count at baseline was 342 cells/mm^3 (IQR 248–476). Figure 2 shows that this indicator increased progressively for those who remained in the programme. The median viral load over this period however remained the same (25, IQR 25–40).

The GP model showed similar treatment outcome when the probability of survival of cohorts initiated to treatment at different times for a minimum of 60 months (five years) using logrank test (p>0.05) was compared. Figure 3 shows the cumulative incidence of mortality across the treatment initiation cohorts by year of treatment initiation.

The survival functions at six (6) and 48 months are 99.6% (95% CI: 99.3%–99.9%) and 89.0% (95% CI: 87.1%–90.7%) respec-

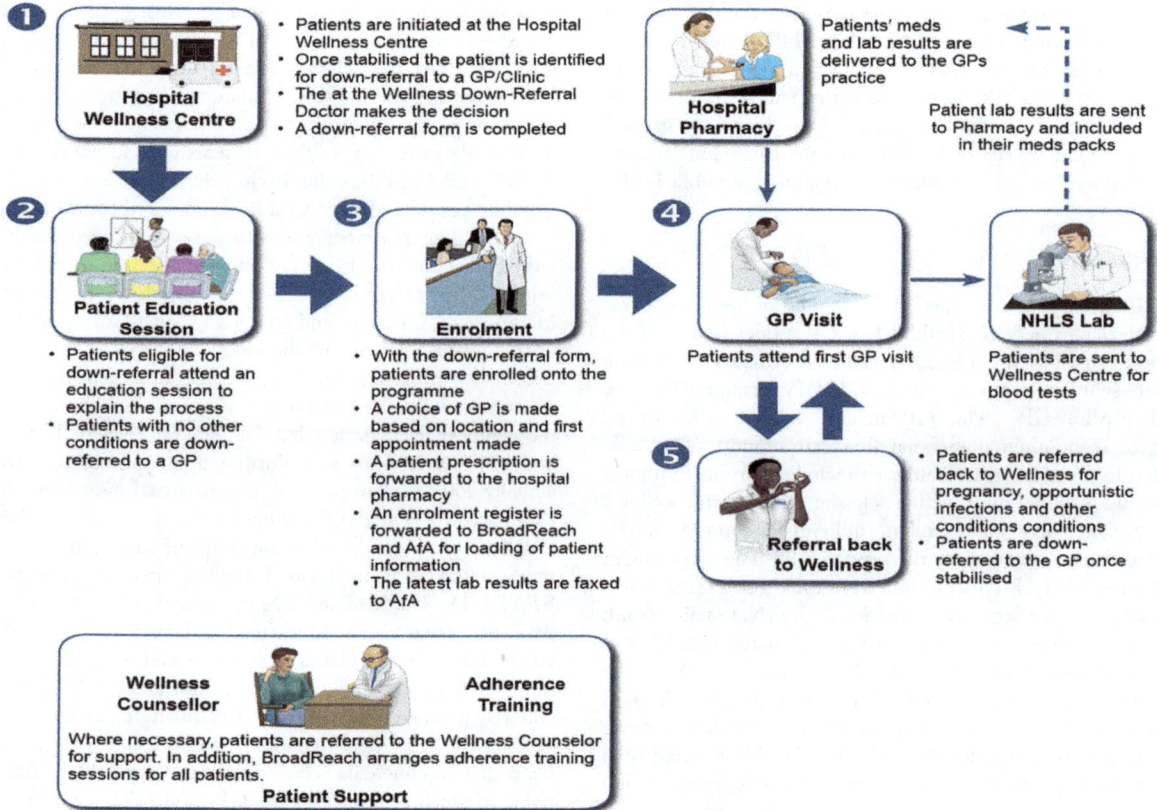

Figure 1. Model implementation process and components.

tively. The retention function at six (6) and 48 months are 100% and 94.5% (95% CI: 93.0%–95.7%) respectively. Survival and retention rates at 6, 12, 24 and 48 months are also shown in Figure 4. The median time to death for patients who died in the model was 21 months (IQR: 12.3–38.1) and the median time to attrition for patients who were lost to follow up was 29 months (IQR: 19.7–45.7).

Discussion

The study findings demonstrate the ability of the private sector to successfully absorb and retain public sector patients over time. The GP model therefore presents an opportunity to significantly

reduce the growing burden of HIV/AIDS care on the public sector. Leveraging more GPs for public sector patients or marginally decreasing doctor-patient ratio could further improve treatment coverage, decongest the public sector and obtain good patient retention and treatment outcomes [8,11].

Unlike most HIV/AIDS programmes, this model only caters for patients who have been stabilized through public sector programmes. This makes it difficult to compare its outcomes with the outcomes of other programmes that enrol all patients irrespective of their viral load. Whilst a direct comparison may be spurious, patient progression noted after down-referral into the GP model is similar to the progression among patients initiated to treatment at CD4 cell counts of between 350 cells/mm^3 and 500 cells/mm^3

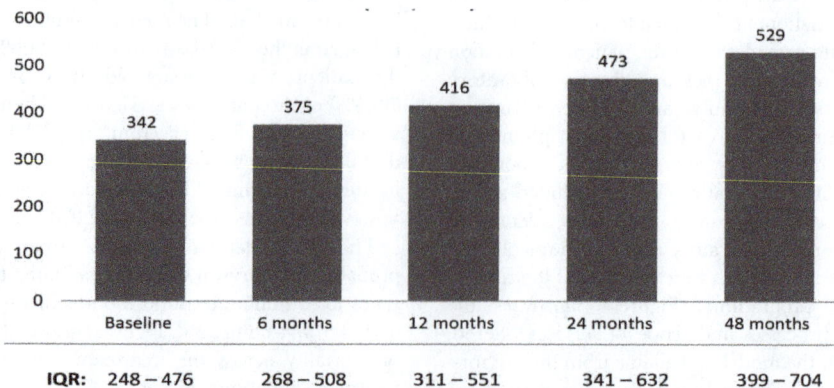

Figure 2. Median CD4 cell counts (cells/mm^3) from baseline at down-referral to 48 months in the GP model.

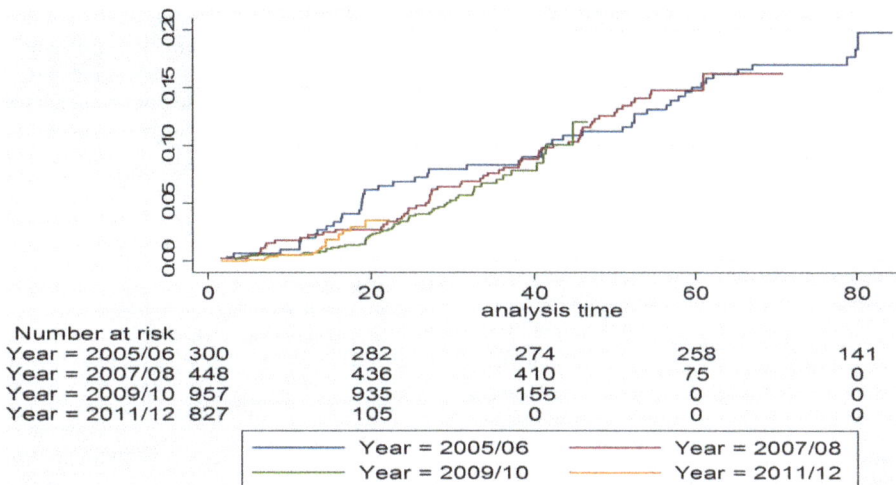

Figure 3. Cumulative incidence of mortality by year of treatment initiation.

[12]. Other studies have found linkages between treatment outcome and year of treatment initiation with improvements in successive years [13]. This trend has been associated with the advances in ART and improved access to services. This study noted significant differences when probability of survival was disaggregated into groups based on their year of enrolment into the GP model. This pattern may have resulted from improvements in psychosocial adjustment to living with HIV and adherence to treatment over time among people who have been in programme for a long time [14]. This proposition may also be a factor of progressively improved immunologic stability and durability of virologic suppression with time [15–17].

The successes reported in this study may also be attributed to the combination of established strengths of both public and private sector HIV/AIDS programmes. The GP model on the one hand harnesses public sector experience and regulations, and on the other leverages the private sector human resources and infrastructure to ensure patient retention and decongestion of public sector facilities. With this, the GP model proposes a complemen-

tary model that harnesses the arguments of both the proponents of universal state-based health care and the advocates of using the private sector to provide health services in areas where the public sector does not have capacity [18].

The private sector in general is often criticized for its high cost and inefficiencies in terms of unnecessary diagnostic tests and treatment options [18]. To address these, patient treatment and testing in the GP model was provided by government pharmacies and laboratories using standard government guidelines. An earlier cost-effectiveness study on this model found it to be relatively cost-effective when compared to down-referring patients to public sector clinics [19]. Concerns about the quality of care in the private sector have also been raised by previous studies [20,21]. Other studies have found diagnostic inaccuracies and sub-therapeutic clinical management to be more profound in the private sector in comparison to the public sector [22–26]. In this regard, the GP model is guided and monitored using government regulations and other support mechanisms including quarterly meetings with public hospital clinicians to discuss cases. These

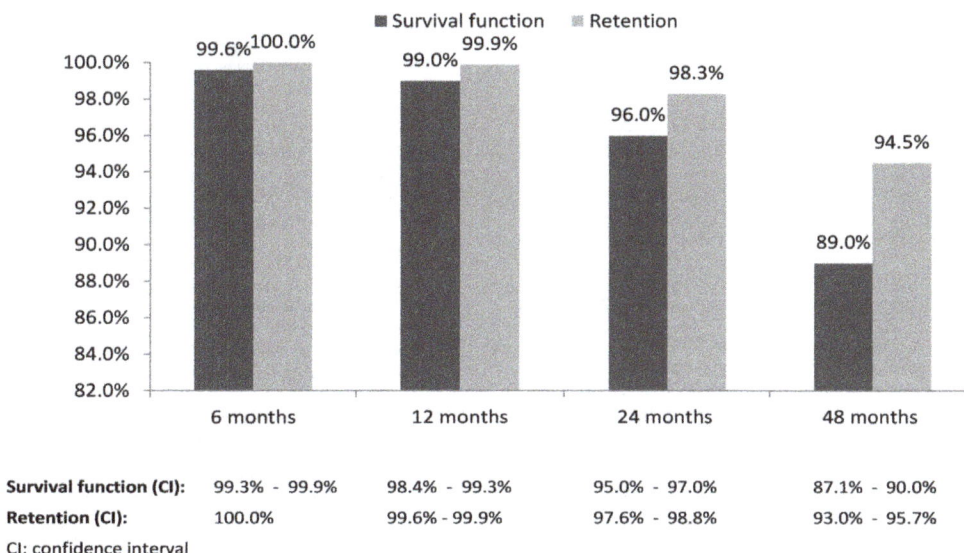

	6 months	12 months	24 months	48 months
Survival function (CI):	99.3% - 99.9%	98.4% - 99.3%	95.0% - 97.0%	87.1% - 90.0%
Retention (CI):	100.0%	99.6% - 99.9%	97.6% - 98.8%	93.0% - 95.7%

CI: confidence interval

Figure 4. Survival and retention rates at different points.

measures and the electronic support systems help to better assure adherence to the prescribed minimum diagnostic and therapeutic guidelines [25]. A combination of adherence support measures were used in the model. The use of such multiple adherence support strategies is also known to improve and better guarantee adherence to treatment and patient retention both of which are critical for optimum treatment outcome [6,27]. Treatment discontinuation due to stock-out has been shown to result in treatment interruption and increased risk of death [28–30]. The GP model's data management system promotes efficient stock management and treatment availability and this is pivotal in dealing with the common drug shortages in the public sector [31].

The limitation of this study was its exclusion of patients transferred-out of the GP programme for a variety of reasons. Following-up patients who have been transferred-out of a programme remains a major problem for many treatment programmes [32]. Consequently, the large scale of the South African epidemic and treatment programme plus the vital importance of uninterrupted treatment and patient retention should necessitate solutions that track individual patients across different points of service uptake and treatment programmes.

In conclusion, the GP model demonstrates the ability of an assisted private sector treatment programme to retain patients and maintain immunologic and virologic outcomes. This model offers lessons to guide strategic and operational decisions, specifically on how to use private sector resources to target defined health concerns or key populations or serve as a stop-gap measure to meet urgent health needs.

Acknowledgments

We are thankful to all those who supported the development of the article in various ways including Aid for AIDS (AfA) staff and the North West Provincial Department of Health. The implementation of the model was made possible by the support of the American People through the U.S. Agency for International Development (USAID) under the Cooperative Agreement No. 674-A-00-08-00008-00. As our disclaimer, the contents of this paper are the responsibility of BroadReach Healthcare and do not necessarily reflect the views of USAID or the United States Government.

Author Contributions

Conceived and designed the experiments: JI SP SR WT JS ED. Performed the experiments: JI SP SR WT JS ED. Analyzed the data: JI SP. Wrote the paper: JI SP SR WT JS ED.

References

1. Shisana O (2013) HIV/AIDS in South Africa: At last the glass is half full. Human Science Research Council. Available: http://www.hsrc.ac.za/en/media-briefs/hiv-aids-stis-and-tb/plenary-session-3-20-june-2013-hiv-aids-in-south-africa-at-last-the-glass-is-half-full. Accessed 2014 Sept 29.
2. Department of Health (2011) The 2011 National Antenatal Sentinel HIV & Syphilis Prevalence Survey in South Africa. Pretoria: National Department of Health.
3. World Health Organisation (2013) Consolidated guidelines on the use of antiretroviral drugs for treating and preventing HIV infection: summary of key features and recommendations, HIV/AIDS Programme. Geneva: World Health Organization.
4. Joint United Nations Programme on HIV/AIDS (2012) World AIDS Day Report. Geneva: UNAIDS.
5. Johnson L (2012) Access to antiretroviral treatment in South Africa, 2004–2011. Southern African Journal of HIV Medicine 13: 22–27.
6. Igumbor JO, Scheepers E, Ebrahim R, Jason A, Grimwood A (2011) An evaluation of the impact of a community-based adherence support programme on ART outcomes in selected government HIV treatment sites in South Africa. AIDS Care 23: 231–236.
7. MacPherson P, Moshabela M, Martinson N, Pronyk P(2009) Mortality and loss to follow-up among HAART initiators in rural South Africa. Trans R Soc Trop Med Hyg 103: 588–93.
8. Fatti G, Grimwood A, Mothibi E, Shea J (2011) The effect of patient load on antiretroviral treatment programmatic outcomes at primary health care facilities in South Africa: a multicohort study. J Acquir Immune Defic Syndr 58: 17–9.
9. Nglazi MD, Lawn SD, Kaplan R, Kranzer K, Orrell C (2011) Changes in programmatic outcomes during 7 years of scale-up at a community-based antiretroviral treatment service in South Africa. J Acquir Immune Defic Syndr 56: 1–8.
10. Stevens WS, Marshall TM (2010) Challenges in implementing HIV load testing in South Africa. J Infect Dis 201: 78–84.
11. Chaix B, Merlo J, Chauvin P (2005) Comparison of a spatial approach with the multilevel approach for investigating place effects on health: the example of healthcare utilisation in France. Journal of Epidemiology and Community Health 59: 517–526.
12. Kitahata MM, Gange SJ, Abraham AG, Merriman B, Saag MS, et al. (2009) Effect of early versus deferred antiretroviral therapy for HIV on survival. N Engl J Med 360: 1815–26.
13. Cornell M, Grimsrud A, Fairall L, Fox MP, van Cutsem G, et al. (2010) Temporal changes in programme outcomes among adult patients initiating antiretroviral therapy across South Africa, 2002–2007. AIDS 24: 2263–70.
14. Igumbor J, Stewart A, Holzemer W (2012) Factors contributing to the health-related quality of life of people living with HIV and their experiences with care and support services in Limpopo Province, South Africa: health and fitness. AJPHERD 18: 812–840.
15. Lok JJ, Bosch RJ, Benson CA, Collier AC, Robbin GK, et al. (2010) Long-term increase in CD4+ T-cell counts during combination antiretroviral therapy for HIV-1 infection. AIDS 24: 1867–76.
16. Johnson LF, Mossong J, Dorrington RE, Schomaker M, Hoffmann CJ, et al. (2013) Life Expectancies of South African Adults Starting Antiretroviral Treatment: Collaborative Analysis of Cohort Studies. PLOS Med 10: e1001418.
17. Nash D, Katyal M, Brinkhof MW, Keiser O, May M, et al. (2008) Long-term immunologic response to antiretroviral therapy in low-income countries: a collaborative analysis of prospective studies. AIDS 22: 2291–302.
18. Basu S, Andrew J, Kishore S, Panjabi R, Stucker D (2012) Comparative Performance of Private and Public Healthcare Systems in Low- and Middle-Income Countries: A Systematic Review. PLOS Med 9: e1001244.
19. Navario P (2009) Implementation of a Novel Model to Enhance Routine HIV Care and Treatment Capacity in South Africa: Outcomes, Costs, and Cost-effectiveness. PhD Thesis, University of Cape Town.
20. Schneider H, Chabikuli N, Blaauw D, Funani I, Brugah R (2005) Sexually transmitted infection: factors associated with quality of care among private general practitioners. S Afr Med J 782–5.
21. Chabikuli N, Schneider H, Blaauw D, Zwi AB, Brugha R (2002) Quality and equity of private sector care for sexually transmitted diseases in South Africa. Health Policy Plan 17: 40–6.
22. Udwadia ZF, Pinto LM, Uplekar MW (2010) Tuberculosis Management by Private Practitioners in Mumbai, India: Has Anything Changed in Two Decades? PLOS ONE 5: e12023.
23. Vandan N, Ali M, Prasad R, Kuroiwa C (2009) Assessment of doctors' knowledge regarding tuberculosis management in Lucknow, India: a public-private sector comparison. Public Health 123: 484–9.
24. Dato MI, Imaz MS (2009) Tuberculosis control and the private sector in a low incidence setting in Argentina. Revista de Salud Pública 11: 370–382.
25. Gbotosho GO, Happi CT, Gaiyu A, Ogundahunsi OA, Sowunmi A, et al. (2009) Potential contribution of prescription practices to the emergence and spread of chloroquine resistance in south-west Nigeria: caution in the use of artemisinin combination therapy. Malaria Journal 8: 1–8.
26. Auer C, Lagahid JY, Tanner M, Weiss MG (2006) Diagnosis and management of tuberculosis by private practitioners in Manila, Philippines. Health policy 77: 172–181.
27. Enriquez M, McKinsey DS (2011) Strategies to improve HIV treatment adherence in developed countries: clinical management at the individual level. HIV AIDS 3: 45–51.
28. Pasquet A, Messou E, Gabillard D, Minga A, Depoulosky A, et al. (2010) Impact of Drug Stock-Outs on Death and Retention to Care among HIV-Infected Patients on Combination Antiretroviral Therapy in Abidjan, Côte d'Ivoire. PLOS ONE 5: e13414.
29. Diabaté S, Alary M, Koffi CK (2007) Determinants of adherence to highly active antiretroviral therapy among HIV-1-infected patients in Cote d'Ivoire. AIDS 21: 1799–1803.
30. Eholie SP, Tanon A, Polneau S, Ouiminga M, Djadji A, et al. (2007) Field adherence to highly active antiretroviral therapy in HIV-infected adults in Abidjan, Cote d'Ivoire. J Acquir Immune Defic Syndr 45: 355–8.
31. Makuch MY, Petta CA, Osis MJ, Bahamondes L (2010) Low priority level for infertility services within the public health sector: a Brazilian case study. Hum Reprod 25: 430–5.
32. Boulle A, Bock P, Osler M, Cohen K, Channing L, et al. (2008) Antiretroviral therapy and early mortality in South Africa. Bull World Health Organ 86: 678–87.

Permissions

The contributors of this book come from diverse backgrounds, making this book a truly international effort. This book will bring forth new frontiers with its revolutionizing research information and detailed analysis of the nascent developments around the world.

We would like to thank all the contributing authors for lending their expertise to make the book truly unique. They have played a crucial role in the development of this book. Without their invaluable contributions this book wouldn't have been possible. They have made vital efforts to compile up to date information on the varied aspects of this subject to make this book a valuable addition to the collection of many professionals and students.

This book was conceptualized with the vision of imparting up-to-date information and advanced data in this field. To ensure the same, a matchless editorial board was set up. Every individual on the board went through rigorous rounds of assessment to prove their worth. After which they invested a large part of their time researching and compiling the most relevant data for our readers.

The editorial board has been involved in producing this book since its inception. They have spent rigorous hours researching and exploring the diverse topics which have resulted in the successful publishing of this book. They have passed on their knowledge of decades through this book. To expedite this challenging task, the publisher supported the team at every step. A small team of assistant editors was also appointed to further simplify the editing procedure and attain best results for the readers.

Apart from the editorial board, the designing team has also invested a significant amount of their time in understanding the subject and creating the most relevant covers. They scrutinized every image to scout for the most suitable representation of the subject and create an appropriate cover for the book.

The publishing team has been an ardent support to the editorial, designing and production team. Their endless efforts to recruit the best for this project, has resulted in the accomplishment of this book. They are a veteran in the field of academics and their pool of knowledge is as vast as their experience in printing. Their expertise and guidance has proved useful at every step. Their uncompromising quality standards have made this book an exceptional effort. Their encouragement from time to time has been an inspiration for everyone.

The publisher and the editorial board hope that this book will prove to be a valuable piece of knowledge for researchers, students, practitioners and scholars across the globe.

List of Contributors

Julia R. G. Raifman and Günther Fink
Department of Global Health and Population, Harvard School of Public Health, Boston, MA, United States of America

Heather E. Lanthorn
Harvard School of Public Health, Boston, MA, United States of America

Slawa Rokicki
Department of Health Policy, Harvard Graduate School of Arts and Sciences, Cambridge, MA, United States of America

Wei Chen, Li-qiong Wang, Jun Ren, Wen-jing Xiong, Fang Lu and Jian-ping Liu
Centre for Evidence-Based Chinese Medicine, Beijing University of Chinese Medicine, Beijing, China

George Lewith
Primary care and population Sciences, Medical School, University of Southampton, Southampton, United Kingdom

Wenhua Liang, Xuan Wu., Shaodong Hong, Yaxiong Zhang, Shiyang Kang, Wenfeng Fang, Tao Qin, Yan Huang, Hongyun Zhao and Li Zhang
Sun Yat-sen University Cancer Center, State Key Laboratory of Oncology in South China, Collaborative Innovation Center for Cancer Medicine, Guangzhou, China

Damrus Tresukoso
Division of Cardiology, Department of Internal Medicine, Faculty of Medicine, Siriraj Hospital, Mahidol University, Siriraj, Bangkoknoi, Bangkok, Thailand

Bhoom Suktitipat
Department of Biochemistry, Faculty of Medicine, Siriraj Hospital, Mahidol University, Siriraj, Bangkoknoi, Bangkok, Thailand
Integrative Computation BioScience Center (ICBS), Mahidol University, Salaya, Nakhon Prathom, Thailand

Ruttakarn Kamkaew, Saiphon Poldee and Atip Likidlilid
Department of Biochemistry, Faculty of Medicine, Siriraj Hospital, Mahidol University, Siriraj, Bangkoknoi, Bangkok, Thailand

Saowalak Hunnangkul and Boonrat Tassaneetrithep
Department of Health Research and Development, Faculty of Medicine, Siriraj Hospital, Mahidol University, Siriraj, Bangkoknoi, Bangkok, Thailand

Makoto Yamaguchi, Shinichi Akiyama, Sawako Kato, Takayuki Katsuno, Tomoki Kosugi, Waichi Sato, Naotake Tsuboi, Yoshinari Yasuda, Masashi Mizuno, Yasuhiko Ito, Seiichi Matsuo and Shoichi Maruyama
Department of Nephrology, Nagoya University Graduate School of Medicine, Nagoya, Japan

Masahiko Ando
Center for Advanced Medicine and Clinical Research, Nagoya University Hospital, Nagoya, Japan

Ryohei Yamamoto
Department of Geriatric Medicine and Nephrology, Osaka University Graduate School of Medicine, Suita, Japan

Zhenhong Zou and Yuming Jiang
Department of General Surgery, Nanfang Hospital, Southern Medical University, Guangzhou City, Guangdong Province, China

Mingjia Xiao
Department of Hepatobiliary Surgery, Wuxi People's Hospital of Nanjing Medical University, Wuxi, Jiangsu Province, China

Ruiyao Zhou
Department of General Surgery, The Third Affiliated Hospital of Wenzhou Medical University, Ruian City, Zhejiang Province, China

Yarong Liu, Jinxu Fang and Kye-Il Joo
Mork Family Department of Chemical Engineering and Materials Science, University of Southern California, Los Angeles, California, United States of America

Michael K. Wong
Division of Medical Oncology, Norris Comprehensive Cancer Center, Keck School of Medicine, University of Southern California, Los Angeles, California, United States of America

Pin Wang
Mork Family Department of Chemical Engineering and Materials Science, University of Southern California, Los Angeles, California, United States of America
Department of Biomedical Engineering, University of Southern California, Los Angeles, California, United States of America
Department of Pharmacology and Pharmaceutical Sciences, University of Southern California, Los Angeles, California, United States of America

Chinwoke Isiguzo and Chinazo Ujuju
Research and Evaluation Division, Society for Family Health, Abuja, Nigeria

Jennifer Anyanti
Technical Services Division, Society for Family Health, Abuja, Nigeria

Ernest Nwokolo
Global Fund Malaria Division, Society for Family Health, Abuja, Nigeria

Anna De La Cruz, Eric Schatzkin and Jenny Liu
The Global Health Group, University of California San Francisco, San Francisco, California, United States of America

Sepideh Modrek
General Medical Disciplines, Stanford University School of Medicine, Palo Alto, California, United States of America

Dominic Montagu
Epidemiology and Biostatistics, University of California San Francisco, San Francisco, California, United States of America

Melissa Ehman
Tuberculosis Control Branch, Division of Communicable Disease Control, Center for Infectious Diseases, California Department of Public Health, Richmond, California, United States of America
Institute of Global Health, Global Health Sciences, University of California San Francisco, San Francisco, California, United States of America

Jennifer Flood and Pennan M. Barry
Tuberculosis Control Branch, Division of Communicable Disease Control, Center for Infectious Diseases, California Department of Public Health, Richmond, California, United States of America

Po-Chun Chen
Department of Radiation Oncology, Pingtung Christian Hospital, Pingtung, Taiwan

Ching-Chieh Yang
Department of Radiation Oncology, Chi-Mei Medical Center, Tainan, Taiwan

Cheng-Jung Wu
Department of Otolaryngology, Kaohsiung Veterans General Hospital, Kaohsiung, Taiwan

Wen-Shan Liu and Wei-Lun Huang
Department of Radiation Oncology, Kaohsiung Veterans General Hospital, Kaohsiung, Taiwan

Ching-Chih Lee
Department of Otolarygology, Dalin Tzu Chi Hospital, Buddhist Tzu Chi Medical Foundation, Chiayi, Taiwan
Cancer Center, Dalin Tzu Chi Hospital, Buddhist Tzu Chi Medical Foundation, Chiayi, Taiwan
School of Medicine, Tzu Chi University, Hualin, Taiwan

Rong-Sen Yang
Department of Orthopedic Surgery, National Taiwan University Hospital, Taipei, Taiwan

I-Shan Hsieh and Wen-Mei Fu
Department of Pharmacology, College of Medicine, National Taiwan University, Taipei, Taiwan

Yingying Su, Fujie Zhang, Huixin Liu, Lin Zhu, Jing Wu and Ning Wang
National Center for AIDS/STD Control and Prevention, Chinese Center for Disease Control and Prevention, Beijing, China

M. Kumi Smith
Department of Epidemiology, University of North Carolina, Chapel Hill, North Carolina, United States of America

Wei Li, Xiaoyuan Gong, Mingyuan Sun, Xingli Zhao, Benfa Gong, Hui Wei and Yingchang Mi
Leukemia Diagnosis and Treatment Center, Institute of Hematology and Blood Disease Hospital, Chinese Academy of Medical Sciences and Peking Union of Medical College, Tianjin, China

Jianxiang Wang
Leukemia Diagnosis and Treatment Center, Institute of Hematology and Blood Disease Hospital, Chinese Academy of Medical Sciences and Peking Union of Medical College, Tianjin, China
State Key Laboratory of Experimental Hematology, Institute of Hematology and Blood Disease Hospital, Chinese Academy of Medical Sciences and Peking Union of Medical College, Tianjin, China

Gary Mo
Department of Pharmaceutical Sciences, University at Buffalo, Buffalo, New York, United States of America
DMPK Modeling and Simulation, Oncology, iMED, AstraZeneca, Waltham, Massachusetts, United States of America

Frank Gibbons and Patricia Schroeder
DMPK Modeling and Simulation, Oncology, iMED, AstraZeneca, Waltham, Massachusetts, United States of America

Wojciech Krzyzanski
Department of Pharmaceutical Sciences, University at Buffalo, Buffalo, New York, United States of America

Stephanie Seah, Abu Bakar Ali Asad and Chih-Liang Chin
Imaging, Merck & Co. Inc., West Point, Pennsylvania, United States of America
Translational Medicine Research Centre, MSD, Singapore, Singapore

Richard Baumgartner and Dai Feng
Biostatistics and Research Decision Sciences, Merck & Co. Inc., Rahway, New Jersey, United States of America

Donald S. Williams and Jeffrey L. Evelhoch
Imaging, Merck & Co. Inc., West Point, Pennsylvania, United States of America

Elaine Manigbas and John D. Beaver
Imaging, Maccine Pte Ltd, Singapore, Singapore

Torsten Reese and Brian Henry
Translational Medicine Research Centre, MSD, Singapore, Singapore

Maxim L. Bychkov, Marine E. Gasparian, Dmitry A. Dolgikh and Mikhail P. Kirpichnikov
Department of Bioengineering, Shemyakin and Ovchinnikov Institute of Bioorganic Chemistry, Moscow, Russia

Lena Novack and Larisa Gimpelevich
Department of Epidemiology, Faculty of Health Sciences, Ben-Gurion University of the Negev, Beer-Sheva, Israel

Slava Kogan and Victor Novack
Clinical Research Center, Soroka University Medical Center, Ben-Gurion University of the Negev, Beer-Sheva, Israel

Michael Howell
The University of Chicago Medicine, Chicago, Illinois, United States of America

Abraham Borer
Infectious Diseases Unit, Soroka University Medical Center, Beer-Sheva, Israel

Ciarán P. Kelly
Division of Gastroenterology, Beth Israel Deaconess Medical Center, Harvard Medical School, Boston, Massachusetts, United States of America

Daniel A. Leffler
The Celiac Center at BIDMC, Division of Gastroenterology, Beth Israel Deaconess Medical Center, Boston, Massachusetts, United States of America

Donald J. Scholten II
Michigan State University College of Human Medicine, Grand Rapids, Michigan, United States of America
Van Andel Research Institute, Grand Rapids, Michigan, United States of America

Christine M. Timmer
Michigan State University College of Human Medicine, Grand Rapids, Michigan, United States of America

Jacqueline D. Peacock and Bart O. Williams
Van Andel Research Institute, Grand Rapids, Michigan, United States of America

Dominic W. Pelle and Matthew R. Steensma
Michigan State University College of Human Medicine, Grand Rapids, Michigan, United States of America
Van Andel Research Institute, Grand Rapids, Michigan, United States of America
Helen DeVos Childen's Hospital, Spectrum Health System, Grand Rapids, Michigan, United States of America

Cong Dai, Wei-Xin Liu, Min Jiang, Ming-Jun Sun
Department of Gastroenterology, First Affiliated Hospital, China Medical University, Shenyang City, Liaoning Province, China

Meng Ling Choong, Shan Ho Tan, Sravanthy Manesh, Anna Ngo, Jacklyn W. Y. Yong and May Ann Lee
Experimental Therapeutics Centre, Agency for Science Technology and Research, Singapore, Singapore

Tuan Zea Tan and Henry He Yang
Bioinformatics Core, Cancer Science Institute of Singapore, National University of Singapore, Singapore

Aneta Novotná, Iveta Bartoňková, Martina Korhoňová and Zdeněk Dvořák
Regional Centre of Advanced Technologies and Materials, Faculty of Science, Palacky University, Olomouc, Czech Republic

Kristýna Krasulová and Pavel Anzenbacher
Institute of Pharmacology, Faculty of Medicine and Dentistry, Palacky University, Olomouc, Czech Republic

Petr Bachleda
2nd Department of Surgery, University Hospital Olomouc, Olomouc, Czech Republic

Shuabe Rajap
Operations Department, BroadReach Healthcare, Cape Town, South Africa

Patrizia Maria Carrieri, Caroline Lions, Julien Cohen, Marion Mora, Fabienne Marcellin, Bruno Spire and Perrine Roux
INSERM UMR912 (SESSTIM), Marseille, France
Aix Marseille Université, UMR_S912, Marseille, France
ORS PACA, Observatoire Régional de la Santé Provence Alpes Côte d'Azur, Marseille, France

Alain Morel
Oppelia, Paris, France

Laurent Michel
INSERM, Research Unit 669, Paris, France
Univ Paris-Sud and Univ Paris Descartes, UMR-S0669, Paris, France
Centre Pierre Nicole, Paris, France

Muriel Vray
Unité de Recherche et d'Expertise en Epidémiologie des Maladies Emergentes, Institut Pasteur, Paris, France
Institut National de la Santé et de la Recherche Médicale (INSERM), Paris, France

Christian Tudorache
Institute Biology Leiden, Leiden University, Leiden, The Netherlands

Erik Burgerhout
Institute Biology Leiden, Leiden University, Leiden, The Netherlands
NewCatch B.V., Leiden, The Netherlands

Sebastiaan Brittijn and Guido van den Thillart
NewCatch B.V., Leiden, The Netherlands

Jude Igumbor, Sophie Pascoe
Research and Development Department, BroadReach Healthcare, Cape Town, South Africa

Index

www.ingramcontent.com/pod-product-compliance
Lightning Source LLC
Chambersburg PA
CBHW061241190326
41458CB00011B/3543